W9-DDE-697

INTRODUCTION TO MEDICAL TERMINOLOGY

Second Edition

INTRODUCTION TO MEDICAL TERMINOLOGY

Second Edition

ANN EHRLICH
CAROL L. SCHROEDER

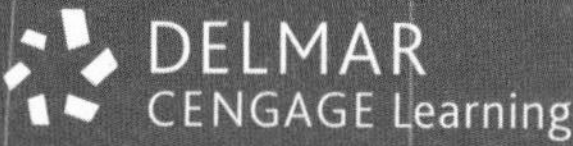

Australia Brazil Japan Korea Mexico Singapore Spain United Kingdom United States

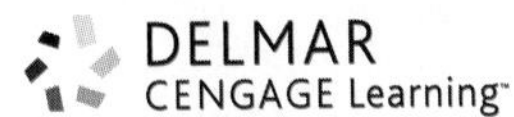

Introduction to Medical Terminology, Second Edition
by Ann Ehrlich and Carol L. Schroeder

Vice President, Career and
Professional Editorial: Dave Garza

Director of Learning Solutions: Matthew Kane

Acquisitions Editor: Matthew Seeley

Managing Editor: Marah Bellegarde

Senior Product Manager: Debra Myette-Flis

Editorial Assistant: Megan Tarquinio

Vice President, Career and
Professional Marketing: Jennifer McAvey

Senior Marketing Manager: Michele McTighe

Production Director: Carolyn S. Miller

Content Project Manager: Thomas Heffernan

Senior Art Director: Jack Pendleton

Technology Project Manager: Benjamin Knapp

Production Technology Analyst: Tom Stover

Library of Congress Control Number: 2008926571

ISBN-13: 978-1-4180-3017-9
ISBN-10: 1-4180-3017-1

Delmar Cengage Learning
5 Maxwell Drive
Clifton Park, NY 12065-2919
USA

Cengage Learning products are represented in Canada by Nelson Education, Ltd.

For your lifelong learning solutions, visit **delmar.cengage.com**
Visit our corporate web site at **cengage.com.**

NOTICE TO THE READER

Publisher does not warrant or guarantee any of the products described herein or perform any independent analysis in connection with any of the product information contained herein. Publisher does not assume, and expressly disclaims, any obligation to obtain and include information other than that provided to it by the manufacturer. The reader is expressly warned to consider and adopt all safety precautions that might be indicated by the activities described herein and to avoid all potential hazards. By following the instructions contained herein, the reader willingly assumes all risks in connection with such instructions. The publisher makes no representations or warranties of any kind, including but not limited to, the warranties of fitness for particular purpose or merchantability, nor are any such representations implied with respect to the material set forth herein, and the publisher takes no responsibility with respect to such material. The publisher shall not be liable for any special, consequential, or exemplary damages resulting, in whole or part, from the readers' use of, or reliance upon, this material.

Printed in the United States of America
2 3 4 5 6 7 12 11 10 09

Contents

Chapter 5: The Cardiovascular System 94

Chapter 6: The Lymphatic and Immune Systems 125

Chapter 7: The Respiratory System 150

Preface

Welcome to the world of medical terminology! Learning this special language is an important step in preparing for your career as a health care professional. Here's good news: Learning medical terms is much easier than learning a foreign language because you are already familiar with quite a few of the words—such as *appendicitis* and *tonsillectomy*. Understanding new words becomes easier with the discovery that many of these terms are made up of interchangeable word parts that are used in different combinations. Once you understand this, you'll be well on your way to translating even the most difficult medical terms, including words you have never seen before. You'll be amazed to see how quickly your vocabulary will grow!

This book and the accompanying teaching materials are designed to make the process as simple as possible. Review the introductory sections at the beginning of the book, including "How to Use This Book" and "How to Use StudyWARE™," so you can find your way around easily. Once you get comfortable with the format, you'll discover you are learning faster than you ever imagined possible.

CHAPTER ORGANIZATION

The text is organized into 15 chapters, 2 appendices, and an index. Each chapter includes special features designed to help you master the medical terms included in this text.

Throughout the text, **primary terms** are shown in bold. These are the most important terms that you need to learn in each chapter. Only these terms are used as correct answers in the exercises and tests.

Secondary terms appear in *orange* italics. These terms, which are included to clarify the meaning of a primary term, are used as distractors in exercises or tests; however, they are never used as correct answers.

Introductory Chapters

Chapters 1 and 2 provide the foundation that enables you to master the rest of the book. Chapter 1 introduces key word parts—the building blocks of most medical terms. Chapter 2 introduces more word parts and provides an overview of basic terms used throughout the health field.

After studying these chapters, complete the Word Part Review that follows Chapter 2 in your student workbook. These practice activities and the test will help you determine whether you've mastered the concept of these all-important building blocks. If you are having trouble here, it is important to put more effort into learning these basics.

Body System Chapters

Chapters 3 through 14 are organized by body system. Because each body system stands alone, you can study these chapters in any sequence. Each chapter begins with an overview of the structures and functions of that system so you can relate these to the specialists, pathology, and diagnostic and treatment procedures that follow.

Chapter 15 introduces basic diagnostic procedures, examination positions, imaging techniques, laboratory tests, and pharmacology. This chapter can be studied at any point in the course.

Appendices

Appendix A: Prefixes, Combining Forms, and Suffixes is a convenient alphabetic reference for medical word parts. When you don't recognize a word part, you can look it up here.

Appendix B: Abbreviations and Their Meanings is an extensive list of commonly used abbreviations and their meanings. Abbreviations are important in medicine and using them *accurately* is essential!

StudyWARE™ CD-ROM

The interactive StudyWARE™ CD-ROM offers an exciting way to gain additional practice in working with medical terms. The exercises and games help you remember even the most difficult terms. See "How to Use StudyWARE™ on page xviii for details.

STUDENT WORKBOOK TO ACCOMPANY INTRODUCTION TO MEDICAL TERMINOLOGY

The Student Workbook contains many features to make learning medical terminology easier. In addition to containing a chapter in the workbook to accompany each textbook chapter, this workbook also contains additional study tools.

Learning Exercises

Your workbook includes Learning Exercises to help you learn the terms presented in each chapter. To provide additional reinforcement, the questions require that you write the short answer. Follow your teacher's instructions about submitting and correcting the completed exercises.

Word Part Review Section

This section, which is included after Chapter 2, helps you evaluate how well you are mastering the word parts.

Comprehensive Medical Terminology Review

This section, which follows Chapter 15, is designed to help you prepare for your final examination. It includes study tips, practice exercises, and a simulated final test.

Flash Cards

Improve your knowledge and test your mastery by using the flash cards in the last section of the workbook. Review the suggestions for games and activities for using these, then carefully remove the pages from the workbook and separate the cards.

Acknowledgments

Special thanks to Don Jacobsen for his help in "pronouncing" the terms in this text, to Katrina Schroeder and Laura Ehrlich for their work on the "Human Touch" stories, and to Winnie Yu, Dr. Shabir Bhimji and Dr. Patrick McKenna for their contributions to the case studies and medical mysteries in the Instructor's Manual. Thanks also to the editorial and production staff of Delmar Cengage Learning for their very professional assistance in making this revision possible, and to the health occupations instructors who continue to be a valuable resource in guiding this book as it evolves.

We are particularly grateful to the individuals who shared their life stories for the Career Profiles in this text and to the Reviewers. Their insights, comments, suggestion, and attention to detail were very important in making certain that this book is "on target" for health career students.

Ann Ehrlich
Carol L. Schroeder

REVIEWERS

Richard T. Boan, PhD
Coordinator of Allied Health Sciences
Health Sciences Department
Midlands Technical College
Columbia, South Carolina

Gerry A. Brasin, CMA, AS, CPC
Education Coordinator
Premier Education Group
Springfield, Massachusetts

Betty Earp, BSN, RN
Nurse Assistant Coordinator
Mesa Community College
Mesa, Arizona

Deborah Babb Huber, BAAS
Medical Transcription Instructor
Pulaski Technical College
North Little Rock, Arkansas

Jane W. Dumas, MSN
Allied Health Department Chairperson
Remington College—Cleveland West Campus
North Olmsted, Ohio

Darlene Kenny, MLT (ASCP)
Allied Health Instructor
Tri-State Business Institute
Erie, Pennsylvania

Laurie Post, RN, MSN
Nursing and Business Instructor
Blue Mountain Community College
Pendleton, Oregon

Jane Zaccardi, MA, RNCS
Adjunct Faculty Evening/Weekend PN Program
Johnson County Community College
Area Vocational Schools
Overland Park, Kansas

How to Use This Book

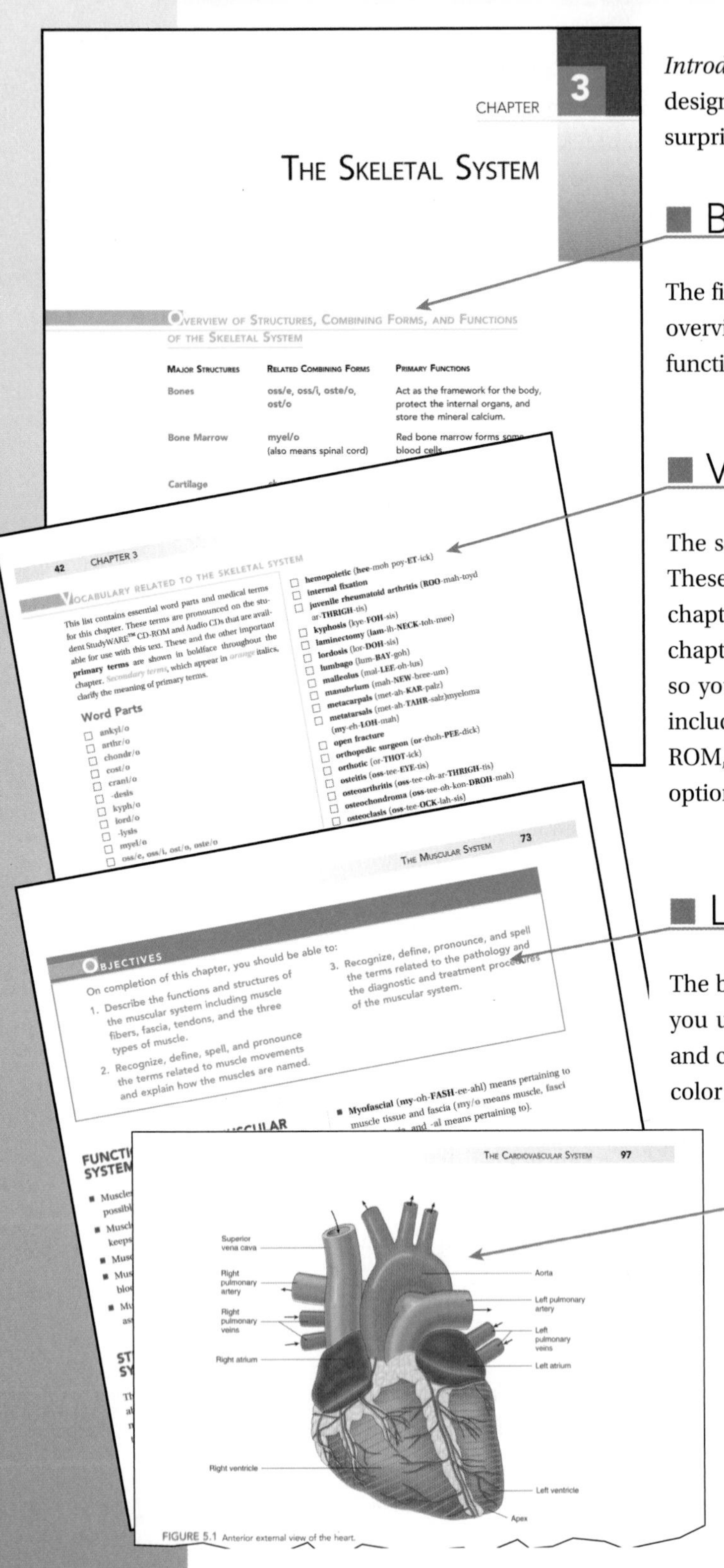

Introduction to Medical Terminology, Second Edition, is designed to help you learn and remember medical terms with surprising ease. The key lies in the following features.

BODY SYSTEM OVERVIEW

The first page of each body system chapter is a chart giving an overview of the structures, related combining forms, and functions most important to that system.

VOCABULARY LIST

The second page of each chapter is a 75-item vocabulary list. These are 15 key word parts and 60 important terms for the chapter. This immediately alerts you to the key terms in the chapter and acts as a review guide. Next to each term is a box so you can check off each term as you've learned it. This list includes the 60 terms pronounced on the StudyWARE™ CD-ROM, which is included with the book, as well as on the optional Audio CDs.

LEARNING OBJECTIVES

The beginning of each chapter lists learning objectives to help you understand what is expected of you as you read the text and complete the exercises. These objectives are set off with a color bar for easy identification.

ILLUSTRATIONS

The book's full-color illustrations help to clarify the text and contain important additional information. Review each illustration and read its caption carefully for easy and effective learning.

SOUNDS-LIKE PRONUNCIATION SYSTEM

The "sounds-like" pronunciation system makes pronunciation easy by respelling the word with syllables you can understand—and say—at a glance. Simply pronounce the term just as it appears in parentheses, accenting the syllables as follows:

- **Primary** (strongest) **accent:** capital letters and bold type
- **Secondary accent:** lowercase letters and bold type

WORD PARTS

Because word parts are so important to learning medical terminology, whenever a term made up of word parts is introduced, the definition is followed (in parentheses) by the word parts highlighted in **magenta** and defined.

PRIMARY AND SECONDARY TERMS

- **Primary terms** are the most important medical words in a chapter. When first introduced, the term appears in boldface and, if appropriate, is followed by the "sounds-like" pronunciation. These are the words you need to concentrate on learning. Only primary terms are used as correct answers in the exercises and tests.
- *Secondary terms* appear in *orange* italics. These terms are included to clarify the meaning of a primary term. Although used as distracters in exercises, the secondary terms are not used as correct answers in exercises or tests.

and tendons, making possible the wide variety of body movements. (Muscles and tendons are discussed in Chapter 4.)

- Calcium, which is required for normal nerve and muscle function, is stored in bones.
- Red bone marrow, which has an important function in the formation of blood cells, is located within spongy bone.

THE STRUCTURE OF BONES

Bone is the form of connective tissue that is the second hardest tissue in the human body. Only dental enamel is harder than bone.

The Tissues of Bone

Although it is a dense and rigid tissue, bone is also capable of growth, healing, and reshaping itself (Figure 3.1).

- **Periosteum** (**pehr**-ee-**OSS**-tee-um) is the tough, fibrous tissue that forms the outermost covering of bone (**peri-** means surrounding, **oste** means bone, and -um is ... ending).
- **Compact b**... bone that ...

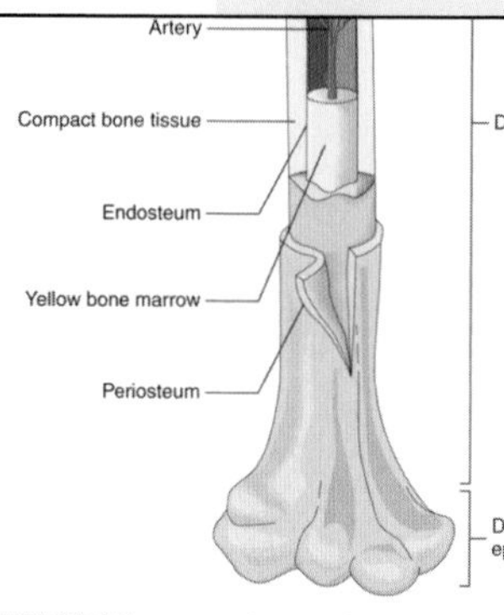

FIGURE 3.1 Anatomic features of a typical long bone.

- **Spongy bone** is lighter, and not as strong, as compac bone. This type of bone is commonly found in the ends and inner portions of long bones such as the femur. Red bone marrow is located within this spong ...

... very strong (burs means bursa, and -itis means inflammation).

- **Chondromalacia** (**kon**-droh-mah-**LAY**-shee-ah) is the abnormal softening of cartilage (chondr/o means cartilage, and -malacia means abnormal softening).
- A **chondroma** (kon-**DROH**-mah) is a slow-growing benign tumor derived from cartilage cells (chondr means cartilage, and -oma means tumor).
- **Costochondritis** (**kos**-toh-kon-**DRIGH**-tis) is an inflammation of the cartilage that connects a rib to the sternum (cost/o means rib, chondr means cartilage, and -itis means inflammation).
- **Hallux valgus** (**HAL**-ucks **VAL**-guss), also known as a *bunion*, is an abnormal enlargement of the joint at the base of the great toe (*hallux* means big toe, and *valgus* means bent).
- **Hemarthrosis** (**hem**-ar-**THROH**-sis) is blood within a joint (hem means blood, arthr means joint, and -osis means abnormal condition or disease). This condition is frequently due to a joint injury. It also can occur spontaneously in patients taking blood-thinning medications or those having a blood clotting disorder such as hemophilia (see Chapters 2 and 5).
- **Synovitis** (sin-oh-**VYE**-tiss) is inflammation of the synovial membrane that results in swelling and pain of the affected joint (synov means synovial membrane, and -itis means inflammation). This condition can be caused by arthritis, trauma, infection, or irritation produced by damaged cartilage.

Dislocation

- **Dislocation**, also known as *luxation* (luck-**SAY**-shun), is the total displacement of a bone from its joint (Figure 3.18).
- **Subluxation** (**sub**-luck-**SAY**-shun) is the partial displacement of a bone from its joint.

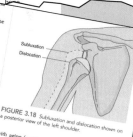

Subluxation
Dislocation

FIGURE 3.18 Subluxation and dislocation shown on a posterior view of the left shoulder.

with aging (oste/o means bone, arthr means joint, and -itis means inflammation) (Figure 3.19).

- This condition is described as a *degenerative joint disease* because it is characterized by the wearing away of the articular cartilage within the joints. *Degenerative* means the breaking down or impairment of a body part.
- **Spondylosis** (**spon**-dih-**LOH**-sis), which is also known as *spinal osteoarthritis*, is a degenerative disorder that can cause the loss of normal spinal structure and function (spondyl means vertebrae, and -osis means abnormal condition or disease).

Gouty Arthritis

Gouty arthritis (**GOW**-tee ar-**THRIGH**-tis), also known as *gout*, is a type of arthritis characterized by deposits of uric acid in the joints. *Uric acid* is a byproduct that is normally excreted by the kidneys. Gout develops when excess uric acid, which is present in the blood, forms crystals in the joints of the feet and legs.

Rheumatoid Arthritis

- The two **temporal bones** form the sides and base of the cranium.
- The **sphenoid bone** (**SFEE**-noid) forms part of the base of the skull and parts of the floor and sides of the orbit. The *orbit* is the bony socket that surrounds and protects the eyeball.
- The **ethmoid bone** (**ETH**-moid) forms part of the posterior portion of the nose, the orbit, and the floor of the cranium.

Auditory Ossicles

The six tiny bones of the middle ear, known as the **auditory ossicles** (**OSS**-ih-kulz), are discussed in Chapter 11.

- The **external auditory meatus** (mee-**AY**-tus), which is located in the temporal bone on each side of the skull, is the opening of the external auditory canal of the outer ear. A *meatus* is the external opening of a canal.

Bones of the Face

The face is made up of the following 14 bones:

- The two **nasal bones** that form the upper part of the bridge of the nose.
- The two **zygomatic bones** (**zye**-goh-**MAT**-ick), also known as the *cheekbones*, articulate with the frontal bone (forehead).
- The two **maxillary bones** (**MACK**-sih-**ler**-ee), also known as the *maxillae*, form most of the upper jaw (singular, *maxilla*).
- The two **palatine bones** (**PAL**-ah-tine) form part of the hard palate of the mouth and the floor of the nose

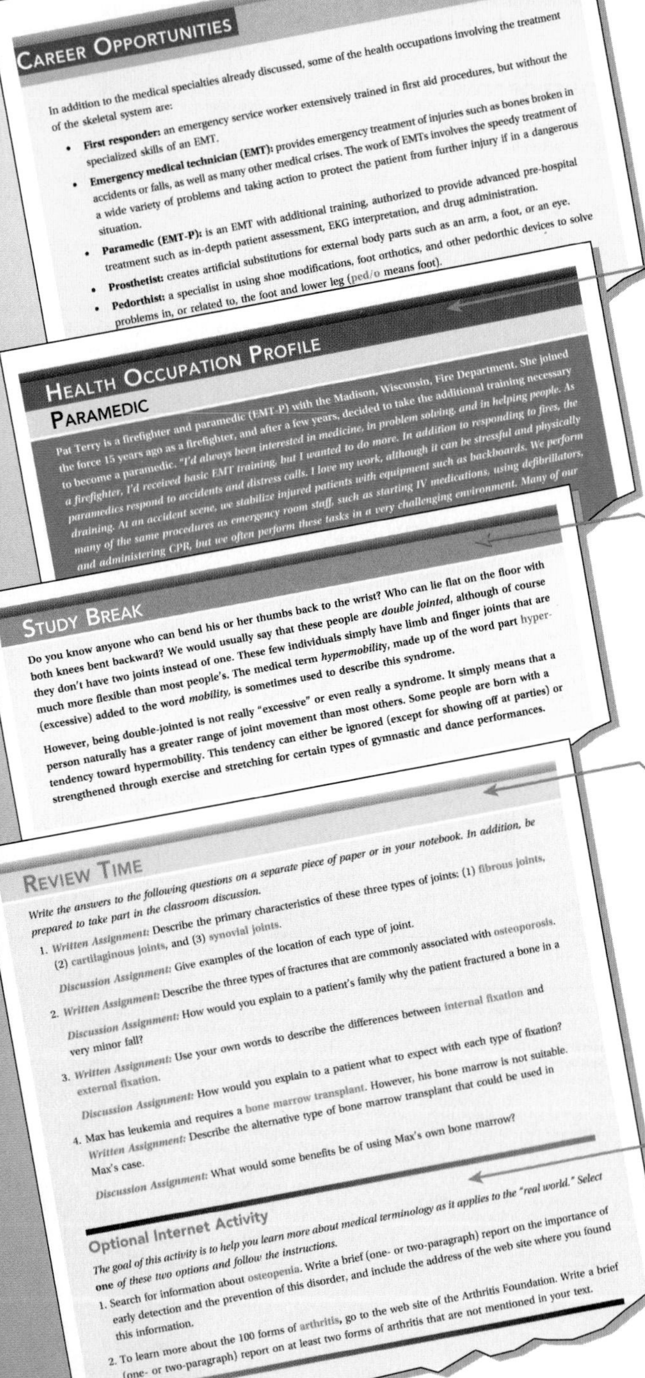

Career Opportunities

In addition to the medical specialties already discussed, some of the health occupations involving the treatment of the skeletal system are:

- **First responder:** an emergency service worker extensively trained in first aid procedures, but without the specialized skills of an EMT.
- **Emergency medical technician (EMT):** provides emergency treatment of injuries such as bones broken in accidents or falls, as well as many other medical crises. The work of EMTs involves the speedy treatment of a wide variety of problems and taking action to protect the patient from further injury if in a dangerous situation.
- **Paramedic (EMT-P):** is an EMT with additional training, authorized to provide advanced pre-hospital treatment such as in-depth patient assessment, EKG interpretation, and drug administration.
- **Prosthetist:** creates artificial substitutions for external body parts such as an arm, a foot, or an eye.
- **Pedorthist:** a specialist in using shoe modifications, foot orthotics, and other pedorthic devices to solve problems in, or related to, the foot and lower leg (ped/o means foot).

Health Occupation Profile

Paramedic

Pat Terry is a firefighter and paramedic (EMT-P) with the Madison, Wisconsin, Fire Department. She joined the force 15 years ago as a firefighter, and after a few years, decided to take the additional training necessary to become a paramedic. *"I'd always been interested in medicine, in problem solving, and in helping people. As a firefighter, I'd received basic EMT training, but I wanted to do more. In addition to responding to fires, the paramedics respond to accidents and distress calls. I love my work, although it can be stressful and physically draining. At an accident scene, we stabilize injured patients with equipment such as backboards. We perform many of the same procedures as emergency room staff, such as starting IV medications, using defibrillators, and administering CPR, but we often perform these tasks in a very challenging environment. Many of our*

Study Break

Do you know anyone who can bend his or her thumbs back to the wrist? Who can lie flat on the floor with both knees bent backward? We would usually say that these people are *double jointed*, although of course they don't have two joints instead of one. These few individuals simply have limb and finger joints that are much more flexible than most people's. The medical term *hypermobility*, made up of the word part hyper- (excessive) added to the word *mobility*, is sometimes used to describe this syndrome.

However, being double-jointed is not really "excessive" or even really a syndrome. It simply means that a person naturally has a greater range of joint movement than most others. Some people are born with a tendency toward hypermobility. This tendency can either be ignored (except for showing off at parties) or strengthened through exercise and stretching for certain types of gymnastic and dance performances.

Review Time

Write the answers to the following questions on a separate piece of paper or in your notebook. In addition, be prepared to take part in the classroom discussion.

1. *Written Assignment:* Describe the primary characteristics of these three types of joints: (1) fibrous joints, (2) cartilaginous joints, and (3) synovial joints.
   Discussion Assignment: Give examples of the location of each type of joint.
2. *Written Assignment:* Describe the three types of fractures that are commonly associated with osteoporosis.
   Discussion Assignment: How would you explain to a patient's family why the patient fractured a bone in a very minor fall?
3. *Written Assignment:* Use your own words to describe the differences between internal fixation and external fixation.
   Discussion Assignment: How would you explain to a patient what to expect with each type of fixation?
4. Max has leukemia and requires a bone marrow transplant. However, his bone marrow is not suitable.
   Written Assignment: Describe the alternative type of bone marrow transplant that could be used in Max's case.
   Discussion Assignment: What would some benefits be of using Max's own bone marrow?

Optional Internet Activity

The goal of this activity is to help you learn more about medical terminology as it applies to the "real world." Select **one** *of these two options and follow the instructions.*

1. Search for information about osteopenia. Write a brief (one- or two-paragraph) report on the importance of early detection and the prevention of this disorder, and include the address of the web site where you found this information.
2. To learn more about the 100 forms of arthritis, go to the web site of the Arthritis Foundation. Write a brief (one- or two-paragraph) report on at least two forms of arthritis that are not mentioned in your text.

CAREER OPPORTUNITIES

As you learn medical terminology, you will want to give some thought as to what career you might want to pursue after graduation. This section, near the end of each chapter, will give you some ideas to consider.

HEALTH OCCUPATION PROFILE

Read the real-life experiences of health care workers to find out how they selected their career, what they do, and how they like it. Their words may inspire your own career choice!

STUDY BREAK

Put down your pencil—there is no quiz on this one. The Study Break is just a brief and amusing pause in your studies before you go on to review the important information in the chapter.

REVIEW TIME

At the end of each chapter, there is a review exercise section with five questions. Each requires a written response and a discussion response. These review exercises give you opportunities to practice communicating with patients (using lay terms) and communicating with other health care professionals (using correct medical terminology). As you progress through the text these exercises become increasingly challenging.

OPTIONAL INTERNET EXERCISES

There are also two Internet exercises at the end of each chapter. One requires you to go to a specific web site. The other requires you to search a particular topic relating to the chapter.

THE HUMAN TOUCH: CRITICAL THINKING EXERCISE

A "real-life" mini story and related critical thinking questions at the end of each chapter involving patients and pathology to help you apply what you are learning to the real world. There are no right or wrong answers, just questions to get you started thinking about and using the new terms you have learned.

THE HUMAN TOUCH: CRITICAL THINKING ACTIVITY

The following story and questions are designed to stimulate critical thinking through class discussion or as a brief essay response. There are no right or wrong answers to these questions.

Hilary Keiser, 15, was having fun on her family's skiing trip until halfway down the slope, her ski struck a piece of debris. As she fell, she heard a snap, felt her left leg twist, and was in severe pain as she landed in the snow.

Steve, a member of the ski patrol, arrived to find Hilary lying in the snow and sobbing miserably while another skier tried to comfort her. Like all ski patrol members, Steve was trained as an EMT. He introduced himself, and then asked how she had fallen and where it hurt. Hilary answered his questions, keeping her leg very still to minimize the pain as Steve began his assessment. She listened as he phoned for help.

The backup team soon arrived, immobilized her leg, and quickly transported her down the mountain. When Hilary was in the warm first aid room, Steve stayed with her and continued his assessment while they waited for the ambulance. When he cut her ski pants leg away to reveal the injury, it was easy to see that she had a fracture: one end of the bone was almost poking through the skin, and there was swelling throughout her lower leg.

Suggested Discussion Topics

1. Discuss the most likely treatment options for Hilary's spiral fracture. Do you think Hilary is too young to be included in decisions about what to do?
2. Skiing can be dangerous, even for an experienced skier. Is the owner and operator of this ski slope in any way responsible for the fact that Hilary broke her leg?

How to Use

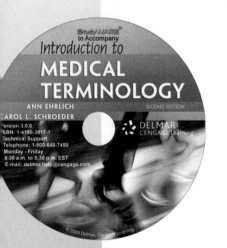

STUDYWARE™ TO ACCOMPANY *INTRODUCTION TO MEDICAL TERMINOLOGY*, SECOND EDITION

MINIMUM SYSTEM REQUIREMENTS

- Operating system: Microsoft Windows 2000, Windows XP, Windows Vista
- Processor: Pentium PC 500 MHz or higher (750 Mhz recommended)
- Memory: 64 MB of RAM (128 MB recommended)
- Screen resolution: 800 × 600 pixels
- Color depth: 16-bit color (thousands of colors)
- Macromedia Flash Player 9. The Macromedia Flash Player is free, and can be downloaded from http://www.adobe.com/products/flashplayer/

INSTALLATION INSTRUCTIONS

1. Insert disc into CD-ROM drive. The StudyWARE™ installation program should start automatically. If it does not, go to step 2.
2. From My Computer, double-click the icon for the CD drive.
3. Double-click the *setup.exe* file to start the program.

TECHNICAL SUPPORT

Telephone: 1-800-648-7450; Monday–Friday 8:30 A.M.–5:30 P.M. Eastern Time
E-mail: delmar.help@cengage.com

StudyWARE™ is a trademark used herein under license.

Microsoft® and Windows® are registered trademarks of the Microsoft Corporation.

Pentium® is a registered trademark of the Intel Corporation.

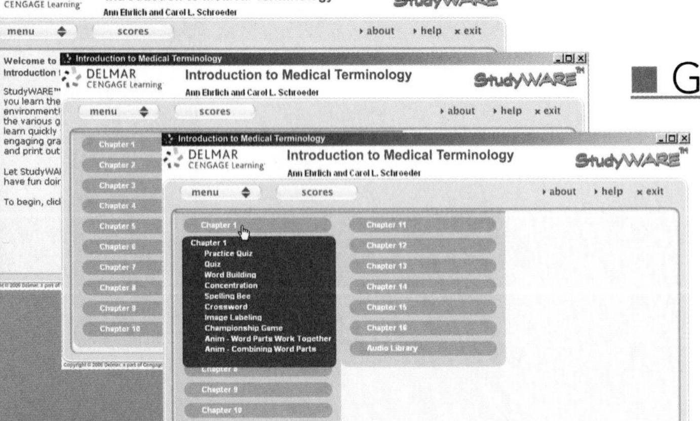

GETTING STARTED

The StudyWARE™ software helps you learn terms and concepts in *Introduction to Medical Terminology*, Second Edition. As you study each chapter in the text, be sure to explore the activities in the corresponding chapter in the software. Use StudyWARE™ as your own private tutor to help you learn the material in your *Introduction to Medical Terminology*, Second Edition textbook.

Getting started is easy. Install the software by inserting the CD-ROM into your computer's CD-ROM drive and following the on-screen instructions. When you open the software, enter your first and last name so the software can store your quiz results. Then choose a chapter from the menu to take a quiz or explore one of the activities.

■ MENUS

You can access the menus from wherever you are in the program. The menus include Quizzes, Activities, and Scores.

Quizzes. Quizzes include multiple choice, true/false, fill-in-the-blank, and word-building questions. You can take the quizzes in both practice mode and quiz mode. Use practice mode to improve your mastery of the material. You have multiple tries to get the answers correct. Instant feedback tells you whether you're right or wrong and helps you learn quickly by explaining why an answer was correct or incorrect. Use quiz mode when you are ready to test yourself and keep a record of your scores. In quiz mode, you have one try to get the answers right, but you can take each quiz as many times as you want.

Scores. You can view your last scores for each quiz and print your results to hand in to your instructor.

Activities. Activities include image labeling, spelling bee, concentration, crossword puzzles, and Championship game. Have fun while increasing your knowledge!

Animations. Animations help you visualize key concepts.

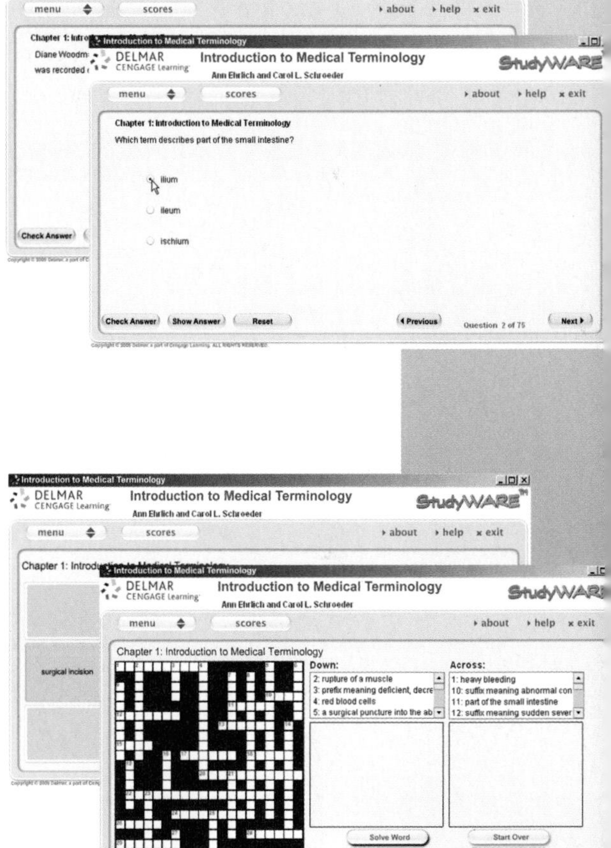

Audio Library. The StudyWARE™ Audio Library is a reference that includes audio pronunciations and definitions for over 900 medical terms! Use the audio library to practice pronunciation and review definitions for medical terms. You can browse terms by chapter or search by key word. Listen to pronunciations of the terms you select, or listen to an entire list of terms.

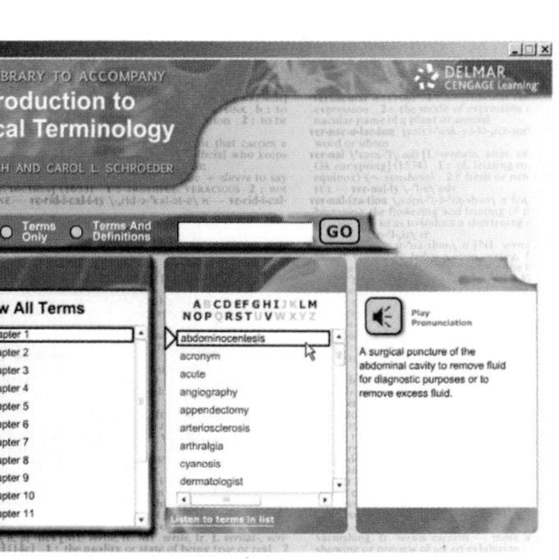

CHAPTER 1

Introduction to Medical Terminology

Overview of Introduction to Medical Terminology

Primary Medical Terms	Primary terms are a new feature in this edition to enable you to prioritize terms in your study of medical terminology.
Word Parts Are the Key	Introduction to word parts and how they create complex medical terms.
Word Roots	The word parts that usually, but not always, indicate the part of the body involved. When a vowel, usually the letter "o," is added to the end of a word root, this is now referred to as a "combining form."
Suffixes	The word part attached at the end of a word that usually, but not always, indicates the procedure, condition, disorder, or disease.
Prefixes	The word part attached at the beginning of a word that usually, but not always, indicates location, time, number, or status.
Determining Meanings on the Basis of Word Parts	Knowledge of word parts helps to decipher medical terms.
Medical Dictionary Use	Guidelines to make the use of a medical dictionary easier.
Pronunciation	Using the easy-to-use "sounds-like" pronunciation system.
Spelling Is Always Important	A one-letter spelling error can change the entire meaning of a term.
Using Abbreviations	Caution is always important when using abbreviations.
Singular and Plural Endings	Unusual singular and plural endings used in medical terms.
Basic Medical Terms	Terms used to describe disease conditions.
Look-Alike Sound-Alike Terms and Word Parts	Clarification of confusing terms that look or sound alike.

VOCABULARY RELATED TO THE INTRODUCTION TO MEDICAL TERMINOLOGY

This list contains essential word parts and medical terms for this chapter. These terms are pronounced on the student StudyWARE™ CD-ROM and Audio CDs that are available for use with this text. These and the other important **primary terms** are shown in boldface throughout the chapter. *Secondary terms*, which appear in *orange* italics, clarify the meaning of primary terms.

Word Parts

- ☐ **-algia**
- ☐ **dys-**
- ☐ **-ectomy**
- ☐ **hyper-**
- ☐ **hypo-**
- ☐ **-itis**
- ☐ **-osis**
- ☐ **-ostomy**
- ☐ **-otomy**
- ☐ **-plasty**
- ☐ **-rrhage**
- ☐ **-rrhaphy**
- ☐ **-rrhea**
- ☐ **-rrhexis**
- ☐ **-sclerosis**

Medical Terms

- ☐ **abdominocentesis** (ab-**dom**-ih-noh-sen-**TEE**-sis)
- ☐ **acronym** (**ACK**-roh-nim)
- ☐ **acute**
- ☐ **angiography** (**an**-jee-**OG**-rah-fee)
- ☐ **appendectomy** (**ap**-en-**DECK**-toh-mee)
- ☐ **arteriosclerosis** (ar-**tee**-ree-oh-skleh-**ROH**-sis)
- ☐ **arthralgia** (ar-**THRAL**-jee-ah)
- ☐ **colostomy** (koh-**LAHS**-toh-mee)
- ☐ **cyanosis** (**sigh**-ah-**NOH**-sis)
- ☐ **dermatologist** (**der**-mah-**TOL**-oh-jist)
- ☐ **diagnosis** (**dye**-ag-**NOH**-sis)
- ☐ **diarrhea** (**dye**-ah-**REE**-ah)
- ☐ **edema** (eh-**DEE**-mah)
- ☐ **endarterial** (**end**-ar-**TEE**-ree-al)
- ☐ **eponym** (**EP**-oh-nim)
- ☐ **erythrocyte** (eh-**RITH**-roh-sight)
- ☐ **fissure** (**FISH**-ur)
- ☐ **fistula** (**FIS**-tyou-lah)
- ☐ **gastralgia** (gas-**TRAL**-jee-ah)
- ☐ **gastritis** (gas-**TRY**-tis)
- ☐ **gastroenteritis** (**gas**-troh-en-ter-**EYE**-tis)
- ☐ **gastrosis** (gas-**TROH**-sis)
- ☐ **hemorrhage** (**HEM**-or-idj)
- ☐ **hepatomegaly** (**hep**-ah-toh-**MEG**-ah-lee)
- ☐ **hypertension** (**high**-per-**TEN**-shun)
- ☐ **hypotension** (**high**-poh-**TEN**-shun)
- ☐ **infection** (in-**FECK**-shun)
- ☐ **inflammation** (**in**-flah-**MAY**-shun)
- ☐ **interstitial** (**in**-ter-**STISH**-al)
- ☐ **intramuscular** (**in**-trah-**MUS**-kyou-lar)
- ☐ **laceration** (**lass**-er-**AY**-shun)
- ☐ **lesion** (**LEE**-zhun)
- ☐ **mycosis** (my-**KOH**-sis)
- ☐ **myelopathy** (my-eh-**LOP**-ah-thee)
- ☐ **myopathy** (my-**OP**-ah-thee)
- ☐ **myorrhexis** (**my**-oh-**RECK**-sis)
- ☐ **natal** (**NAY**-tal)
- ☐ **neonatology** (**nee**-oh-nay-**TOL**-oh-jee)
- ☐ **neuritis** (new-**RYE**-tis)
- ☐ **otorhinolaryngology** (**oh**-toh-**rye**-noh-**lar**-in-**GOL**-oh-jee)
- ☐ **palpation** (pal-**PAY**-shun)
- ☐ **palpitation** (**pal**-pih-**TAY**-shun)
- ☐ **pathology** (pah-**THOL**-oh-jee)
- ☐ **phalanges** (fah-**LAN**-jeez)
- ☐ **poliomyelitis** (**poh**-lee-oh-**my**-eh-**LYE**-tis)
- ☐ **prognosis** (prog-**NOH**-sis)
- ☐ **prostate** (**PROS**-tayt)
- ☐ **pyoderma** (**pye**-oh-**DER**-mah)
- ☐ **pyrosis** (pye-**ROH**-sis)
- ☐ **remission**
- ☐ **sign**
- ☐ **supination** (**soo**-pih-**NAY**-shun)
- ☐ **suppuration** (**sup**-you-**RAY**-shun)
- ☐ **supracostal** (**sue**-prah-**KOS**-tal)
- ☐ **symptom** (**SIMP**-tum)
- ☐ **syndrome** (**SIN**-drohm)
- ☐ **tonsillitis** (**ton**-sih-**LYE**-tis)
- ☐ **trauma** (**TRAW**-mah)
- ☐ **triage** (tree-**AHZH**)
- ☐ **viral** (**VYE**-ral)

OBJECTIVES

On completion of this chapter, you should be able to:

1. Identify the roles of the four types of word parts used in forming medical terms.
2. Using your knowledge of word parts, analyze unfamiliar medical terms.
3. Describe the steps in locating a term in a medical dictionary.
4. Define the commonly used prefixes, word roots, combining forms, and suffixes introduced in this chapter.
5. Pronounce medical terms correctly using the "sounds-like" system.
6. Recognize the importance of always spelling medical terms correctly.
7. State why caution is important when using abbreviations.
8. Recognize, define, spell, and pronounce the medical terms in this chapter.

PRIMARY MEDICAL TERMS

In this book, you will be introduced to many medical terms; however, mastering them will be easier than you anticipate because this book has this new feature to make learning easier:

- **Primary terms** appear in boldface. Learning these terms should be your highest priority as only primary terms are used as correct answers in the Learning Exercises and tests.
- *Secondary terms* appear in *orange* italics. Some of these terms are the "also known as" names for conditions or procedures. Other secondary terms clarify words used in the definitions of primary terms.

WORD PARTS ARE THE KEY

Learning medical terminology is much easier once you understand how word parts work together to form medical terms. This book includes many aids to help you continue reinforcing your word building skills.

- The types of word parts and the rules for their use are explained in this chapter. Learn these rules and follow them.
- When a term is made up of recognizable word parts, these word parts and their meanings are included with the definition of that term. These word parts appear in **magenta**.
- The Learning Exercises for each chapter include a "Challenge Word Building" section to help develop your skills in working with word parts.
- After Chapter 2, there is a Word Part Review. This section provides additional word part practice and enables you to evaluate your progress toward mastering the meaning of these word parts.

The Four Types of Word Parts

Four types of word parts may be used to create medical terms. Guidelines for their use are shown in Table 1.1.

- **A word root** contains the basic meaning of the term. This word part usually, *but not always*, indicates the involved body part. For example, the word root meaning stomach is **gastr**.
- A **combining form** is a word root with a vowel at the end so that a suffix beginning with a consonant can be added. When a combining form appears alone, it is shown with a slash (/) between the word root and the combining vowel. For example, the combining form meaning stomach is **gastr/o**.

TABLE 1.1
WORD PART GUIDELINES

1. A word root cannot stand alone. A suffix must be added to complete the term.
2. The rules for creating a combining form by adding a vowel apply when a suffix beginning with a consonant is added to a word root. These rules are explained in Table 1.3.
3. When a prefix is necessary, it is always placed at the beginning of the word.

- A **suffix** usually, *but not always*, indicates the procedure, condition, disorder, or disease. A suffix *always* comes at the end of a word.
- **A prefix** usually, *but not always*, indicates location, time, number, or status. A prefix *always* comes at the beginning of a word.

WORD ROOTS

Word roots act as the foundation of most medical terms. They usually, *but not always*, describe the part of the body that is involved (Figure 1.1). As shown in Table 1.2, some word roots indicate color.

Combining Form Vowels

A combining form vowel is added to the end of a word root under certain conditions to make the resulting medical term easier to pronounce. The rules for the use of combining form vowels are explained in Table 1.3.

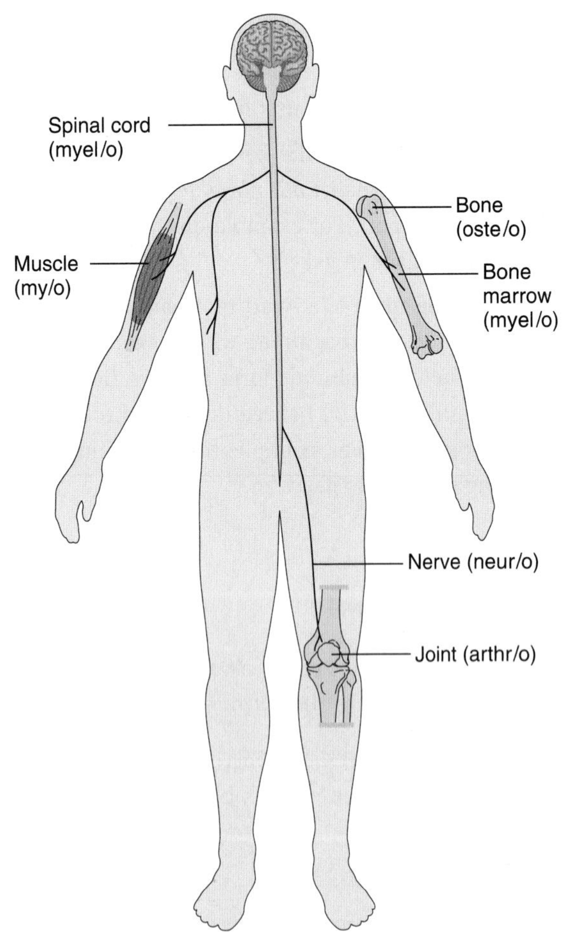

FIGURE 1.1 Word roots, shown here as combining forms, usually indicate the involved body part.

- The letter "o" is the most commonly used combining vowel.
- When a word root is shown alone as a combining form, it includes a slash (/) and the combining vowel.

SUFFIXES

A suffix is a word part that is added to the end of a word to complete that term. In medical terminology, suffixes usually, *but not always*, indicate a procedure, condition, disorder, or disease. For example, **tonsill/o** means tonsils. The suffix that is added completes the term and tells what is happening to the tonsils (Figure 1.2).

- **Tonsillitis** (**ton**-sih-**LYE**-tis) is an inflammation of the tonsils (**tonsill** means tonsils, and **-itis** means inflammation).
- A **tonsillectomy** (**ton**-sih-**LECK**-toh-mee) is the surgical removal of the tonsils (**tonsill** means tonsils, and **-ectomy** means surgical removal).

Suffixes as Noun Endings

A *noun* is a word that is the name of a person, place, or thing. In medical terminology, some suffixes change the word root into a noun. For example, the **cranium** (**KRAY**-nee-um) is the portion of the skull that encloses the brain (**crani** means skull, and **-um** is a noun ending). Other suffixes complete the term by changing the word root into a noun. Suffixes that are commonly used as "Noun Endings" are listed in a table at the beginning of Appendix A.

Suffixes Meaning "Pertaining To"

An *adjective* is a word that defines or describes a thing. In medical terminology, many suffixes meaning "pertaining to" change the word root into an adjective. For example, the term **cardiac** is an adjective that means pertaining to the heart (**cardi** means heart, and **-ac** means pertaining to). Commonly used suffixes meaning "pertaining to" are listed in a table at the beginning of Appendix A.

Suffixes Meaning Abnormal Condition

In medical terminology, many suffixes, such as **-osis**, mean "abnormal condition or disease." For example, **gastrosis** (gas-**TROH**-sis) means any disease of the stomach (**gastr** means stomach, and **-osis** means abnormal condition or disease). These suffixes are also listed in a table at the beginning of Appendix A.

TABLE 1.2

WORD ROOTS/COMBINING FORMS INDICATING COLOR

cyan/o means blue	**Cyanosis** (**sigh**-ah-**NOH**-sis) is blue discoloration of the skin caused by a lack of adequate oxygen in the blood (**cyan** means blue, and **-osis** means abnormal condition or disease).
erythr/o means red	An **erythrocyte** (eh-**RITH**-roh-sight) is a mature red blood cell (**erythr/o** means red, and **-cyte** means cell).
leuk/o means white	A **leukocyte** (**LOO**-koh-sight) is a white blood cell (**leuk/o** means white, and **-cyte** means cell).
melan/o means black	**Melanosis** (**mel**-ah-**NOH**-sis) is any condition of unusual deposits of black pigment in body tissues or organs (**melan** means black, and **-osis** means abnormal condition or disease).
poli/o means gray	**Poliomyelitis** (**poh**-lee-oh-**my**-eh-**LYE**-tis) is a viral infection of the gray matter of the spinal cord (**poli/o** means gray, **myel** means spinal cord, and **-itis** means inflammation).

TABLE 1.3

RULES FOR USING COMBINING FORM VOWELS

1. **A combining vowel *is used* when the suffix begins with a consonant.**
   For example, when **neur/o** (nerve) is joined with the suffix **-plasty** (surgical repair), the combining vowel "o" *is used* because-**plasty** begins with a consonant.
   Neuroplasty (**NEW**-roh-**plas**-tee) is the surgical repair of a nerve (**neur/o** means nerve, and **-plasty** means surgical repair).

2. **A combining vowel *is not used* when the suffix begins with a vowel (a, e, i, o, u).**
   For example, when **neur/o** (nerve) is joined with the suffix **-itis** (inflammation), no combining vowel is used because **-itis** begins with a vowel.
   Neuritis (new-**RYE**-**tis**) is inflammation of a nerve or nerves (**neur** means nerve, and **-itis** means inflammation).

3. **A combining vowel *is used* when two or more word roots are joined.**
   For example, gastroenteritis combines two word roots with a suffix. When **gastr/o** (stomach) is joined with **enter/o** (small intestine), the combining vowel *is used* with **gastr/o.** A combining vowel *is not used* with **enter/o** because it is joining the suffix **-itis**, which begins with a vowel.
   Gastroenteritis (**gas**-troh-en-ter-**EYE**-tis) is an inflammation of the stomach and small intestine (**gastr/o** means stomach, **enter** means small intestine, and **-itis** means inflammation).

Suffixes Related to Pathology

Pathology (pah-**THOL**-oh-jee) is the study of all aspects of diseases (**path** means disease, and **-ology** means study of). Suffixes related to pathology describe specific disease conditions.

- **-algia** means pain and suffering. **Gastralgia** (gas-**TRAL**-jee-ah), also known as *stomach ache*, means pain in the stomach (**gastr** means stomach, and **-algia** means pain).
- **-dynia** also means pain. **Gastrodynia** (**gas**-troh-**DIN**-ee-ah) also means pain in the stomach (**gastr/o** means stomach, and **-dynia** means pain). Although **-dynia** has the same meaning as **-algia**, it is not used as commonly.

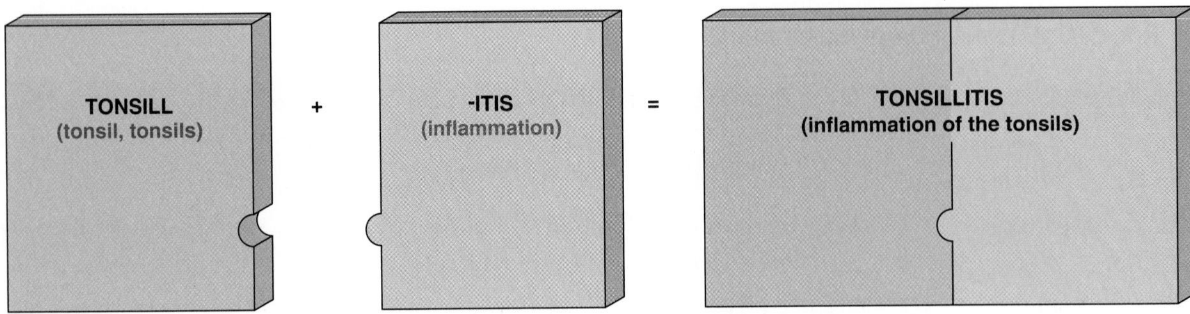

FIGURE 1.2 The term tonsillitis is created by adding the suffix -itis to the word root tonsill.

- **-itis** means inflammation. **Gastritis** (gas-**TRY**-tis) is an inflammation of the stomach (**gastr** means stomach, and **-itis** means inflammation).
- **-malacia** means abnormal softening. **Arteriomalacia** (ar-**tee**-ree-oh-mah-**LAY**-shee-ah) is the abnormal softening of the walls of an artery or arteries (**arteri/o** means artery, and **-malacia** means abnormal softening). Notice that **-malacia** is the opposite of **-sclerosis**.
- **-megaly** means enlargement. **Hepatomegaly** (**hep**-ah-toh-**MEG**-ah-lee) is abnormal enlargement of the liver (**hepat/o** means liver, and **-megaly** means enlargement).
- **-necrosis** means tissue death. **Arterionecrosis** (ar-**tee**-ree-oh-neh-**KROH**-sis) is the tissue death of an artery or arteries (**arteri/o** means artery, and **-necrosis** means tissue death).
- **-sclerosis** means abnormal hardening. **Arteriosclerosis** (ar-**tee**-ree-oh-skleh-**ROH**-sis) is the abnormal hardening of the walls of an artery or arteries (**arteri/o** means artery, and **-sclerosis** means abnormal hardening). Notice that **-sclerosis** is the opposite of **-malacia**.
- **-stenosis** means abnormal narrowing. **Arteriostenosis** (ar-**tee**-ree-oh-steh-**NOH**-sis) is the abnormal narrowing of an artery or arteries (**arteri/o** means artery, and **-stenosis** means abnormal narrowing.)

Suffixes Related to Procedures

Some suffixes identify the procedure that is performed on the body part identified by the word root.

- **-centesis** is a surgical puncture to remove fluid for diagnostic purposes or to remove excess fluid. **Abdominocentesis** (ab-**dom**-ih-noh-sen-**TEE**-sis) is the surgical puncture of the abdominal cavity to remove fluid (**abdomin/o** means abdomen, and **-centesis** means a surgical puncture to remove fluid).
- **-graphy** means the process of producing a picture or record. **Angiography** (**an**-jee-**OG**-rah-fee) is the process of producing a radiographic (x-ray) study of the blood vessels after the injection of a contrast medium to make these blood vessels visible (**angi/o** means blood vessel, and **-graphy** means the process of recording).
- **-gram** means a picture or record. An **angiogram** (**AN**-jee-oh-**gram**) is the film produced by angiography (**angi/o** means blood vessel, and **-gram** means a picture or record).
- **-plasty** means surgical repair. **Myoplasty** (**MY**-oh-**plas**-tee) is the surgical repair of a muscle (**myo** means muscle, and **-plasty** means surgical repair).
- **-scopy** means visual examination. **Arthroscopy** (ar-**THROS**-koh-pee) is the visual examination of the internal structure of a joint (**arthr/o** means joint, and **-scopy** means visual examination).

The "Double R" Suffixes

Suffixes beginning with two "Rs," which are often referred to as the "double RRs," can be particularly confusing. They are grouped together here to help you understand the word parts and to remember the differences.

- **-rrhage** and **-rrhagia** mean bleeding; however, they are most often used to describe sudden, severe bleeding. A **hemorrhage** (**HEM**-or-idj) is the loss of a large amount of blood in a short time (**hem/o** means blood, and **-rrhage** means bursting forth of blood).
- **-rrhaphy** means surgical suturing to close a wound and includes the use of sutures, staples, or surgical glue. **Myorrhaphy** (my-**OR**-ah-fee) is the surgical suturing of a muscle wound (**my/o** means muscle, and **-rrhaphy** means surgical suturing).
- **-rrhea** means flow or discharge and refers to the flow of most body fluids. **Diarrhea** (**dye**-ah-**REE**-ah) is the frequent flow of loose or watery stools (**dia-** means through, and **-rrhea** means flow or discharge).

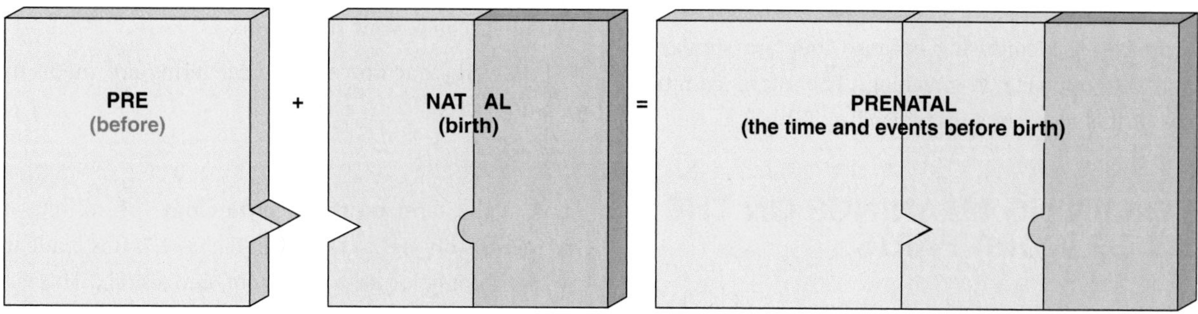

FIGURE 1.3 The term prenatal is created by joining the suffix -al to the word root nat and then adding the prefix pre-.

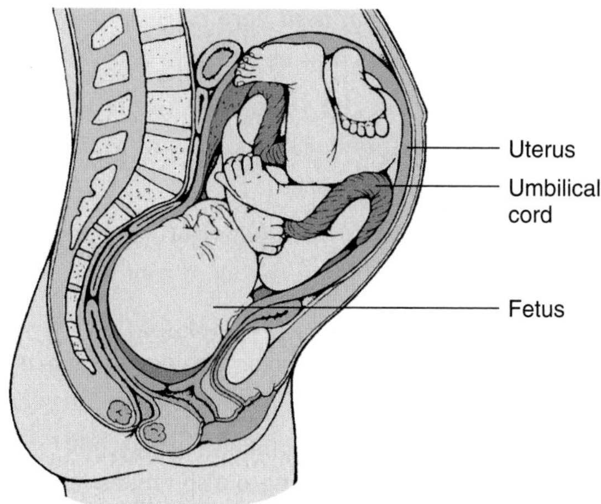

FIGURE 1.4 Shown here, as a diagram, is the *prenatal* development of a fetus (baby).

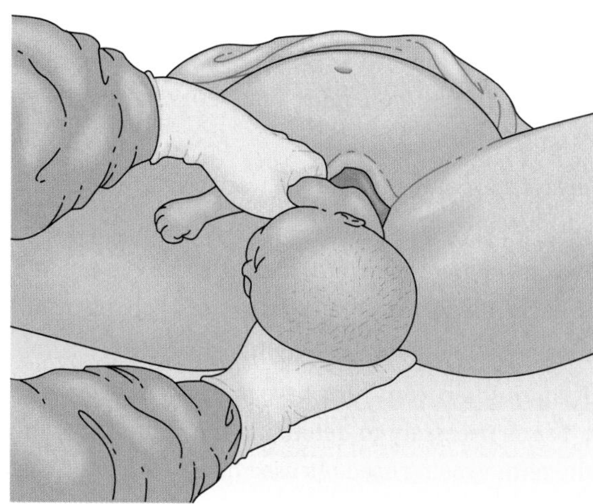

FIGURE 1.5 Shown here is a *perinatal* event of the baby's head emerging during a normal birth.

- **-rrhexis** means rupture. **Myorrhexis** (**my**-oh-**RECK**-sis) is the rupture of a muscle (**my/o** means muscle, and **-rrhexis** means rupture).

PREFIXES

A prefix is added to the beginning of a word to influence the meaning of that term. Prefixes usually, *but not always*, indicate location, time, or number. The term **natal** (**NAY**-tal) means pertaining to birth (**nat** means birth, and **-al** means pertaining to). The following examples show how prefixes change the meaning of this term (Figures 1.3–1.6).

- **Prenatal** (pre-**NAY**-tal) means the time and events before birth (**pre-** means before, **nat** means birth, and **-al** means pertaining to).
- **Perinatal** (**pehr**-ih-**NAY**-tal) refers to the time and events surrounding birth (**peri-** means surrounding, **nat** means birth, and **-al** means pertaining to). This is the time just before, during, and just after birth.

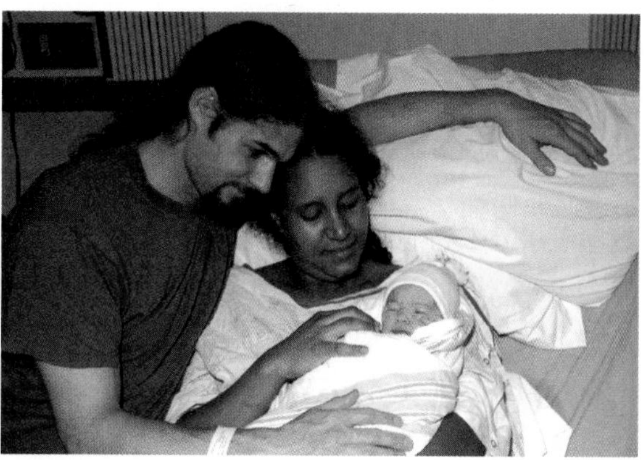

FIGURE 1.6 A joyful *postnatal* event as the new parents bond with their new baby.

- **Postnatal** (pohst-**NAY**-tal) refers to the time and events after birth (**post-** means after, **nat** means birth, and **-al** means pertaining to).

Contrasting and Confusing Prefixes

Some prefixes are confusing because they are similar in spelling, but opposite in meaning. The more common prefixes of this type are summarized in Table 1.4.

DETERMINING MEANINGS ON THE BASIS OF WORD PARTS

Knowing the meaning of the word parts often makes it possible to figure out the definition of an unfamiliar medical term.

Taking Terms Apart

To determine a word's meaning by looking at the component pieces, you must first separate it into word parts.

- Always start at the end of the word, with the suffix, and work toward the beginning.
- As you separate the word parts, identify the meaning of each. Identifying the meaning of each part should give you a definition of the term.
- Because some word parts have more than one meaning, it also is necessary to determine the context in which the term is being used. As used here, *context* means to determine which body system this term is referring to.
- If you have any doubt, use your medical dictionary to double-check your definition.
- Be aware that not all medical terms are made up of word parts.

An Example

Look at the term **otorhinolaryngology** (**oh**-toh-**rye**-noh-**lar**-in-**GOL**-oh-jee) as shown in Figure 1.7. It is made up of two combining forms, a word root, and a suffix. This is how it looks when the word parts have been separated by working from the end to the beginning.

- The suffix **-ology** means the study of.
- The word root **laryng** means larynx and throat. The combining vowel *is not used* here because the word root is joining a suffix that begins with a vowel.
- The combining form **rhin/o** means nose. The combining vowel *is used* here because the word root **rhin** is joining another word root.
- The combining form **ot/o** means ear. The combining vowel *is used* here because the word root **ot** is joining another word root.
- Together they form otorhinolaryngology, which is the study of the ears, nose, and throat (**ot/o** means ear, **rhin/o** means nose, **laryng** means throat, and **-ology** means study of). Note: Laryng/o also means larynx and this is discussed in Chapter 7.

TABLE 1.4

CONTRASTING PREFIXES

ab- means away from. **Abnormal** means not normal or away from normal.	**ad-** means toward or in the direction of. **Addiction** means drawn toward or a strong dependence on a drug or substance.
dys- means bad, difficult, or painful. **Dysfunctional** means an organ or body part that is not working properly.	**eu-** means good, normal, well, or easy. **Euthyroid** (you-**THIGH**-roid) means a normally functioning thyroid gland.
hyper- means excessive or increased. **Hypertension** (**high**-per-**TEN**-shun) is higher than normal blood pressure.	**hypo-** means deficient or decreased. **Hypotension** (**high**-poh-**TEN**-shun) is lower than normal blood pressure.
inter- means between or among. **Interstitial** (**in**-ter-**STISH**-al) means between, but not within, the parts of a tissue.	**intra-** means within or inside. **Intramuscular** (**in**-trah-**MUS**-kyou-lar) means within the muscle.
sub- means under, less, or below. **Subcostal** (sub-**KOS**-tal) means below a rib or ribs.	**super-, supra-** mean above or excessive. **Supracostal** (**sue**-prah-**KOS**-tal) means above or outside the ribs.

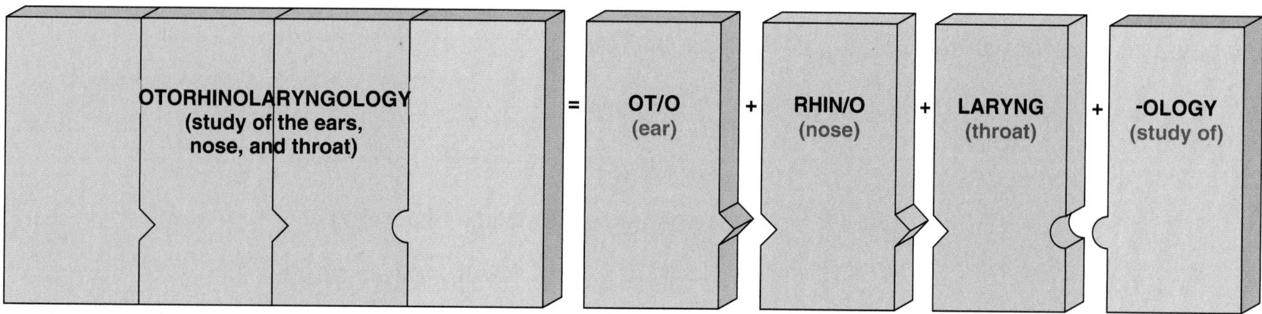

FIGURE 1.7 To determine the meaning of a medical term, the word parts are separated beginning at the end of the word and working toward the front.

- Because this is such a long name, this specialty is frequently referred to as *ENT* (ears, nose, and throat). A shortened version of this term is **otolaryngology** (**oh**-toh-**lar**-in-**GOL**-oh-jee), which is the study of the ears and larynx or throat (**ot/o** means ears, **larynx** means larynx, and **-ology** means study of).

Guessing at Meanings

When you are able to guess at the meaning of a term on the basis of word parts that it is made up of, you must always double-check for accuracy because some terms have more than one meaning. For example, look at the term **lithotomy** (lih-**THOT**-oh-mee):

- On the basis of word parts, a **lithotomy** is a surgical incision for the removal of a stone (**lith** means stone, and **-otomy** means a surgical incision). This meaning is discussed further in Chapter 9.
- However, **lithotomy** is also the name of an examination position in which the patient is lying on the back with the feet and legs raised and supported in stirrups. The term is used to describe this position because in the early days, this was the preferred position for lithotomy surgery. This term is discussed further in Chapter 15.
- This type of possible confusion is one of the many reasons why a medical dictionary is an important medical terminology tool.

MEDICAL DICTIONARY USE

Learning to use a medical dictionary and other resources to find the definition of a term is an important part of mastering the correct use of medical terms. The following tips for dictionary use apply whether you are working with a traditional book-form dictionary or with electronic dictionary software on your computer.

If You Know How to Spell the Word

When starting to work with an unfamiliar print dictionary, spend a few minutes reviewing its user guide, table of contents, and appendices. The time you spend reviewing now will be saved later when you are looking up unfamiliar terms.

- On the basis of the first letter of the word, start in the appropriate section of the dictionary. Look at the top of the page for clues. The top left word is the first term on the page. The top right word is the last term on that page.
- Next, look alphabetically for words that start with the first and second letters of the word you are researching. Continue looking through each letter until you find the term you are looking for.
- When you think you have found it, check the spelling very carefully, letter by letter, working from left to right. Terms with similar spellings have very different meanings.
- When you find the term, carefully check *all* of the definitions.

If You Do Not Know How to Spell the Word

Listen carefully to the term and write it down. If you cannot find the word on the basis of your spelling, start looking for alternative spellings based on the beginning sound as shown in Table 1.5. Note: All of these examples are in this text. However, you could practice looking them up in the dictionary!

TABLE 1.5

Guidelines to Looking Up the Spelling of Unfamiliar Terms

If it sounds like	It may begin with	Example
F	F	**flatus** (**FLAY**-tus) [see Chapter 8]
	PH	**phlegm** (**FLEM**) [see Chapter 7]
J	G	**gingivitis** (**jin**-jih-**VYE**-tis) [see Chapter 8]
	J	**jaundice** (**JAWN**-dis) [see Chapter 8]
K	C	**crepitus** (**KREP**-ih-tus) [see Chapter 3]
	CH	**cholera** (**KOL**-er-ah) [see Chapter 8]
	K	**kyphosis** (kye-**FOH**-sis) [see Chapter 3]
	QU	**quadriplegia** (**kwad**-rih-**PLEE**-jee-ah) [see Chapter 4]
S	C	**cytology** (sigh-**TOL**-oh-jee) [see Chapter 2]
	PS	**psychologist** (sigh-**KOL**-oh-jist) [see Chapter 10]
	S	**serum** (**SEER**-um) [see Chapter 5]
Z	X	**xeroderma** (zee-roh-**DER**-mah) [see Chapter 12]
	Z	**zygote** (**ZYE**-goht) [see Chapter 14]

Look Under Categories

Most print dictionaries use categories such as *Diseases* and *Syndromes* to group disorders with these terms in their titles. For example:

- *Venereal disease* would be found under *Disease, venereal.* These sexually transmitted diseases are discussed further in Chapter 14.
- *Fetal alcohol syndrome* would be found under *Syndrome, fetal alcohol.* This condition is discussed further in Chapter 2.
- When you come across a term such as one of these and cannot find it listed by the first word, the next step is to look under the appropriate category.

Multiple Word Terms

When you are looking for a term that includes more than one word, begin your search with the last term. If you do not find it there, move forward to the next word.

- For example, *congestive heart failure* is sometimes listed under *heart failure, congestive.* This term is discussed in Chapter 5.

Searching for Definitions on the Internet

Internet search engines are valuable resources in finding definitions and details about medical conditions and terms; however, it is important that you rely on a site, such as the National Institutes of Health (NIH) web site (www.nih.gov), which is known to be a reputable information source. For better results, an Internet search should include visits to at least two different sites. If there is a major difference in the definitions here, go on to a third site.

PRONUNCIATION

A medical term is easier to understand, and remember, when you know how to pronounce it properly. To help you master the pronunciation of new terms, a commonly accepted pronunciation of that word appears (in parentheses) next to the term. Audio for the terms on the vocabulary list is available on the student StudyWARE™ CD-ROM.

The "sounds-like" pronunciation system is used in this textbook. Here the word is respelled using normal

English letters to create sounds that are familiar. To pronounce a new word, just say it as it is spelled in the parentheses.

- The part of the word that receives the primary (most) emphasis when you say it is shown in uppercase boldface letters. For example, **edema** (eh-**DEE**-mah) describes swelling caused by excess fluid in the body tissues.
- A part of the word that receives secondary (less) emphasis when you say it is shown in boldface lowercase letters.
  For example, **appendicitis** (ah-**pen**-dih-**SIGH**-tis) means an inflammation of the appendix (**appendic** means appendix, and **-itis** means inflammation).

A Word of Caution

Frequently, there is more than one correct way to pronounce a medical term.

- The pronunciation of many medical terms is based on their Greek, Latin, or other foreign origin. However, there is a trend toward pronouncing terms as they would sound in English.
- The result is more than one "correct" pronunciation for a term. The text shows the most commonly accepted pronunciation.
- If your instructor prefers an alternative pronunciation, follow the instructions you are given.

SPELLING IS ALWAYS IMPORTANT

Accuracy in spelling medical terms is extremely important!

- Changing just one or two letters can completely change the meaning of a word—and this difference literally could be a matter of life or death for the patient.
- The section "Look-Alike Sound-Alike Terms and Word Parts" later in this chapter will help you become aware of some terms and word parts that are frequently confused.
- The spelling shown in this text is commonly accepted in the United States (US). You may encounter alternative spellings used in England, Australia, and Canada.

USING ABBREVIATIONS

Abbreviations are frequently used as a shorthand way to record long and complex medical terms; Appendix B contains an alphabetized list of many of the more commonly used medical abbreviations.

- Abbreviations can also lead to confusion and errors! Therefore, it is important that you be very careful when using or interpreting an abbreviation.
- For example, the abbreviation *BE* means both "below elbow" (as in amputation) and "barium enema." Just imagine what a difference a mix-up here would make for the patient!
- Most clinical agencies have policies for accepted abbreviations. It is important to follow this list for the facility where you are working.
- If there is any question in your mind about which abbreviation to use, always follow this rule: *When in doubt, spell it out.*

SINGULAR AND PLURAL ENDINGS

Many medical terms have Greek or Latin origins. As a result of these different origins, there are unusual rules for changing a singular word into a plural form. In addition, English endings have been adopted for some commonly used terms.

- Table 1.6 provides guidelines to help you better understand how these plurals are formed.
- Also, throughout the text, when a term with an unusual singular or plural form is introduced, both forms are included. For example, the **phalanges** (fah-**LAN**-jeez) are the bones of the fingers and toes (singular, *phalanx*) (Figure 1.8).

BASIC MEDICAL TERMS TO DESCRIBE DISEASES

Some of the basic medical terms used to describe diseases and disease conditions are shown in Table 1.7.

LOOK-ALIKE SOUND-ALIKE TERMS AND WORD PARTS

This section highlights some frequently used terms and word parts that are confusing because they look and sound alike. However, the meanings are very different, and it is important that you pay close attention to these terms and word parts as you encounter them in the text.

arteri/o, ather/o, and arthr/o

- **arteri/o** means artery. **Endarterial** (**end**-ar-**TEE**-ree-al) means pertaining to the interior or lining of an artery (**end-** means within, **arteri** means artery, and **-al** means pertaining to). See Chapter 5.

TABLE 1.6

GUIDELINES TO UNUSUAL PLURAL FORMS

Guideline	Singular	Plural
1. If the singular term ends in the suffix **-a**, the plural is usually formed by changing the ending to **-ae**.	bursa vertebra	bursae vertebrae
2. If the singular term ends in the suffix **-ex** or **-ix**, the plural is usually formed by changing these endings to **-ices**.	appendix index	appendices indices
3. If the singular term ends in the suffix **-is**, the plural is usually formed by changing the ending to **-es**.	diagnosis metastasis	diagnoses metastases
4. If the singular term ends in the suffix **-itis**, the plural is usually formed by changing the **-is** ending to **-ides**.	arthritis meningitis	arthritides meningitides
5. If the singular term ends in the suffix **-nx**, the plural is usually formed by the **-x** ending to **-ges**.	phalanx meninx	phalanges meninges
6. If the singular term ends in the suffix **-on**, the plural is usually formed by changing the ending to **-a**.	criterion ganglion	criteria ganglia
7. If the singular term ends in the suffix **-um**, the plural usually is formed by changing the ending to **-a**.	diverticulum ovum	diverticula ova
8. If the singular term ends in the suffix **-us**, the plural is usually formed by changing the ending to **-i**.	alveolus malleolus	alveoli malleoli

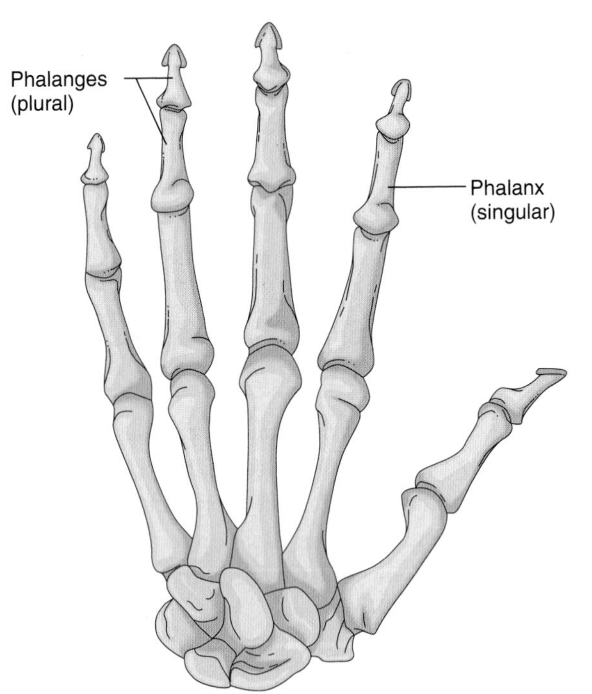

FIGURE 1.8 Singular and plural endings. A phalanx is one finger or toe bone. Phalanges are more than one finger or toe bones.

- **ather/o** means plaque or fatty substance. An **atheroma** (**ath**-er-**OH**-mah) is a fatty deposit within the wall of an artery (**ather** means fatty substance, and **-oma** means tumor). See Chapter 5.
- **arthr/o** means joint. **Arthralgia** (ar-**THRAL**-jee-ah) means pain in a joint or joints (**arthr** means joint, and **-algia** means pain). See Chapter 3.

-ectomy, -ostomy and -otomy

- **-ectomy** means surgical removal. An **appendectomy** (**ap**-en-**DECK**-toh-mee) is the surgical removal of the appendix (**append** means appendix, and **-ectomy** means surgical removal). See Chapter 8.
- **-ostomy** means the surgical creation of an artificial opening to the body surface. A **colostomy** (koh-**LAHS**-toh-mee) is the surgical creation of an artificial excretory opening between the colon and the body surface (**col** means colon, and **-ostomy** means the creation of an artificial opening). See Chapter 8.

TABLE 1.7

Basic Medical Terms to Describe Disease Conditions

A **sign** is objective evidence of disease such as a fever. *Objective* means the sign can be evaluated or measured by the patient or others.	A **symptom** (**SIMP**-tum) is subjective evidence of a disease, such as pain or a headache. *Subjective* means that it can be evaluated or measured only by the patient.	A **syndrome** (**SIN**-drohm) is a set of the signs and symptoms that occur together as part of a specific disease process.
A **diagnosis** (**dye**-ag-**NOH**-sis) is the identification of a disease (plural, *diagnoses*). To *diagnose* is the process of reaching a diagnosis.	A **differential diagnosis**, which is also known as to *rule out* (R/O) is an attempt to determine which one of several diseases can be producing the signs and symptoms that are present.	A **prognosis** (prog-**NOH**-sis) is a prediction of the probable course and outcome of a disorder (plural, *prognoses*).
An **acute** condition has a rapid onset, a severe course, and a relatively short duration.	A **chronic** condition is of long duration. Although such diseases can be controlled, they are rarely cured.	A **remission** is the temporary, partial, or complete disappearance of the symptoms of a disease without having achieved a cure.
A **disease** is a condition in which one or more body parts are not functioning normally. Some diseases are named for their signs and symptoms. For example, *chronic fatigue syndrome* is a persistent overwhelming fatigue of unknown origin (see Chapter 4).	An **eponym** (**EP**-oh-nim) is a disease, structure, operation, or procedure named for the person who discovered or described it first. For example, *Alzheimer's disease* is named for German neurologist Alois Alzheimer (see Chapter 10).	An **acronym** (**ACK**-roh-nim) is a word formed from the initial letter of the major parts of a compound term. For example, the acronym **laser** stands for **l**ight **a**mplification by **s**timulated **e**mission of **r**adiation (see Chapter 12).

- **-otomy** means cutting or a surgical incision. A **colotomy** (koh-**LOT**-oh-mee) is a surgical incision into the colon (**col** means colon, and **-otomy** means a surgical incision). See Chapter 8.

Fissure and Fistula

- A **fissure** (**FISH**-ur) is a groove or crack-like sore of the skin (see Chapter 12). This term also describes normal folds in the contours of the brain (see Chapter 10).
- A **fistula** (**FIS**-tyou-lah) is an abnormal passage, usually between two internal organs, or leading from an organ to the surface of the body. A fistula may be due to surgery, injury, or the draining of an abscess.

Ileum and Ilium

- The **ileum** (**ILL**-ee-um) is the last and longest portion of the small intestine. *Memory aid:* il**e**um is spelled with an ***e*** as in int**e**stine. See Chapter 8.
- The **ilium** (**ILL**-ee-um) is part of the hip bone. *Memory aid:* il**i**um is spelled with an ***i*** as in h**i**p. See Chapter 3.

Infection and Inflammation

- An **infection** (in-**FECK**-shun) is the invasion of the body by a pathogenic (disease producing) organism. The infection can remain localized (near the point of entry) or can be systemic (affecting the entire body). Signs and symptoms of infection include malaise, chills and fever, redness, heat and swelling, or exudate from a wound. *Malaise* is a feeling of general discomfort or uneasiness that is often the first indication of an infection or other disease. An *exudate* is fluid, such as pus, that leaks out of an infected wound.
- **Inflammation** (**in**-flah-**MAY**-shun) is a localized response to an injury or destruction of tissues. The

cardinal signs (indications) of inflammation are (1) *erythema* (redness), (2) *hyperthermia* (heat), (3) *edema* (swelling), and (4) *pain*. These are caused by extra blood flowing into the area as part of the healing process.

- Although the suffix **-itis** means inflammation, it also is commonly used to indicate infection.

Laceration and Lesion

- A **laceration** (**lass**-er-**AY**-shun) is a torn or jagged wound or an accidental cut wound. See Chapter 12.
- A **lesion** (**LEE**-zhun) is a pathologic change of the tissues due to disease or injury. See Chapter 12.

Mucous and Mucus

- The adjective **mucous** (**MYOU**-kus) describes the specialized mucous membranes that line the body cavities. See Chapter 7.
- The noun **mucus** (**MYOU**-kus) is the name of the fluid secreted by the mucous membranes. See Chapter 7.

myc/o, myel/o, and my/o

- **myc/o** means fungus. **Mycosis** (my-**KOH**-sis) describes any abnormal condition or disease caused by a fungus (**myc** means fungus, and **-osis** means abnormal condition or disease).
- **myel/o** means bone marrow *or* spinal cord. The term **myelopathy** (my-eh-**LOP**-ah-thee) describes any pathologic change or disease in the spinal cord (**myel/o** means spinal cord or bone marrow, and **-pathy** means disease).
- **my/o** means muscle. The term **myopathy** (my-**OP**-ah-thee) describes any pathologic change or disease of muscle tissue (**my/o** means muscle, and **-pathy** means disease).

-ologist and -ology

- **-ologist** means specialist. A **dermatologist** (**der**-mah-**TOL**-oh-jist) is a physician who specializes in diagnosing and treating disorders of the skin (**dermat** means skin, and **-ologist** means specialist).
- **-ology** means the study of. **Neonatology** (**nee**-oh-nay-**TOL**-oh-jee) is the study of disorders of the newborn (**neo-** means new, **nat** means birth, and **-ology** means study of).

Palpation and Palpitation

- **Palpation** (pal-**PAY**-shun) is an examination technique in which the examiner's hands are used to feel the texture, size, consistency, and location of certain body parts. See Chapter 15.
- **Palpitation** (**pal**-pih-**TAY**-shun) is a pounding or racing heart. See Chapter 5.

Prostate and Prostrate

- The **prostate** (**PROS**-tayt) is a male gland that lies under the urinary bladder and surrounds the urethra.
- **Prostrate** (**PROS**-trayt) means to collapse and be lying flat or to be overcome with exhaustion.

pyel/o, py/o, and pyr/o

- **pyel/o** means renal pelvis, which is part of the kidney. **Pyelitis** (**pye**-eh-**LYE**-tis) is an inflammation of the renal pelvis (**pyel** means renal pelvis, and **-itis** means inflammation). See Chapter 9.
- **py/o** means pus. **Pyoderma** (**pye**-oh-**DER**-mah) is any acute, inflammatory, pus-forming bacterial skin infection such as impetigo (**py/o** means pus, and **-derma** means skin). See Chapter 12.
- **pyr/o** means fever or fire. **Pyrosis** (pye-**ROH**-sis), also known as *heartburn*, is discomfort due to the regurgitation of stomach acid upward into the esophagus (**pyr** means fever or fire, and **-osis** means abnormal condition or disease). See Chapter 8.

Supination and Suppuration

- **Supination** (**soo**-pih-**NAY**-shun) is the act of rotating the arm so that the palm of the hand is forward or upward. See Figure 4.7 in Chapter 4.
- **Suppuration** (**sup**-you-**RAY**-shun) is the formation or discharge of pus. See Chapter 9.

Triage and Trauma

- **Triage** (tree-**AHZH**) is the medical screening of patients to determine their relative priority of need and the proper place of treatment. For example, emergency personnel arriving on an accident scene must identify which of the injured require care first and determine where they can be treated most effectively.

- **Trauma** (**TRAW**-mah) means wound or injury. These are the types of injuries that might occur in an accident, shooting, natural disaster, or fire.

Viral and Virile

- **Viral** (**VYE**-ral) means pertaining to a virus (**vir** means virus or poison, and **-al** means pertaining to).
- **Virile** (**VIR**-ill) means having the nature, properties, or qualities of an adult male.

ABBREVIATIONS RELATED TO THE INTRODUCTION TO MEDICAL TERMINOLOGY

Table 1.8 presents an overview of the abbreviations related to the terms introduced in this chapter. Note: To avoid errors or confusion, always be cautious when using abbreviations.

TABLE 1.8

ABBREVIATIONS RELATED TO THE INTRODUCTION TO MEDICAL TERMINOLOGY

appendectomy or appendicitis = AP	**AP** = appendectomy or appendicitis
chronic fatigue syndrome = CFS	**CFS** = chronic fatigue syndrome
diagnosis = DG, Dg, Diag, diag, DX, Dx	**DG, Dg, Diag, diag, DX, Dx** = diagnosis
differential diagnosis = D/D, DD, DDx, diaf. Diag	**D/D, DD, DDx, diaf. diag** =differential diagnosis
hemorrhage = He	**He** = hemorrhage
inflammation = Inflam, Inflamm	**Inflam, Inflamm** = inflammation
intramuscular = IM	**IM** = intramuscular
pathology = PA, Pa, path	**Pa, PA, Path** = pathology
postnatal = PN	**PN** = postnatal
prognosis = prog, progn, Prx, Px	**prog, progn, Prx, Px** = prognosis

Career Opportunities: Setting Your Goals

Learning about medical terminology is essential to a wide range of health occupations, from transplant surgeon to dance therapist. As you learn about the different body systems and fields of medical care, think about which jobs sound most appealing to you. Look in the library and on the Internet for detailed information about careers you might want to pursue.

Some health occupations require only a high school diploma and a willingness to learn on the job, whereas others require a college degree plus many years of postgraduate study. Table 1.9 can help you plan your future in the health occupation you choose.

In the chapters to come, there will be many career ideas for you to consider. While most involve direct contact with patients, others deal with vital behind-the-scenes work, such as keeping accurate medical records and maintaining complex life-saving equipment. A few examples of these careers are:

- **Medical records administrator:** plans and maintains systems for storing and obtaining medical records
- **Medical records** or **health information technician:** organizes and codes patient records, gathers statistical or research data, and records information
- **Medical records clerk:** files and retrieves patient records
- **Medical billing clerk:** sends invoices to patients and insurance companies, listing the procedures and tests that have been performed
- **Medical transcriptionist:** works with doctors and other health professionals to key in text from dictated recordings to prepare reports and correspondence
- **Medical illustrator, photographer** or **writer:** helps create books, newspaper and magazine articles, informational brochures for patients, and other print and Internet materials in the medical field
- **Health unit clerk:** performs administrative and secretarial tasks in a health care facility such as a hospital, clinic or nursing home
- **Administrative medical assistant:** works in a physician's office or clinic as a receptionist or office manager
- **Insurance underwriter** or **assistant:** analyzes information to process insurance applications and evaluate claims for medical treatment and disability coverage
- **Biomedical equipment technician** or **precision instrument repairer:** installs, tests, services, and maintains the various types of equipment essential for medical diagnosis and treatment, such as x-ray machines, incubators, dialysis machines, heart-lung machines, and respirators
- **Biomedical researcher:** works in a laboratory setting to explore and test new drug therapies
- **Pharmaceutical sales representative:** provides drug information and samples to medical personnel on behalf of the manufacturer
- **Mortuary worker:** prepares bodies for burial or cremation, plans funeral services, and helps console the bereaved

TABLE 1.9

EDUCATION AND LEVELS OF TRAINING

Career Level	Educational Requirement	Examples
Aide or Assistant	One or more years of course study and/or on-the-job training	• Dental assistant • Medical assistant • Nurse assistant
Nurse (LPN, LVN) or Technician	Two-year associate degree, special health occupations education, or 3–4 years of on-the-job training	• Dental hygienist • Medical laboratory technician • Surgical technician • Physical therapy assistant
Registered Nurse (RN) or Technologist	Four-year college bachelor's degree	• Medical laboratory technologist • Registered nurse
Therapist	A 1- or 2-year postgraduate master's degree	• Physical therapist • Occupational therapist • Speech therapist
Professional	Postgraduate education in medical specialty (master's or doctorate degree)	• Dentist • Medical doctor • Occupational therapist • Psychologist • Speech therapist

HEALTH OCCUPATION PROFILE

ADMINISTRATIVE MEDICAL ASSISTANT

Brad Hamilton is a certified medical assistant (CMA). ***"My introduction to medical assisting began when I took a health occupations course in high school. I knew I wanted a career in health care, but I didn't know whether I wanted to work with patients or if I would like an administrative role better. Since medical assistants are trained in both areas, after graduation I enrolled in a medical assisting program. For me, this was a great career choice. (Being one of the few guys in the class wasn't bad either!)***

"My first job was working as a clinical assistant in a private practice. I enjoyed working with patients; but I liked the administrative side of the job best, so I started taking business courses in the evenings. This educational background, plus my work experience, helped me move into a supervisory position at a large private clinic. I love what I'm doing and feel that my job gives me the best of both worlds in health care."

Study Break

Learning word parts can help you understand more than just medical words. It might come in handy to know that intramural sports are those played within the walls, or confines, of the school (intra- means within, and mural means pertaining to walls). You could point out that extracurricular activities take place after classes end (extra- means outside, and curricular means the course).

Try making up a few silly words to play around with word parts and amuse your friends. Start by figuring out the meaning of these made-up words:

- **Hyperhungry**
- **Rhinobop**
- **Leukomelano TV**

You could even try your hand at untangling the longest word in the dictionary, pneumonoultramicroscopicsilicovolcanokoniosis. (Hint: it's a lung disease.)

Review Time

Write the answers to the following questions on a separate piece of paper or in your notebook. In addition, be prepared to take part in the classroom discussion.

1. ***Written Assignment:*** Describe the differences between a **sign** and a **symptom**.

   Discussion Assignment: Why are both types of observations important diagnostic indicators?

2. ***Written Assignment:*** Use your own words to define the term **triage**.

   Discussion Assignment: What are the kinds of situations in which triage would be important?

3. ***Written Assignment:*** Use your word part skills to determine the meaning of the term **cardiopulmonary** (**pulmon/o** means lungs) and then state the definition and identify the word parts that make up this term.

   Discussion Assignment: What rules relating to the use of combining vowels are used in this term?

4. ***Written Assignment:*** Use your medical dictionary to research the eponym **Graves' disease** and report on the name, and dates, of the physician for whom this disease is named.

   Discussion Assignment: What is an **eponym**?

5. ***Written Assignment:*** Compare the terms **diagnosis** and **prognosis**.

   Discussion Assignment: How is information about both the diagnosis and prognosis important to the patient and to his or her family?

continues

Optional Internet Activity

The goal of this activity is to help you learn more about medical terminology as it applies to the "real world." Select ***one*** *of these two options below and follow the instructions.*

1. Search for information about the Health Occupations Students of America (HOSA). Write a brief (one- or two-paragraph) report on something new you learned here and include the address of the web site where you found this information.

2. The U.S Department of Labor Bureau of Labor Statistics maintains a web site (www.bis.gov) that provides an Occupational Outlook Handbook with training requirements and opportunities for many different health occupations. Select a health occupation of interest to you and write a brief (one- or two-paragraph) report on something new you learned here. Be certain to include in your report the name of the occupation you researched.

THE HUMAN TOUCH: CRITICAL THINKING EXERCISE

The following story and questions are designed to stimulate critical thinking through class discussion or as a brief essay response. There are no right or wrong answers to these questions.

"Next week on* Triage*: Can Dr. Cloud save Diana from bacterial endocarditis? Will Dr. Hart be forced to perform an emergency tracheotomy? And find out what the Triage team does when an entire cruise ship comes down with gastroenteritis."

Rose switched off the TV. She had no idea what the announcer's words had meant, but it sounded exciting and she couldn't wait for next week's episode. She had initially watched* Triage *more for the love story between Dr. Cloud and the clumsy Diana (who was always ending up in the emergency room and consequently in Dr. Cloud's arms) than for the medical details. However, after watching the show so much, she was inspired to pursue a career in medicine.

She had signed up for the medical terminology class offered at her high school and was thrilled when her first assignment was to watch an episode of* Triage*—imagine that, a TV show as homework! She looked down at the sheet of paper in her lap at all of the unfamiliar terms she had written down during the show. Now her job was to look up all of the words that she didn't understand. She got out her new textbook, cracked the binding, and got to work. There were so many words on the page, she initially felt overwhelmed, but then she remembered what her teacher had said: **"Break the word into word parts in order to understand the meaning."**

She began with endocarditis. Starting at the end as her teacher had suggested, she looked up -itis, meaning inflamed. Then she worked out that card means heart. That left only the endo-, meaning inner. So putting it all together, she figured out that next week on the show, Diana will come to Dr. Cloud with an inflammation of the inner walls of her heart. **"Hey, that wasn't so hard!"** ***she thought to herself and moved on to "tracheotomy."***

continues

Suggested Discussion Topics

1. Do you think that TV shows represent medical situations accurately? If not, what do you think is exaggerated or incorrect?
2. Do you think that most people understand all the medical terms they hear on the radio or TV, or read in the newspaper or magazines? What advantages will you have when you've learned about medical terminology?
3. Rose is unsure as to what kind of medical career she wants to pursue. Discuss ways in which she might learn more about different medical careers.
4. Discuss the factors that will influence Rose's career choice. Include in your discussion post-high school options that she might pursue before making a final career choice.

STUDENT WORKBOOK AND StudyWARE™ CD-ROM

1. Go to your **Student Workbook** and complete the Learning Exercises for this chapter.

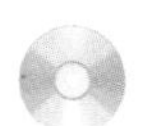

2. Go to the **StudyWARE™ CD-ROM** and have fun with the exercises and games for this chapter.

CHAPTER 2

THE HUMAN BODY IN HEALTH AND DISEASE

OVERVIEW OF THE HUMAN BODY IN HEALTH AND DISEASE

Anatomic Reference Systems	Terms used to describe the location of body planes, directions, and cavities.
Structures of the Body	The cells, tissues, and glands that form the body systems that work together to enable the body to function properly.
Genetics	The genetic components that transfer characteristics from parents to their children.
Tissues	A group of similarly specialized cells that work together to perform specific functions.
Glands	A group of specialized cells that are capable of producing secretions.
Body Systems and Related Organs	Organs are somewhat independent parts of the body that perform specific functions. Organs with related functions are organized into body systems.
Pathology	The study of the nature and cause of disease that involve changes in structure and function.

Vocabulary Related to the Human Body in Health and Disease

This list contains essential word parts and medical terms for this chapter. These terms are pronounced on the student StudyWARE™ CD-ROM and Audio CDs that are available for use with this text. These and the other important **primary terms** are shown in boldface throughout the chapter. *Secondary terms*, which appear in *orange* italics, clarify the meaning of primary terms.

Word Parts

- ☐ **aden/o**
- ☐ **adip/o**
- ☐ **anter/o**
- ☐ **caud/o**
- ☐ **cephal/o**
- ☐ **cyt/o**
- ☐ **endo-**
- ☐ **exo-**
- ☐ **hist/o**
- ☐ **-ologist**
- ☐ **-ology**
- ☐ **path/o**
- ☐ **-plasia**
- ☐ **poster/o**
- ☐ **-stasis**

Medical Terms

- ☐ **abdominal cavity** (ab-**DOM**-ih-nal)
- ☐ **adenectomy** (**ad**-eh-**NECK**-toh-mee)
- ☐ **adenocarcinoma** (**ad**-eh-noh-**kar**-sih-**NOH**-mah)
- ☐ **adenoma** (**ad**-eh-**NOH**-mah)
- ☐ **adenomalacia** (**ad**-eh-noh-mah-**LAY**-shee-ah)
- ☐ **adenosclerosis** (**ad**-eh-noh-skleh-**ROH**-sis)
- ☐ **anaplasia** (**an**-ah-**PLAY**-zee-ah)
- ☐ **anatomy** (ah-**NAT**-oh-mee)
- ☐ **anomaly** (ah-**NOM**-ah-lee)
- ☐ **anterior** (an-**TEER**-ee-or)
- ☐ **aplasia** (ah-**PLAY**-zee-ah)
- ☐ **bloodborne transmission**
- ☐ **caudal** (**KAW**-dal)
- ☐ **cephalic** (seh-**FAL**-ick)
- ☐ **chromosomes** (**KROH**-moh-sohmes)
- ☐ **communicable disease** (kuh-**MEW**-nih-kuh-bul)
- ☐ **congenital disorder** (kon-**JEN**-ih-tahl)
- ☐ **cytoplasm** (**SIGH**-toh-plazm)
- ☐ **distal** (**DIS**-tal)
- ☐ **dorsal** (**DOR**-sal)
- ☐ **dysplasia** (dis-**PLAY**-see-ah)
- ☐ **endemic** (en-**DEM**-ick)
- ☐ **endocrine glands** (**EN**-doh-krin)
- ☐ **epidemic** (**ep**-ih-**DEM**-ick)
- ☐ **epigastric region** (**ep**-ih-**GAS**-trick)
- ☐ **etiology** (**ee**-tee-**OL**-oh-jee)
- ☐ **exocrine glands** (**ECK**-soh-krin)
- ☐ **functional disorder**
- ☐ **genetic disorder**
- ☐ **geriatrician** (**jer**-ee-ah-**TRISH**-un)
- ☐ **hemophilia** (**hee**-moh-**FILL**-ee-ah)
- ☐ **histology** (hiss-**TOL**-oh-jee)
- ☐ **homeostasis** (**hoh**-mee-oh-**STAY**-sis)
- ☐ **hyperplasia** (**high**-per-**PLAY**-zee-ah)
- ☐ **hypertrophy** (high-**PER**-troh-fee)
- ☐ **hypogastric region** (**high**-poh-**GAS**-trick)
- ☐ **hypoplasia** (**high**-poh-**PLAY**-zee-ah)
- ☐ **iatrogenic illness** (eye-**at**-roh-**JEN**-ick)
- ☐ **idiopathic disorder** (**id**-ee-oh-**PATH**-ick)
- ☐ **infectious disease** (in-**FECK**-shus)
- ☐ **inguinal** (**ING**-gwih-nal)
- ☐ **medial** (**MEE**-dee-al)
- ☐ **mesentery** (**MESS**-en-**terr**-ee)
- ☐ **midsagittal plane** (mid-**SADJ**-ih-tal)
- ☐ **nosocomial infection** (**nos**-oh-**KOH**-mee-al in-**FECK**-shun)
- ☐ **pandemic** (pan-**DEM**-ick)
- ☐ **pelvic cavity** (**PEL**-vick)
- ☐ **peritoneum** (**pehr**-ih-toh-**NEE**-um)
- ☐ **peritonitis** (**pehr**-ih-toh-**NIGH**-tis)
- ☐ **phenylketonuria** (**fen**-il-**kee**-toh-**NEW**-ree-ah)
- ☐ **physiology** (**fiz**-ee-**OL**-oh-jee)
- ☐ **posterior** (pos-**TEER**-ee-or)
- ☐ **proximal** (**PROCK**-sih-mal)
- ☐ **retroperitoneal** (**ret**-roh-**pehr**-ih-toh-**NEE**-al)
- ☐ **stem cells**
- ☐ **thoracic cavity** (thoh-**RAS**-ick)
- ☐ **transverse plane** (trans-**VERSE**)
- ☐ **umbilicus** (um-**BILL**-ih-kus)
- ☐ **vector-borne transmission**
- ☐ **ventral** (**VEN**-tral)

OBJECTIVES

On completion of this chapter, you should be able to:

1. Define anatomy and physiology and the uses of anatomic reference systems to identify the anatomic position plus body planes, directions, and cavities.
2. Recognize, define, spell, and pronounce the terms related to cells, and genetics.
3. Recognize, define, spell, and pronounce the terms related to the structure, function, pathology, and procedures of tissues, and glands.
4. Identify the major organs and functions of the body systems.
5. Recognize, define, spell, and pronounce the terms used to describe pathology, the modes of transmission, and the types of diseases.

ANATOMIC REFERENCE SYSTEMS

Anatomic reference systems are used to describe the locations of the structural units of the body. The simplest anatomic reference is the one we learn in childhood: our right hand is on the right, and our left hand on the left.

In medical terminology, there are several additional ways to describe the location of different body parts. These anatomical reference systems include:

- Body planes
- Body directions
- Body cavities
- Structural units

When body parts function together to perform a related function they are grouped together and are known as a body system (see Table 2.1).

Anatomy and Physiology Defined

- **Anatomy** (ah-**NAT**-oh-mee) is the study of the structures of the body.
- **Physiology** (**fiz**-ee-**OL**-oh-jee) is the study of the functions of the structures of the body (**physi** means nature or physical, and **-ology** means study of).

The Anatomic Position

The **anatomic position** describes the body assuming that the individual is standing in the standard position that includes:

- Standing up straight so that the body is erect and facing forward.
- Holding the arms at the sides with the hands turned with the palms turned toward the front. This position is shown in Figure 2.1.

The Body Planes

Body planes are imaginary vertical and horizontal lines used to divide the body into sections for descriptive purposes (Figures 2.1 and 2.2). These planes are aligned to a body standing in the anatomic position.

The Vertical Planes

A **vertical plane** is an up-and-down plane that is a right angle to the horizon.

- The **midsagittal plane** (mid-**SADJ**-ih-tal), also known as the *midline*, is the sagittal plane that divides the body into *equal* left and right halves (see Figure 2.1).
- A **sagittal plane** (**SADJ**-ih-tal) is a vertical plane that divides the body into *unequal* left and right portions.
- A **frontal plane** is a vertical plane that divides the body into anterior (front) and posterior (back) portions. Also known as the *coronal plane*, it is located at right angles to the sagittal plane (see Figure 2.2).

The Horizontal Plane

A **horizontal plane** is a flat crosswise plane, such as the horizon.

- A **transverse plane** (trans-**VERSE**) is a horizontal plane that divides the body into superior (upper) and inferior (lower) portions. A transverse plane can be at the waist or at any other level across the body (see Figure 2.2).

Body Direction Terms

The relative location of sections of the body, or of an organ, can be described through the use of pairs of contrasting body direction terms. These terms are illustrated in Figures 2.3 and 2.4.

TABLE 2.1

Major Body Systems

Body System	Major Structures	Major Functions
Skeletal System (Chapter 3)	bones, joints, and cartilage	Supports and shapes the body. Protects the internal organs. Forms some blood cells and stores minerals.
Muscular System (Chapter 4)	muscles, fascia, and tendons	Holds the body erect. Makes movement possible. Moves body fluids and generates body heat.
Cardiovascular System (Chapter 5)	heart, arteries, veins, capillaries, and blood	Blood circulates throughout the body to transport oxygen and nutrients to cells, and to carry waste products to the kidneys where waste is removed by filtration.
Lymphatic System (Chapter 6)	lymph, lymphatic vessels, and lymph nodes	Removes and transports waste products from the fluid between the cells. Destroys harmful substances such as pathogens and cancer cells in the lymph nodes. Returns the filtered lymph to the bloodstream where it becomes plasma again.
Immune System (Chapter 6)	tonsils, spleen, thymus, skin, and specialized blood cells	Defends the body against invading pathogens and allergens.
Respiratory System (Chapter 7)	nose, pharynx, trachea, larynx, and lungs	Brings oxygen into the body for transportation to the cells. Removes carbon dioxide and some water waste from the body.
Digestive System (Chapter 8)	mouth, esophagus, stomach, small intestines, large intestines, liver, and pancreas	Digests ingested food so it can be absorbed into the bloodstream. Eliminates solid waste.
Urinary System (Chapter 9)	kidneys, ureters, urinary bladder, and urethra	Filters blood to remove waste. Maintains the electrolyte and fluid balance within the body.
Nervous System (Chapter 10)	nerves, brain, and spinal cord	Coordinates the reception of stimuli. Transmits messages throughout the body.
Special Senses (Chapter 11)	eyes and ears	Receive visual and auditory information and transmit it to the brain.
Integumentary System (Chapter 12)	skin, sebaceous glands, and sweat glands	Protects the body against invasion by bacteria. Aids in regulating the body temperature and water content.
Endocrine System (Chapter 13)	adrenal glands, gonads, pancreas, parathyroids, pineal, pituitary, thymus, and thyroid	Integrates all body functions.
Reproductive Systems (Chapter 14)	Male: penis and testicles Female: ovaries, uterus, and vagina	Produces new life.

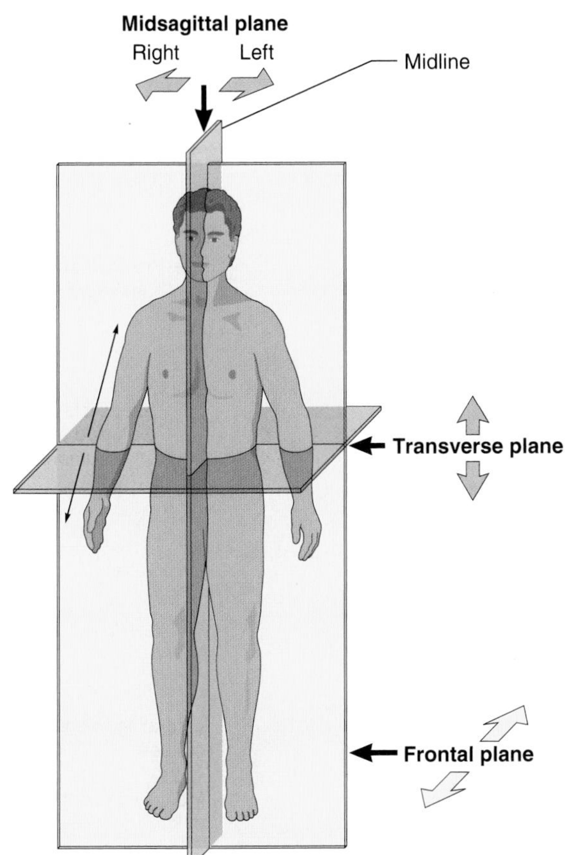

FIGURE 2.1 Body planes are imaginary lines used to divide the body for descriptive purposes. The midsagittal plane, shown in blue, divides the body into *equal* left and right halves.

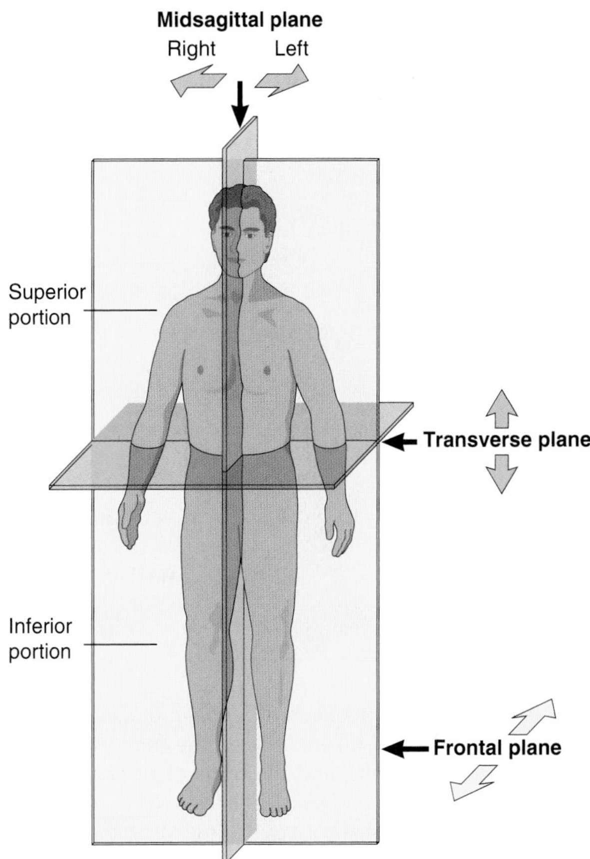

FIGURE 2.2 The transverse plane, shown in orange, divides the body into superior (upper) and inferior (lower) portions. The frontal plane, shown in yellow, divides the body into anterior (front) and posterior (back) portions.

- **Ventral** (**VEN**-tral) refers to the front, or belly side, of the organ or body (**ventr** means belly side of the body, and **-al** means pertaining to). Ventral is the opposite of *dorsal.*
- **Dorsal** (**DOR**-sal) refers to the back of the organ or body (**dors** means back of the body, and **-al** means pertaining to). Dorsal is the opposite of *ventral.*
- **Anterior** (an-**TEER**-ee-or) means situated in the front. It also means on the front or forward part of an organ (**anter** means front or before, and **-ior** means pertaining to). For example, the stomach is located anterior to (in front of) the pancreas. Anterior is also used in reference to the ventral surface of the body. Anterior is the opposite of *posterior.*
- **Posterior** (pos-**TEER**-ee-or) means situated in the back. It also means on the back part of an organ (**poster** means back or toward the back, and **-ior** means pertaining to). For example, the pancreas is located posterior to (behind) the stomach. The term posterior is also used in reference to the dorsal surface of the body. Posterior is the opposite of *anterior.*
- **Superior** means uppermost, above, or toward the head. For example, the lungs are located superior to (above) the diaphragm. Superior is the opposite of *inferior.*
- **Inferior** means lowermost, below, or toward the feet. For example, the stomach is located inferior to (below) the diaphragm. Inferior is the opposite of *superior.*
- **Cephalic** (seh-**FAL**-ick) means toward the head (**cephal** means head, and **-ic** means pertaining to). Cephalic is the opposite of *caudal.*
- **Caudal** (**KAW**-dal) means toward the lower part of the body (**caud** means tail or lower part of the body, and **-al** means pertaining to). Caudal is the opposite of *cephalic.*
- **Proximal** (**PROCK**-sih-mal) means situated nearest the midline or beginning of a body structure. For example, the proximal end of the humerus (bone of the upper arm) forms part of the shoulder. Proximal is the opposite of *distal.*
- **Distal** (**DIS**-tal) means situated farthest from the midline or beginning of a body structure. For example,

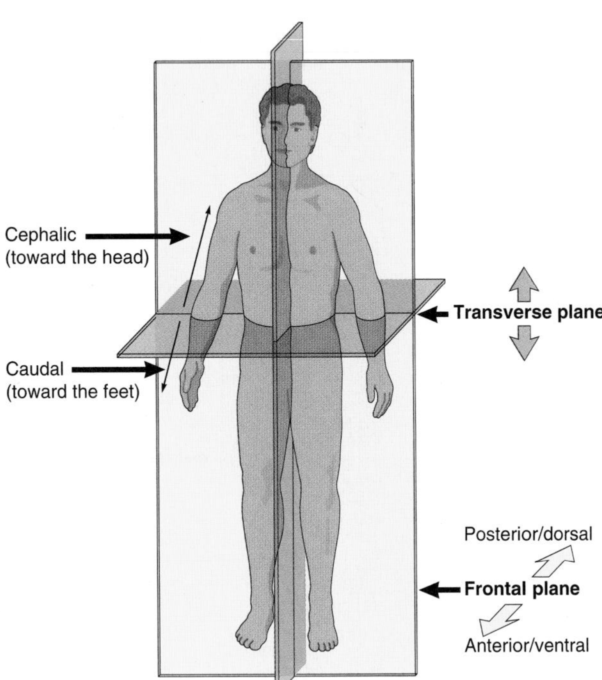

FIGURE 2.3 Body directions: *Cephalic* means toward the head, and *caudal* means toward the feet. *Anterior* means toward the front, and the front of the body is known as the *ventral surface. Posterior* means toward the back, and the back of the body is known as the *dorsal surface.*

the distal end of the humerus forms part of the elbow (see Figure 2.4). Distal is the opposite of *proximal.*

- **Medial** (**MEE**-dee-al) means the direction toward, or nearer, the midline. For example, the medial ligament of the knee is near the inner surface of the leg (see Figure 2.4). Medial is the opposite of *lateral.*
- **Lateral** means the direction toward or nearer the side and away from the midline. For example, the lateral ligament of the knee is near the side of the leg. Lateral is the opposite of *medial. Bilateral* means relating to, or having, two sides.

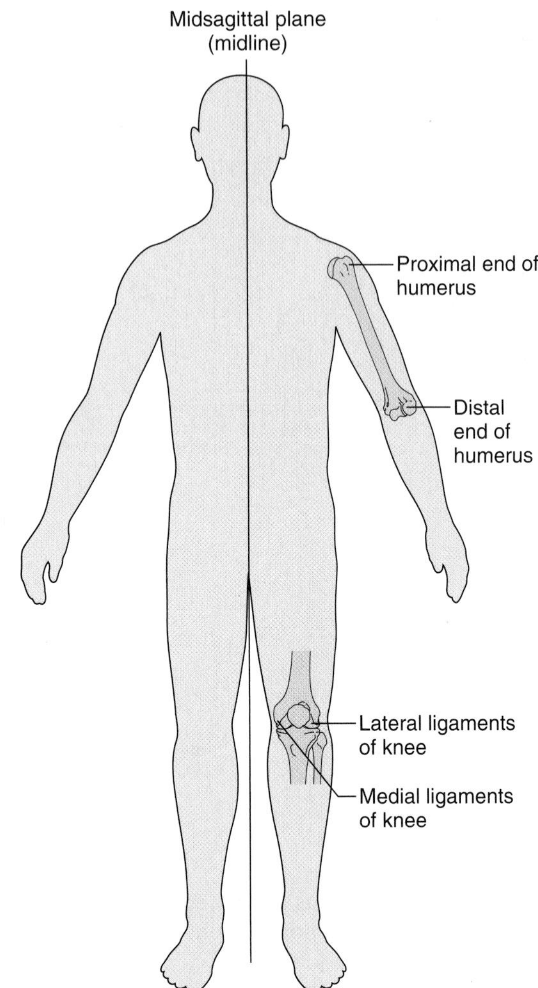

FIGURE 2.4 Body directions: *Proximal* means situated nearest the midline, and *distal* means situated farthest from the midline. *Medial* means toward or nearer the midline, and *lateral* means toward the side and away from the midline.

Major Body Cavities

The two major **body cavities**, which are the dorsal and the ventral cavities, are spaces within the body that contain and protect internal organs (Figure 2.5).

The Dorsal Cavity

The **dorsal cavity**, which is located along the back of the body and head, contains organs of the nervous system that coordinate body functions and is divided into two portions:

- The **cranial cavity**, which is located within the skull, surrounds and protects the brain. *Cranial* means pertaining to the skull.
- The **spinal cavity**, which is located within the spinal column, surrounds and protects the spinal cord.

The Ventral Cavity

The **ventral cavity**, which is located along the front of the body, contains the body organs that maintain homeostasis. **Homeostasis** (**hoh**-mee-oh-**STAY**-sis) is the processes through which the body maintains a constant internal environment (**home/o** means constant, and **-stasis** means control).

- The **thoracic cavity** (thoh-**RAS**-ick), also known as the *chest cavity* or *thorax*, surrounds and protects the

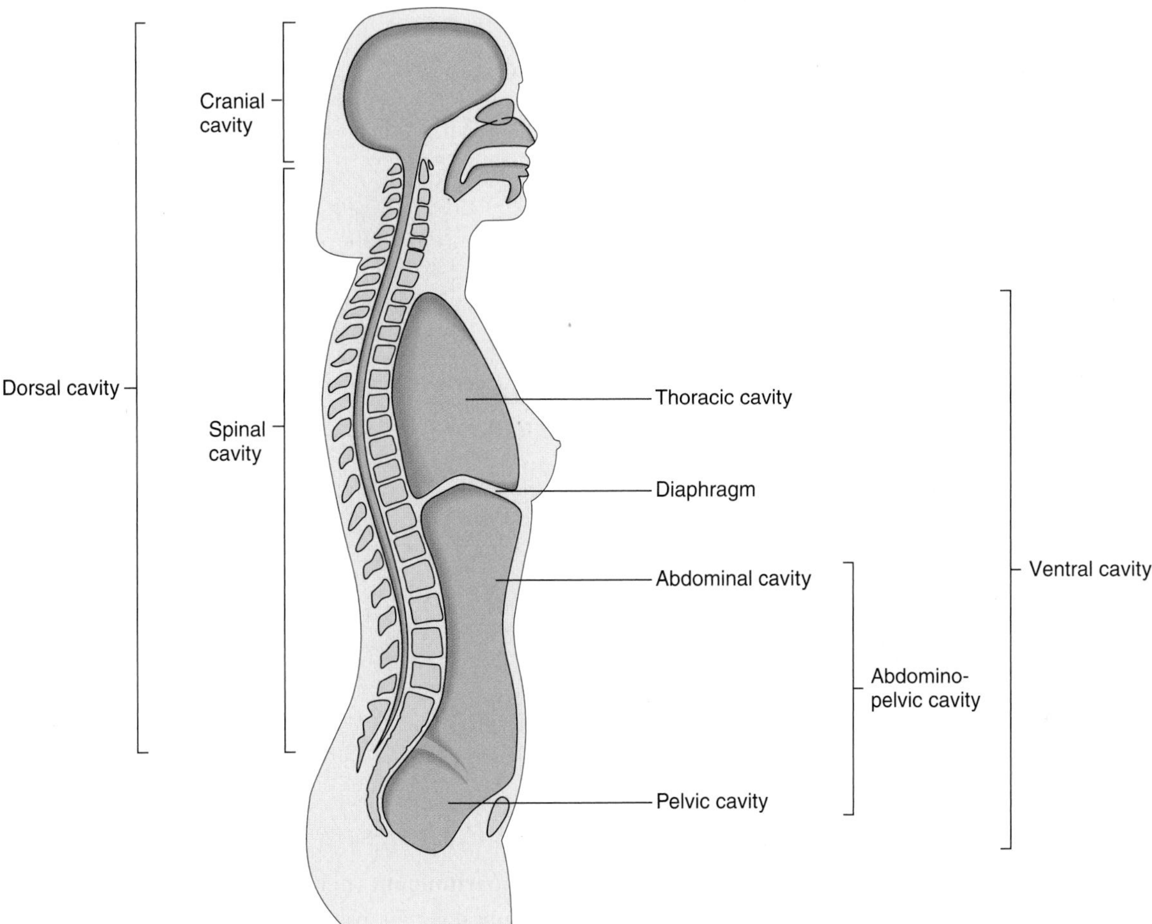

FIGURE 2.5 The major body cavities.

heart and the lungs. The *diaphragm* is a muscle that separates the thoracic and abdominal cavities.

- The **abdominal cavity** (ab-**DOM**-ih-nal) contains primarily the major organs of digestion. This cavity is frequently referred to simply as the **abdomen** (**AB**-doh-men).
- The **pelvic cavity** (**PEL**-vick) is the space formed by the hip bones and it contains primarily the organs of the reproductive and excretory systems.
- There is no physical division between the abdominal and pelvic cavities. The term **abdominopelvic cavity** (ab-**dom**-ih-noh-**PEL**-vick) refers to these two cavities as a single unit (**abdomin/o** means abdomen, **pelv** means pelvis, and **-ic** means pertaining to).
- The term **inguinal** (**ING**-gwih-nal), which means relating to the groin, refers to the entire lower area of the abdomen. This includes the *groin* which is the crease at the junction of the trunk with the upper end of the thigh.

Regions of the Thorax and Abdomen

Regions of the thorax and abdomen are a descriptive system that divides the abdomen and lower portion of the thorax into nine parts (Figure 2.6).

- The **hypochondriac regions** (**high**-poh-**KON**-dree-ack) are located on the left and right sides of the body and are covered by the lower ribs (**hypo-** means below, **chondr/i** means cartilage, and **-ac** means pertaining to). As used here, the term *hypochondriac* means below the ribs. This term also describes an individual with an abnormal concern about his or her health (see Chapter 10).
- The **epigastric region** (**ep**-ih-**GAS**-trick) is located above the stomach (**epi-** means above, **gastr** means stomach, and **-ic** means pertaining to).
- The **lumbar regions** (**LUM**-bar) are located on the left and right sides near the inward curve of the spine (**lumb** means lower back, and **-ar** means pertaining to). The term *lumbar* describes the part of the back between the ribs and the pelvis.

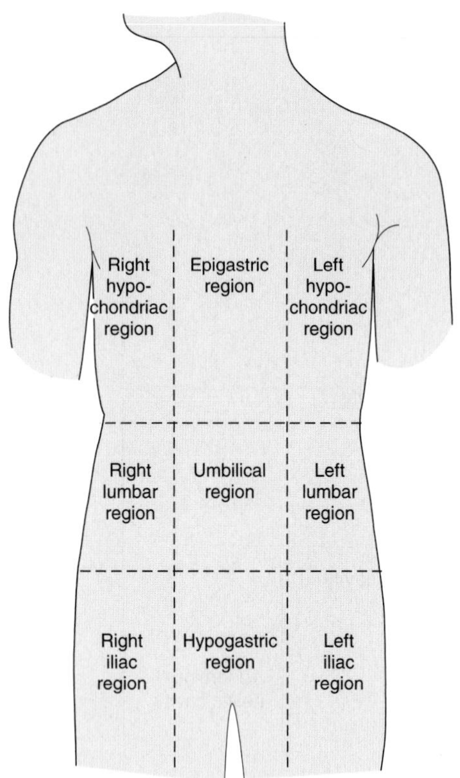

FIGURE 2.6 Regions of the thorax and abdomen.

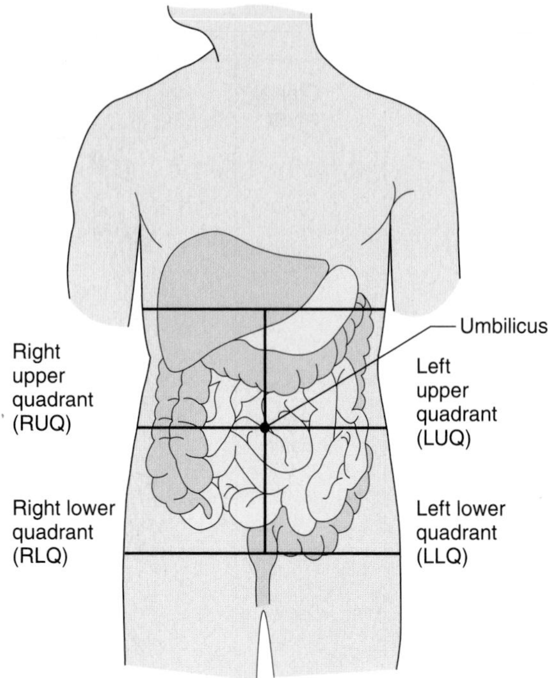

FIGURE 2.7 Division of the abdomen into quadrants.

- The **umbilical region** (um-**BILL**-ih-kal) surrounds the **umbilicus** (um-**BILL**-ih-kus) which is commonly known as the *belly button* or *navel*. This pit in the center of the abdominal wall marks the point where the umbilical cord was attached before birth.
- The **iliac regions** (**ILL**-ee-ack) are located on the left and right sides over the hip bones (**ili** means hip bone, and **-ac** means pertaining to). The iliac region is named for the wide portion of the hip bone.
- The **hypogastric region** (**high**-poh-**GAS**-trick) is located below the stomach (**hypo-** means below, **gastr** means stomach, and **-ic** means pertaining to).

Quadrants of the Abdomen

Describing where an abdominal organ or pain is located is made easier by dividing the abdomen into four imaginary quadrants. The term **quadrant** means divided into four. As shown in Figure 2.7 the quadrants of the abdomen are the:

- Right upper quadrant (RUQ)
- Left upper quadrant (LUQ)
- Right lower quadrant (RLQ)
- Left lower quadrant (LLQ)

The Peritoneum

The **peritoneum** (**pehr**-ih-toh-**NEE**-um) is a multilayered membrane that protects and holds the organs in place within the abdominal cavity. A *membrane* is a thin layer of tissue that covers a surface, lines a cavity, or divides a space or organ.

- The **parietal peritoneum** (pah-**RYE**-eh-tal **pehr**-ih-toh-**NEE**-um) is the outer layer of the peritoneum that lines the interior of the abdominal wall. *Parietal* means cavity wall.
- The **visceral peritoneum** (**VIS**-er-al **pehr**-ih-toh-**NEE**-um) is the inner layer of the peritoneum that surrounds the organs of the abdominal cavity. *Visceral* means relating to the internal organs.
- The **mesentery** (**MESS**-en-**terr**-ee) is a fused double layer of the parietal peritoneum that attaches parts of the intestine to the interior abdominal wall.
- **Retroperitoneal** (**ret**-roh-**pehr**-ih-toh-**NEE**-al) means located behind the peritoneum (**retro-** means behind, **periton** means peritoneum, and **-eal** means pertaining to). For example, the location of the kidneys is retroperitoneal with one on each side of the spinal column.
- **Peritonitis** (**pehr**-ih-toh-**NIGH**-tis) is inflammation of the peritoneum (**periton** means peritoneum, and **-itis** means inflammation).

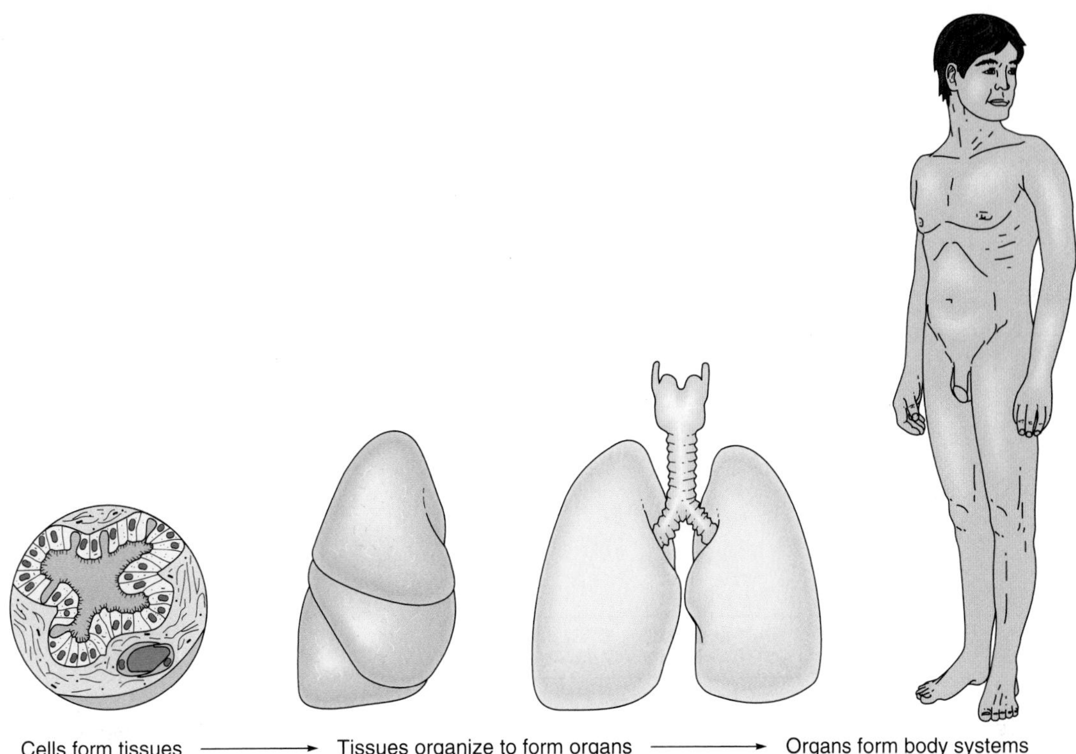
Cells form tissues
Tissues organize to form organs
Organs form body systems

FIGURE 2.8 The human body is highly organized, from the single cell to the total organism.

STRUCTURES OF THE BODY

The body is made up of increasing larger, and more complex, structural units. From smallest to largest these are: cells, tissues, organs, and the body systems (Figure 2.8). Working together, these structures form the complete body and enable it to function properly.

CELLS

Cells are the basic structural and functional units of the body. Cells are specialized and grouped together to form tissues and organs.

- **Cytology** (sigh-**TOL**-oh-jee) is the study of the anatomy, physiology, pathology, and chemistry of the cell (**cyt** means cell, and **-ology** means study of).

The Structure of Cells

- The **cell membrane** (**MEM**-brain) is the tissue that surrounds and protects the contents of the cell by separating them from its external environment (see Figure 2.9).
- **Cytoplasm** (**SIGH**-toh-plazm) is the material within the cell membrane that is *not* part of the nucleus (**cyt/o** means cell, and **-plasm** means formative material of cells).
- The **nucleus** (**NEW**-klee-us), which is surrounded by the nuclear membrane, is a structure within the cell that has two important functions: (1) it controls the activities of the cell, and (2) it helps the cell divide.

Stem Cells

Stem cells differ from other kinds of cells in the body because of two characteristics:

- **Stem cells** are unspecialized cells that are able to renew themselves for long periods of time by cell division. This is in contrast to other types of cells that have a specialized role and die after a determined lifespan.
- Under certain conditions stem cells can be transformed into cells with special functions such as the cells of the heart muscle that make the heartbeat possible or the specialized cells of the pancreas that are capable of producing insulin.

Adult Stem Cells

Adult stem cells, also known as *somatic stem cells*, are undifferentiated cells found among differentiated cells in a tissue or organ. Normally the primary role of these cells is

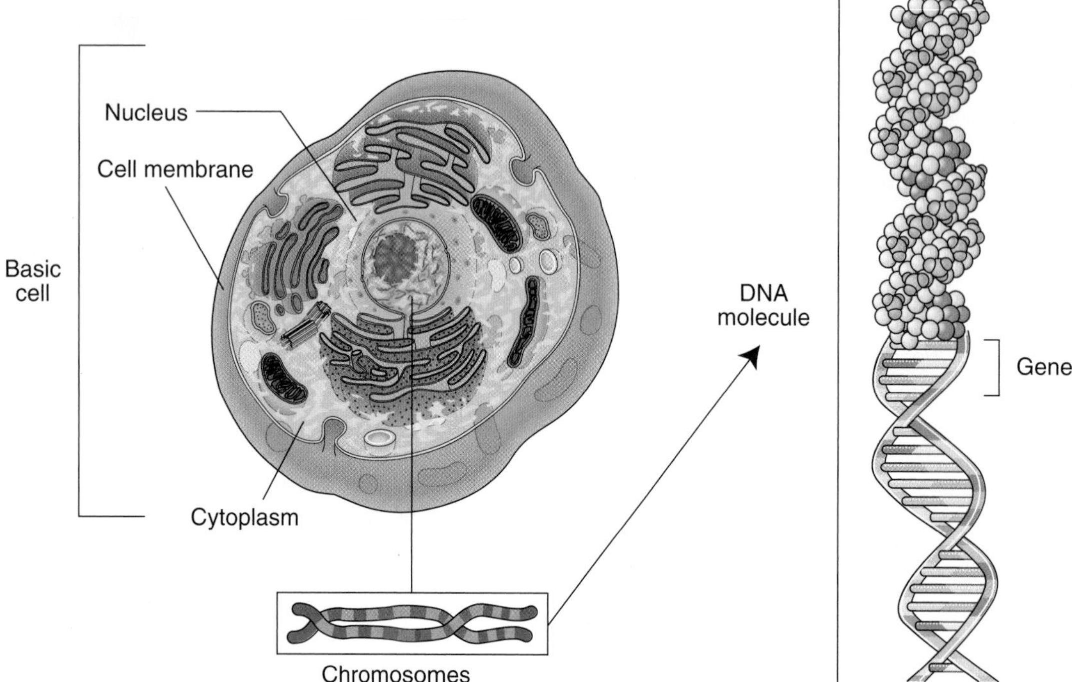

FIGURE 2.9 Basic cell and DNA molecule.

to maintain and repair the tissue in which they are found. The term *undifferentiated* means not having a specialized function or structure. In contrast the term *differentiated* means having a specialized function or structure.

Stem cells potentially have many therapeutic uses, including being transplanted from one individual to another. Cells for this purpose are harvested from the *hemopoietic* (blood forming) tissue of the donor's bone marrow. However unless there is an excellent match between the donor and recipient, there is the possibility of rejection known as *graft versus host disease*.

Embryonic Stem Cells

Embryonic stem cells are undifferentiated cells that are unlike any specific adult cell; however, they have the important ability to form *any* adult cell.

- These cells can proliferate (grow rapidly) indefinitely in a laboratory, and could therefore potentially provide a source for adult muscle, liver, bone, or blood cells.
- Because these cells are more primitive than adult stem cells, an embryonic stem cell transplant does not require as perfect a match between the patient and donor as the transplantation of adult stem cells.
- Embryonic stem cells come from the *cord blood* found in the umbilical cord and placenta of a newborn infant. Embryonic stem cells from cord blood can be harvested at the time of birth without danger to mother or child. These cells are kept frozen until needed for treatment purposes.
- Embryonic stem cells can also be obtained from surplus embryos produced by in vitro (test tube) fertilization (see Chapter 14). With the informed consent of the donor couple, stem cells obtained in this manner are being used for important medical and scientific research.

GENETICS

A **gene** is a fundamental physical and functional unit of heredity. Genes control hereditary disorders and all physical traits such as hair, skin, and eye color.

Genetics is the study of how genes are transferred from parents to their children and the role of genes in health and disease (**gene** means producing, and **-tics** means pertaining to). A specialist in this field is known as a **geneticist** (jeh-**NET**-ih-sist).

Dominant and Recessive Genes

Each newly formed individual receives two genes of each genetic trait: one from the father and one from the mother.

- When a **dominant gene** is inherited from either parent, the offspring *will* inherit that genetic condition or characteristic. For example, freckles are a physical trait that is transmitted by a dominant gene. So too is the hereditary disorder Huntington's disease which is discussed later in this chapter.

- When the same **recessive gene** is inherited from both parents, the offspring *will have* that condition. For example, *sickle cell anemia* is a group of inherited red blood cell disorders that are transmitted by a recessive gene. When this gene is transmitted by both parents, the child *will have* sickle cell anemia.
- When a **recessive gene** is inherited from only one parent, and a normal gene is inherited for the other parent, the offspring *will not have* the condition. Although this child will not develop sickle cell anemia, he or she does have *sickle cell anemia trait*. Children with this trait can transmit the sickle cell gene to their offspring. Sickle cell anemia is discussed further in Chapter 5.

The Human Genome

A **genome** (JEE-nohm) is the complete set of genetic information of an individual. The Human Genome Project was formed to study this genetic code in all people, and found that it is over 99% identical among humans throughout the world. The first complete mapping of the human genome was just published in 2003. Having access to this data is a very important step in studying the use of genetics in health and science.

Chromosomes

Chromosomes (**KROH**-moh-sohmes) are the genetic structures located within the nucleus of each cell (see Figure 2.9). These chromosomes are made up of the DNA molecules containing the body's genes. Packaging genetic information into chromosomes helps a cell keep a large amount of genetic information neat, organized, and compact. Each chromosome contains about 100,000 genes.

- A *somatic cell* is any cell in the body except the gametes (sex cells). *Somatic* means pertaining to the body in general. Somatic cells contain 46 chromosomes arranged into 23 pairs. There are 22 identical pairs of chromosomes, plus another pair. In a typical female, this pair consists of XX chromosomes. In a typical male, this pair consists of an XY chromosome pair. It is this chromosome pair that determines the sex of the individual.
- A *sex cell* (sperm or egg), also known as a *gamete*, is the only type of cell that *does not* contain 46 chromosomes. Instead each ovum (egg) or sperm has 23 single chromosomes. In a female, one of these will be an X chromosome. In a male one of these will be either an X or a Y chromosome. When a sperm and ovum join, the newly formed offspring receives 23 chromosomes from each parent, for a total of 46.
- It is the X or Y chromosome from the father that determines the gender of the child.
- A defect in chromosomes can lead to birth defects. For example, individuals with Down syndrome have 47 chromosomes instead of the usual 46. Down syndrome is discussed later in this chapter.

DNA

DNA is the abbreviation for *deoxyribonucleic acid*. The basic structure of the DNA molecule, which is located on the pairs of chromosomes in the nucleus of each cell, is the same for all living organisms. Human DNA contains thousands of genes that provide the information essential for heredity, determining our physical appearance, disease risks, and other traits (see Figure 2.9).

- DNA is packaged in a chromosome as two spiraling strands that twist together to form a double helix. A *helix* is a shape twisted like a spiral staircase. A *double helix* consists of two of these strands twisted together.
- DNA is found in the nucleus of all types of cells except erythrocytes (red blood cells). The difference here is due to the fact that erythrocytes do not have a nucleus.
- The DNA for each individual is different and no two DNA patterns are exactly the same. The only exception to this rule is identical twins, which are formed from one fertilized egg that divides. Although their DNA is identical, these twins do develop fingerprints and other characteristics that make each of them unique.
- A very small sample of DNA, such as from human hair or tissue can be used to identify individuals in criminal investigations, paternity suits, or genealogy research.

Genetic Mutation

A **genetic mutation** is a change of the sequence of a DNA molecule. Potential causes of genetic mutation include exposure to radiation or environmental pollution.

- A *somatic cell mutation* is a change within the cells of the body. These changes affect the individual but *cannot* be transmitted to the next generation.
- A *gametic cell mutation* is a change within the genes in a gamete (sex cell) that *can* be transmitted by a parent to his or her children.

- *Genetic engineering* is the manipulating or splicing of genes for scientific or medical purposes. The production of human insulin from modified bacteria is an example of one result of genetic engineering.

Genetic Disorders

A **genetic disorder**, also known as a *hereditary disorder*, is a pathological condition caused by an absent or defective gene. Some genetic disorders are obvious at birth. Other may manifest (become evident) at any time in life. The following are examples of genetic disorders.

- **Cystic fibrosis** (CF) is a genetic disorder that is present at birth and affects both the respiratory and digestive systems (see Chapter 7).
- **Down syndrome** (DS) is a genetic variation that is associated with characteristic facial appearance, learning disabilities, and physical abnormalities such as heart valve disease.
- **Hemophilia** (**hee**-moh-**FILL**-ee-ah) is a group of hereditary bleeding disorders in which a blood-clotting factor is missing. This blood coagulation disorder is characterized by spontaneous hemorrhages or severe bleeding following an injury.
- **Huntington's disease** (HD) is a genetic disorder that is passed from parent to child. Each child of a parent with the gene for Huntington's disease has a 50-50 chance of inheriting this defective gene. This condition causes nerve degeneration with symptoms that most often appear in midlife. (*Degeneration* means worsening condition.) This damage eventually results in uncontrolled movements and the loss of some mental abilities.
- **Muscular dystrophy** (**DIS**-troh-fee) is the term used to describe a group of genetic diseases that are characterized by progressive weakness and degeneration of the skeletal muscles that control movement (see Chapter 4).
- **Phenylketonuria** (**fen**-il-**kee**-toh-**NEW**-ree-ah), which is commonly known as *PKU*, is a genetic disorder in which the essential digestive enzyme phenylalanine hydroxylase is missing. PKU can be detected by a blood test performed on infants at birth. With careful dietary supervision, children born with PKU can lead normal lives. Without early detection and treatment, PKU causes severe mental retardation.
- **Tay-Sachs disease** (**TAY SAKS**) is a fatal genetic disorder in which harmful quantities of a fatty substance build up in tissues and nerve cells in the brain. Both parents must carry the mutated gene in order to have an affected child. The most common form of the disease affects babies who appear healthy at birth and seem to develop normally for the first few months. Development then slows and a relentless deterioration of mental and physical abilities results in progressive blindness, paralysis, and early death.

TISSUES

A **tissue** is a group or layer of similarly specialized cells that join together to perform certain specific functions. The four main types of tissue are epithelial, connective, muscle, and nerve.

- **Histology** (hiss-**TOL**-oh-jee) is the study of the structure, composition, and function of tissues (**hist** means tissue, and **-ology** means a study of).
- A **histologist** (hiss-**TOL**-oh-jist) is a specialist in the study of the organization of tissues at all levels (**hist** means tissue, and **-ologist** means specialist).

Epithelial Tissues

Epithelial tissues (**ep**-ih-**THEE**-lee-al) form a protective covering for all of the internal and external surfaces of the body. These tissues also form glands.

- **Epithelium** (**ep**-ih-**THEE**-lee-um) is the specialized epithelial tissue that forms the epidermis of the skin and the surface layer of mucous membranes. The *epidermis*, which is the outer layer of the skin, is discussed in Chapter 12.
- **Endothelium** (**en**-doh-**THEE**-lee-um) is the specialized epithelial tissue that lines the blood and lymph vessels, body cavities, glands, and organs.

Connective Tissues

Connective tissues support and connect organs and other body tissues. The four kinds of connective tissue are:

- **Dense connective tissues**, such as bone and cartilage, form the joints and framework of the body (see Chapter 3).
- **Adipose tissue**, also known as *fat*, provides protective padding, insulation, and support (**adip** means fat, and **-ose** means pertaining to).
- **Loose connective tissue** surrounds various organs and supports both nerve cells and blood vessels.

- **Liquid connective tissues**, which are blood (Chapter 5) and lymph (Chapter 6), transport nutrients and waste products throughout the body.

Muscle Tissue

Muscle tissue contains cells with the specialized ability to contract and relax (see Chapter 4).

Nerve Tissue

Nerve tissue contains cells with the specialized ability to react to stimuli and to conduct electrical impulses (see Chapter 10).

Pathology of Tissue Formation

Disorders of the tissues, which are frequently due to unknown causes, can occur before birth as the tissues are forming or appear later in life.

Incomplete Tissue Formation

- **Aplasia** (ah-**PLAY**-zee-ah) is the defective development, or the congenital absence, of an organ or tissue (**a**- means without, and **-plasia** means formation). Compare aplasia with *hypoplasia.*
- **Hypoplasia** (**high**-poh-**PLAY**-zee-ah) is the incomplete development of an organ or tissue usually due to a deficiency in the number of cells (**hypo**- means deficient, and **-plasia** means formation). Compare hypoplasia with *aplasia.*

Abnormal Tissue Formation

- **Anaplasia** (**an**-ah-**PLAY**-zee-ah) is a change in the structure of cells and in their orientation to each other (**ana**- means excessive, and **-plasia** means formation). This abnormal cell development is characteristic of tumor formation in cancers. Contrast anaplasia with *hypertrophy.*
- **Dysplasia** (dis-**PLAY**-see-ah) is abnormal development or growth of cells, tissues, or organs (**dys**- means bad, and **-plasia** means formation).
- **Hyperplasia** (**high**-per-**PLAY**-zee-ah) is the enlargement of an organ or tissue because of an abnormal increase in the number of cells in the tissues (**hyper**- means excessive, and **-plasia** means formation). Contrast hyperplasia with *hypertrophy.*
- **Hypertrophy** (high-**PER**-troh-fee) is a general increase in the bulk of a body part or organ that is due to an increase in the size, but not in the number, of cells in the tissues (**hyper**- means excessive, and **-trophy** means development). This enlargement is not due to tumor formation. Contrast hypertrophy with *anaplasia* and *hyperplasia.*

GLANDS

A **gland** is a group of specialized epithelial cells that are capable of producing secretions. A *secretion* is the substance produced by a gland. The two major types of glands are exocrine and endocrine glands (Figure 2.10).

- **Exocrine glands** (**ECK**-soh-krin), such as sweat glands, secrete chemical substances into ducts that lead either to other organs or out of the body (**exo**- means out of, and **-crine** means to secrete). See Chapter 12.
- **Endocrine glands** (**EN**-doh-krin), which produce hormones, do not have ducts (**endo**- means within, and **-crine** means to secrete). These hormones are secreted directly into the bloodstream, which are then transported to organs and structures throughout the body (see Chapter 13).

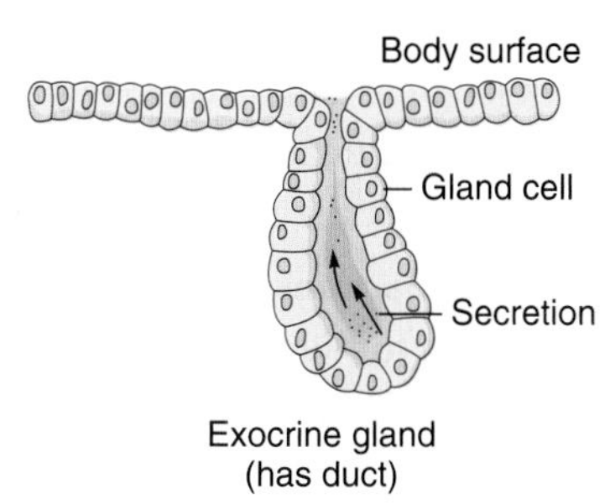

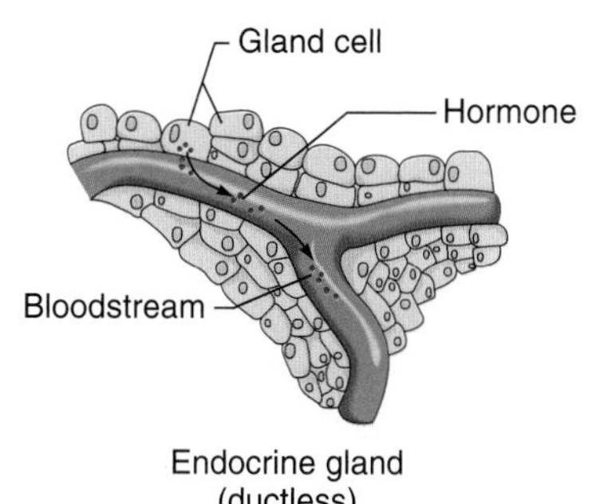

FIGURE 2.10 *Exocrine glands* secrete their chemical substances into ducts that lead either to other organs or out of the body. *Endocrine glands* pour their secretions directly into the bloodstream.

Pathology and Procedures of the Glands

- **Adenitis** (**ad**-eh-**NIGH**-tis) is the inflammation of a gland (**aden** means gland, and **-itis** means inflammation).
- An **adenocarcinoma** (**ad**-eh-noh-**kar**-sih-**NOH**-mah) is a malignant tumor that originates in glandular tissue (**aden/o** means gland, **carcin** means cancerous, and **-oma** means tumor). *Malignant* means harmful, capable of spreading, and potentially life threatening.
- An **adenoma** (**ad**-eh-**NOH**-mah) is a benign tumor that arises in, or resembles, glandular tissue (**aden** means gland, and **-oma** means tumor). *Benign* means not life threatening.
- **Adenomalacia** (**ad**-eh-noh-mah-**LAY**-shee-ah) is the abnormal softening of a gland (**aden/o** means gland, and **-malacia** means abnormal softening). Adenomalacia is the opposite of *adenosclerosis.*
- **Adenosis** (**ad**-eh-**NOH**-sis) is any disease condition of a gland (**aden** means gland, and **-osis** means an abnormal condition or disease).
- **Adenosclerosis** (**ad**-eh-noh-skleh-**ROH**-sis) is the abnormal hardening of a gland (**aden/o** means gland, and **-sclerosis** means abnormal hardening). Adenosclerosis is the opposite of *adenomalacia.*
- An **adenectomy** (**ad**-eh-**NECK**-toh-mee) is the surgical removal of a gland (**aden** means gland, and **-ectomy** means surgical removal).

BODY SYSTEMS AND RELATED ORGANS

A body **organ** is a somewhat independent part of the body that performs a specific function. For purposes of description, the related tissues and organs are described as being organized into body systems with specialized functions. These body systems are explained in Table 2.1.

PATHOLOGY

Pathology (pah-**THOL**-oh-jee) is the study of the nature and cause of disease that involves changes in structure and function. Pathology also means a condition produced by disease. The word root (combining form) **path/o** and the suffix **-pathy** mean disease; however, they also mean suffering, feeling, and emotion.

- A **pathologist** (pah-**THOL**-oh-jist) specializes in the laboratory analysis of tissue samples to confirm or establish a diagnosis (**path** means disease, and **-ologist** means specialist). These tissue specimens can be removed in biopsies, during operations, or in postmortem examinations. *Postmortem* means after death and a postmortem examination is also known as an **autopsy** (**AW**-top-see).
- **Etiology** (**ee**-tee-**OL**-oh-jee) is the study of the causes of diseases (**eti-** means cause, and **-ology** means study of). Disease-producing organisms are discussed further in Chapter 6.

Disease Transmission

A *pathogen* is a disease-producing microorganism such as a virus. *Transmission* is the spread of a disease. *Contamination* means that a pathogen is possibly present. Contamination occurs through a lack of proper hygiene standards or by failure to take appropriate infection control precautions.

- A **communicable disease** (kuh-**MEW**-nih-kuh-bul), also known as a *contagious disease*, is any condition that is transmitted from one person to another either by direct or by indirect contact with contaminated objects. *Communicable* means capable of being transmitted.
- **Indirect contact transmission** refers to situations in which a susceptible person is infected by contact with a contaminated surface.
- **Bloodborne transmission** is the spread of a disease through contact with blood or other body fluids that are contaminated with blood. Examples of bloodborne transmission are human immunodeficiency virus (HIV), hepatitis B, and most sexually transmitted diseases (STDs). These disorders are discussed in Chapters 6 and 14.
- **Airborne transmission** occurs through contact with contaminated respiratory droplets spread by a cough or sneeze. Examples include tuberculosis, flu, colds, and measles (see Chapter 7).
- **Food-borne and waterborne transmission**, also known as *fecal-oral transmission*, is caused by eating or drinking contaminated food or water that has not been properly treated to remove contamination or kill pathogens that are present (see Chapter 8).
- **Vector-borne transmission** is the spread of certain disease due to the bite of a vector. As used here, the term *vector* describes insects or animals such as flies, mites, fleas, ticks, rats, and dogs that are capable of transmitting a disease. Mosquitoes are the most common vectors, and the diseases they transmit include malaria and West Nile virus.

Outbreaks of Diseases

An **epidemiologist** (**ep**-ih-**dee**-mee-**OL**-oh-jist) is a specialist in the study of outbreaks of disease within a population group (**epi-** means above, **dem** means population, and **-ologist** means specialist).

- **Endemic** (en-**DEM**-ick) refers to the ongoing presence of a disease within a population, group, or area (**en-** means within, **dem** means population, and **-ic** means pertaining to). For example, the common cold is endemic because it is always present within the general population.
- An **epidemic** (**ep**-ih-**DEM**-ick) is a sudden and widespread outbreak of a disease within a specific population group or area (**epi-** means above, **dem** means population, and **-ic** means pertaining to). For example, a sudden widespread outbreak of measles is an epidemic.
- **Pandemic** (pan-**DEM**-ick) refers to an outbreak of a disease occurring over a large geographic area, possibly worldwide (**pan-** means entire, **dem** means population, and **-ic** means pertaining to). For example, the worldwide spread of AIDS is pandemic.

Types of Diseases

- A **functional disorder** produces symptoms for which no physiological or anatomical cause can be identified. For example, a panic attack is a functional disorder (see Chapter 10).
- An **iatrogenic illness** (eye-**at**-roh-**JEN**-ick) is an unfavorable response due to prescribed medical treatment. For example, severe burns resulting from radiation therapy are iatrogenic.
- An **idiopathic disorder** (**id**-ee-oh-**PATH**-ick) is an illness without known cause (**idi/o** means peculiar to the individual, **path** means disease, and **-ic** means pertaining to). *Idiopathic* means without known cause.
- An **infectious disease** (in-**FECK**-shus) is an illness caused by living pathogenic organisms such as bacteria and viruses (see Chapter 6).
- A **nosocomial infection** (**nos**-oh-**KOH**-mee-al in-**FECK**-shun) is a disease acquired in a hospital or clinical setting. *Nosocomial* means hospital-acquired. For example, MRSA infections are often spread in hospitals (see Chapter 6).
- An **organic disorder** (or-**GAN**-ick) produces symptoms caused by detectable physical changes in the body. For example, chickenpox, which has a characteristic rash, is an organic disorder caused by a virus (see Chapter 6).

Congenital Disorders

A **congenital disorder** (kon-**JEN**-ih-tahl) is an abnormal condition that exists at the time of birth. *Congenital* means existing at birth. These conditions can be caused by a developmental disorder before birth, prenatal influences, premature birth, or injuries during the birth process.

Developmental Disorders

A **developmental disorder**, also known as a *birth defect*, can result in an anomaly or malformation such as the absence of a limb or the presence of an extra toe. An **anomaly** (ah-**NOM**-ah-lee) is a deviation from what is regarded as normal.

- The term **atresia** (at-**TREE**-zee-ah) describes the congenital absence of a normal opening or the failure of a structure to be tubular. For example, an *anal atresia* is the congenital absence of the opening at the bottom end of the anus.

Prenatal Influences

Prenatal influences are the mother's health, behavior, and the prenatal medical care she does, or does not, receive before delivery.

- An example of a problem with the mother's health is a *rubella* infection. Birth defects often develop if a pregnant woman contracts this viral infection early in her pregnancy (see Chapter 6).
- An example of a problem caused by the mother's behavior is **fetal alcohol syndrome** (FAS) which is caused by the mother's consumption of alcohol during the pregnancy. This resulting condition of the baby is characterized by physical and behavioral traits, including growth abnormalities, mental retardation, brain damage, and socialization difficulties.
- An example of a problem caused by the lack of adequate prenatal medical care is premature delivery or a low birth-weight baby.

Premature Birth and Birth Injuries

- *Premature birth*, which is a birth that occurs earlier than 37 weeks of development, can cause serious health problems because the baby's body systems have not had time to form completely. Breathing difficulties and heart problems are common in premature babies.

- *Birth injuries* are congenital disorders that were not present before the events surrounding the time of birth. For example, *cerebral palsy*, which is the result of brain damage, can be caused by premature birth or inadequate oxygen to the brain during the birth process (see Chapter 10).

AGING

Aging is the normal progression of the life cycle that will eventually end in death. During the latter portion of life, individuals become increasingly at higher risk of developing health problems that are chronic or eventually fatal. As the average life span is becoming longer, a larger portion of the population is affected by such disorders related to aging.

- The study of the medical problem and care of the aged is known as **geriatrics** (jer-ee-**AT**-ricks) or as *gerontology*. Both of these terms have the same meaning; however, geriatrics is the preferred term.
- A physician who specializes in the care of older people is known as a **geriatrician** (**jer**-ee-ah-**TRISH**-un) or as a *gerontologist*. Both of these terms have the same meaning; however, geriatrician is the preferred term.

ABBREVIATIONS RELATED TO THE HUMAN BODY IN HEALTH AND DISEASE

Table 2.2 presents an overview of the abbreviations related to the terms introduced in this chapter. Note: To avoid errors or confusion, always be cautious when using abbreviations.

TABLE 2.2

ABBREVIATIONS RELATED TO THE HUMAN BODY IN HEALTH AND DISEASE

anterior = A	**A** = anterior
abdomen = Abd, Abdo	**Abd, Abdo** = abdomen
anatomy = anat	**anat** = anatomy
communicable disease = CD	**CD** = communicable disease
chromosome or chromosomes = CH, chr	**CH, chr** = chromosome or chromosomes
cytology, cytoplasm = cyt	**cyt** = cytology, cytoplasm
dorsal = D	**D** = dorsal
epidemic = epid	**epid** = epidemic
hemophilia = HEM, hemo	**HEM, hemo** = hemophilia
histology = HIS, Histo, histol	**HIS, Histo, histol** = histology
physiology, posterior = P	**P** = physiology, posterior
umbilical = umb	**umb** = umbilical
ventral = V, vent, ventr	**V, vent, ventr** = ventral

CAREER OPPORTUNITIES

In addition to medical specialties requiring advanced graduate degrees, such as an MD, there are many interesting health occupations to consider that require a shorter course of education. Some of these jobs specialize primarily with one body system, such as a dental assistant or a respiratory therapist. (These are listed at the end of each of the body system chapters.) Others treat the patient's general health care needs, including:

- **Medical assistant:** prepares patients for examination, takes vital signs and medical history, performs basic laboratory tests, and cleans and maintains equipment. May also fill an administrative role such as the position of receptionist or office manager.
- **Nurse assistant, nurse's aide, patient care technician (PCT)**, or **orderly:** provides basic and essential patient care such as bathing, bed making, and feeding.
- **Registered nurse (RN), licensed practical nurse (LPN)**, and **licensed vocational nurse (LVN):** state-licensed to provide and manage patient care. An RN is authorized to provide specialized services, including administering medications, teaching, and supervising other staff members. An LPN or LVN provides for patients' needs under the supervision of an RN or physician. There are many nursing specialties, including:

  Community health nurse
  Critical care nurse
  Flight nurse
  Hospice nurse
  Infectious disease nurse
  IV therapy nurse
  Nurse anesthetist
  Private duty nurse
  School nurse
  Surgery scrub nurse

- **Nurse practitioner (NP):** an RN with advanced training in the diagnosis and treatment of illness. An NP provides primary care for patients, often in collaboration with a physician, and in some states, the NP may write prescriptions.
- **Physician assistant (PA):** performs routine medical examinations and diagnostic tests, and treats minor injuries and diseases under the supervision of a physician. In many states, a PA may prescribe medications.
- **Medical Translator:** provides bilingual assistance for accurate communications between health care providers and non-English-speaking patients. A medical translator must know medical terminology in English and a second language.

Health Occupation Profile
Emergency Room Technician

Vicky Edwards is an emergency room technician at a hospital in St. Louis. *"My years of working for doctors in their offices (ENT, internal medicine, and general surgery) gave me a good background for the interesting and intense work I do at the hospital. My duties include aiding with triage (screening patients to determine the priority of treatment), head-to-toe patient assessment, phlebotomy (taking blood), and all point-of-care procedures such as inserting catheters and taking blood sugar tests, EKGs, and vital signs. Emergency trauma situations are frequent in a big city hospital, and it is exhilarating when we are able to save a life. But caring for all our patients and giving them that little extra TLC are just as important."*

Study Break

What is the most common infectious disease on earth? Hint: You would have to live in a small, very isolated community, or perhaps in the frozen wastelands of Antarctica to avoid it, and yet no one has ever found a cure.

Answer: **the common cold. We do know that this contagious condition is usually caused by one of over 100 types of rhinovirus (rhino means nose, plus *virus*) and that it is spread through sneezing, coughing, and inadequate hand washing.**

The common cold is sometimes confused with the flu (influenza), which can be fatal. In the deadliest flu outbreak on record, over 21 million people died worldwide in just 2 years (1918 and 1919). The flu is a viral infection characterized by a fever in addition to cold-like symptoms. It is very contagious and usually occurs in epidemics rather than isolated cases.

Review Time

Write the answers to the following questions on a separate piece of paper or in your notebook. In addition, be prepared to take part in the classroom discussion.

1. ***Written Assignment:*** Using terms a layperson would understand, state the differences between **congenital** and **genetic disorders** and give an example of each.

   Discussion Assignment: How do you think genetic counseling would affect a young couple who are at risk for transmitting cystic fibrosis to their children?

2. ***Written Assignment:*** What is the difference between an **organic disorder** and a **functional disorder**?

   Discussion Assignment: Give examples of these two disorders.

3. ***Written Assignment:*** What is the difference between an **iatrogenic illness** and a **nosocomial infection**?

   Discussion Assignment: Describe the differences between the causes of these conditions.

continues

4. ***Written Assignment:*** Using your own words, describe the differences between **sagittal, frontal,** and **transverse planes.**

   Discussion Assignment: Where is each of these planes located?

5. ***Written Assignment:*** Identify the **two dorsal** and **three ventral body cavities.**

   Discussion Assignment: How would you describe to a patient which organs are protected by each cavity?

Optional Internet Activity

The goal of this activity is to help you learn more about medical terminology as it applies to the "real world." Select ***one*** *of these two options and follow the instructions.*

1. Search for information about **Down syndrome**. Write a brief (one- or two-paragraph) report on something new that you learned here and include the address of the web site where you found this information.
2. To learn more about **Tay-Sachs disease**, look for the web site of the NINDS (National Institute of Neurological Disorders and Strokes). Write a brief (one- or-two paragraph) report on something new you learned here.

THE HUMAN TOUCH: CRITICAL THINKING ACTIVITY

The following story and questions are designed to stimulate critical thinking through class discussion or as a brief essay response. There are no right or wrong answers to these questions.

The sign in the fifth floor restroom read,* "Dirty hands spread disease. Always use soap." *Dave rinsed his hands with water, gave his hair a quick finger-through, and then rushed into the hallway, already late for biology class.

***There was an overwhelming smell as he entered the classroom, and he could immediately tell why: on each counter was sitting the day's project, a fetal pig.* "Do these things have to stink?" *he asked his teacher.* "Well, Dave, if they didn't 'stink' of the formaldehyde, they would be rotting and could be spreading diseases. Now let's get started," *the teacher said. At the end of class period, they were told,* "Be sure to wash your hands thoroughly before leaving this classroom."**

This reminded Dave of the lectures they had earlier in the semester about diseases caused by pathogens and how these diseases are spread. As he looked around the classroom, Dave was aware of the other students. Most were gathering up their books to go directly to lunch without washing their hands, Gail and Susan were sharing a bottle of water, Beth was rubbing her eyes, and Jim was coughing without covering his mouth! Suddenly, Dave had a mental image of pathogens everywhere: crawling on hands, lying on counter tops, floating in the air—and all of these pathogens were looking for someone to infect! Dave shook his head to get rid of this mental image. Then he went to the sink and carefully washed his hands again—this time with soap and hot water.

continues

Suggested Discussion Topics

1. Identify and discuss the examples of potential methods of disease transmission that are included in Dave's story and describe what should have been done to eliminate these risks.
2. Describe how bloodborne, airborne, and food-borne diseases are transmitted and give an example of each type of transmission.
3. Discuss what might happen in a school if a cafeteria worker has a food-borne disease, and at the end of a trip to the lavatory, did not wash his or her hands. Instead, the worker went right back to work without putting on gloves preparing salads and putting fresh fruit out for lunch.
4. When treating a bloody wound, the caregiver is required to wear protective gloves. Discuss the possible reasons for this. Is this step taken to protect the patient against diseases on the caregiver's hands? Is this step required to protect the caregiver from a bloodborne disease that the patient might have?

STUDENT WORKBOOK AND StudyWARE™ CD-ROM

1. Go to your **Student Workbook** and complete the Learning Exercises for this chapter plus the **Word Part Review** activities.

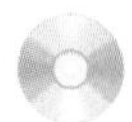

2. Go to the **StudyWARE™ CD-ROM** and have fun with the exercises and games for this chapter.

CHAPTER 3

THE SKELETAL SYSTEM

OVERVIEW OF STRUCTURES, COMBINING FORMS, AND FUNCTIONS OF THE SKELETAL SYSTEM

MAJOR STRUCTURES	RELATED COMBINING FORMS	PRIMARY FUNCTIONS
Bones	oss/e, oss/i, oste/o, ost/o	Act as the framework for the body, protect the internal organs, and store the mineral calcium.
Bone Marrow	myel/o (also means spinal cord)	Red bone marrow forms some blood cells. Yellow bone marrow stores fat.
Cartilage	chondr/o	Creates a smooth surface for motion within the joints and protects the ends of the bones.
Joints	arthr/o	Work with the muscles to make a variety of motions possible.
Ligaments	ligament/o	Connect one bone to another.
Synovial Membrane	synovi/o, synov/o	Forms the lining of synovial joints and secretes synovial fluid.
Synovial Fluid	synovi/o, synov/o	Lubricant that makes smooth joint movements possible.
Bursa	burs/o	Cushions areas subject to friction during movement.

VOCABULARY RELATED TO THE SKELETAL SYSTEM

This list contains essential word parts and medical terms for this chapter. These terms are pronounced on the student StudyWARE™ CD-ROM and Audio CDs that are available for use with this text. These and the other important **primary terms** are shown in boldface throughout the chapter. *Secondary terms*, which appear in *orange* italics, clarify the meaning of primary terms.

Word Parts

- ☐ **ankyl/o**
- ☐ **arthr/o**
- ☐ **chondr/o**
- ☐ **cost/o**
- ☐ **crani/o**
- ☐ **-desis**
- ☐ **kyph/o**
- ☐ **lord/o**
- ☐ **-lysis**
- ☐ **myel/o**
- ☐ **oss/e, oss/i, ost/o, oste/o**
- ☐ **scoli/o**
- ☐ **spondyl/o**
- ☐ **synovi/o, synov/o**
- ☐ **-um**

Medical Terms

- ☐ **acetabulum** (**ass**-eh-**TAB**-you-lum)
- ☐ **allogenic** (**al**-oh-**JEN**-ick)
- ☐ **ankylosing spondylitis** (**ang**-kih-**LOH**-sing **spon**-dih-**LYE**-tis)
- ☐ **arthrodesis** (**ar**-throh-**DEE**-sis)
- ☐ **arthrolysis** (ar-**THROL**-ih-sis)
- ☐ **arthroscopy** (ar-**THROS**-koh-pee)
- ☐ **autologous** (aw-**TOL**-uh-guss)
- ☐ **chondroma** (kon-**DROH**-mah)
- ☐ **chondromalacia** (**kon**-droh-mah-**LAY**-shee-ah)
- ☐ **comminuted fracture** (**KOM**-ih-**newt**-ed)
- ☐ **compression fracture**
- ☐ **costochondritis** (**kos**-toh-kon-**DRIGH**-tis)
- ☐ **craniostenosis** (**kray**-nee-oh-steh-**NOH**-sis)
- ☐ **crepitation** (**krep**-ih-**TAY**-shun)
- ☐ **dual x-ray absorptiometry** (ab-**sorp**-shee-**OM**-eh-tree)
- ☐ **fibrous dysplasia** (dis-**PLAY**-see-ah)
- ☐ **hallux valgus** (**HAL**-ucks **VAL**-guss)
- ☐ **hemarthrosis** (**hem**-ar-**THROH**-sis)
- ☐ **hemopoietic** (**hee**-moh poy-**ET**-ick)
- ☐ **internal fixation**
- ☐ **juvenile rheumatoid arthritis** (**ROO**-mah-toyd ar-**THRIGH**-tis)
- ☐ **kyphosis** (kye-**FOH**-sis)
- ☐ **laminectomy** (**lam**-ih-**NECK**-toh-mee)
- ☐ **lordosis** (lor-**DOH**-sis)
- ☐ **lumbago** (lum-**BAY**-goh)
- ☐ **malleolus** (mal-**LEE**-oh-lus)
- ☐ **manubrium** (mah-**NEW**-bree-um)
- ☐ **metacarpals** (met-ah-**KAR**-palz)
- ☐ **metatarsals** (met-ah-**TAHR**-salz)myeloma (**my**-eh-**LOH**-mah)
- ☐ **open fracture**
- ☐ **orthopedic surgeon** (**or**-thoh-**PEE**-dick)
- ☐ **orthotic** (or-**THOT**-ick)
- ☐ **osteitis** (**oss**-tee-**EYE**-tis)
- ☐ **osteoarthritis** (**oss**-tee-oh-ar-**THRIGH**-tis)
- ☐ **osteochondroma** (**oss**-tee-oh-kon-**DROH**-mah)
- ☐ **osteoclasis** (**oss**-tee-**OCK**-lah-sis)
- ☐ **osteomalacia** (**oss**-tee-oh-mah-**LAY**-shee-ah)
- ☐ **osteomyelitis** (**oss**-tee-oh-**my**-eh-**LYE**-tis)
- ☐ **osteonecrosis** (**oss**-tee-oh-neh-**KROH**-sis)
- ☐ **osteopenia** (**oss**-tee-oh-**PEE**-nee-ah)
- ☐ **osteoporosis** (**oss**-tee-oh-poh-**ROH**-sis)
- ☐ **osteoporotic hip fracture** (**oss**-tee-oh-pah-**ROT**-ick)
- ☐ **osteorrhaphy** (**oss**-tee-**OR**-ah-fee)
- ☐ **Paget's disease** (**PAJ**-its)
- ☐ **pathologic fracture**
- ☐ **percutaneous vertebroplasty** (**per**-kyou-**TAY**-nee-us **VER**-tee-broh-**plas**-tee)
- ☐ **periostitis** (**pehr**-ee-oss-**TYE**-tis)
- ☐ **podiatrist** (poh-**DYE**-ah-trist)
- ☐ **prosthesis** (pros-**THEE**-sis)
- ☐ **rheumatoid arthritis** (**ROO**-mah-toyd ar-**THRIGH**-tis)
- ☐ **rickets** (**RICK**-ets)
- ☐ **scoliosis** (**skoh**-lee-**OH**-sis)
- ☐ **spina bifida** (**SPY**-nah **BIF**-ih-dah)
- ☐ **spiral fracture**
- ☐ **spondylolisthesis** (**spon**-dih-loh-liss-**THEE**-sis)
- ☐ **spondylosis** (**spon**-dih-**LOH**-sis)
- ☐ **subluxation** (**sub**-luck-**SAY**-shun)
- ☐ **synovectomy** (sin-oh-**VECK**-toh-mee)
- ☐ **vertebrae** (**VER**-teh-bray)

OBJECTIVES

On completion of this chapter, you should be able to:

1. Identify and describe the major functions and structures of the skeletal system.
2. Describe three types of joints.
3. Differentiate between the axial and appendicular skeletons.
4. Identify the medical specialists who treat disorders of the skeletal system.
5. Recognize, define, spell, and pronounce terms related to the pathology and the diagnostic and treatment procedures of the skeletal system.

STRUCTURES AND FUNCTIONS OF THE SKELETAL SYSTEM

The **skeletal system** consists of the bones, bone marrow, cartilage, joints, ligaments, synovial membrane, synovial fluid, and bursa. This body system also has many important functions:

- Bones act as the framework of the body.
- Bones support and protect the internal organs.
- Joints work in conjunction with muscles, ligaments, and tendons, making possible the wide variety of body movements. (Muscles and tendons are discussed in Chapter 4.)
- Calcium, which is required for normal nerve and muscle function, is stored in bones.
- Red bone marrow, which has an important function in the formation of blood cells, is located within spongy bone.

THE STRUCTURE OF BONES

Bone is the form of connective tissue that is the second hardest tissue in the human body. Only dental enamel is harder than bone.

The Tissues of Bone

Although it is a dense and rigid tissue, bone is also capable of growth, healing, and reshaping itself (Figure 3.1).

- **Periosteum** (**pehr**-ee-**OSS**-tee-um) is the tough, fibrous tissue that forms the outermost covering of bone (**peri-** means surrounding, **oste** means bone, and **-um** is a noun ending).
- **Compact bone** is the dense, hard, and very strong bone that forms the protective outer layer of bones.

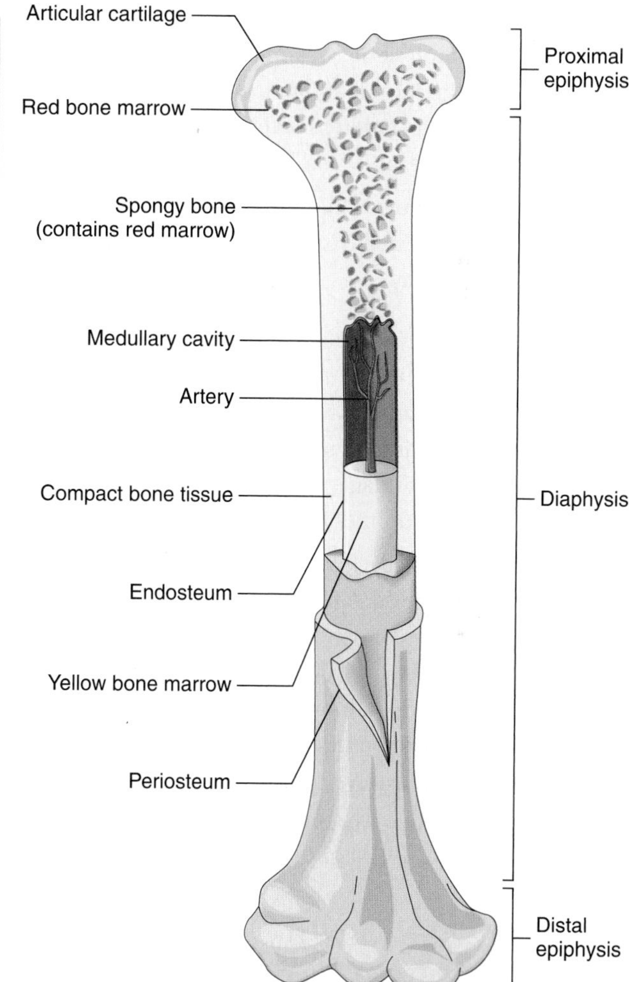

FIGURE 3.1 Anatomic features of a typical long bone.

- **Spongy bone** is lighter, and not as strong, as compact bone. This type of bone is commonly found in the ends and inner portions of long bones such as the femur. Red bone marrow is located within this spongy bone.

- The **medullary cavity** (**MED**-you-**lehr**-ee) is located in the shaft of a long bone and is surrounded by compact bone. *Medullary* means pertaining to the inner section.
- The **endosteum** (en-**DOS**-tee-um) is the tissue that lines the medullary cavity (**end-** means within, **oste** means bone, and **-um** is a noun ending).

Bone Marrow

- **Red bone marrow**, which is located within the spongy bone, is hemopoietic tissue that manufactures red blood cells, hemoglobin, white blood cells, and thrombocytes. These types of cells are discussed in Chapter 5. **Hemopoietic** (**hee**-moh poy-**ET**-ick) means pertaining to the formation of blood cells (**hem/o** means blood, and **-poietic** means pertaining to formation). This term is also spelled *hematopoietic*.
- **Yellow bone marrow**, which functions as a fat storage area, is composed chiefly of fat cells and is located in the medullary cavity.

Cartilage

- **Cartilage** (**KAR**-tih-lidj) is the smooth, rubbery, blue-white connective tissue that acts as a shock absorber between bones. Cartilage, which is more elastic than bone, also makes up the flexible parts of the skeleton such as the outer ear and the tip of the nose.
- **Articular cartilage** (ar-**TICK**-you-lar **KAR**-tih-lidj) covers the surfaces of bones where they come together to form joints. This cartilage makes smooth joint movement possible and protects the bones from rubbing against each other (see Figures 3.1 and 3.4).
- The **meniscus** (meh-**NIS**-kus) is the curved fibrous cartilage found in some joints, such as the knee and the temporomandibular joint of the jaw (see Figure 3.5).

Anatomic Landmarks of Bones

- The **diaphysis** (dye-**AF**-ih-sis) is the shaft of a long bone (see Figure 3.1).
- The **epiphysis** (eh-**PIF**-ih-sis), which is covered with articular cartilage, is the wide end of a long bone. The *proximal epiphysis* is the end of the bone located nearest to the midline of the body. The *distal epiphysis* is the end of the bone located farthest away from the midline.
- A **foramen** (foh-**RAY**-men) is an opening in a bone through which blood vessels, nerves, and ligaments pass (plural, *foramina*). For example, the spinal cord passes through the *foramen magnum* of the occipital bone.
- A **process** is a normal projection on the surface of a bone that serves as an attachment for muscles and tendons. For example, the *mastoid process* is the bony projection located on temporal bones just behind the ears (see Figure 3.7).

JOINTS

Joints, which are also known as *articulations*, are the place of union between two or more bones. Joints are classified according to either their construction or based on the degree of movement they allow.

Fibrous Joints

Fibrous joints, consisting of inflexible layers of dense connective tissue, hold the bones tightly together. In adults these joints, which are also known as *sutures*, do not allow any movement (see Figure 3.7). In newborns and very young children some fibrous joints are movable before they have solidified.

- The **fontanelles** (**fon**-tah-**NELLS**), also known as the *soft spots*, are normally present on the skull of a newborn (Figure 3.2). These flexible soft spots facilitate the passage of the infant through the birth canal. They also allow for the growth of the skull during the first year. As the child matures, and the sutures close, the fontanelles gradually harden.

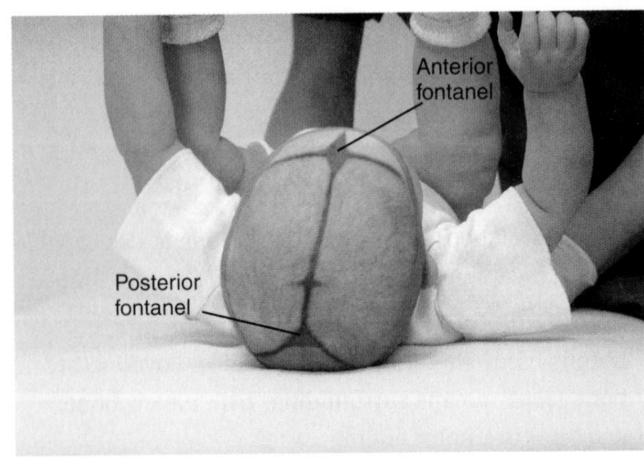

FIGURE 3.2 *Fontanelles* of an infant's skull provide the flexibility required during birth and the first year of growth.

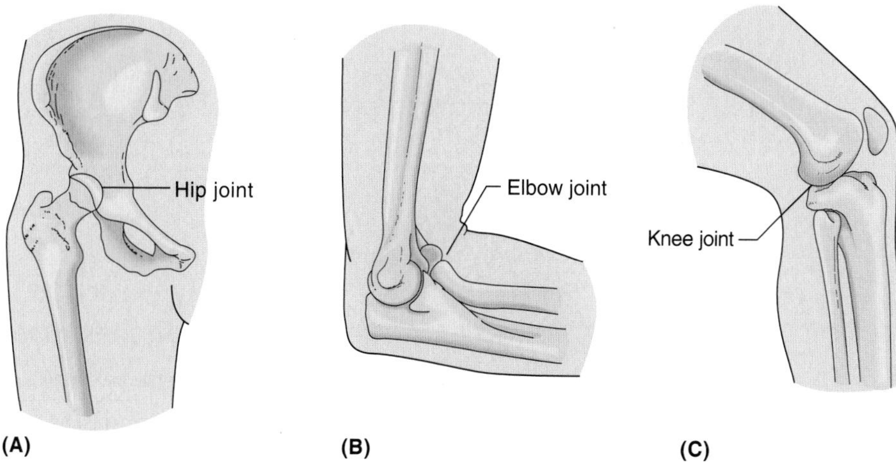

FIGURE 3.3 Examples of *synovial joints.* (A) Ball and socket joint of the hip. (B) Hinge joint of the elbow. (C) Hinge joint of the knee.

Cartilaginous Joints

Cartilaginous joints (**kar**-tih-**LADJ**-ih-nus) allow only slight movement and consist of bones connected entirely by cartilage. Examples include:

- Cartilaginous joints, such as where the ribs connect to the sternum (breast bone), are shown in Figure 3.10. These joints allow movement during breathing.
- The **pubic symphysis** (**PEW**-bick **SIM**-fih-sis) is the cartilaginous joint known that allows some movement to facilitate childbirth. This joint is located between the pubic bones in the anterior (front) of the pelvis as shown in Figure 3.14.

Synovial Joints

A **synovial joint** (sih-**NOH**-vee-al) is created where two bones articulate to permit a variety of motions. As used here the term *articulate* means to come together. These joints are also described based on their type of motion (Figure 3.3).

- *Ball and socket joints*, such as the hips and shoulders, allow a wide range of movement in many directions (Figure 3.3A).
- *Hinge joints*, such as the knees and elbows, are synovial joints that allow movement primarily in one direction or plane (Figure 3.3B and 3.3C).

Components of Synovial Joints

Synovial joints consist of several components that make complex movements possible (Figure 3.4).

- The **synovial capsule** is the outermost layer of strong fibrous tissue that resembles a sleeve as it surrounds the joint.

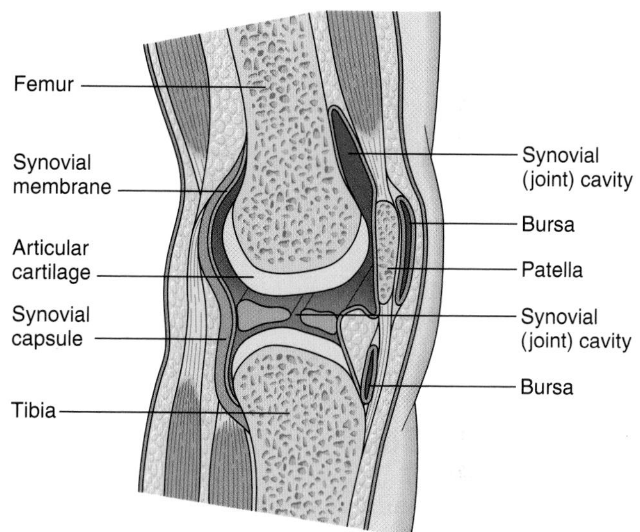

FIGURE 3.4 A lateral view of the knee showing the structures of a *synovial joint* and *bursa.*

- **Synovial membrane** lines the capsule and secretes synovial fluid.
- **Synovial fluid**, which flows within the synovial cavity, acts as a lubricant to make the smooth movement of the joint possible.
- **Ligaments** (**LIG**-ah-mentz) are bands of fibrous tissue that form joints by connecting one bone to another bone, or joining a bone to cartilage. Complex hinge joints, such as the knee, are made up of a series of ligaments that permit movement in different directions (see Figure 3.5).
- A **bursa** (**BER**-sah) is a fibrous sac that acts as a cushion to ease movement in areas that are subject to

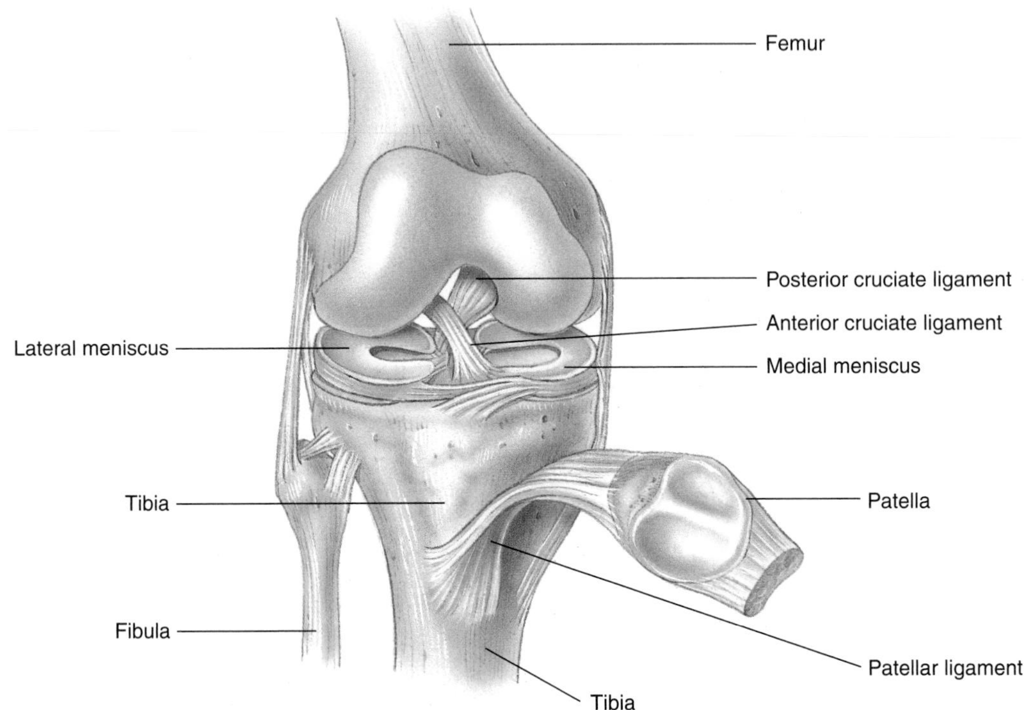

FIGURE 3.5 Major ligaments of the knee. This anterior view of the knee shows the complex system of ligaments that make its movements possible.

friction such as in the shoulder, elbow, and knee joints where a tendon passes over a bone (plural, *bursae*).

THE SKELETON

The typical adult human skeleton consists of approximately 206 bones as shown in Figure 3.6. Depending upon the age of the individual, the exact number of ranges from 206 to 350 bones. For descriptive purposes, the skeleton is divided into the axial and appendicular skeletal systems.

Axial Skeleton

The **axial skeleton** protects the major organs of the nervous, respiratory, and circulatory systems. *Axial* means pertaining to an axis, which is an imaginary line that runs lengthwise through the center of the body.

The axial skeleton consists of 80 bones including those of the skull; the ribs, sternum, and thoracic vertebrae of the thoracic cavity; and the other vertebrae of the spinal column.

Appendicular Skeleton

The **appendicular skeleton** makes body movement possible and also protects the organs of digestion, excretion, and reproduction. The term *appendicular* means referring to an appendage. An *appendage* is anything that is attached to a major part of the body.

The appendicular skeleton consists of 126 bones that are organized into the *upper extremities* (shoulders, arms, forearms, wrists, and hands) and the *lower extremities* (hips, thighs, legs, ankles, and feet).

Bones of the Skull

The **skull** consists of the eight bones that form the cranium, 14 bones that form the face, and six bones in the middle ear. As you study the following bones of the skull, refer to Figures 3.7 and 3.8.

Bones of the Cranium

The **cranium** (**KRAY**-nee-um), which is made up of the following eight bones, is the portion of the skull that encloses the brain (**crani** means skull, and **-um** is a noun ending).

- The **frontal bone** forms the forehead.
- The two **parietal bones** (pah-**RYE**-eh-tal) form most of the roof and upper sides of the cranium.
- The **occipital bone** (ock-**SIP**-ih-tal) forms the posterior floor and walls of the cranium.

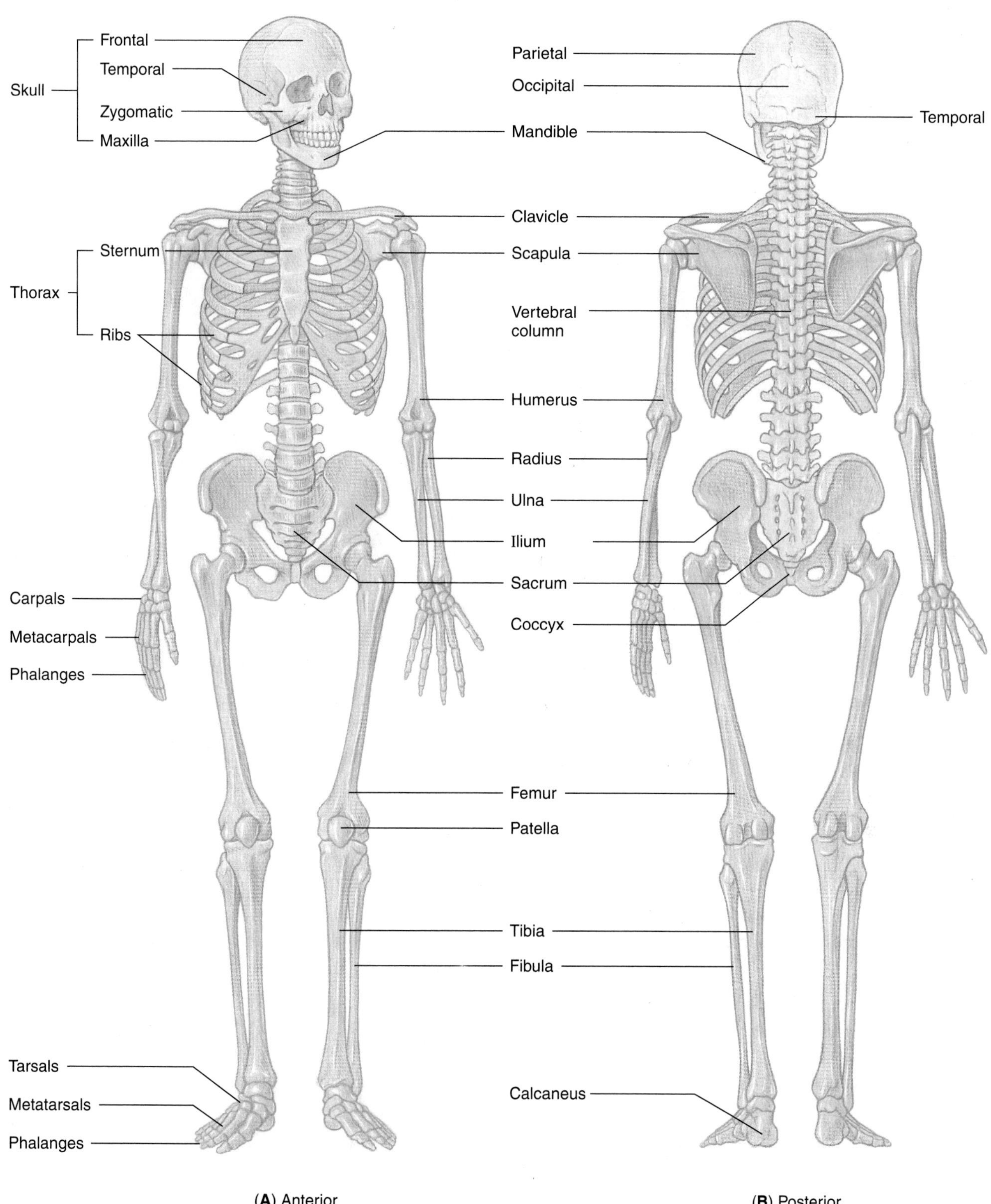

FIGURE 3.6 Anterior and posterior views of the human skeleton.

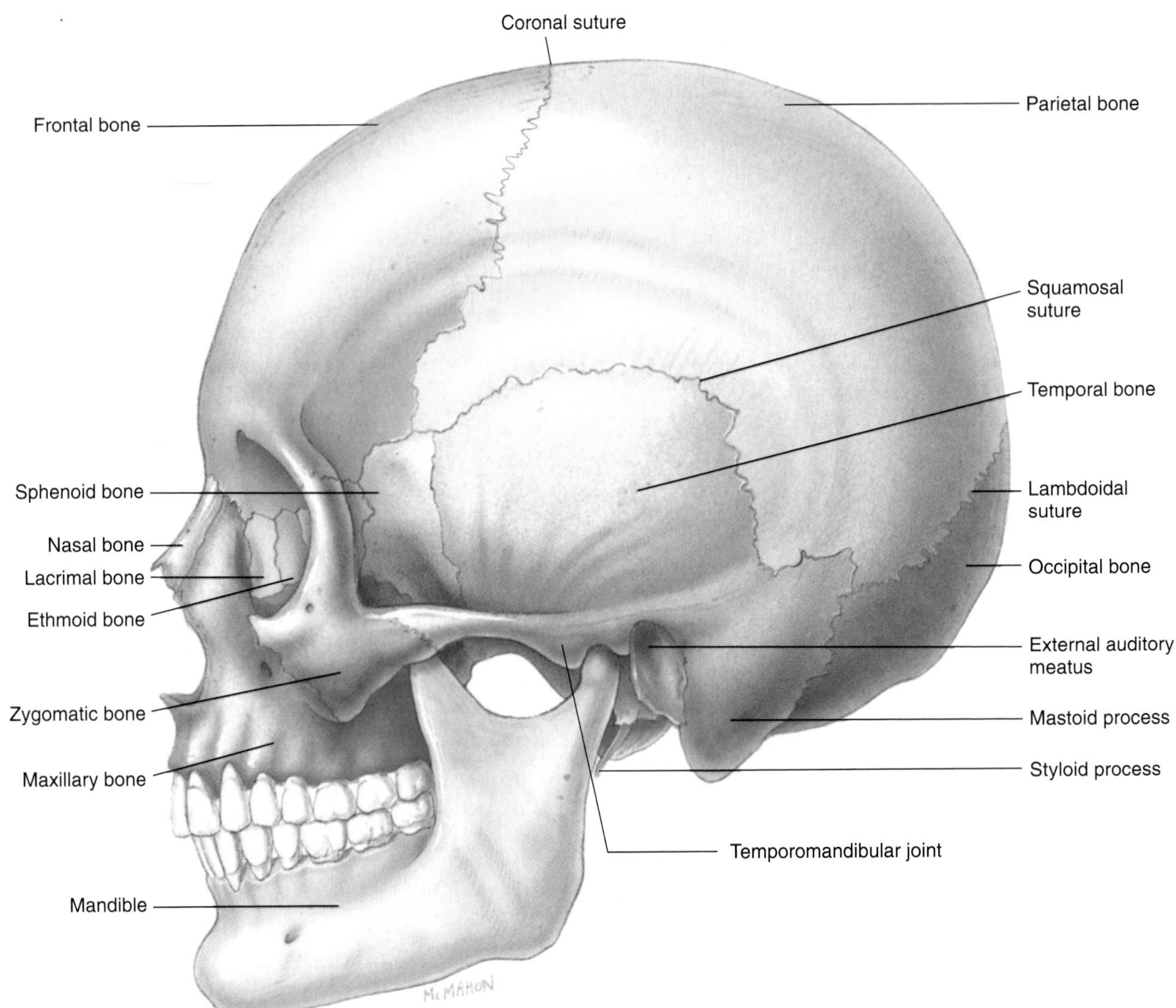

FIGURE 3.7 Lateral view of the adult human skull.

- The two **temporal bones** form the sides and base of the cranium.
- The **sphenoid bone** (**SFEE**-noid) forms part of the base of the skull and parts of the floor and sides of the orbit. The *orbit* is the bony socket that surrounds and protects the eyeball.
- The **ethmoid bone** (**ETH**-moid) forms part of the posterior portion of the nose, the orbit, and the floor of the cranium.

Auditory Ossicles

The six tiny bones of the middle ear, known as the **auditory ossicles** (**OSS**-ih-kulz), are discussed in Chapter 11.

- The **external auditory meatus** (mee-**AY**-tus), which is located in the temporal bone on each side of the skull, is the opening of the external auditory canal of the outer ear. A *meatus* is the external opening of a canal.

Bones of the Face

The face is made up of the following 14 bones:

- The two **nasal bones** that form the upper part of the bridge of the nose.
- The two **zygomatic bones** (**zye**-goh-**MAT**-ick), also known as the *cheekbones*, articulate with the frontal bone (forehead).
- The two **maxillary bones** (**MACK**-sih-**ler**-ee), also known as the *maxillae*, form most of the upper jaw (singular, *maxilla*).
- The two **palatine bones** (**PAL**-ah-tine) form part of the hard palate of the mouth and the floor of the nose.

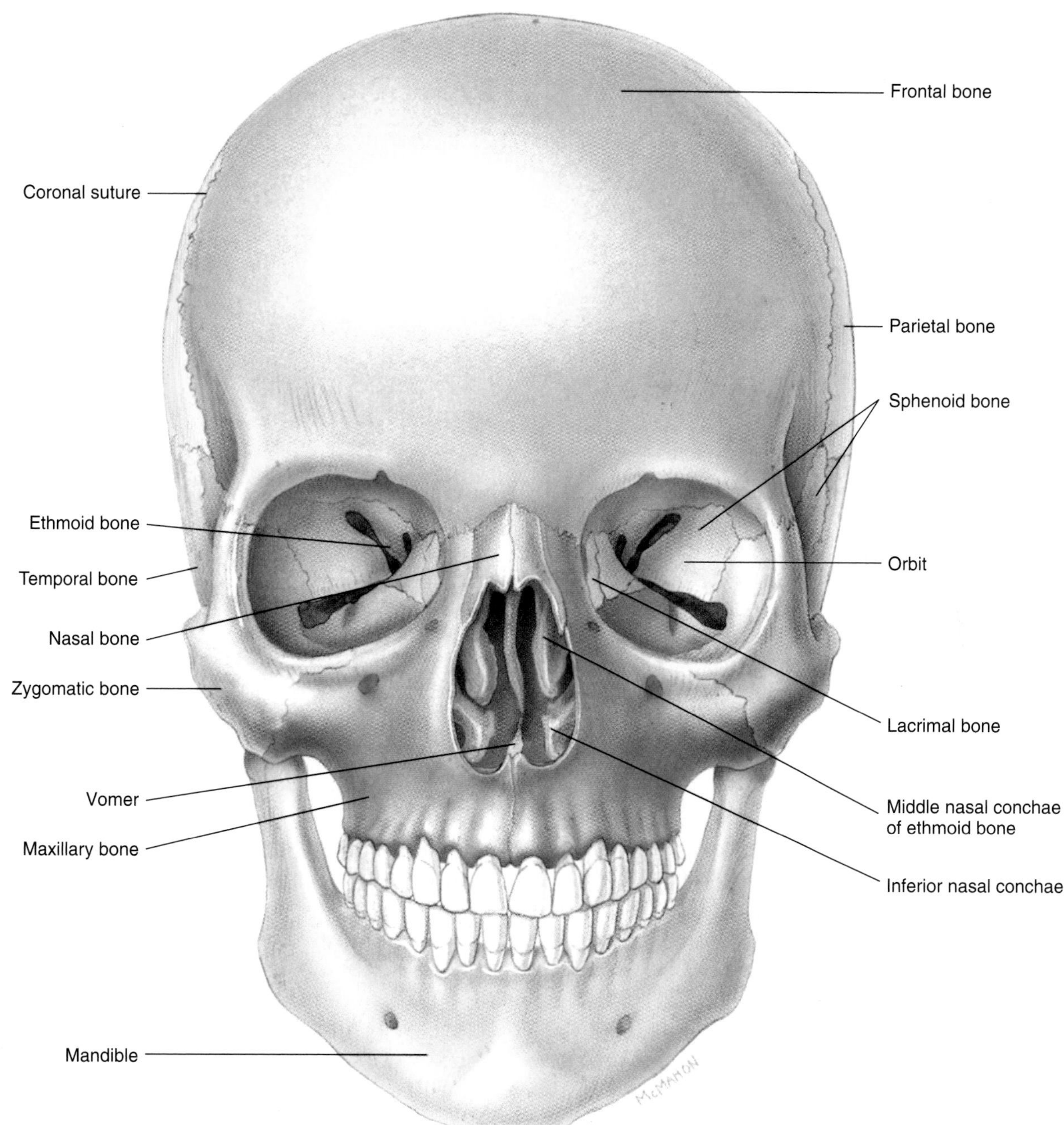

FIGURE 3.8 Anterior view of the adult human skull.

- The two **lacrimal bones** (**LACK**-rih-mal) make up part of the orbit at the inner angle of the eye.
- The two **inferior conchae** (**KONG**-kee *or* **KONG**-kay) are the thin, scroll-like bones that form part of the interior of the nose (singular, *concha*).
- The **vomer bone** (**VOH**-mer) forms the base for the nasal septum. The *nasal septum* is the cartilage wall that divides the two nasal cavities.
- The **mandible** (**MAN**-dih-bul), also known as the *jawbone*, is the only movable bone of the skull. The mandible is attached to the skull at the **temporomandibular joint** (**tem**-poh-roh-man-**DIB**-you-lar), which is also known as the *TMJ* (see Figure 3.7).

Thoracic Cavity

The **thoracic cavity** (thoh-**RAS**-ick), also known as the *rib cage*, is the bony structure that protects the heart and lungs. It consists of the ribs, sternum, and upper portion of the spinal column extending from the neck to the diaphragm, not including the arms (Figure 3.9).

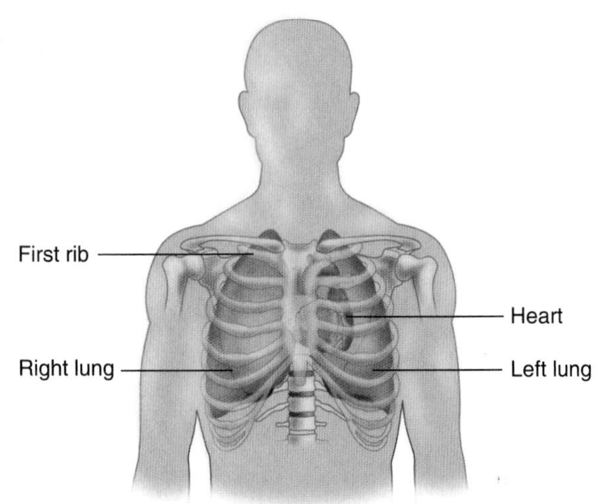

FIGURE 3.9 The *thoracic cavity* protects the heart and lungs.

Ribs

The 12 pairs of **ribs**, which are also known as *costals*, attach posteriorly to the thoracic vertebrae (**cost** means rib, and **-al** means pertaining to) (Figure 3.10).

- The first seven pairs of ribs, called *true ribs*, are attached anteriorly to the sternum.
- The next three pairs of ribs, called *false ribs*, are attached anteriorly to cartilage that joins with the sternum.
- The last two pairs of ribs, called *floating ribs*, are only attached posteriorly.

Sternum

The **sternum** (**STER**-num), also known as the *breastbone*, forms the middle of the front of the rib cage and is divided into three parts (see Figure 3.10).

- The **manubrium** (mah-**NEW**-bree-um) is the bony structure that forms the upper portion of the sternum.
- The **body of the sternum** is the bony structure that forms the middle portion of the sternum.
- The **xiphoid process** (**ZIF**-oid) is the structure made of cartilage that forms the lower portion of the sternum.

Shoulders

The shoulders form the **pectoral girdle** (**PECK**-toh-rahl), which supports the arms and hands; this also known as the *shoulder girdle*. As used here, the term *girdle* means a structure that encircles the body. As you study the bones of the shoulder, refer to Figures 3.6 and 3.10.

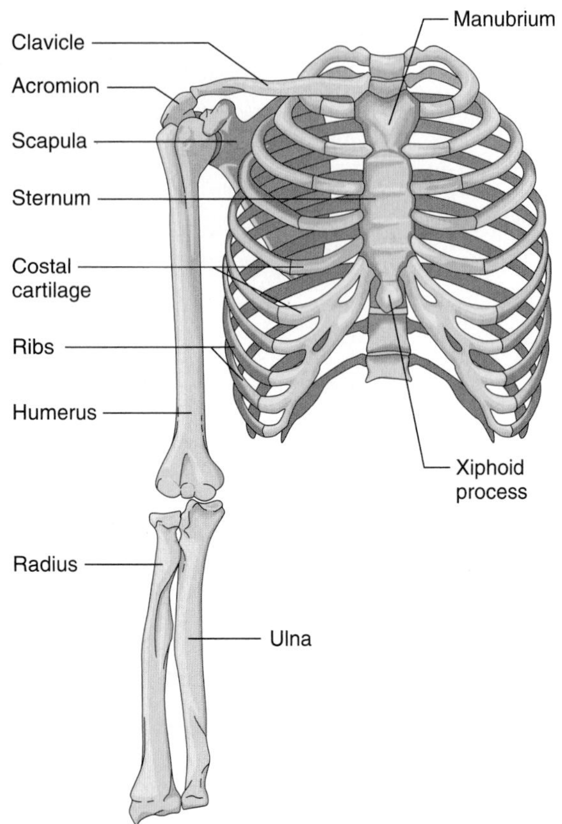

FIGURE 3.10 Anterior view of the ribs, shoulder, and arm. (Cartilaginous structures are shown in blue.)

- The **clavicle** (**KLAV**-ih-kul), also known as the *collar bone*, is a slender bone that connects the manubrium of the sternum to the scapula.
- The **scapula** (**SKAP**-you-lah) is also known as the *shoulder blade* (plural, *scapulae*).
- The **acromion** (ah-**KROH**-mee-on) is an extension of the scapula that forms the high point of the shoulder.

Arms

As you study the following bones of the arms, refer to Figures 3.6 and 3.10.

- The **humerus** (**HEW**-mer-us) is the bone of the upper arm (plural, *humeri*).
- The **radius** (**RAY**-dee-us) is the smaller and shorter bone in the forearm. The radius runs up the thumb side of the forearm.
- The **ulna** (**ULL**-nah) is the larger and longer bone of the forearm. The proximal end of the ulna articulates

with the distal end of the humerus to form the elbow joint.

- The **olecranon process** (oh-**LEK**-rah-non), commonly known as the *funny bone*, is a large projection on the upper end of the ulna. This forms the point of the elbow and exposes a nerve that tingles when struck.

Wrists, Hands, and Fingers

As you study the following bones of the wrist and hand, refer to Figure 3.11.

- The eight **carpals** (**KAR**-palz) are the bones that form the wrist. These bones form the carpal tunnel, a narrow bony passage through which passes the median nerve and the tendons of the fingers. Carpal tunnel syndrome is described in Chapter 4.
- The **metacarpals** (met-ah-**KAR**-palz) are the five bones that form the palms of the hand.
- The **phalanges** (fah-**LAN**-jeez) are the 14 bones of the fingers (singular, *phalanx*). The bones of the toes are also known as phalanges.
- Each of the four fingers has three bones. These are the distal (outermost), middle, and proximal (nearest the hand) phalanges.
- The thumb has two bones. These are the distal and proximal phalanges.

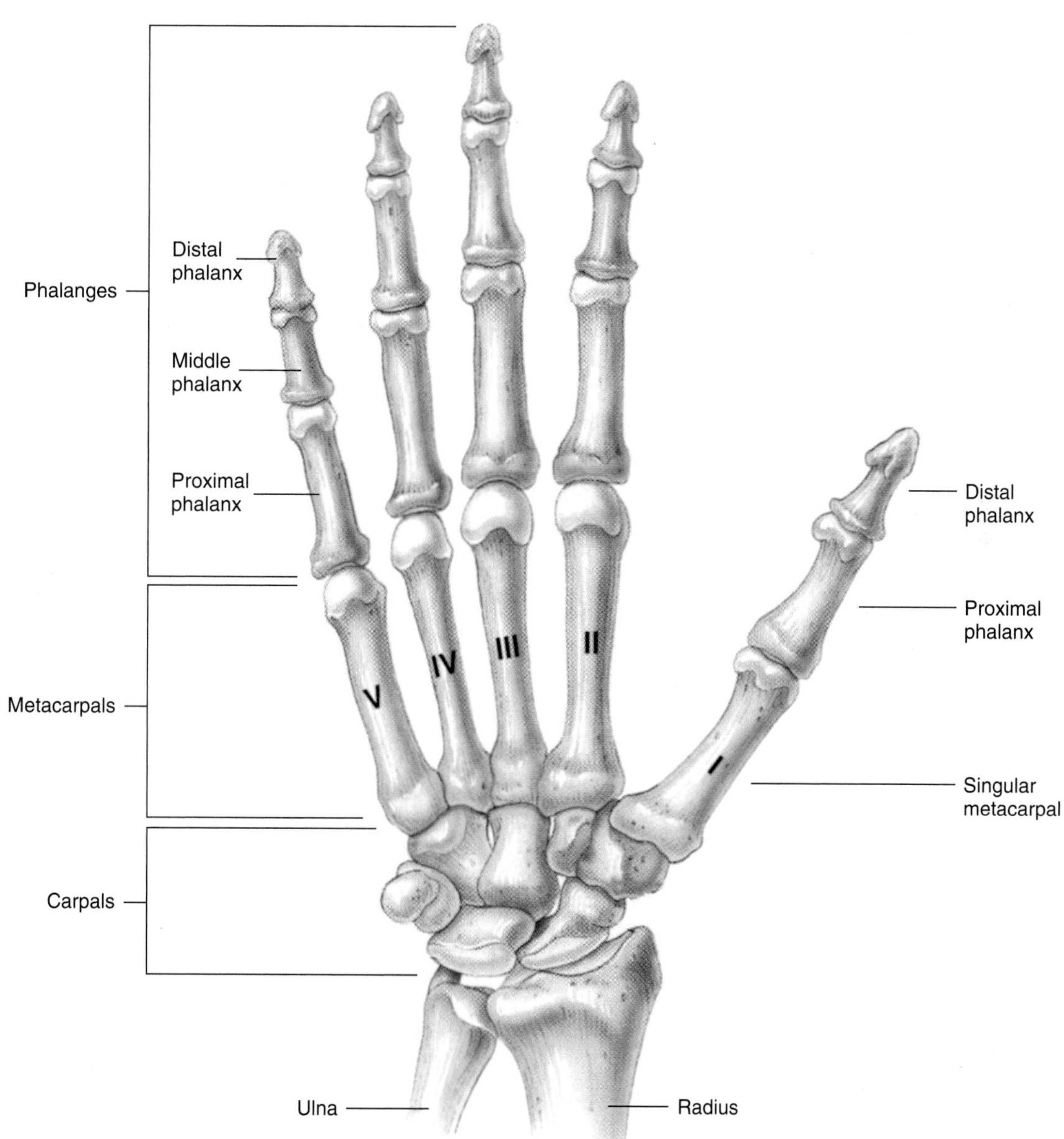

FIGURE 3.11 Superior view of the bones of the lower left arm, wrist, and hand.

The Spinal Column

The **spinal column**, also known as the *vertebral column*, supports the head and body, and protects the spinal cord. This structure consists of 26 **vertebrae** (**VER**-teh-bray). A vertebra is a single segment of the spinal column. *Vertebral* means pertaining to the vertebrae.

Structures of a Vertebra

The **vertebrae** (**VER**-teh-bray) are the bony structure units of the spinal column. As you study the following structures, refer to Figure 3.12.

- The *body of the vertebra* is the solid anterior portion.
- The *lamina* (**LAM**-ih-nah) is the posterior portion of a vertebra (plural, *laminae*). The transverse and spinous processes extend from this area.
- The *vertebral foramen* is the opening in the middle of the vertebra. The spinal cord passes through this opening.

Types of Vertebrae

As you study the types of vertebrae refer to Figure 3.13.

- The **cervical vertebrae** (**SER**-vih-kal) are the first set of seven vertebrae that form the neck. They are also known as **C1** through **C7.** *Cervical* means pertaining to the neck.
- The **thoracic vertebrae** (thoh-**RASS**-ick) make up the second set of 12 vertebrae. They form the outward curve of the spine and are known as **T1** through **T12**. *Thoracic* means pertaining to the thoracic cavity.
- The **lumbar vertebrae** (**LUM**-bar) make up the third set of five vertebrae and form the inward curve of the lower spine. They are known as **L1** through **L5**. The lumbar vertebrae are the largest and strongest of the vertebrae and bear most of the body's weight. *Lumbar* means relating to the part of the back and sides between the ribs and the pelvis.

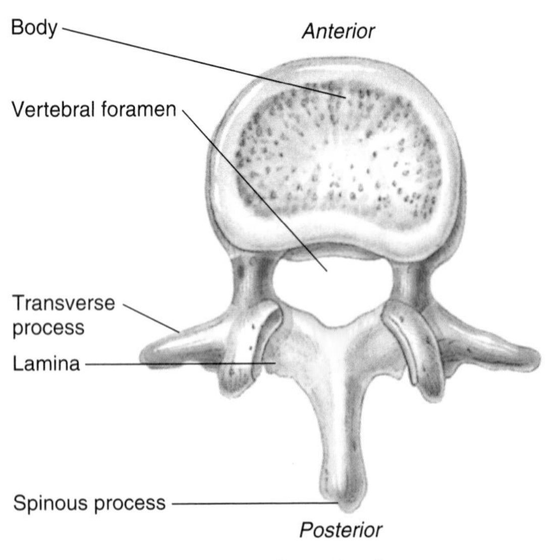

FIGURE 3.12 Characteristics of a typical vertebra.

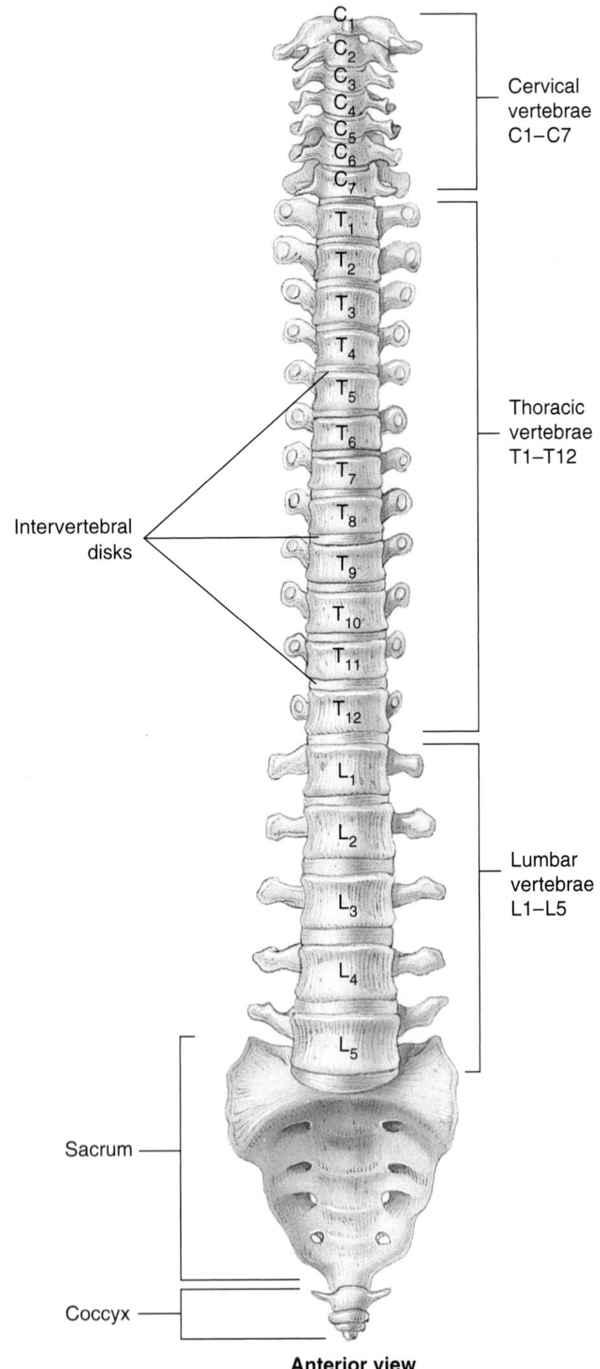

FIGURE 3.13 Anterior view of the vertebral column.

Sacrum and Coccyx

The remaining two vertebrae are the sacrum and coccyx. As you study these structures, refer to Figures 3.13 and 3.14.

- The **sacrum** (**SAY**-krum) is the slightly curved, triangular-shaped bone near the base of the spine that forms the lower portion of the back. At birth, the sacrum is composed of five separate bones; however they fuse together in the young child to form a single bone.
- The **coccyx** (**KOCK**-sicks), also known as the *tailbone*, forms the end of the spine and is actually made up of four small vertebrae that are fused together.

Intervertebral Disks

The **intervertebral disks** (**in**-ter-**VER**-teh-bral), which are made of cartilage, separate and cushion the vertebrae from each other. These disks act as shock absorbers and allow for movement of the spinal column (see Figure 3.20A).

Pelvic Girdle

The **pelvic girdle**, which protects internal organs and supports the lower extremities, is also known as the *pelvis* or *hips*. The pelvis is a cup-shaped ring of bone at the lower end of the trunk that consists of the *ilium, ischium,* and *pubis* (see Figures 3.14 and 3.16).

- The **ilium** (**ILL**-ee-um) is the broad blade-shaped bone that forms the back and sides of the pubic bone.
- The **sacroiliac** (**say**-kroh-**ILL**-ee-ack) is the slightly movable articulation between the sacrum and posterior portion of the ilium (**sacr/o** means sacrum, **ili** means ilium, and **-ac** means pertaining to).
- The **ischium** (**ISS**-kee-um), which forms the lower posterior portion of the pubic bone, bears the weight of the body when sitting.
- The **pubis** (**PEW**-bis), which forms the anterior portion of the pubic bone, is located just below the urinary bladder.
- The ileum, ischium, and pubis are separate at birth; however, they fuse to form the left and right **pubic bones**. These bones are held securely together by the pubic symphysis.
- The **acetabulum** (**ass**-eh-**TAB**-you-lum), also known as the *hip socket*, is the large circular cavity in each side of the pelvis that articulates with the head of the femur to form the hip joint (see Figures 3.14 and 3.16).

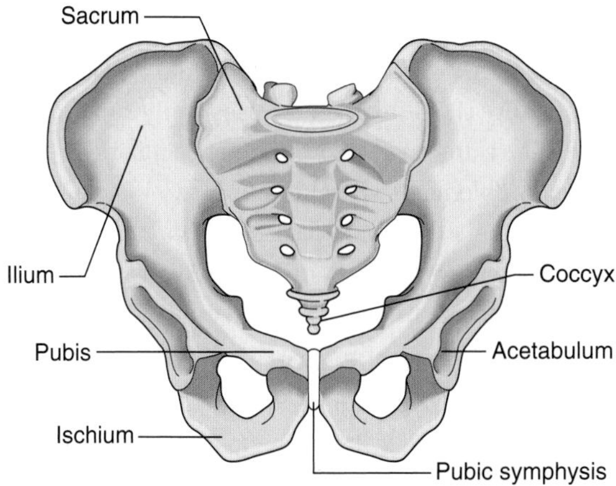

FIGURE 3.14 Anterior view of the pelvis.

Legs and Knees

As you study the following bones, refer to Figures 3.15 and 3.16.

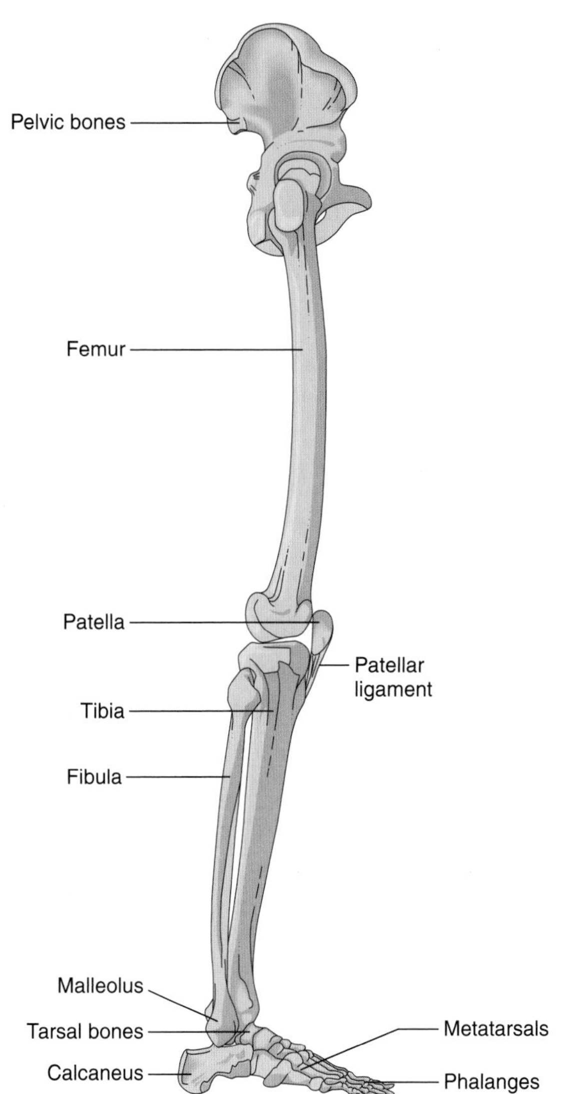

FIGURE 3.15 Lateral view of bones of the lower extremity.

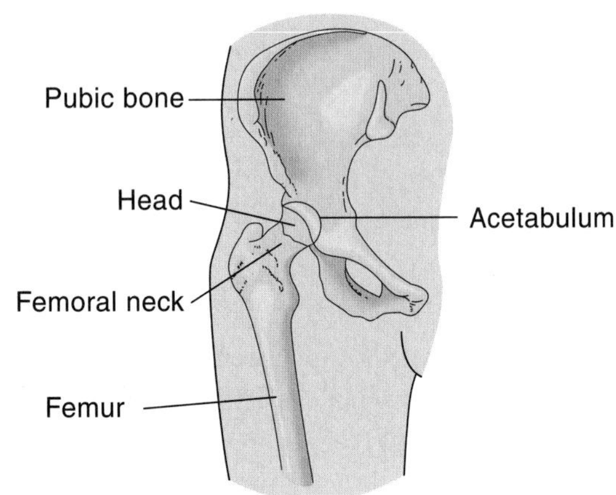

FIGURE 3.16 Structures of the proximal end of the femur and the acetabulum (hip socket).

Femur

The **femur** (**FEE**-mur) is the upper leg bone. Also known as the *thigh bone*, it is the largest bone in the body.

- The *head of the femur* articulates with the acetabulum (hip socket).
- The *femoral neck* is the narrow area just below the head of the femur. *Femoral* means pertaining to the femur.

Knees

The **knees** are the complex joints that make possible movement between the upper and lower leg (see Figure 3.5).

- The **patella** (pah-**TEL**-ah), also known as the *kneecap*, is the bony anterior portion of the knee.
- The term **popliteal** (pop-**LIT**-ee-al) means referring to the posterior space behind the knee where the ligaments, vessels, and muscles related to this joint are located.
- The **cruciate ligaments** (**KROO**-shee-ayt), which are shown in Figure 3.5, make possible the movements of the knee. These are known as the *anterior* and *posterior cruciate ligaments* because they are shaped like a cross.

Lower Leg

The lower leg is made up of two bones: the *tibia* and the *fibula* (see Figure 3.15).

- The **tibia** (**TIB**-ee-ah), also known as the *shinbone*, is the larger weight-bearing bone in the anterior of the lower leg.
- The **fibula** (**FIB**-you-lah) is the smaller of the two bones of the lower leg.
- The **malleolus** (mal-**LEE**-oh-lus) is the rounded bony protuberance on each side of the ankle (plural, *malleoli*).

The Ankles

The **ankles**, which form the joint between the lower leg and the foot, are each made up of seven short **tarsal** (**TAHR**-sal) bones. These bones are similar to the bones of the wrist, but are larger in size (Figure 3.17).

- The **talus** (**TAY**-luss) is the anklebone that articulates with the tibia and fibula (see Figures 3.15 and 3.17).
- The **calcaneus** (kal-**KAY**-nee-uss), also known as the *heel bone*, is the largest of the tarsal bones (Figures 3.15 and 3.17).

The Feet and Toes

The feet and toes are made up of the following bones.

- The five **metatarsals** (met-ah-**TAHR**-salz) form that part of the foot to which the toes are attached.
- The **phalanges** are the bones of the toes. The great toe has two phalanges. Each of the other toes has three phalanges. The bones of the fingers are also called phalanges.

MEDICAL SPECIALTIES RELATED TO THE SKELETAL SYSTEM

- A **chiropractor** (**KYE**-roh-**prack**-tor) holds a Doctor of Chiropractic degree and specializes in the manipulative treatment of disorders originating from misalignment of the spine. *Manipulative treatment* involves manually adjusting the positions of the bones.
- An **orthopedic surgeon** (**or**-thoh-**PEE**-dick), also known as an *orthopedist*, is a physician who specializes in diagnosing and treating diseases and disorders involving the bones, joints, and muscles.
- An **osteopath** (**oss**-tee-oh-**PATH**) holds a Doctor of Osteopathy (DO) degree and uses traditional forms of medical treatment in addition to specializing in treating health problems by spinal manipulation (**oste/o** means bone, and **-path** means disease). This type of medical practice is known as *osteopathy*; however, that term is also used to mean any bone disease.
- A **podiatrist** (poh-**DYE**-ah-trist) holds a Doctor of Podiatry (DP) or Doctor of Podiatric Medicine (DPM) degree and specializes in diagnosing and treating disorders of the foot (**pod** mean foot, and **-iatrist** means specialist).

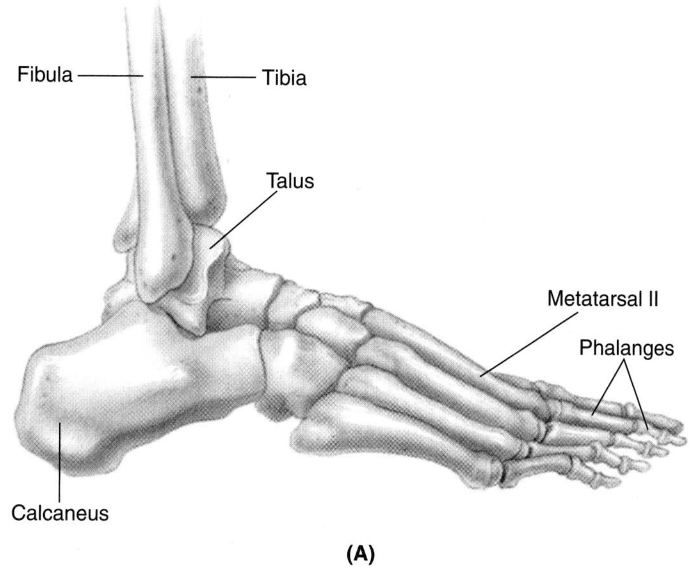

(A)

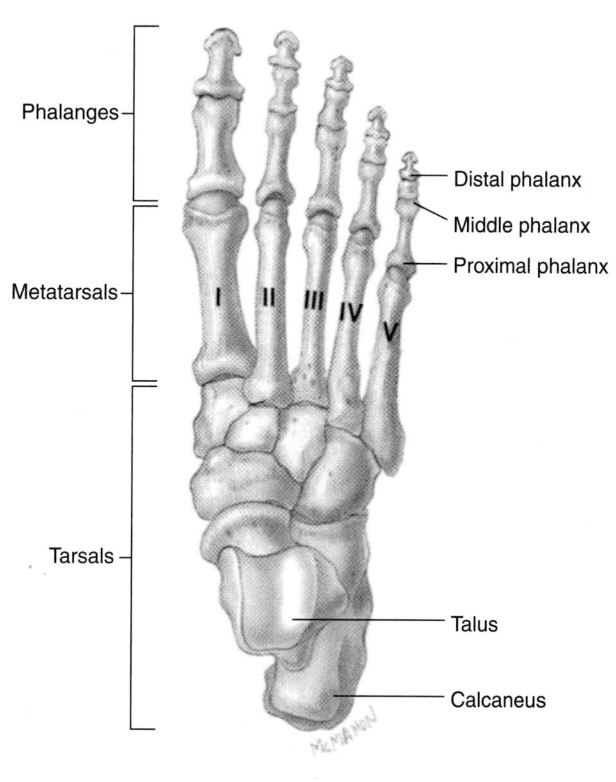

(B)

FIGURE 3.17 Bones of the right ankle and foot. (A) Lateral view. (B) Superior view.

PATHOLOGY OF THE SKELETAL SYSTEM

Joints

- **Ankylosis** (**ang**-kih-**LOH**-sis) is the loss, or absence, of mobility in a joint due to disease, injury, or a surgical procedure (**ankyl** means crooked, bent, or stiff, and **-osis** means abnormal condition or disease). *Mobility* means being capable of movement.
- **Arthrosclerosis** (**ar**-throh-skleh-**ROH**-sis) is stiffness of the joints, especially in the elderly (**arthr/o** means joint, and **-sclerosis** means abnormal hardening).

- **Bursitis** (ber-**SIGH**-tis) is an inflammation of a bursa (**burs** means bursa, and **-itis** means inflammation).
- **Chondromalacia** (**kon**-droh-mah-**LAY**-shee-ah) is the abnormal softening of cartilage (**chondr/o** means cartilage, and **-malacia** means abnormal softening).
- A **chondroma** (kon-**DROH**-mah) is a slow-growing benign tumor derived from cartilage cells (**chondr** means cartilage, and **-oma** means tumor).
- **Costochondritis** (**kos**-toh-kon-**DRIGH**-tis) is an inflammation of the cartilage that connects a rib to the sternum (**cost/o** means rib, **chondr** means cartilage, and **-itis** means inflammation).
- **Hallux valgus** (**HAL**-ucks **VAL**-guss), also known as a *bunion*, is an abnormal enlargement of the joint at the base of the great toe (*hallux* means big toe, and *valgus* means bent).
- **Hemarthrosis** (**hem**-ar-**THROH**-sis) is blood within a joint (**hem** means blood, **arthr** means joint, and **-osis** means abnormal condition or disease). This condition is frequently due to a joint injury. It also can occur spontaneously in patients taking blood-thinning medications or those having a blood clotting disorder such as hemophilia (see Chapters 2 and 5).
- **Synovitis** (sin-oh-**VYE**-tiss) is inflammation of the synovial membrane that results in swelling and pain of the affected joint (**synov** means synovial membrane, and **-itis** means inflammation). This condition can be caused by arthritis, trauma, infection, or irritation produced by damaged cartilage.

Dislocation

- **Dislocation**, also known as *luxation* (luck-**SAY**-shun), is the total displacement of a bone from its joint (Figure 3.18).
- **Subluxation** (**sub**-luck-**SAY**-shun) is the partial displacement of a bone from its joint.

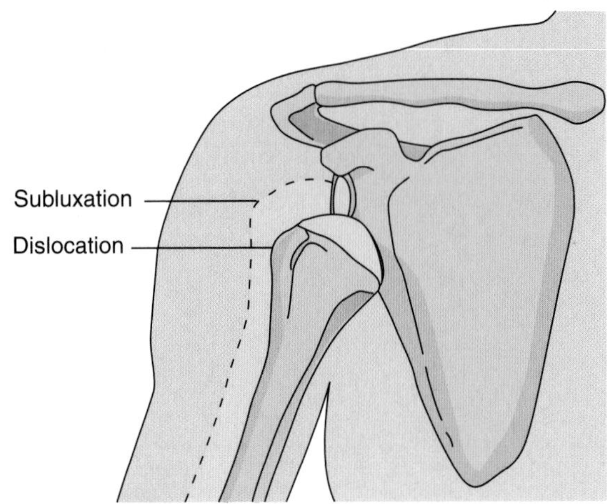

FIGURE 3.18 *Subluxation* and *dislocation* shown on a posterior view of the left shoulder.

Arthritis

Arthritis (ar-**THRIGH**-tis) is an inflammatory condition of one or more joints (**arthr** means joint, and **-itis** means inflammation). There are many different forms and causes of arthritis. *Rheumatism* is an obsolete term for arthritis to describe any painful disorder of the joints; however, in lay language, this word is still in use.

Osteoarthritis

Osteoarthritis (**oss**-tee-oh-ar-**THRIGH**-tis), also known as *wear-and-tear arthritis*, is most commonly associated with aging (**oste/o** means bone, **arthr** means joint, and **-itis** means inflammation) (Figure 3.19).

- This condition is described as a *degenerative joint disease* because it is characterized by the wearing away of the articular cartilage within the joints. *Degenerative* means the breaking down or impairment of a body part.
- **Spondylosis** (**spon**-dih-**LOH**-sis), which is also known as *spinal osteoarthritis*, is a degenerative disorder that can cause the loss of normal spinal structure and function (**spondyl** means vertebrae, and **-osis** means abnormal condition or disease).

Gouty Arthritis

Gouty arthritis (**GOW**-tee ar-**THRIGH**-tis), also known as *gout*, is a type of arthritis characterized by deposits of uric acid in the joints. *Uric acid* is a byproduct that is normally excreted by the kidneys. Gout develops when excess uric acid, which is present in the blood, forms crystals in the joints of the feet and legs.

Rheumatoid Arthritis

Rheumatoid arthritis (**ROO**-mah-toyd ar-**THRIGH**-tis), commonly known by its abbreviation RA, is a chronic autoimmune disorder in which the joints and some organs of other body systems are attacked. *Autoimmune disorders* are described in Chapter 6.

- As RA progressively attacks the synovial membranes they inflamed and thickened so that the joints are increasingly swollen, painful, and immobile.

Ankylosing Spondylitis

Ankylosing spondylitis (**ang**-kih-**LOH**-sing **spon**-dih-**LYE**-tis) is a form of rheumatoid arthritis that primarily causes inflammation of the joints between the vertebrae. *Ankylosing* means the progressive stiffening of a joint or joints, and *spondylitis* means inflammation of the vertebrae.

Juvenile Rheumatoid Arthritis

Juvenile rheumatoid arthritis is an autoimmune disorder that affects children aged 16 years or less with symptoms that include stiffness, pain, joint swelling, skin rash, fever, slowed growth, and fatigue.

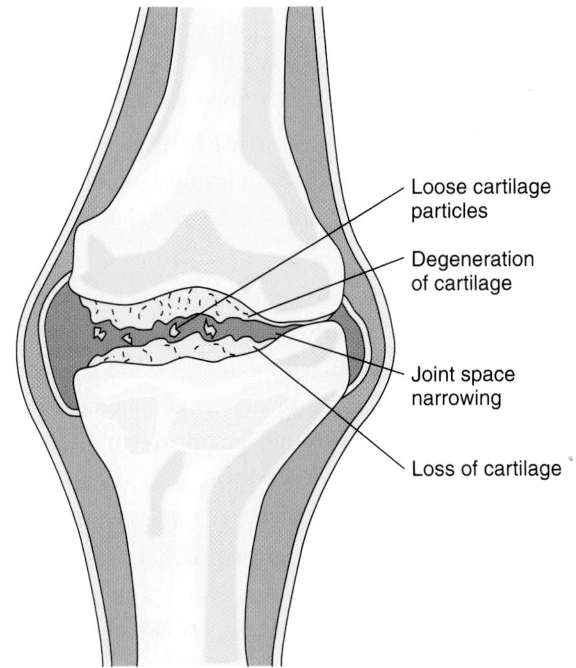

FIGURE 3.19 Damage to the knee joint caused by *osteoarthritis.*

The Spinal Column

- A **herniated disk** (**HER**-nee-**ayt**-ed), also known as a *slipped* or *ruptured disk*, is the breaking apart of an intervertebral disk that results in pressure on spinal nerve roots (Figure 3.20B).
- **Lumbago** (lum-**BAY**-goh), also known as *low back pain*, is pain of the lumbar region of the spine (**lumb** means lumbar, and **-ago** means diseased condition).
- **Spondylolisthesis** (**spon**-dih-loh-liss-**THEE**-sis) is the forward slipping movement of the body of one of the lower lumbar vertebrae on the vertebra or sacrum below it (**spondyl/o** means vertebrae, and **-listhesis** means slipping).
- **Spina bifida** (**SPY**-nah **BIF**-ih-dah) is a congenital defect that occurs during early pregnancy when the spinal canal fails to close completely around the spinal cord to protect it. *Spina* means pertaining to the spine. *Bifida* means split. Some cases of spina bifida are due to a lack of the nutrient folic acid during the early stages of pregnancy.

Curvatures of the Spine

- **Kyphosis** (kye-**FOH**-sis) is an abnormal increase in the outward curvature of the thoracic spine as viewed from the side (**kyph** means hump and **-osis** means abnormal condition or disease). This condition, also known as

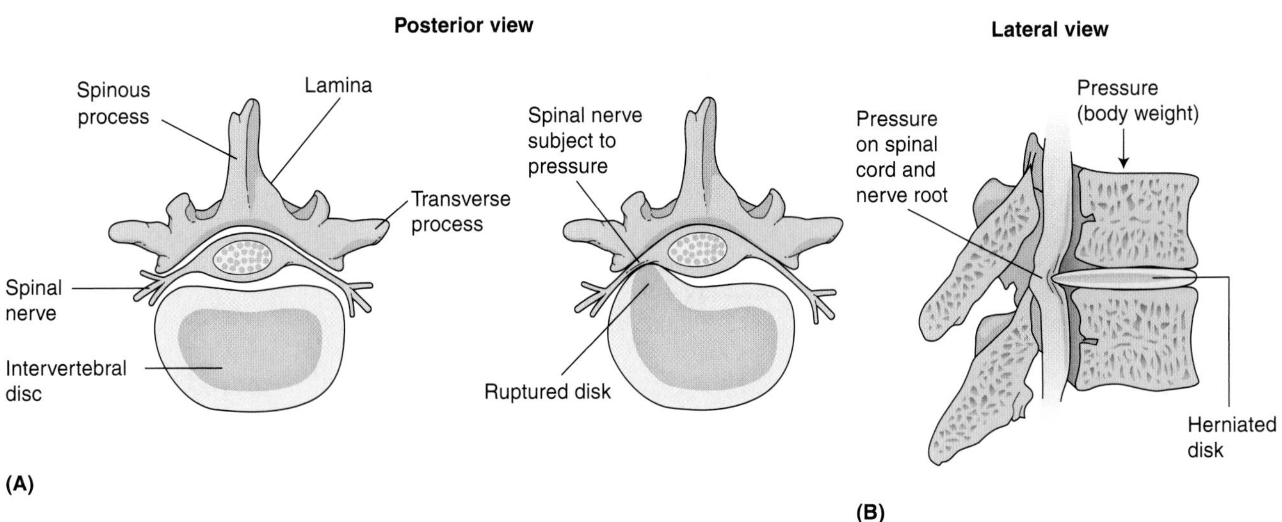

FIGURE 3.20 (A) Superior view of a normal intervertebral disk. (B) Superior and lateral views of a ruptured disk causing pressure on a spinal nerve.

humpback or *dowager's hump*, is frequently associated with aging (see Figure 3.21A).

- **Lordosis** (lor-**DOH**-sis) is an abnormal increase in the forward curvature of the lumbar spine (**lord** means bent backward, and **-osis** means abnormal condition or disease). This condition is also known as *swayback* (see Figure 3.21B).
- **Scoliosis** (**skoh**-lee-**OH**-sis) is an abnormal lateral (sideways) curvature of the spine (**scoli** means curved, and **-osis** means abnormal condition or disease) (see Figure 3.21C).

Bones

- **Craniostenosis** (**kray**-nee-oh-steh-**NOH**-sis) is a malformation of the skull due to the premature closure of the cranial sutures (**crani/o** means skull, and **-stenosis** means abnormal narrowing).
- **Fibrous dysplasia** (dis-**PLAY**-see-ah) is a bone disorder of unknown cause that destroys normal bone structure and replaces it with fibrous (scar-like) tissue. This leads to uneven growth, brittleness, and deformity of the affected bones.
- **Ostealgia** (**oss**-tee-**AL**-jee-ah), also known as *osteodynia*, mean pain in a bone (**oste** means bone, and **-algia** means pain).
- **Osteitis** (**oss**-tee-**EYE**-tis), also spelled *ostitis*, is an inflammation of bone (**oste** means bone, and **-itis** means inflammation).
- **Osteomalacia** (**oss**-tee-oh-mah-**LAY**-shee-ah), also known as *adult rickets*, is abnormal softening of bones in adults (**oste/o** means bone, and **-malacia** means abnormal softening). This condition is usually caused by a deficiency of vitamin D, calcium, and/or phosphate. Compare with *rickets*.
- **Osteomyelitis** (**oss**-tee-oh-**my**-eh-**LYE**-tis) is an inflammation of the bone marrow and adjacent bone (**oste/o** means bone, **myel** means bone marrow, and **-itis** means inflammation). The bacterial infection that causes osteomyelitis often originates in another part of the body and spreads to the bone via the blood.
- **Osteonecrosis** (**oss**-tee-oh-neh-**KROH**-sis) is the death of bone tissue due to a lack of insufficient blood supply (**oste/o** means bone, and **-necrosis** means tissue death).
- **Paget's disease** (**PAJ**-its), also known as *osteitis deformans*, is a bone disease of unknown cause. This condition is characterized by the excessive breakdown of bone tissue, followed by abnormal bone formation. The new bone is structurally enlarged, but weakened and filled with new blood vessels.
- **Periostitis** (**pehr**-ee-oss-**TYE**-tis) is an inflammation of the periosteum (**peri-** means surrounding, **ost** means bone, and **-itis** means inflammation). This condition is often associated with shin splints which are discussed in Chapter 4.
- **Rickets** (**RICK**-ets), also known as *infantile osteomalacia*, is a deficiency disease occurring in children. This

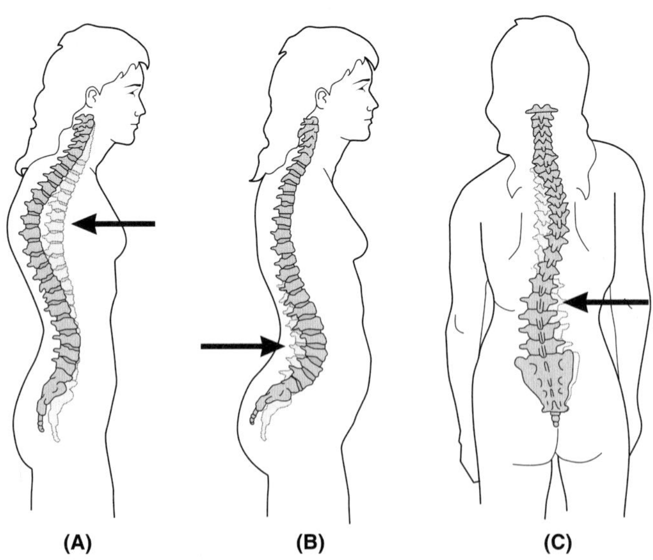

FIGURE 3.21 Abnormal curvatures of the spine. (A) *Kyphosis.* (B) *Lordosis.* (C) *Scoliosis.* (Normal curvatures are shown in shadow.)

condition, which is characterized by defective bone growth, results from a vitamin D deficiency that is sometimes due to insufficient exposure to sunlight.

- **Short stature**, formerly known as *dwarfism*, is condition resulting from the failure of the bones of the limbs to grow to an appropriate length. The average adult height is no more than 4'10" and these individuals are appropriately referred to as "*little people*."
- The term **talipes** (**TAL**-ih-peez), also known as *clubfoot*, describes any congenital deformity of the foot involving the talus (ankle bones).

Bone Tumors

- **Primary bone cancer** is a relatively rare malignant tumor that originates in a bone. *Malignant* means becoming progressively worse and life-threatening. As an example, *Ewing's sarcoma* is a tumor that occurs in the bones of the upper arm, legs, pelvis, or rib. The peak incidence is between ages 10 and 20 years.
- The term **secondary bone cancer** describes tumors that have metastasized (spread) to bones from other organs such as the breasts and lungs. Additional malignancies and tumors are discussed in Chapter 6.
- A **myeloma** (**my**-eh-**LOH**-mah) is a type of cancer that occurs in blood-making cells found in the red bone marrow (**myel** means bone marrow, and **-oma** means tumor). This condition can cause pathologic fractures and is often fatal.
- An **osteochondroma** (**oss**-tee-oh-kon-**DROH**-mah) is a benign bony projection covered with cartilage (**oste/o** means bone, **chondr** means cartilage, and **-oma** means tumor). *Benign* means something that is not life threatening and does not recur. This type of tumor is also known as an *exostosis* (plural, *exostoses*).

Osteoporosis

Osteoporosis (**oss**-tee-oh-poh-**ROH**-sis) is a marked loss of bone density and an increase in bone porosity that is frequently associated with aging (**oste/o** means bone, **por** means small opening, and **-osis** means abnormal condition or disease).

- **Osteopenia** (**oss**-tee-oh-**PEE**-nee-ah) is thinner than average bone density in a young person (**oste/o** means bone, and **-penia** means deficiency). This term is used to describe the condition of someone who does not yet have osteoporosis, but is at risk for developing it.

Osteoporosis Related Fractures

Osteoporosis is primarily responsible for three types of fractures:

- A **compression fracture**, also known as a *vertebral crush fracture*, occurs when the bone is pressed together (compressed) on itself. These fractures are sometimes caused by the spontaneous collapse of weakened vertebrae or can be due to an injury. This results in pain, loss of height, and development of the spinal curvature known as *dowager's hump* (Figure 3.22).
- A **Colles' fracture**, which is named for the Irish surgeon Abraham Colles, is also known as a *fractured wrist*. This fracture occurs at the lower end of the radius when a person tries to stop a fall by landing on his or her hands. The impact of this fall causes the bone weakened by osteoporosis to break (Figure 3.23).
- An **osteoporotic hip fracture** (**oss**-tee-oh-pah-**ROT**-ick), also known as a *broken hip*, is usually caused by weakening of the bones due to osteoporosis and can occur either spontaneously or as the result of a fall. Complications from these fractures can result in the loss of function, mobility, independence, or death. *Osteoporotic* means pertaining to or caused by the porous condition of bones.

Fractures

A **fracture**, which is a *broken bone*, is described in terms of its complexity (Figure 3.24).

- A **closed fracture**, also known as a *simple fracture* or a *complete fracture*, is one in which the bone is broken, but there is no open wound in the skin (see also Figure 3.25).
- An **open fracture**, also known as a *compound fracture*, is one in which the bone is broken and there is an open wound in the skin.
- A **comminuted fracture** (**KOM**-ih-**newt**-ed) is one in which the bone is splintered or crushed. *Comminuted* means crushed into small pieces.
- A **greenstick fracture**, or *incomplete fracture*, is one in which the bone is bent and only partially broken. This type of fracture occurs primarily in children.
- An **oblique fracture** occurs at an angle across the bone.
- A **pathologic fracture** occurs when a weakened bone breaks under normal strain. This is due to bones being

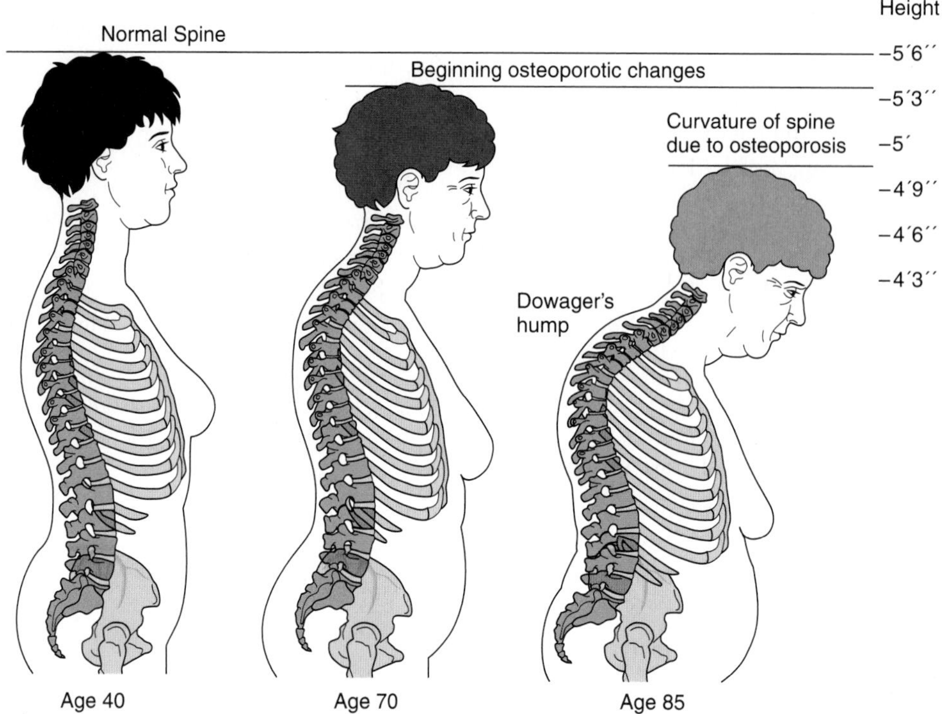

FIGURE 3.22 Curvature of the spine and related body changes due to osteoporosis.

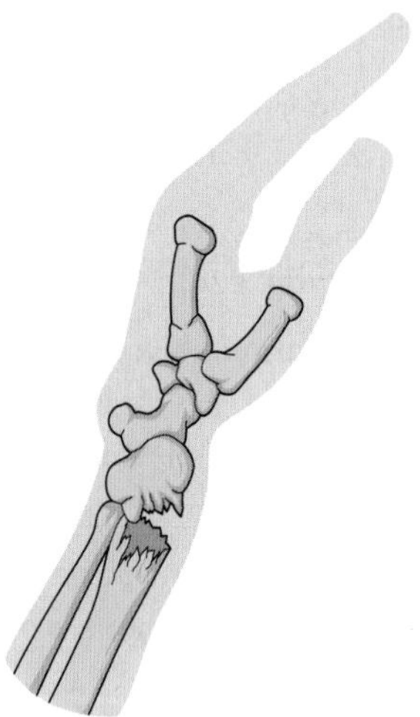

FIGURE 3.23 A *Colles' fracture* of the left wrist.

weakened by osteoporosis or to a disease process such as cancer.

- A **spiral fracture** is a fracture in which the bone has been twisted apart. This type of fracture occurs as the result of a severe twisting motion such as in a sports injury.
- A **stress fracture**, which is an overuse injury, is a small crack in the bone that often develops from chronic, excessive impact. Additional overuse and sports injuries are discussed in Chapter 4.
- A **transverse fracture** occurs straight across the bone.

Additional Terms Associated with Fractures

- A **fat embolus** (**EM**-boh-lus) can form when a long bone is fractured and fat cells from yellow bone marrow are released into the blood. An *embolus* is any foreign matter circulating in the blood that can become lodged and block the blood vessel.
- **Crepitation** (**krep**-ih-**TAY**-shun), also known as *crepitus*, is the grating sound heard when the ends of a broken bone move together. This term also describes the crackling sound heard in lungs affected with pneumonia and the clicking sound heard in the movements of some joints.
- As the bone heals, a **callus** (**KAL**-us) forms as a bulging deposit around the area of the break. This tissue eventually becomes bone. A *callus* is also a thickening of the skin caused by repeated rubbing.

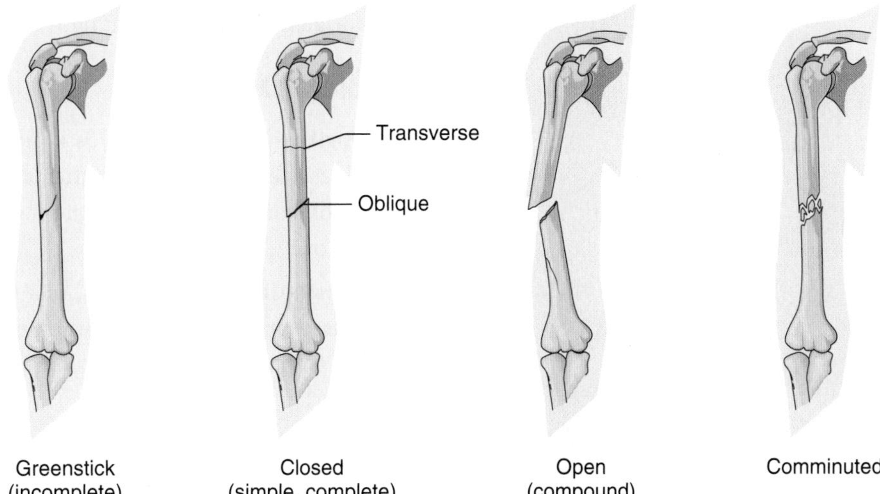

FIGURE 3.24 Types of bone *fractures.*

DIAGNOSTIC PROCEDURES OF THE SKELETAL SYSTEM

- A **radiograph**, also known as an *x-ray*, is the use of x-radiation to visualize bone fractures and other abnormalities (Figure 3.25).
- **Arthroscopy** (ar-**THROS**-koh-pee) is the visual examination of the internal structure of a joint (**arthr/o** means joint, and **-scopy** means visual examination) using an *arthroscope*.
- A **bone marrow biopsy** is a diagnostic test that may be necessary after abnormal types or numbers of red or white blood cells are found in a complete blood count test.
- *Bone marrow aspiration* is the use of a syringe to withdraw the liquid bone marrow. This procedure is used to obtain tissue for diagnostic purposes or to collect bone marrow for medical procedures such as stem cell transplantation.
- **Magnetic resonance imaging** (MRI) is used to image soft tissue structures such as the interior of complex joints. It is not the most effective method of imaging hard tissues such as bone.
- *Bone scans*, a form of nuclear medicine, and *arthrocentesis* are discussed in Chapter 15.

Bone Density Testing

Bone density testing is used to determine losses or changes in bone density. These tests are used to diagnose conditions such as osteoporosis, osteomalacia, osteopenia, and Paget's disease.

- **Ultrasonic bone density testing** is a screening test for osteoposoris or other conditions that cause a loss of bone mass. In this procedure, sound waves are used to take measurements of the calcenaeous (heel) bone. If the results indicate risks, more definitive testing is indicated.
- **Dual x-ray absorptiometry** (ab-**sorp**-shee-**OM**-eh-tree) is a low-exposure radiographic measurement of the spine and hips to measure bone density. This test produces more accurate results than ultrasonic bone density testing.

TREATMENT PROCEDURES OF THE SKELETAL SYSTEM

Bone Marrow Transplants

A **bone marrow transplant** (BMT) is used to treat certain types of cancers, such as leukemia and lymphomas, that affect bone marrow. Leukemia is discussed in Chapter 5, and lymphomas are discussed in Chapter 6.

- In this treatment, initially both the cancer cells and the patient's bone marrow are destroyed with high-intensity radiation and chemotherapy.
- Next, healthy bone marrow stem cells are transfused into the recipient's blood. These cells migrate to the spongy bone, where they multiply to form cancer-free red bone marrow.

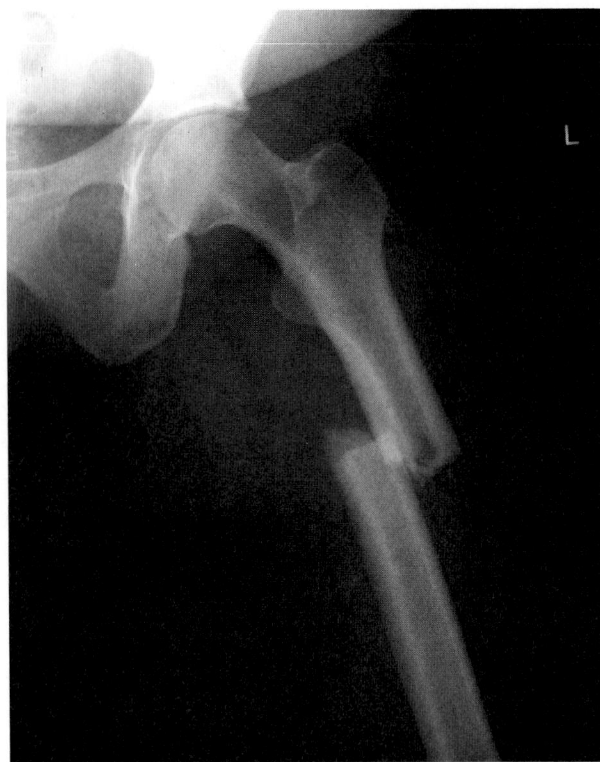

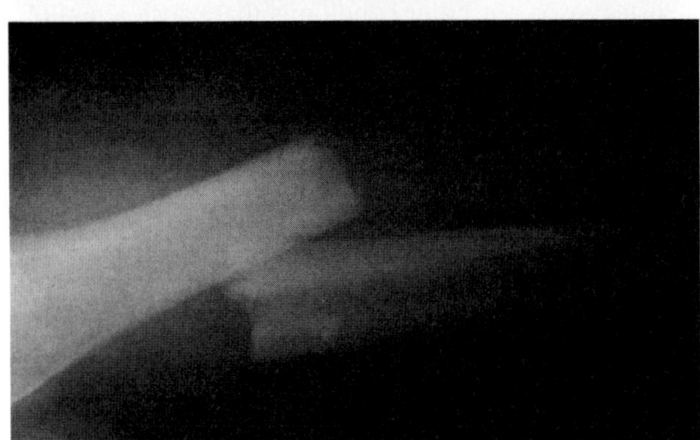

FIGURE 3.25 Radiographs of a *closed fracture* of the femur. Top: an anteroposterior (AP) view. Bottom: a lateral view of the same fracture. This view more exactly locates the ends of the fracture.

Allogenic Bone Marrow Transplant

An **allogenic bone marrow transplant** uses healthy bone marrow cells from a compatible donor, often a sibling. However, unless this is a perfect match, there is the danger that the recipient's body will reject the transplant. **Allogenic** (**al**-oh-**JEN**-ick) means originating within another.

Autologous Bone Marrow Transplant

In an **autologous bone marrow transplant**, the patient receives his own bone marrow cells which have been harvested, cleansed, treated, and then stored before the remaining bone marrow is destroyed. **Autologous** (aw-**TOL**-uh-guss) means originating within an individual.

Medical Devices

- An **orthotic** (or-**THOT**-ick) is a mechanical appliance, such as a leg brace or splint, that is specially designed to control, correct, or compensate for impaired limb function.
- A **prosthesis** (pros-**THEE**-sis) is a substitute for a diseased or missing body part, such as a leg that has been amputated (plural, *prostheses*).

Joints

- **Arthrodesis** (**ar**-throh-**DEE**-sis), also known as *surgical ankylosis*, is the surgical fusion (joining together) of two bones to stiffen a joint, such as an ankle, elbow, or shoulder (**arthr/o** means joint, and **-desis** means surgical fixation of bone or joint). This procedure is performed to treat severe arthritis or a damaged joint. Compare with *arthrolysis*.
- **Arthrolysis** (ar-**THROL**-ih-sis) is the surgical loosening of an ankylosed joint (**arthr/o** means joint, and **-lysis** means loosening or setting free). Note: The suffix **-lysis** also means breaking down or destruction and may indicate either a pathologic state or a therapeutic procedure. Compare with *arthrodesis*.
- **Arthroscopic surgery** (**ar**-throh-**SKOP**-ick) is a minimally invasive procedure for the treatment of the interior of a joint. For example, torn cartilage can be removed with the use of an arthroscope and instruments inserted through small incisions (see Figure 3.26).
- A **bursectomy** (ber-**SECK**-toh-mee) is the surgical removal of a bursa (**burs** means the bursa, and **-ectomy** means surgical removal).
- **Chondroplasty** (**KON**-droh-**plas**-tee) is the surgical repair of damaged cartilage (**chondr/o** means cartilage, and **-plasty** means surgical repair).
- A **synovectomy** (sin-oh-**VECK**-toh-mee) is the surgical removal of a synovial membrane from a joint (**synov** means synovial membrane, and **-ectomy** means surgical removal). One use of this procedure, which can be performed endoscopically, is to repair joint damage caused by rheumatoid arthritis.

Joint Replacement

Based on its word parts, the term **arthroplasty** (**AR**-throh-**plas**-tee) means the surgical repair of a damaged joint (**arthr/o** means joint, and **-plasty** means surgical repair);

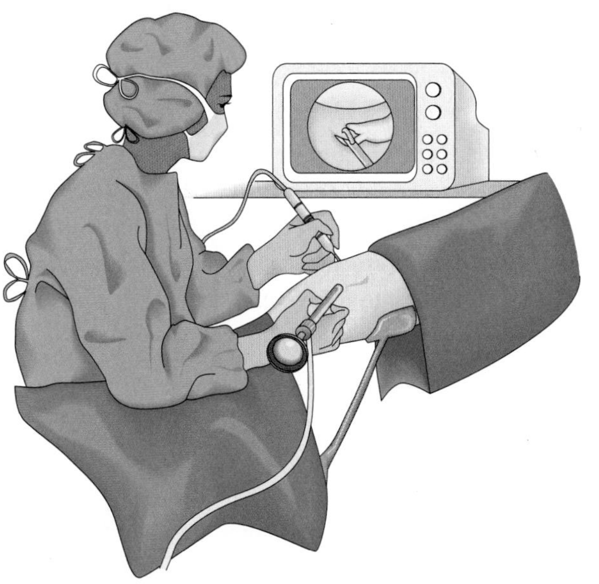

(A) Arthroscope in use

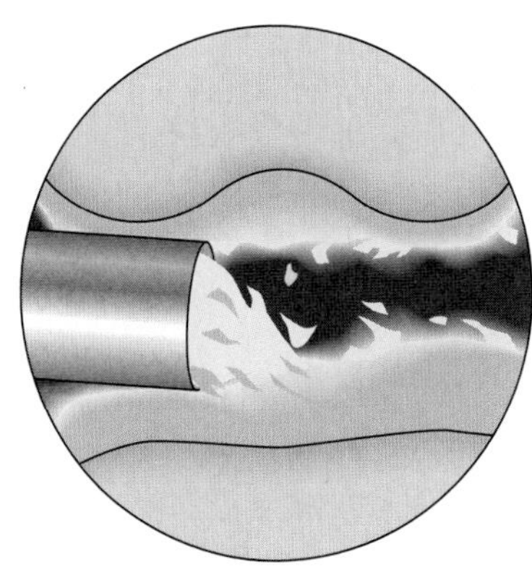

(B) Internal view of the knee during arthroscopy

FIGURE 3.26 *Arthroscopic surgery.* (A) The physician views progress on a monitor. (B) Internal view as diseased tissue is removed during surgery.

however, this term has come to mean the surgical placement of an artificial joint. These procedures are named for the involved joint and the amount of the joint that is replaced (see Figures 3.27 and 3.28).

- The joint replacement part is a prosthesis that this is commonly referred to as an *implant*.
- A **total knee replacement** (TKR) means that all of the parts of the knee were replaced. This procedure is also known as a *total knee arthroplasty* (Figure 3.27).
- A **partial knee replacement** (PKR) describes a procedure in which only part of the knee is replaced.
- A **total hip replacement** (THR), also known as a *total hip arthroplasty*, is performed to restore a damaged hip to full function. During the surgery, a plastic lining is fitted into the acetabulum to restore a smooth surface. The head of the femur is removed and replaced with a metal ball attached to a metal shaft that is fitted into the femur. These smooth surfaces restore the function of the hip joint.
- **Bone-conserving hip resurfacing** is an alternative to removing the head of the femur. Function is restored to the hip by placing a metal cap over the head of the femur to allow it to move smoothly over a metal lining in the acetabulum (see Figure 3.28).
- **Revision surgery** is the replacement of a worn or failed implant.

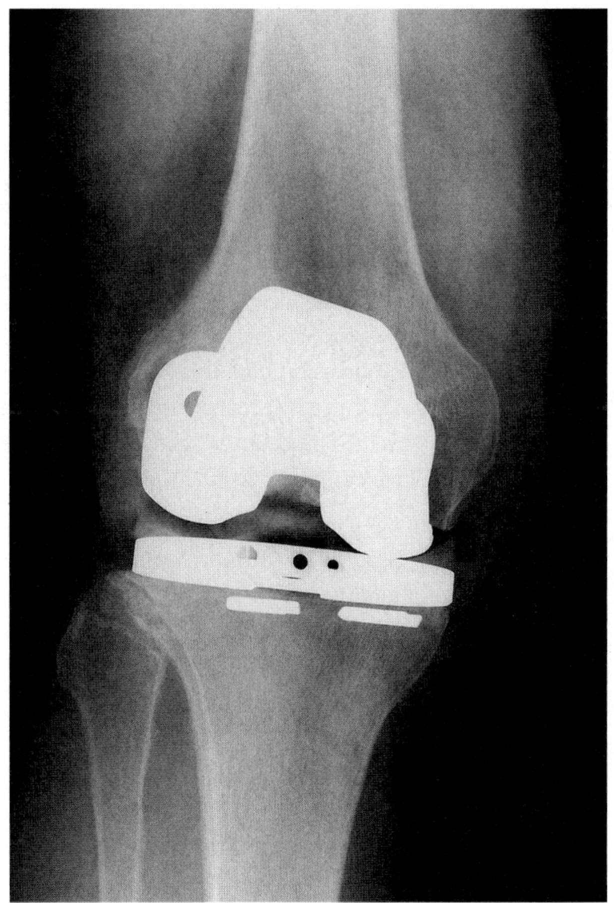

FIGURE 3.27 Radiograph (x-ray) of a *total knee replacement.* On the film the metallic components appear brighter than the bone.

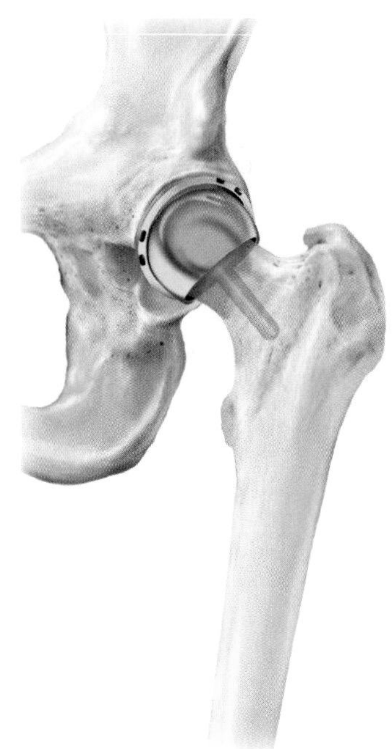

FIGURE 3.28 Bone-conserving hip resurfacing. (Courtesy of Birmingham HIP Resurfacing System.)

Spinal Column

- A **percutaneous diskectomy** (**per**-kyou-**TAY**-nee-us dis-**KECK**-toh-mee) is performed to treat a herniated intervertebral disk. In this procedure, a thin tube is inserted through the skin of the back to suction out the ruptured disk or to vaporize it with a laser. *Percutaneous* means performed through the skin.
- A **percutaneous vertebroplasty** (**per**-kyou-**TAY**-nee-us **VER**-tee-broh-**plas**-tee) is performed to treat osteoporosis-related compression fractures (**vertebr/o** means vertebra, and **-plasty** means surgical repair). In this minimally invasive procedure, bone cement is injected to stabilize compression fractures within the spinal column.
- A **laminectomy** (**lam**-ih-**NECK**-toh-mee) is the surgical removal of a lamina, or posterior portion, of a vertebra (**lamin** means lamina, and **-ectomy** means surgical removal) (see Figure 3.20A).
- **Spinal fusion** is a technique to immobilize part of the spine by joining together (fusing) two or more vertebrae. *Fusion* means to join together.

Bones

- A **craniectomy** (**kray**-nee-**EK**-toh-mee) is the surgical removal of a portion of the skull (**crani** means skull, and **-ectomy** means surgical removal). This procedure is performed to treat craniostenosis or to relieve increased intracranial pressure due to swelling of the brain. The term *intracranial pressure* describes the amount of pressure inside the skull.
- A **craniotomy** (**kray**-nee-**OT**-oh-mee) is a surgical incision or opening into the skull (**crani** means skull, and **-otomy** means a surgical incision). This procedure is performed to gain access to the brain to remove a tumor, to relieve intracranial pressure, or to obtain access for other surgical procedures.
- A **cranioplasty** (**KRAY**-nee-oh-**plas**-tee) is the surgical repair of the skull (**crani/o** means skull, and **-plasty** means surgical repair).
- **Osteoclasis** (**oss**-tee-**OCK**-lah-sis) is the surgical fracture of a bone to correct a deformity (**oste/o** means bone, and **-clasis** means to break).
- An **ostectomy** (oss-**TECK**-toh-mee) is the surgical removal of bone (**ost** means bone, and **-ectomy** means the surgical removal).
- **Osteoplasty** (**OSS**-tee-oh-**plas**-tee) is the surgical repair of a bone or bones (**oste/o** means bone, and **-plasty** means surgical repair).
- **Osteorrhaphy** (**oss**-tee-**OR**-ah-fee) is the surgical suturing, or wiring together, of bones (**oste/o** means bone, and **-rrhaphy** means surgical suturing).
- **Osteotomy** (**oss**-tee-**OT**-oh-mee) is a surgical incision or sectioning of a bone (**oste** means bone, and **-otomy** means a surgical incision).
- A **periosteotomy** (**pehr**-ee-**oss**-tee-**OT**-oh-mee) is an incision through the periosteum to the bone (**peri-** means surrounding, **oste** means bone, and **-otomy** means surgical incision).

Treatment of Fractures

- **Closed reduction**, also known as *manipulation*, is the attempted realignment of the bone involved in a fracture or joint dislocation. The affected bone is returned to its normal anatomic alignment by manually applied forces and then is usually immobilized to maintain the realigned position during healing (Figure 3.29).
- When a closed reduction is not practical, a surgical procedure known as an *open reduction* is required to realign the bone parts.
- **Immobilization**, also known as *stabilization*, is the act of holding, suturing, or fastening the bone in a fixed position with strapping or a cast.

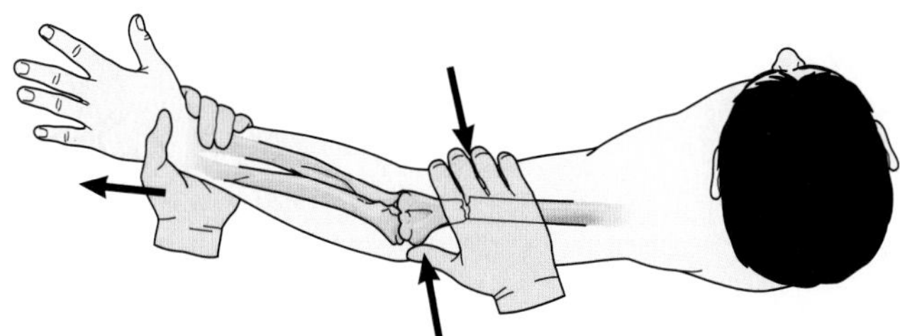

FIGURE 3.29 *Closed reduction* of a fractured left humerus.

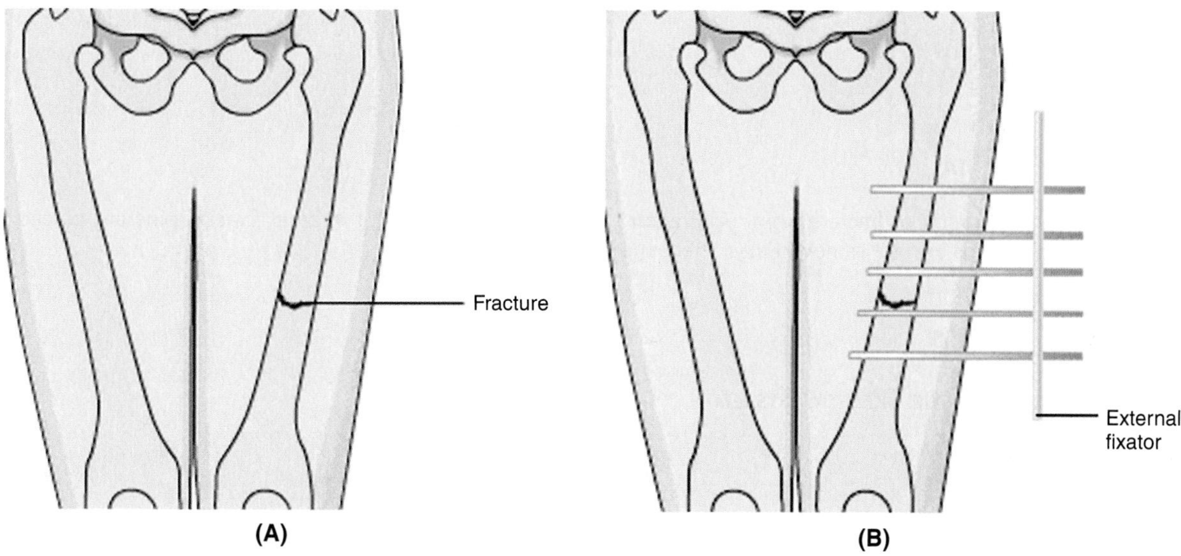

FIGURE 3.30 *External fixation* of the femur. (A) Fracture of the epiphysis of a femur. (B) *External fixation* stabilizes the bone and is removed after the bone has healed.

- **Traction** is a pulling force exerted on a limb in a distal direction in an effort to return the bone or joint to normal alignment.

External and Internal Fixation

- **External fixation** is a fracture treatment procedure in which pins are placed through the soft tissues and bone so that an external appliance can be used to hold the pieces of bone firmly in place during healing. When healing is complete, the appliance is removed (Figure 3.30).
- **Internal fixation**, also known as *open reduction internal fixation* (ORIF), is a fracture treatment in which a plate or pins are placed directly into the bone to hold the broken pieces in place. This form of fixation is *not* usually removed after the fracture has healed (Figure 3.31).

ABBREVIATIONS RELATED TO THE SKELETAL SYSTEM

Table 3.1 presents an overview of the abbreviations related to the terms introduced in this chapter. Note: To avoid errors or confusion, always be cautious when using abbreviations.

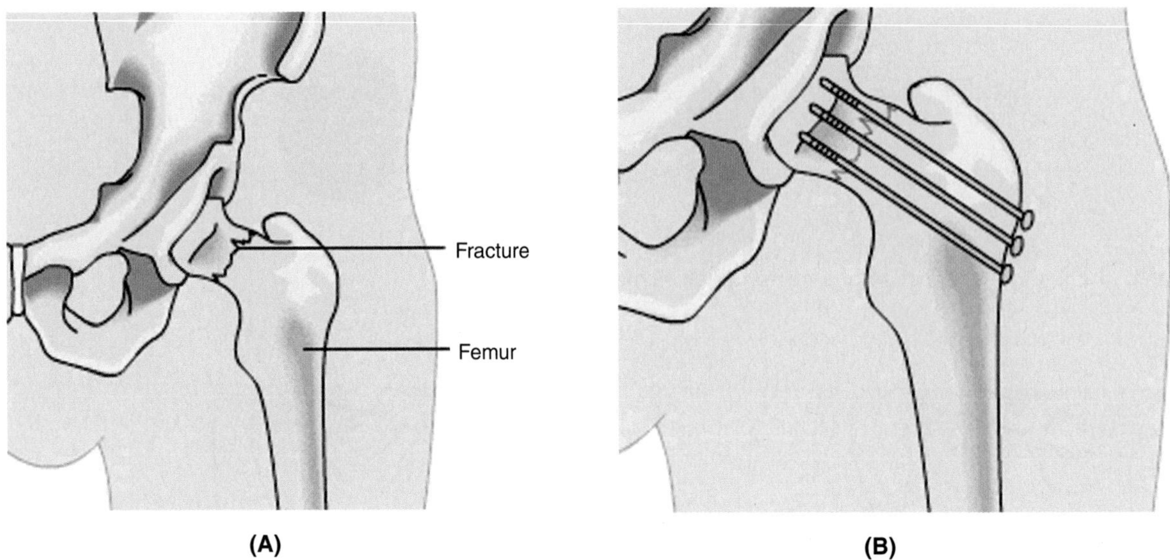

FIGURE 3.31 *Internal fixation* of fractured hip. (A) Fracture of the femoral neck. (B) *Internal fixation* pins are placed to stabilize the bone. These pins are not removed after the bone has healed.

TABLE 3.1

Abbreviations Related to the Skeletal System

bone density testing = BDT	**BDT** = bone density testing
closed reduction = CR	**CR** = closed reduction
fracture = Fx	**Fx** = fracture
osteoarthritis = OA	**OA** = osteoarthritis
osteoporosis = OP	**OP** = osteoporosis
temporomandibular joint = TMJ	**TMJ** = temporomandibular joint
total hip arthroplasty = THA	**THA** = total hip arthroplasty
total joint arthroplasty = TJA	**TJA** = total joint arthroplasty
total knee arthroplasty = TKA	**TKA** = total knee arthroplasty

CAREER OPPORTUNITIES

In addition to the medical specialties already discussed, some of the health occupations involving the treatment of the skeletal system are:

- **First responder:** an emergency service worker extensively trained in first aid procedures, but without the specialized skills of an EMT.
- **Emergency medical technician (EMT):** provides emergency treatment of injuries such as bones broken in accidents or falls, as well as many other medical crises. The work of EMTs involves the speedy treatment of a wide variety of problems and taking action to protect the patient from further injury if in a dangerous situation.
- **Paramedic (EMT-P):** is an EMT with additional training, authorized to provide advanced pre-hospital treatment such as in-depth patient assessment, EKG interpretation, and drug administration.
- **Prosthetist:** creates artificial substitutions for external body parts such as an arm, a foot, or an eye.
- **Pedorthist:** a specialist in using shoe modifications, foot orthotics, and other pedorthic devices to solve problems in, or related to, the foot and lower leg (**ped/o** means foot).
- **Podiatric medical assistant:** makes castings of feet, takes x-rays, and assists the podiatrist in surgery.
- **Orthopedic assistant:** works under the supervision of a physician or therapist in the field of sports medicine or orthopedics, performing diagnostic tests and treating injuries with bandaging, casting, and rehabilitation exercises.

HEALTH OCCUPATION PROFILE

PARAMEDIC

Pat Terry is a firefighter and paramedic (EMT-P) with the Madison, Wisconsin, Fire Department. She joined the force 15 years ago as a firefighter, and after a few years, decided to take the additional training necessary to become a paramedic. ***"I'd always been interested in medicine, in problem solving, and in helping people. As a firefighter, I'd received basic EMT training, but I wanted to do more. In addition to responding to fires, the paramedics respond to accidents and distress calls. I love my work, although it can be stressful and physically draining. At an accident scene, we stabilize injured patients with equipment such as backboards. We perform many of the same procedures as emergency room staff, such as starting IV medications, using defibrillators, and administering CPR, but we often perform these tasks in a very challenging environment. Many of our ambulance calls are from individuals suffering from cardiac arrests, diabetic emergencies, and asthma attacks. I love being able to calm patients and to get them the help they need in time."***

Study Break

Do you know anyone who can bend his or her thumbs back to the wrist? Who can lie flat on the floor with both knees bent backward? We would usually say that these people are *double jointed,* although of course they don't have two joints instead of one. These few individuals simply have limb and finger joints that are much more flexible than most people's. The medical term *hypermobility,* made up of the word part hyper- (excessive) added to the word *mobility,* is sometimes used to describe this syndrome.

However, being double-jointed is not really "excessive" or even really a syndrome. It simply means that a person naturally has a greater range of joint movement than most others. Some people are born with a tendency toward hypermobility. This tendency can either be ignored (except for showing off at parties) or strengthened through exercise and stretching for certain types of gymnastic and dance performances.

Review Time

Write the answers to the following questions on a separate piece of paper or in your notebook. In addition, be prepared to take part in the classroom discussion.

1. ***Written Assignment:*** Describe the primary characteristics of these three types of joints: (1) **fibrous joints**, (2) **cartilaginous joints**, and (3) **synovial joints**.

   Discussion Assignment: Give examples of the location of each type of joint.

2. ***Written Assignment:*** Describe the three types of fractures that are commonly associated with **osteoporosis**.

   Discussion Assignment: How would you explain to a patient's family why the patient fractured a bone in a very minor fall?

3. ***Written Assignment:*** Use your own words to describe the differences between **internal fixation** and **external fixation**.

   Discussion Assignment: How would you explain to a patient what to expect with each type of fixation?

4. Max has leukemia and requires a **bone marrow transplant**. However, his bone marrow is not suitable. ***Written Assignment:*** Describe the alternative type of bone marrow transplant that could be used in Max's case.

   Discussion Assignment: What would some benefits be of using Max's own bone marrow?

5. Mrs. Valdez fell and broke her hip, and her physician said she needs a **THR**. ***Written Assignment:*** Explain this abbreviation and procedure in terms that Mrs. Valdez and her family will understand.

   Discussion Assignment: How is a total hip replacement designed to function like a natural hip?

continues

Optional Internet Activity

The goal of this activity is to help you learn more about medical terminology as it applies to the "real world." Select **one** *of these two options and follow the instructions.*

1. Search for information about **osteopenia**. Write a brief (one- or two-paragraph) report on the importance of early detection and the prevention of this disorder, and include the address of the web site where you found this information.

2. To learn more about the 100 forms of **arthritis**, go to the web site of the Arthritis Foundation. Write a brief (one- or two-paragraph) report on at least two forms of arthritis that are not mentioned in your text.

THE HUMAN TOUCH: CRITICAL THINKING ACTIVITY

The following story and questions are designed to stimulate critical thinking through class discussion or as a brief essay response. There are no right or wrong answers to these questions.

Hilary Keiser, 15, was having fun on her family's skiing trip until halfway down the slope, her ski struck a piece of debris. As she fell, she heard a snap, felt her left leg twist, and was in severe pain as she landed in the snow.

Steve, a member of the ski patrol, arrived to find Hilary lying in the snow and sobbing miserably while another skier tried to comfort her. Like all ski patrol members, Steve was trained as an EMT. He introduced himself, and then asked how she had fallen and where it hurt. Hilary answered his questions, keeping her leg very still to minimize the pain as Steve began his assessment. She listened as he phoned for help.

The backup team soon arrived, immobilized her leg, and quickly transported her down the mountain. When Hilary was in the warm first aid room, Steve stayed with her and continued his assessment while they waited for the ambulance. When he cut her ski pants leg away to reveal the injury, it was easy to see that she had a fracture: one end of the bone was almost poking through the skin, and there was swelling throughout her lower leg.

Hilary's parents rushed in from the slopes as soon as they heard she was hurt. At first, they were upset and not very helpful. Their concern for their daughter made it hard to give calm answers, and they kept getting in the way as they tried to help. But they were reassured by Steve's calm demeanor, and appreciated his offer of a ride to follow the ambulance taking Hilary to the nearest hospital. The x-rays taken there showed a spiral fracture of Hilary's fibula. The staff was not surprised, since spiral fractures are common in skiing accidents. After looking at the x-rays, the ER doctor presented the treatment options to Hilary's parents and gave them time alone with her to reach a decision.

continues

Suggested Discussion Topics

1. Discuss the most likely treatment options for Hilary's spiral fracture. Do you think Hilary is too young to be included in decisions about what to do?
2. Skiing can be dangerous, even for an experienced skier. Is the owner and operator of this ski slope in any way responsible for the fact that Hilary broke her leg?
3. If the skier comforting Hilary after she fell couldn't find a ski patrol member to help, what could she have done?
4. In assessing her injury, Steve asked Hilary and her parents about her medical history and allergies. Discuss why having this information is important and what precautions Hilary might have taken if she had gone skiing without her family.

STUDENT WORKBOOK AND StudyWARE™ CD-ROM

1. Go to your **Student Workbook** and complete the Learning Exercises for this chapter.

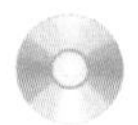

2. Go to the **StudyWARE™ CD-ROM** and have fun with the exercises and games for this chapter.

CHAPTER 4

THE MUSCULAR SYSTEM

OVERVIEW OF STRUCTURES, COMBINING FORMS, AND FUNCTIONS OF THE MUSCULAR SYSTEM

MAJOR STRUCTURES	RELATED COMBINING FORMS	PRIMARY FUNCTIONS
Muscles	**muscul/o, my/o, myos/o**	Make body movement possible, hold body erect, move body fluids, and produce body heat.
Fascia	**fasci/o**	Cover, support, and separate muscles.
Tendons	**ten/o, tend/o, tendin/o**	Attach muscles to bones.

VOCABULARY RELATED TO THE MUSCULAR SYSTEM

This list contains essential word parts and medical terms for this chapter. These terms are pronounced on the student StudyWARE™ CD-ROM and Audio CDs that are available for use with this text. These and the other important **primary terms** are shown in boldface throughout the chapter. *Secondary terms*, which appear in *orange* italics, clarify the meaning of primary terms.

Word Parts

- ☐ **bi-**
- ☐ **-cele**
- ☐ **dys-**
- ☐ **fasci/o**
- ☐ **fibr/o**
- ☐ **-ia**
- ☐ **-ic**
- ☐ **kines/o kinesi/o**
- ☐ **my/o**
- ☐ **-plegia**
- ☐ **-rrhexis**
- ☐ **tax/o**
- ☐ **ten/o, tend/o, tendin/o**
- ☐ **ton/o**
- ☐ **tri-**

Medical Terms

- ☐ **abduction** (ab-**DUCK**-shun)
- ☐ **adduction** (ah-**DUCK**-shun)
- ☐ **adhesion** (ad-**HEE**-zhun)
- ☐ **ataxia** (ah-**TACK**-see-ah)
- ☐ **atonic** (ah-**TON**-ick)
- ☐ **atrophy** (**AT**-roh-fee)
- ☐ **bradykinesia** (**brad**-ee-kih-**NEE**-zee-ah)
- ☐ **carpal tunnel syndrome** (**KAR**-pul)
- ☐ **chronic fatigue syndrome**
- ☐ **circumduction** (**ser**-kum-**DUCK**-shun)
- ☐ **contracture** (kon-**TRACK**-chur)
- ☐ **dorsiflexion** (**dor**-sih-**FLECK**-shun)
- ☐ **dyskinesia** (**dis**-kih-**NEE**-zee-ah)
- ☐ **dystaxia** (dis-**TACK**-see-ah)
- ☐ **dystonia** (dis-**TOH**-nee-ah)
- ☐ **electromyography** (ee-**leck**-troh-my-**OG**-rah-fee)
- ☐ **electroneuromyography** (ee-**leck**-troh-**new**-roh-my-**OG**-rah-fee)
- ☐ **epicondylitis** (**ep**-ih-**kon**-dih-**LYE**-tis)
- ☐ **ergonomics** (er-goh-**NOM**-icks)
- ☐ **exercise physiologist** (**fiz**-ee-**OL**-oh-jist)
- ☐ **fasciitis** (**fas**-ee-**EYE**-tis)
- ☐ **fibromyalgia syndrome** (**figh**-broh-my-**AL**-jee-ah)
- ☐ **ganglion cyst** (**GANG**-glee-on **SIST**)
- ☐ **heel spur**
- ☐ **hemiparesis** (**hem**-ee-pah-**REE**-sis)
- ☐ **hemiplegia** (**hem**-ee-**PLEE**-jee-ah)
- ☐ **hyperkinesia** (**high**-per-kye-**NEE**-zee-ah)
- ☐ **hypertonia** (**high**-per-**TOH**-nee-ah)
- ☐ **hypokinesia** (**high**-poh-kye-**NEE**-zee-ah)
- ☐ **hypotonia** (**high**-poh-**TOH**-nee-ah)
- ☐ **impingement syndrome** (im-**PINJ**-ment **SIN**-drohm)
- ☐ **intermittent claudication** (**klaw**-dih-**KAY**-shun)
- ☐ **muscular dystrophy** (**DIS**-troh-fee)
- ☐ **myasthenia gravis** (**my**-as-**THEE**-nee-ah **GRAH**-vis)
- ☐ **myocele** (**MY**-oh-seel)
- ☐ **myoclonus** (**my**-oh-**KLOH**-nus)
- ☐ **myofascial release** (**my**-oh-**FASH**-ee-ahl)
- ☐ **myolysis** (my-**OL**-ih-sis)
- ☐ **myoparesis** (**my**-oh-**PAR**-eh-sis)
- ☐ **myorrhaphy** (my-**OR**-ah-fee)
- ☐ **myotonia** (**my**-oh-**TOH**-nee-ah)
- ☐ **nocturnal myoclonus** (nock-**TER**-nal **my**-oh-**KLOH**-nus)
- ☐ **oblique** (oh-**BLEEK**)
- ☐ **paralysis** (pah-**RAL**-ih-sis)
- ☐ **paraplegia** (**par**-ah-**PLEE**-jee-ah)
- ☐ **physiatrist** (**fiz**-ee-**AT**-rist)
- ☐ **plantar fasciitis** (**PLAN**-tar **fas**-ee-**EYE**-tis)
- ☐ **polymyositis** (**pol**-ee-**my**-oh-**SIGH**-tis)
- ☐ **pronation** (proh-**NAY**-shun)
- ☐ **quadriplegia** (**kwad**-rih-**PLEE**-jee-ah)
- ☐ **sarcopenia** (**sar**-koh-**PEE**-nee-ah)
- ☐ **shin splint**
- ☐ **singultus** (sing-**GUL**-tus)
- ☐ **spasmodic torticollis** (spaz-**MOD**-ick **tor**-tih-**KOL**-is)
- ☐ **sphincter** (**SFINK**-ter)
- ☐ **sprain**
- ☐ **tenodesis** (ten-**ODD**-eh-sis)
- ☐ **tenodynia** (**ten**-oh-**DIN**-ee-ah)
- ☐ **tenolysis** (ten-**OL**-ih-sis)
- ☐ **tenorrhaphy** (ten-**OR**-ah-fee)

OBJECTIVES

On completion of this chapter, you should be able to:

1. Describe the functions and structures of the muscular system including muscle fibers, fascia, tendons, and the three types of muscle.
2. Recognize, define, spell, and pronounce the terms related to muscle movements and explain how the muscles are named.
3. Recognize, define, pronounce, and spell the terms related to the pathology and the diagnostic and treatment procedures of the muscular system.

FUNCTIONS OF THE MUSCULAR SYSTEM

- Muscles hold the body erect and make movement possible.
- Muscle movement generates nearly 85% of the heat that keeps the body warm.
- Muscles move food through the digestive system.
- Muscle movement, such as walking, aids the flow of blood through veins as it returns to the heart.
- Muscle action moves fluids through the ducts and tubes associated with other body systems.

STRUCTURES OF THE MUSCULAR SYSTEM

The body has more than 600 muscles, which make up about 40%–45% of the body's weight. Skeletal muscles are made up of fibers, are covered with fascia, and are attached to bones by tendons.

Muscle Fibers

Muscle fibers are the long, slender cells that make up muscles. Each muscle consists of a group of fibers that are held together by connective tissue and enclosed in a fibrous sheath.

Fascia

Fascia (**FASH**-ee-ah) is the sheet of fibrous connective tissue that covers, supports, and separates muscles or groups of muscles (plural, *fasciae* or *fascias*). Fascia is flexible to allow muscle movements; however, it does not have elastic properties to accommodate the swelling of the enclosed tissues.

- **Myofascial** (**my**-oh-**FASH**-ee-ahl) means pertaining to muscle tissue and fascia (**my/o** means muscle, **fasci** means fascia, and **-al** means pertaining to).

Tendons

- A **tendon** is a narrow band of nonelastic, dense, fibrous connective tissue that attaches a muscle to a bone. Do not confuse tendons with ligaments, which connect one bone to another bone (Figure 4.1).
- For example, the *Achilles tendon* attaches the gastrocnemius muscle (the major muscle of the calf of the leg) to the heel bone (see Figure 4.11).
- An *aponeurosis* is a sheetlike fibrous connective tissue that resembles a flattened tendon that serves as a fascia to bind muscles together or as a means of connecting muscle to bone (plural, *aponeuroses*). As an example, the abdominal aponeurosis can be seen in Figure 4.10.

TYPES OF MUSCLE TISSUE

The three types of muscle tissue are skeletal, smooth, and myocardial (Figure 4.2). These muscle types are described according to their appearance and function.

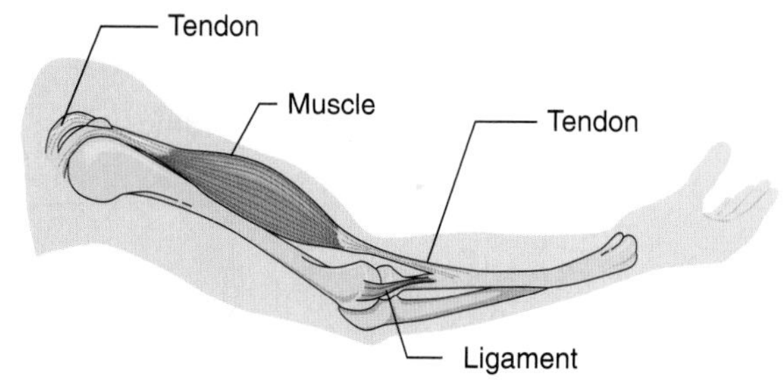

FIGURE 4.1 *Tendons* attach muscle to bone. *Ligaments* join bone to bone.

Skeletal Muscles

- **Skeletal muscles** are attached to the bones of the skeleton and make body motions possible (see Figure 4.2A).
- Skeletal muscles are also known as *voluntary muscles* because we have conscious (voluntary) control over these muscles.
- Skeletal muscles are also known as *striated muscles* because under a microscope, the dark and light bands in the muscle fibers create a striped appearance. *Striated* means striped.

Smooth Muscles

Smooth muscles are located in the walls of internal organs such as the digestive tract, blood vessels, and ducts leading from glands (see Figure 4.2B). Their function is to move and control the flow of fluids through these structures.

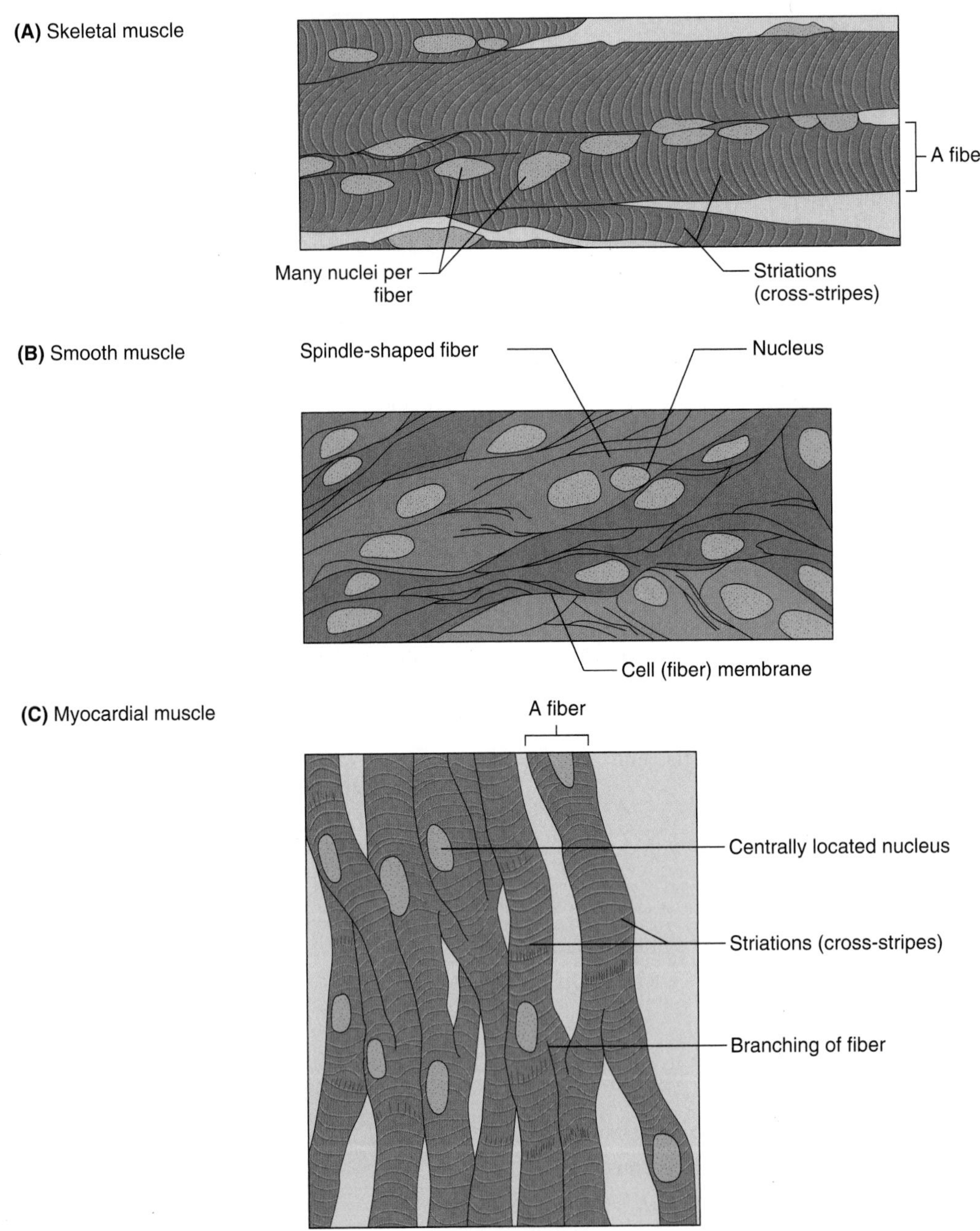

FIGURE 4.2 Types of muscle tissue. (A) Skeletal muscle. (B) Smooth muscle. (C) Myocardial muscle.

- Smooth muscles are also known as *involuntary muscles* because they are under the control of the autonomic nervous system and are *not* under voluntary control. The autonomic nervous system is discussed in Chapter 10.
- Smooth muscles are also known as *unstriated muscles* because they do *not* have the dark and light bands that produce the striped appearance seen in striated muscles.
- Smooth muscles are also known as *visceral muscles* because they are found in the large internal organs (except the heart) and in hollow structures such as those of the digestive and urinary systems. *Visceral* means relating to the internal organs.

Myocardial Muscle

Myocardial muscles (**my**-oh-**KAR**-dee-al), also known as *myocardium* or *cardiac muscle*, form the muscular walls of the heart (**my/o** means muscle, **cardi** means heart, and **-al** means pertaining to) (see Figure 4.2C).

Myocardial muscle is like striated skeletal muscle in appearance, but is similar to smooth muscle in that its action is involuntary. It is the constant contraction and relaxation of the myocardial muscle that causes the heartbeat. This topic is discussed in Chapter 5.

MUSCLE CONTRACTION AND RELAXATION

A wide range of muscle movements are made possible by the combination of specialized muscle types, muscle innervation, and organization into antagonistic muscle pairs.

Muscle Innervation

Muscle innervation (**in**-err-**VAY**-shun) is the stimulation of a muscle by an impulse transmitted by a motor nerve. Motor nerves enable the brain to stimulate a muscle to contract. When the stimulation stops, the muscle relaxes.

If the nerve impulse is disrupted because of injury or disease, the muscle will be unable to function properly or can be paralyzed and unable to contract.

- **Neuromuscular** (**new**-roh-**MUS**-kyou-lar) means pertaining to the relationship between nerve and muscle (**neur/o** means nerve, **muscul** means muscle, and **-ar** means pertaining to).

Antagonistic Muscle Pairs

All muscles are arranged in antagonistic pairs. The term *antagonistic* refers to working in opposition to each other. Muscles within each pair are made up of specialized cells that can change length or shape by contracting and relaxing. When one muscle of a pair contracts, the other muscle of the pair relaxes. It is these contrasting actions that make motion possible.

- **Contraction** is the tightening of a muscle. As the muscle contracts, it becomes shorter, and thicker, causing the belly (center) of the muscle to enlarge.
- **Relaxation** occurs when a muscle returns to its original form. As the muscle relaxes it becomes longer, and thinner, and the belly is no longer enlarged.

As an example, the triceps and biceps work as a pair to make movement of the arm possible (Figure 4.3).

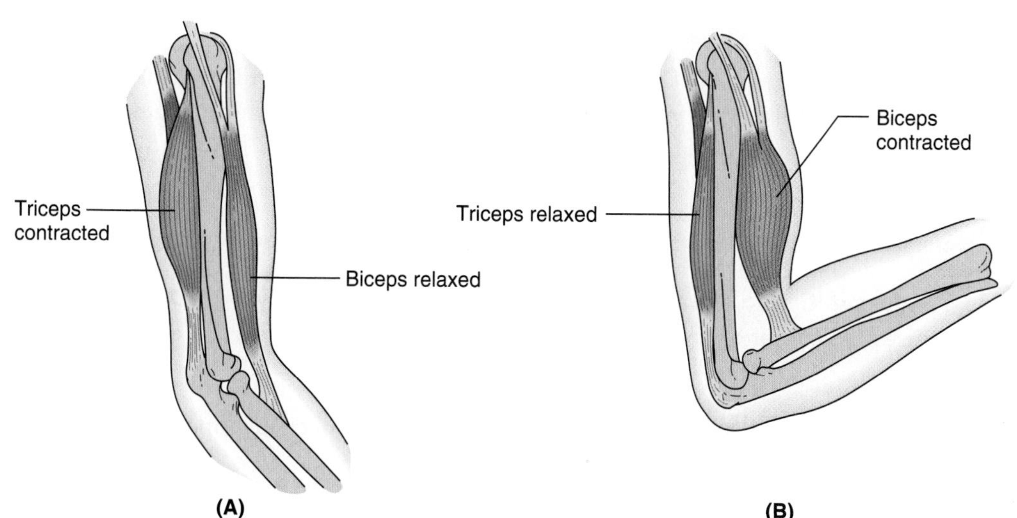

FIGURE 4.3 An antagonistic skeletal muscle pair of the upper arm. (A) During *extension*, the *triceps* is contracted and the biceps is *relaxed*. (B) During *flexion*, the *triceps* is relaxed and the *biceps* is contracted.

CONTRASTING MUSCLE MOTION

These muscle motions, which occur as pairs of opposites, are described in the following text, contrasted in Table 4.1, and illustrated in Figures 4.4 through 4.8.

Abduction and Adduction

Abduction (ab-**DUCK**-shun) is the movement of a limb *away from* the midline of the body (**ab**- means away from, **duct** means to lead, and **-ion** means action). An *abductor* is a muscle that moves a part away from the midline.

In contrast, **adduction** (ah-**DUCK**-shun) is the movement of a limb *toward* the midline of the body (**ad**- means toward, **duct** means to lead, and **-ion** means action). An *adductor* is a muscle that moves a part toward the midline (Figure 4.4).

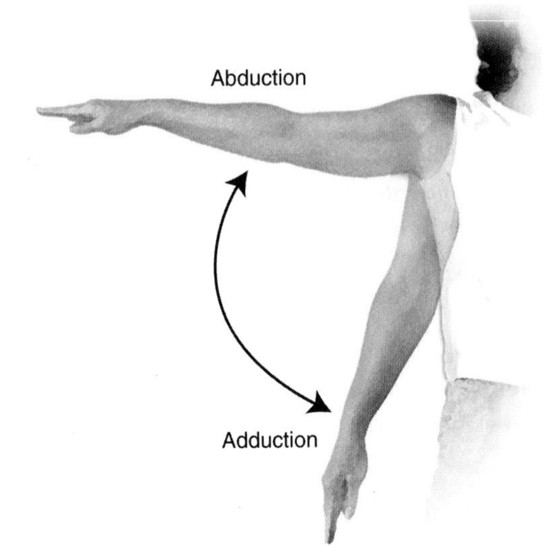

FIGURE 4.4 Abduction moves the arm away from the body. Adduction moves the arm toward the body.

Flexion and Extension

Flexion (**FLECK**-shun) means decreasing the angle between two bones by bending a limb at a joint (**flex** means to bend, and **-ion** means action). A *flexor* is a muscle that bends a limb at a joint.

In contrast, **extension** means increasing the angle between two bones or the straightening of a limb (**ex**- means away from, **tens** means to stretch out, and **-ion** means action). An *extensor* is a muscle that straightens a limb at a joint (Figure 4.5).

- **Hyperextension** is the extreme or overextension of a limb or body part beyond its normal limit. For example, movement of the head far backward or far forward beyond the normal range of motion causes hyperextension of the muscles of the neck.

Elevation and Depression

Elevation is the act of raising or lifting a body part, such as raising the ribs when breathing in (see Chapter 7). A *levator* is a muscle that raises a body part.

In contrast, **depression** is the act of lowering a body part, such as lowering the ribs when breathing out. A *depressor* is a muscle that lowers a body part.

TABLE 4.1
CONTRASTING MUSCLE MOTIONS

Abduction moves away from the midline. During abduction, the arm moves outward away from the side of the body.	**Adduction** moves toward the midline. During adduction, the arm moves inward toward the side of the body.
Flexion decreases an angle, as in bending a joint. During flexion, the knee or elbow are bent.	**Extension** increases an angle, as in straightening a joint. During extension, the knee or elbow are straightened.
Elevation raises a body part. During elevation, the *levator anguli oris* raises the corner of the mouth in a smile.	**Depression** lowers a body part. During depression, the *depressor anguli oris* lowers the corner of the mouth in a frown.
Rotation turns a bone on its own axis.	**Circumduction** is the circular movement at the far end of a limb.
Supination turns the palm of the hand upward or forward.	**Pronation** turns the palm of the hand downward or backward.
Dorsiflexion bends the foot upward at the ankle.	**Plantar flexion** bends the foot downward at the ankle.

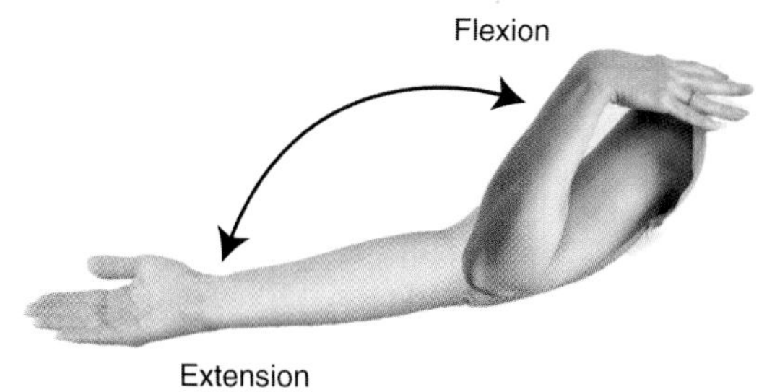

FIGURE 4.5 *Extension* increases the angle of the elbow and moves the hand away from the body. *Flexion* decreases the angle of the elbow and moves the hand toward the body.

Rotation and Circumduction

Rotation is a circular movement around an axis such as the shoulder joint. An *axis* is an imaginary line that runs lengthwise through the center of the body.

In contrast, **circumduction** (**ser**-kum-**DUCK**-shun) is the circular movement of a limb at the far end. An example of circumduction is the swinging motion of the far end of the arm (Figure 4.6).

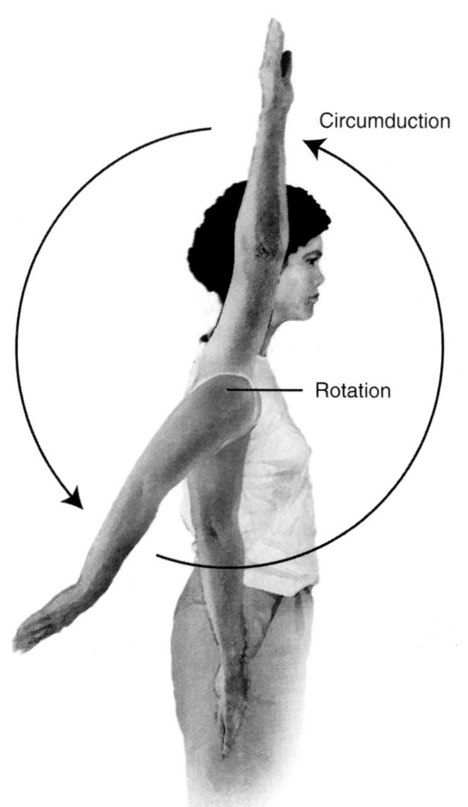

FIGURE 4.6 *Rotation* is a circular movement around an axis such as the shoulder joint. *Circumduction* is the circular movement at the far end of a limb.

- A *rotator muscle* turns a body part on its axis. For example, the head of the humerus (the bone of the upper arm) rotates within the shoulder joint.
- The *rotator cuff* is the group of muscles and their tendons that hold the head of the humerus securely in place as it rotates within the shoulder joint (see Figure 4.13).

Supination and Pronation

Supination (**soo**-pih-**NAY**-shun) is the act of rotating the arm or the leg so that the palm of the hand, or sole of the foot, is turned forward or upward.

In contrast, **pronation** (proh-**NAY**-shun) is the act of rotating the arm or leg so that the palm of the hand or sole of the foot is turned downward or backward (Figure 4.7).

Dorsiflexion and Plantar Flexion

Dorsiflexion (**dor**-sih-**FLECK**-shun) is the movement that bends the foot upward at the ankle. Pointing the toes and foot upward decreases the angle between the top of the foot and the front of the leg.

In contrast, **plantar flexion** (**PLAN**-tar **FLECK**-shun) is the movement that bends the foot downward at the ankle. *Plantar* means pertaining to the sole of the foot. Pointing the toes and foot downward increases the angle between the top of the foot and the front of the leg (Figure 4.8).

HOW MUSCLES ARE NAMED

As you study this section, refer to Figures 4.9 through 4.12. Figures 4.10 and 4.11 show the superficial muscles that are located just under the skin.

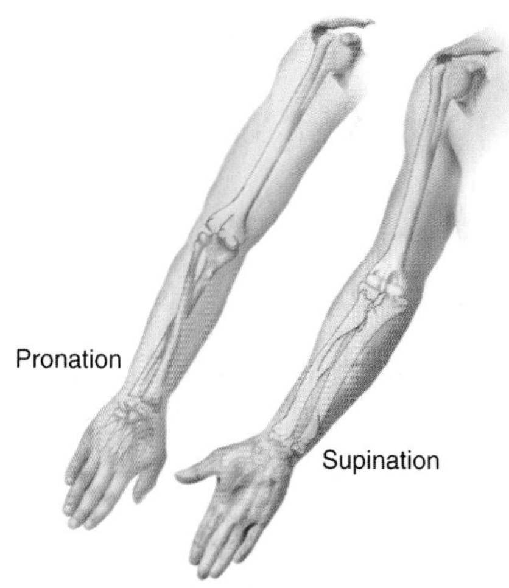

FIGURE 4.7 *Supination* is turning the arm so the palm of the hand is turned upward. *Pronation* is turning the arm so the palm of the hand is turned downward.

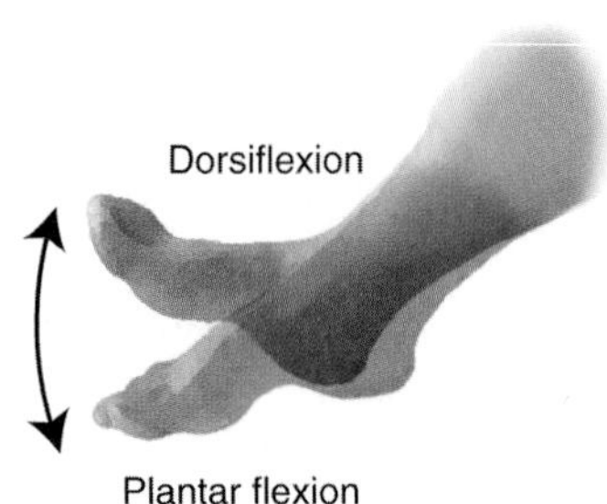

FIGURE 4.8 *Dorsiflexion* bends the foot upward at the ankle. *Plantar flexion* bends the foot downward at the ankle.

Muscles Named for Their Origin and Insertion

The movements of skeletal muscles are made possible by two points of attachment known as the origin and insertion. Some muscles are also named for these points.

- The **origin**, which is the less moveable attachment, is the place where the muscle begins. The origin is located nearest the midline of the body or on a less moveable part of the skeleton.
- The **insertion**, which is the more moveable attachment, is the place where the muscle ends by attaching to a bone or tendon. In contrast to the origin, this that is farthest from the midline of the body.
- For example, the *sternocleidomastoid* muscle, which is shown in Figure 4.9, helps bend the neck and rotate the head. This muscle is named for its two points of origin and one point of insertion. The origins of this muscle are near the midline at the sternum (breastbone) and the clavicle (collar bone). The insertion of this muscle, which is away from the midline, is into the mastoid process of the temporal bone (located just behind the ear).

Muscles Named for Their Action

Some muscles are named for their action, such as flexion or extension.

- For example, the *flexor carpi muscles* and the *extensor carpi muscles* are the pair of muscles that make flexion (bending) and extension (straightening) of the wrist possible (see Figure 4.10). *Carpi* means wrist or wrist bones.

Muscles Named for Their Location

Some muscles are named for their location on the body or the organ they are near:

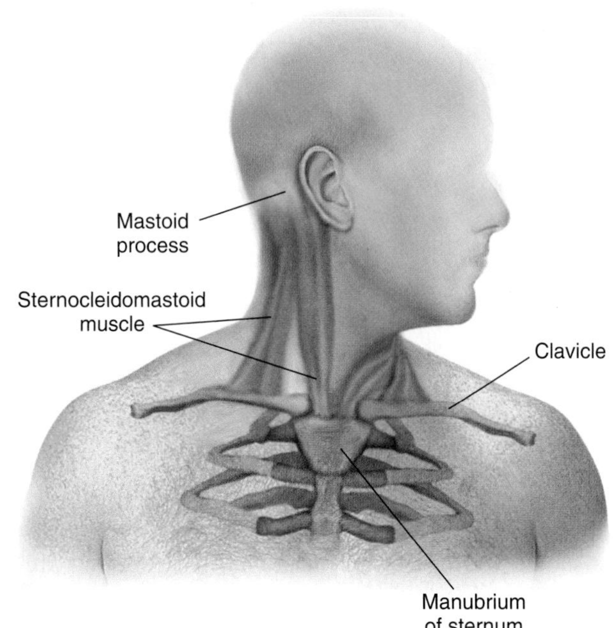

FIGURE 4.9 The sternocleidomastoid muscle is named for its *origins* and *insertion*.

- For example, the *pectoralis major* is a thick, fan-shaped muscle situated on the anterior chest wall (see Figure 4.10). In the male, this muscle makes up the bulk of the chest muscles. In the female, this muscle lies under the breast. *Pectoral* means relating to the chest.
- Other muscles indicate their location by including the terms *lateralis* and *medialis* in their names. *Lateralis* means toward the side. *Medialis* means toward the midline. For example, the *vastus lateralis* and the *vastus medialis* (see Figure 4.10). These muscles flex and extend the leg at the knee.
- Some muscles indicate their location by including external and internal in their names. *External*, or *superficial* mean near the surface and *internal* means deeper location. The *external oblique* and *internal oblique* flex and rotate the spinal column and compress the abdomen.

Muscles Named for Fiber Direction

Some muscles are named for the direction in which their fibers run (Figure 4.12).

- **Oblique** (oh-**BLEEK**) means slanted or at an angle. As an example, the *external oblique* and *internal oblique* muscles have a slanted alignment.

- **Rectus** (**RECK**-tus) means in straight alignment with the vertical axis of the body. As an example, the *rectus abdominis* muscle has a straight alignment.
- A **sphincter** (**SFINK**-ter) is a ring-like muscle that tightly constricts the opening of a passageway. A sphincter is named for the passage involved. As an example, the *anal sphincter* closes the anus.
- **Transverse** (trans-**VERSE**) means in a crosswise direction. An example is the *transverse abdominis* muscle, which has a crosswise alignment.

Muscles Named for Number of Divisions

Muscles may be named according to the number of divisions forming them (see Figure 4.3).

- The **biceps brachii** (**BRAY**-kee-eye), also known as the *biceps*, is formed from two divisions (**bi-** means two, and **-ceps** means head). This muscle of the anterior upper arm flexes the elbow.
- The **triceps brachii** (**BRAY**-kee-eye), also known as the *triceps*, is formed from three divisions (**tri-** means three, and **-ceps** means head). This muscle of the posterior upper arm extends the elbow.

Muscles Named for Their Size or Shape

Some muscles are named because they are broad or narrow or large or small.

- For example, the **gluteus maximus** (**GLOO**-tee-us) is the largest muscle of the buttock (see Figure 4.11).
- Other muscles are named because they are shaped like a familiar object. For example, the **deltoid muscle** is shaped like an inverted triangle or the Greek letter delta. The deltoid forms the muscular cap of the shoulder (see Figures 4.10 and 4.11).

Muscles Named for Strange Reasons

Some muscles, such as the hamstrings, have seemingly strange names. The reason this group of muscles is so named is because these are the muscles by which a butcher hangs a slaughtered pig.

- The **hamstring group**, located at the back of the upper leg, consists of three separate muscles: the *biceps femoris*, *semitendinosus*, and *semimembranosus* muscles. The primary functions of the hamstrings are knee flexion and hip extension (see Figure 4.11).

MEDICAL SPECIALTIES RELATED TO THE MUSCULAR SYSTEM

- An **exercise physiologist** (**fiz**-ee-**OL**-oh-jist) is a specialist who works under the supervision of a physician to develop, implement, and coordinate exercise programs, and administer medical tests to promote physical fitness.
- A **neurologist** (new-**ROL**-oh-jist) is a physician who specializes in treating the causes of paralysis and similar muscular disorders in which there is a loss of function.
- A **physiatrist** (**fiz**-ee-**AT**-rist) is a physician who specializes in physical medicine and rehabilitation with the focus on restoring function. *Rehabilitation* is restoration, following disease, illness, or injury, of the ability to function in a normal or near-normal manner.
- A **rheumatologist** (roo-mah-**TOL**-oh-jist) is a physician who specializes in the diagnosis and treatment of arthritis and disorders such as osteoporosis, fibromyalgia and tendonitis that are characterized by inflammation in the joints and connective tissues.
- A **sports medicine physician** specializes in treating sports-related injuries of the bones, joints, and muscles.

PATHOLOGY OF THE MUSCULAR SYSTEM

Fibers, Fascia, and Tendons

- **Fasciitis** (**fas**-ee-**EYE**-tis), which is also spelled *fascitis*, is inflammation of a fascia (**fasci** means fascia, and **-itis** means inflammation).
- **Fibromyalgia syndrome** (**figh**-broh-my-**AL**-jee-ah) is a debilitating chronic condition characterized by fatigue, diffuse and or specific muscle, joint, or bone pain, and a wide range of other symptoms (**fibr/o** means fibrous connective tissue, **my** means muscle, and **-algia** means pain). *Debilitating* means a condition causing weakness. Contrast fibromyalgia syndrome with *chronic fatigue syndrome.*
- **Tenodynia** (**ten**-oh-**DIN**-ee-ah), also known as *tenalgia*, is pain in a tendon (**ten/o** means tendon, and **-dynia** means pain).
- **Tendinitis** (**ten**-dih-**NIGH**-tis) is an inflammation of the tendons caused by excessive or unusual use of the joint (**tendon** means tendon, and **-itis** means inflammation). The terms *tendonitis*, *tenonitis*, and *tenontitis* all have the same meaning.

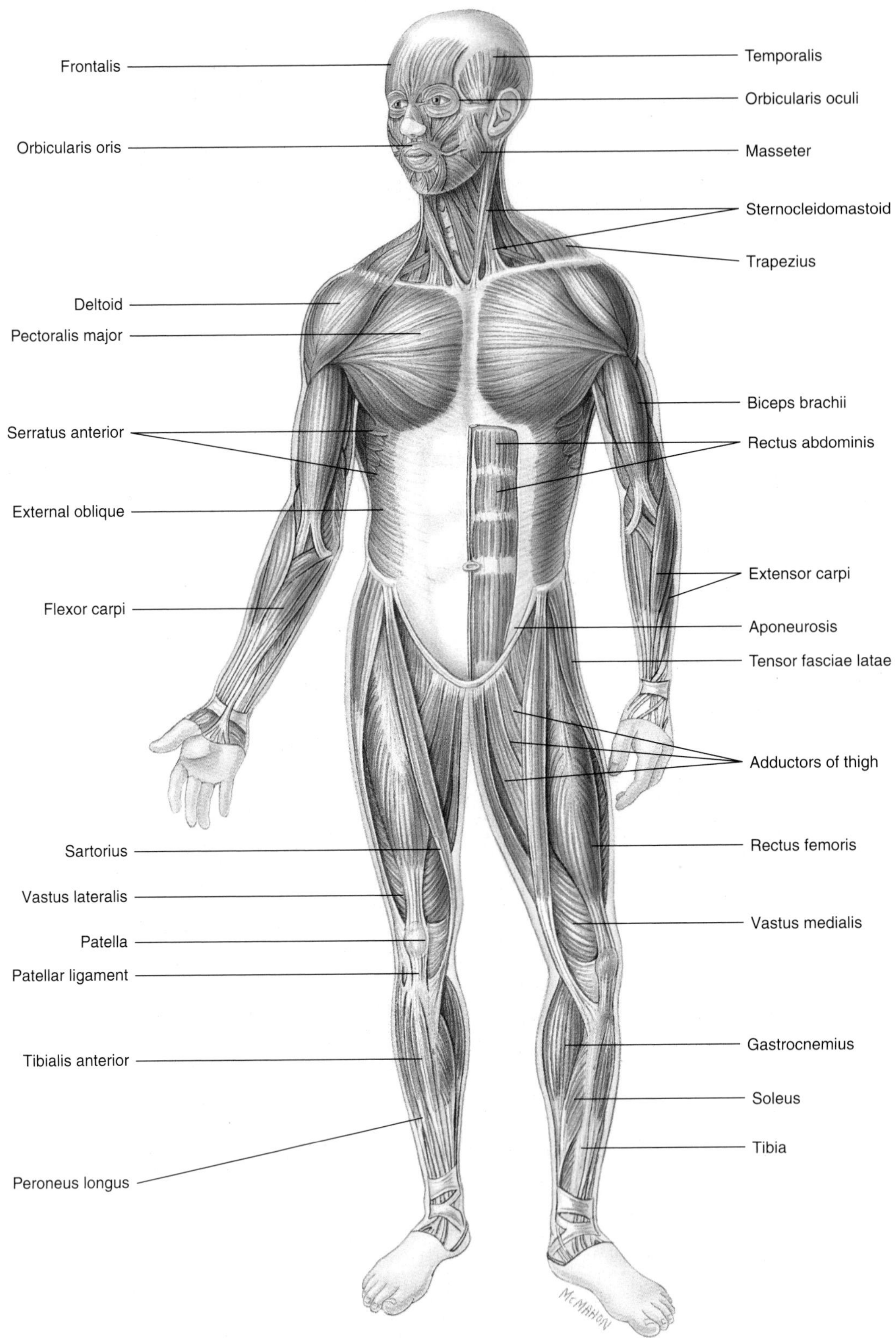

FIGURE 4.10 Superficial muscles of body (anterior view).

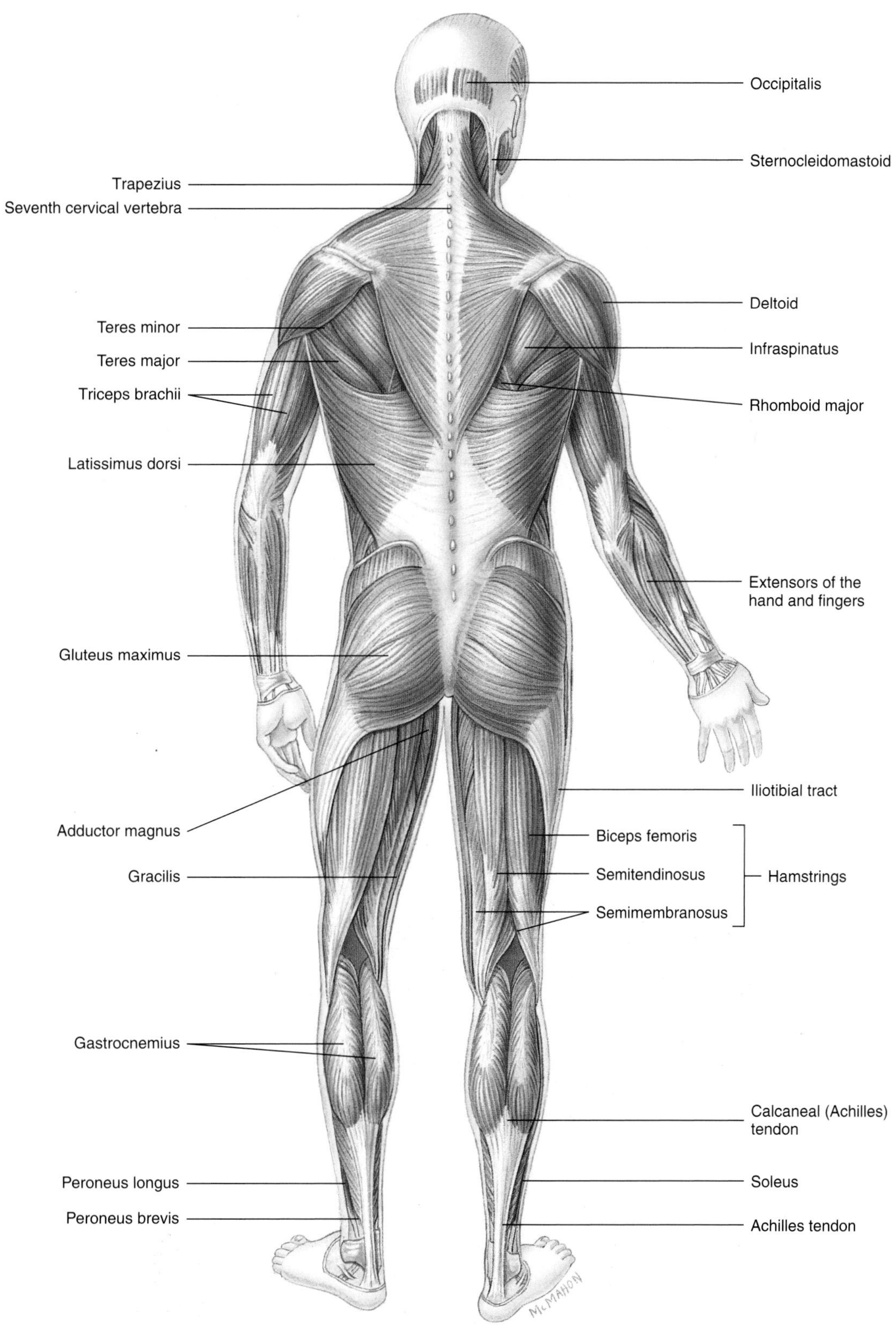

FIGURE 4.11 Superficial muscles of body (posterior view).

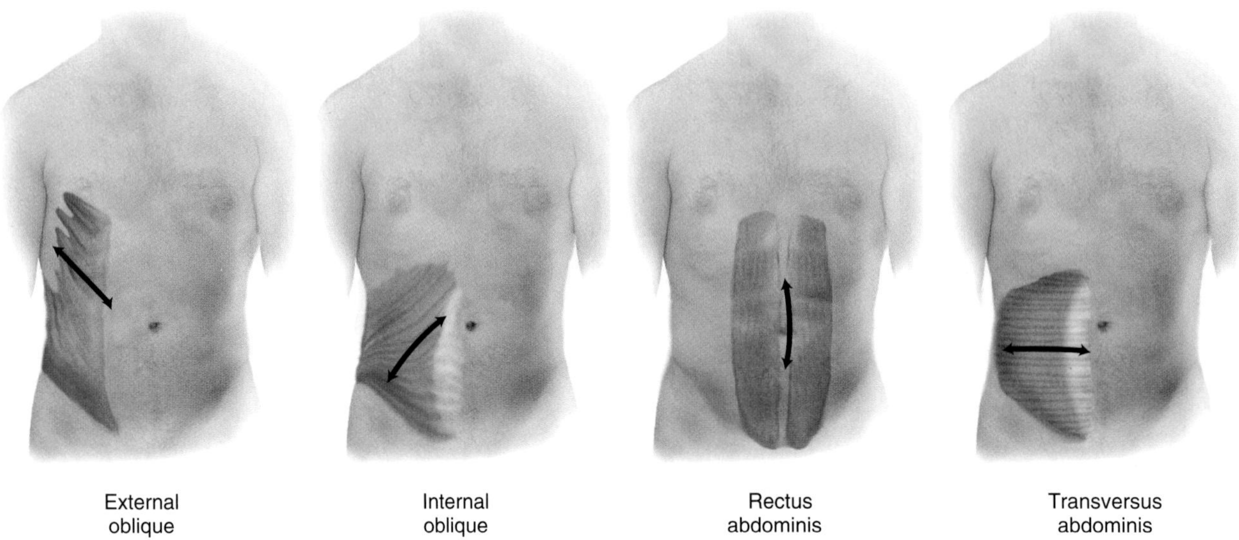

FIGURE 4.12 Examples of muscles named for their direction.

Chronic Fatigue Syndrome

Chronic fatigue syndrome (CFS) is a disorder of unknown cause that affects many body systems. It is discussed in this chapter because many of the symptoms are similar to those of the fibromyalgia syndrome.

- CFS is a debilitating and complex disorder characterized by profound fatigue that is not improved by bed rest and may be made worse by physical or mental activity.
- Those with CFS often function at a much lower level of activity than they were capable of before the beginning of the illness. This persistent overwhelming fatigue lasts more than 2 months and does not improve with bed rest.

Muscle Disorders

- An **adhesion** (ad-**HEE**-zhun) is a band of fibrous tissue that holds structures together abnormally. Adhesions can form in muscles, or in internal organs, as the result of an injury or surgery.
- **Atrophy** (**AT**-roh-fee) means weakness or wearing away of body tissues and structures. Atrophy of a muscle or muscles can be caused by pathology or by disuse of the muscle over a long period of time.
- **Myalgia** (my-**AL**-jee-ah), also known as *myodynia*, is tenderness or pain in the muscles (**my** means muscle, and **-algia** means pain).
- A **myocele** (**MY**-oh-seel) is the herniation (protrusion) of muscle substance through a tear in the fascia surrounding it (**my/o** means muscle, and **-cele** means a hernia). A *hernia* is the protrusion of a part or structure through the tissues normally containing it.
- **Myolysis** (my-**OL**-ih-sis) is the degeneration of muscle tissue (**my/o** means muscle, and **-lysis** means destruction or breaking down in disease). *Degeneration* means deterioration or breaking down. *Deterioration* means the process of becoming worse.
- **Myomalacia** (**my**-oh-mah-**LAY**-shee-ah) is abnormal softening of muscle tissue (**my/o** means muscle, and **-malacia** means abnormal softening).
- **Myorrhexis** (**my**-oh-**RECK**-sis) is the rupture or tearing of a muscle (**my/o** means muscle, and **-rrhexis** means rupture).
- **Polymyositis** (**pol**-ee-**my**-oh-**SIGH**-tis) is a muscle disease characterized by the simultaneous inflammation and weakening of voluntary muscles in many parts of the body (**poly-** means many, **myos** means muscle, and **-itis** means inflammation). The affected muscles are typically those closest to the trunk or torso, and the resulting weakness can be severe.
- **Sarcopenia** (**sar**-koh-**PEE**-nee-ah) is the loss of muscle mass, strength, and function that comes with aging (**sarc/o** means flesh, and **-penia** means deficiency). A weight or resistance training program can significantly improve muscle mass and slow, but not stop this process.

Muscle Tone

Muscle tone, also known as *tonus*, is the state of balanced muscle tension (contraction and relaxation) that makes normal posture, coordination, and movement possible. As used here the term *tonic* means pertaining to muscle tone.

- **Atonic** (ah-**TON**-ick) means lacking normal muscle tone or strength (**a-** means without, **ton** means tone, and **-ic** means pertaining to).
- **Dystonia** (dis-**TOH**-nee-ah) is a condition of abnormal muscle tone that causes the impairment of voluntary muscle movement (**dys-** means bad, **ton** means tone, and **-ia** means condition).
- **Hypertonia** (**high**-per-**TOH**-nee-ah) is a condition of excessive tone of the skeletal muscles (**hyper-** means excessive, **ton** means tone, and **-ia** means condition). Hypertonia is the opposite of *hypotonia*.
- **Hypotonia** (**high**-poh-**TOH**-nee-ah) is a condition in which there is diminished tone of the skeletal muscles (**hypo-** means deficient, **ton** means tone, and **-ia** means condition). Hypotonia is the opposite of *hypertonia*.
- **Myotonia** (**my**-oh-**TOH**-nee-ah) is a neuromuscular disorder characterized by the slow relaxation of the muscles after a voluntary contraction (**my/o** means muscle, **ton** means tone, and **-ia** means condition).

Voluntary Muscle Movement

- **Ataxia** (ah-**TACK**-see-ah) is the inability to coordinate muscle activity during voluntary movement (**a-** means without, **tax** means coordination, and **-ia** means condition). These movements, which are often shaky and unsteady, are most frequently caused by abnormal activity in the cerebellum (see Chapter 10).
- **Dystaxia** (dis-**TACK**-see-ah), also known as *partial ataxia*, is a mild form of ataxia (**dys-** means bad, **tax** means coordination, and **-ia** means condition).
- A **contracture** (kon-**TRACK**-chur) is the permanent tightening of fascia, muscles, tendons, ligaments, or skin that occurs when normally elastic connective tissues are replaced with nonelastic fibrous tissues. The most common causes of contractures are scarring or the lack of use due to immobilization or inactivity.
- **Intermittent claudication** (**klaw**-dih-**KAY**-shun) is pain in the leg muscles that occurs during exercise and is relieved by rest. *Intermittent* means coming and going at intervals, and *claudication* means limping. This condition, which is due to poor circulation, is associated with peripheral vascular disease (see Chapter 5).
- A **spasm** is a sudden, violent, involuntary contraction of one or more muscles.
- A **cramp** is a localized muscle spasm named for its cause, such as a heat cramp or writer's cramp.
- **Spasmodic torticollis** (spaz-**MOD**-ick **tor**-tih-**KOL**-is), also known as *wryneck*, is a stiff neck due to spasmodic contraction of the neck muscles that pull the head toward the affected side. *Spasmodic* means relating to a spasm, and *torticollis* means a contraction, or shortening, of the muscles of the neck.

Muscle Function

- **Bradykinesia** (**brad**-ee-kih-**NEE**-zee-ah) is extreme slowness in movement (**brady-** means slow, **kines** means movement, and **-ia** means condition). This is one of the symptoms of Parkinson's disease, which is discussed in Chapter 10.
- **Dyskinesia** (**dis**-kih-**NEE**-zee-ah) is the distortion or impairment of voluntary movement such as in a tic or spasm (**dys-** means bad, **kines** means movement, and **-ia** means condition). A *tic* is a spasmodic muscular contraction that often involves parts of the face. Although these movements appear purposeful, they are not under voluntary control.
- **Hyperkinesia** (**high**-per-kye-**NEE**-zee-ah), also known as *hyperactivity*, is abnormally increased muscle function or activity (**hyper-** means excessive, **kines** means movement, and **-ia** means condition). Hyperkinesia is the opposite of *hypokinesia*.
- **Hypokinesia** (**high**-poh-kye-**NEE**-zee-ah) is abnormally decreased muscle function or activity (**hypo-** means deficient, **kines** means movement, and **-ia** means condition). Hypokinesia is the opposite of *hyperkinesia*.

Myoclonus

Myoclonus (**my**-oh-**KLOH**-nus) is the sudden, involuntary jerking of a muscle or group of muscles (**my/o** means muscle, **clon** mean violent action, and **-us** is a singular noun ending).

- **Nocturnal myoclonus** (nock-**TER**-nal **my**-oh-**KLOH**-nus) is jerking of the limbs that can occur normally as a person is falling asleep. *Nocturnal* means pertaining to night.
- **Singultus** (sing-**GUL**-tus), also known as *hiccups*, is myoclonus of the diaphragm that causes the characteristic hiccup sound with each spasm.

Myasthenia Gravis

Myasthenia gravis (**my**-as-**THEE**-nee-ah **GRAH**-vis) is a chronic autoimmune disease that affects the neuromuscular junction and produces serious weakness of voluntary muscles. *Myasthenia* means muscle weakness (**my** means muscle, and **-asthenia** means weakness or lack of strength). *Gravis* comes from the Latin meaning grave or serious.

Muscular Dystrophy

The condition commonly known as **muscular dystrophy** (**DIS**-troh-fee) is properly referred to as *muscular dystrophies*. This general term describes a group of more than 30 genetic diseases that are characterized by progressive weakness and degeneration of the skeletal muscles that control movement, without affecting the nervous system. There is no specific treatment to stop or reverse any form of muscular dystrophy. Three of the most common forms are described below.

- *Duchenne muscular dystrophy* (DMD) is the most common form of muscular dystrophy. This condition affects primarily boys with onset between the ages of 3 and 5 years. The disorder progresses rapidly so that most of these boys are unable to walk by age 12 and later need a respirator to breathe.
- *Becker muscular dystrophy* (BMD) is very similar to, but less severe than, Duchenne muscular dystrophy.

Repetitive Stress Disorders

Repetitive stress disorders, also known as *repetitive motion disorders*, are a variety of muscular conditions that result from repeated motions performed in the course of normal work, daily activities, or recreation such as sports. The symptoms caused by these frequently repeated motions involve muscles, tendons, nerves, and joints.

- **Compartment syndrome** involves the compression of nerves and blood vessels due to swelling within the enclosed space created by the fascia that separates groups of muscles. This syndrome can be caused by trauma, tight bandages or casts, or by repetitive activities such as running.
- **Overuse injuries** are minor tissue injuries that have not been given time to heal. Such injuries can be caused by spending hours at the computer keyboard or by lengthy sports training sessions.
- **Overuse tendinitis** (**ten**-dih-**NIGH**-tis), also known as *overuse tendinosis*, is inflammation of tendons caused by excessive or unusual use of a joint (**tendin-** means tendon, and **-itis** means inflammation).
- **Stress fractures**, which are also overuse injuries, are discussed in Chapter 3.

Myofascial Pain Syndrome

Myofascial pain syndrome is a chronic pain disorder that affects muscles and fascia throughout the body. This condition, which is caused by the development of trigger points, produces local and referred muscle pain. *Trigger points* are tender areas that most commonly develop where the fascia comes into contact with a muscle. *Referred pain* describes pain that originates in one area of the body, but felt in another.

Rotator Cuff Injuries

- **Impingement syndrome** (im-**PINJ**-ment) occurs when inflamed and swollen tendons are caught in the narrow space between the bones within the shoulder joint. A common sign of impingement syndrome is discomfort when raising your arm above your head.
- **Rotator cuff tendinitis** (**ten**-dih-**NIGH**-tis) is an inflammation of the tendons of the rotator cuff (Figure 4.13). This condition is often named for the cause, such as *tennis shoulder* or *pitcher's shoulder*.
- A **ruptured rotator cuff** develops when rotator cuff tendinitis is left untreated or if the overuse continues. This occurs as the irritated tendon weakens and tears.

Carpal Tunnel Syndrome

The carpal tunnel is a narrow, bony passage under the carpal ligament that is located one-fourth of an inch below the inner surface of the wrist. *Carpal* means pertaining to the wrist. The median nerve, and the tendons that bend the fingers, pass through this tunnel (Figure 4.14).

Carpal tunnel syndrome symptoms occur when the tendons that pass through the carpal tunnel are chronically overused and become inflamed and swollen.

- This swelling creates pressure on the median nerve as it passes through the carpal tunnel.
- This pressure causes pain, burning, and paresthesia in the thumb, index finger, and middle finger. The ring finger and little finger are not affected because these fingers are innervated by a different nerve. *Paresthesia* is an abnormal sensation such as burning, tingling, or numbness and is discussed in Chapter 10.
- **Carpal tunnel release** is the surgical enlargement of the carpal tunnel or cutting of the carpal ligament to relieve nerve pressure. This treatment is used to relieve the pressure on tendons and nerves in severe cases of carpal tunnel syndrome.

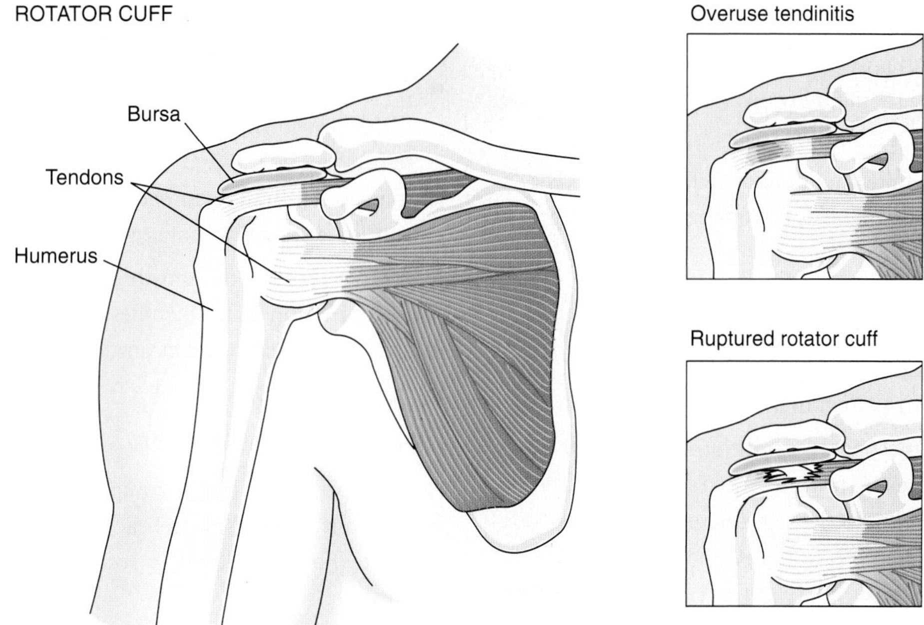

FIGURE 4.13 Diagrammatic views of the *rotator cuff* in health (left) and with injuries (right).

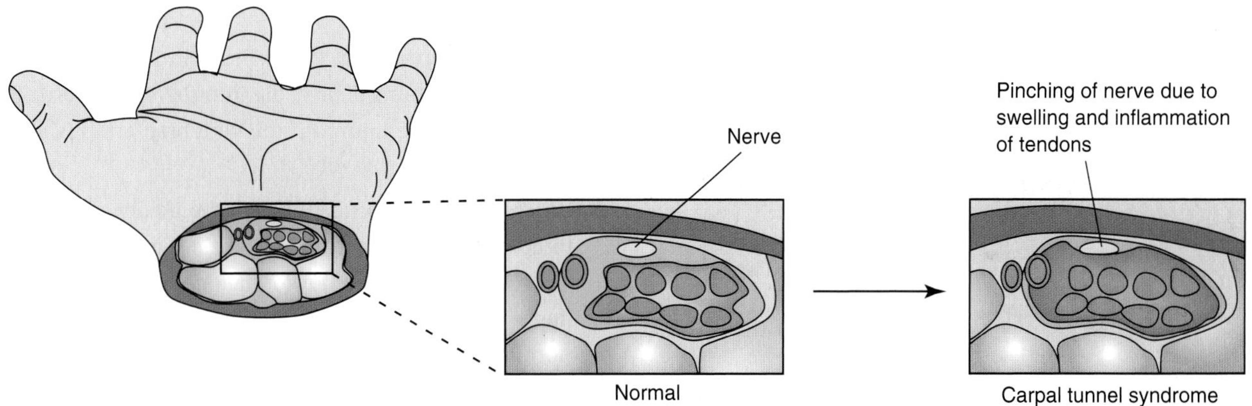

FIGURE 4.14 When the tendons that pass through the carpal tunnel become inflamed and swollen, they pinch the nerve and cause *carpal tunnel syndrome.*

Ganglion Cyst

A **ganglion cyst** (**GANG**-glee-on **SIST**) is a harmless fluid-filled swelling that occurs most commonly on the outer surface of the wrist. This condition, which can be caused by repeated minor injuries, is usually painless and does not require treatment. (Do not confuse this use of the term *ganglion* here with the nerve ganglions described in Chapter 10.)

Epicondylitis

Epicondylitis (**ep**-ih-**kon**-dih-**LYE**-tis) is inflammation of the tissues surrounding the elbow (**epi-** means on, **condyl** means condyle, and **-itis** means inflammation).

- *Lateral epicondylitis*, also known as *tennis elbow*, is characterized by pain on the outer side of the forearm
- *Medial epicondylitis*, also known as *golfer's elbow*, is characterized by pain on the palm-side of the forearm.

Ankle and Foot Problems

- A **heel spur** is a calcium deposit in the plantar fascia near its attachment to the calcaneus (heel) bone that can be one of the causes of *plantar fasciitis.*
- **Plantar fasciitis** (**PLAN**-tar **fas**-ee-**EYE**-tis) is an inflammation of the plantar fascia on the sole of the foot. This condition causes foot or heel pain when walking or running (Figure 4.15).

Sports Injuries

The following injuries are frequently associated with sports overuse; however, some may also be caused by other forms of trauma.

- A **sprain** is an injury to a joint, such as ankle, knee, or wrist that usually involves a stretched or torn ligament (Figure 4.16).
- A **strain** is an injury to the body of the muscle or to the attachment of a tendon. Strains usually are associated with overuse injuries that involve a stretched or torn muscle or tendon attachment.
- A **shin splint** is a painful condition caused by the muscle tearing away from the tibia (shin bone). Shin splints can develop in the anterolateral (front and side) muscles or in the posteromedial (back and middle) muscles of the lower leg (Figures 4.10 and 4.11). This type of injury is usually caused by repeated stress to the lower leg, such as running on hard surfaces.
- A **hamstring injury** can be a strain or tear on any of the three hamstring muscles that straighten the hip and bend the knee. When these muscles contract too quickly, an injury can occur that is characterized by sudden and severe pain in the back of the thigh.
- **Achilles tendinitis** (**ten**-dih-**NIGH**-tis) is a painful inflammation of the Achilles tendon caused by excessive stress being placed on that tendon.

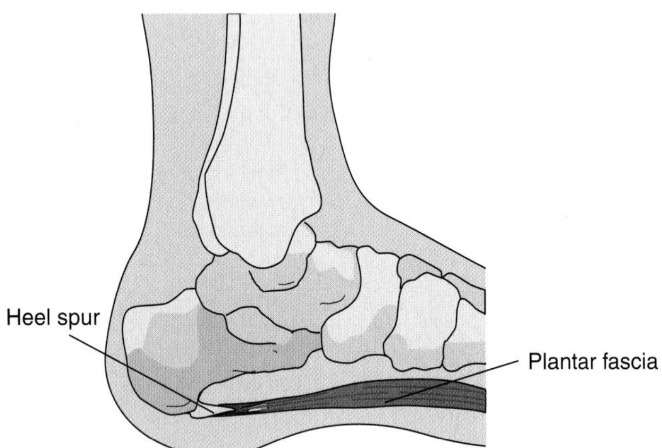

FIGURE 4.15 A *heel spur* and *plantar fasciitis.*

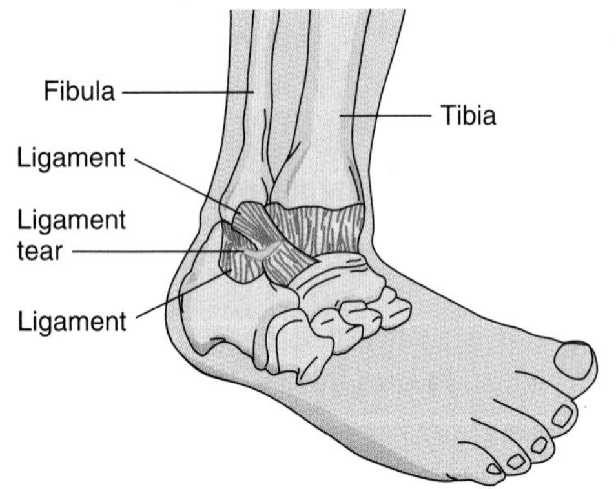

FIGURE 4.16 A *sprained ankle* involves one or more stretched or torn ligaments.

Spinal Cord Injuries

As described in Chapter 3, the spinal cord is surrounded and protected by the bony vertebrae. This protection is essential because the spinal cord is soft, with the consistency of toothpaste.

- The type of paralysis caused by a **spinal cord injury** (SCI) is determined by the level of the vertebra closest to the injury. The higher on the spinal cord the injury occurs, the greater the area of the body that may be affected.
- An injury occurs when a vertebra is broken and a piece of the broken bone is pressing into the spinal cord. The cord can also be injured if the vertebrae are pushed or pulled out of alignment.
- When the spinal cord is injured, the ability of the brain to communicate with the body below the level of the injury may be reduced or lost altogether. When that happens, the affected parts of the body will not function normally.
- An *incomplete injury* means that the person has some function below the level of the injury, even though that function isn't normal.
- A *complete injury* means that there is complete loss of sensation and muscle control below the level of the injury; however, a complete injury does not mean that there is no hope of any improvement.

Types of Paralysis

Paralysis (pah-**RAL**-ih-sis) is the loss of sensation and voluntary muscle movements in a muscle through disease or injury to its nerve supply. Damage can be either temporary or permanent (plural, *paralyses*).

- **Myoparesis** (**my**-oh-**PAR**-eh-sis) is a weakness or slight muscular paralysis (**my/o** means muscle, and **-paresis** means partial or incomplete paralysis).

- **Hemiparesis** (**hem**-ee-pah-**REE**-sis) is slight paralysis or weakness affecting one side of the body (**hemi-** means half, and **-paresis** means partial or incomplete paralysis). Contrast hemiparesis with *hemiplegia*.
- **Hemiplegia** (**hem**-ee-**PLEE**-jee-ah) is total paralysis affecting only one side of the body (**hemi-** means half, and **-plegia** means paralysis). This form of paralysis is usually associated with a stroke or brain damage. Damage to one side of the brain causes paralysis on the opposite side of the body. An individual affected with hemiplegia is known as a *hemiplegic*. Contrast with *hemiparesis*.
- **Paraplegia** (**par**-ah-**PLEE**-jee-ah) is the paralysis of both legs and the lower part of the body. An individual affected with paraplegia is known as a *paraplegic*.
- **Quadriplegia** (**kwad**-rih-**PLEE**-jee-ah) is paralysis of all four extremities (**quadr/i** means four, and **-plegia** means paralysis). An individual affected with quadriplegia is known as a *quadriplegic*.
- **Cardioplegia** (**kar**-dee-oh-**PLEE**-jee-ah), also known as *cardiac arrest*, is paralysis of heart muscle (**cardi/o** means heart, and **-plegia** means paralysis). This can be caused by a direct blow or trauma. Temporary stopping of cardiac activity can be induced by using drugs.

DIAGNOSTIC PROCEDURES OF THE MUSCULAR SYSTEM

- **Deep tendon reflexes** (DTR) are tested with a reflex hammer that is used to strike a tendon (Figure 4.17). A *reflex* is an involuntary response to a stimulus. No response, or an abnormal response, can indicate a disruption of the nerve supply to the involved muscles. Reflexes also are lost in deep coma or because of medication such as heavy sedation.
- **Range of motion testing** (ROM) is a diagnostic procedure to evaluate joint mobility and muscle strength (Figure 4.18). Range of motion exercises are used to increase strength, flexibility, and mobility.
- **Electromyography** (ee-**leck**-troh-my-**OG**-rah-fee) is a diagnostic test that measures the electrical activity within muscle fibers in response to nerve stimulation (**electr/o** means electricity, **my/o** means muscle, and **-graphy** means the process of producing a picture or record). The resulting record is called an *electromyogram*. Electromyography is most frequently used when people have symptoms of weakness, and examination shows impaired muscle strength.
- **Electroneuromyography** (ee-**leck**-troh-**new**-roh-my-**OG**-rah-fee), also known as *nerve conduction studies*,

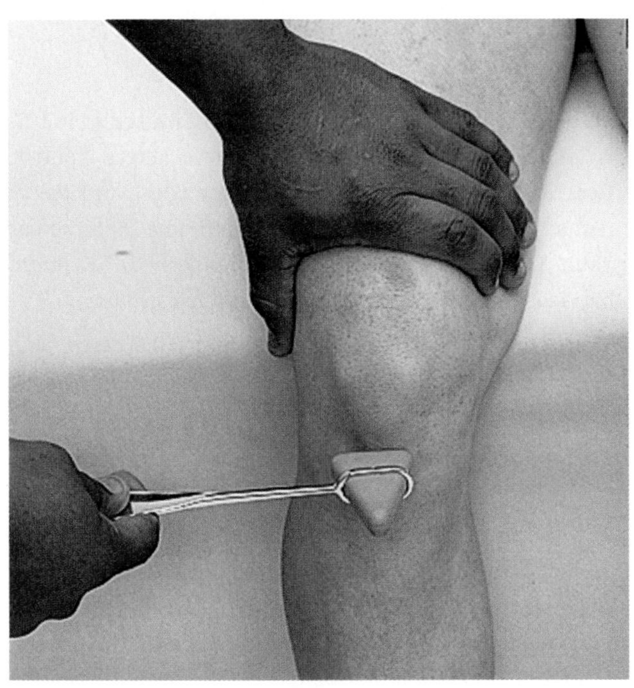

(A)

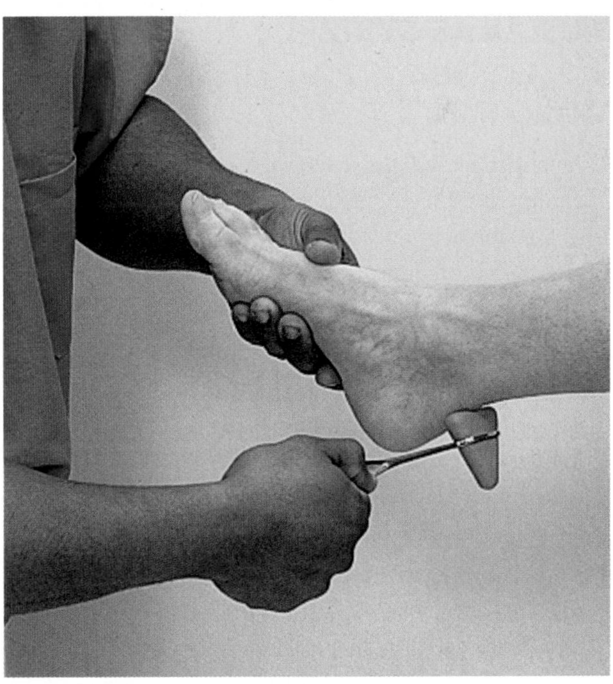

(B)

FIGURE 4.17 Assessment of *deep tendon reflexes*. (A) Testing the *patellar reflex*. (B) Testing the *Achilles tendon reflex*.

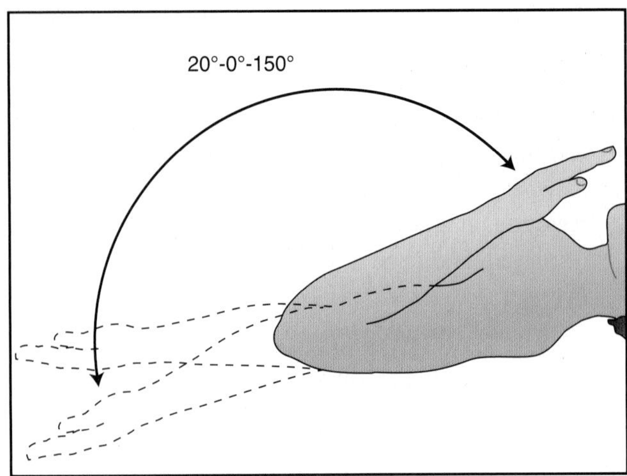

FIGURE 4.18 *Range of motion testing* is used to evaluate joint mobility. The results are expressed in degrees.

is a diagnostic procedure for testing and recording neuromuscular activity by the electric stimulation of the nerve trunk that carries fibers to and from the muscle (**electr/o** means electricity, **neur/o** means nerve, **my/o** means muscle, and **-graphy** means the process of producing a picture or record). The primary goal of this examination is to determine the site of a nerve lesion or of muscle pathology.

TREATMENT PROCEDURES OF THE MUSCULAR SYSTEM

Medications

- An **antispasmodic**, also known as an *anticholingeric*, is administered to suppress smooth muscle contractions of the stomach, intestine, or bladder. For example, *atropine* is an antispasmodic that can be administered preoperatively to relax smooth muscles during surgery.
- A **skeletal muscle relaxant** is administered to relax certain muscles and to relieve the stiffness, pain, and discomfort caused by strains, sprains, or other muscle injuries. These medications act on the central nervous system and may have a negative interaction with alcohol and some antidepressants (see Chapter 10).
- A **neuromuscular blocker**, also known as a *neuromuscular blocking agent*, is a drug that causes temporary paralysis by blocking the transmission of nerve stimuli to the muscles. These drugs are used as an adjunct to anesthesia during surgery to cause skeletal muscles to relax. As used here, *adjunct* means in addition to.

Ergonomics

Ergonomics (er-goh-**NOM**-icks) is the study of the human factors that affect the design and operation of tools and the work environment. This term is usually applied to the design of equipment and workspaces, with the goal of reducing injuries, strain and stress.

Occupational and Physical Therapy

Occupational therapy consists of activities to promote recovery and rehabilitation to assist patients in normalizing their ability to perform the **activities of daily living** (ADL). These activities include bathing, grooming, brushing teeth, eating, and dressing.

Physical therapy is treatment to prevent disability or to restore functioning through the use of exercise, heat, massage, and other methods to improve circulation, flexibility, and muscle strength.

- **Myofascial release** is a specialized soft tissue manipulation technique used to ease the pain of conditions such as fibromyalgia, myofascial pain syndrome, movement restrictions, temporomandibular joint disorders (TMJ), and carpal tunnel syndrome.
- **Therapeutic ultrasound** utilizes high-frequency sound waves to treat muscle injuries by generating heat deep within muscle tissue. This heat eases pain, reduces muscle spasms, and accelerates healing by increasing the flow of blood into the target tissues.

RICE

The most common first aid treatment of muscular injuries is known by the acronym **RICE**. These letters stand for **R**est, **I**ce, **C**ompression, and **E**levation. Rest and ice are recommended for the first few days after the injury to ease pain. Compression, such as wrapping with a stretch bandage, and elevation help to minimize swelling.

After the first few days, as the pain decreases, using heat, accompanied by stretching and light exercises, helps to bring blood to the injured area to speed healing.

Fascia

- A **fasciotomy** (**fash**-ee-**OT**-oh-mee) is a surgical incision through the fascia to relieve tension or pressure (**fasci** means fascia, and **-otomy** means a surgical incision). Without this procedure, the pressure causes a loss of circulation that damages the affected tissues.
- **Fascioplasty** (**FASH**-ee-oh-**plas**-tee) is the surgical repair of fascia (**fasci/o** means fascia, and **-plasty** means surgical repair).

Tendons

- **Tenodesis** (ten-**ODD**-eh-sis) is the surgical suturing of the end of a tendon to a bone (**ten/o** means tendon, and **-desis** means to bind or tie together). Tenodesis is the opposite of *tenolysis*.
- **Tenolysis** (ten-**OL**-ih-sis), also known as *tendolysis*, is the release of a tendon from adhesions (**ten/o** means tendon, and **-lysis** means to set free). Tenolysis is the opposite of *tenodesis*.
- A **tenectomy** (teh-**NECK**-toh-mee), also known as a *tenonectomy*, is the surgical resection of a portion of a tendon or tendon sheath (**ten** means tendon, and **-ectomy** means surgical removal). The term *resection* describes the removal of tissue or part or all of an organ by surgery.
- **Tenoplasty** (**TEN**-oh-**plas**-tee), also known as **tendinoplasty**, is the surgical repair of a tendon (**ten/o** means tendon, and **-plasty** means surgical repair).
- **Tenorrhaphy** (ten-**OR**-ah-fee) is surgical suturing together of the divided ends of a tendon (**ten/o** means tendon, and **-rrhaphy** means surgical suturing).
- A **tenotomy** (teh-**NOT**-oh-mee), also known as a *tendotomy*, is the surgical division of a tendon for relief of a deformity caused by the abnormal shortening of a muscle, such as strabismus (**ten** means tendon, and **-otomy** means surgical incision). *Strabismus* is discussed in Chapter 11.

Muscles

- A **myectomy** (my-**ECK**-toh-mee) is the surgical excision of a portion of a muscle (**my** means muscle, and **-ectomy** means surgical removal). *Excision* means cutting out or removal.
- **Myoplasty** (**MY**-oh-**plas**-tee) is the surgical repair of a muscle (**my/o** means muscle, and **-plasty** means surgical repair).
- **Myorrhaphy** (my-**OR**-ah-fee) is the surgical suturing a muscle wound (**my/o** means muscle, and **-rrhaphy** means surgical suturing).
- A **myotomy** (my-**OT**-oh-mee) is a surgical incision into a muscle (**my** means muscle, and **-otomy** means surgical incision).

ABBREVIATIONS RELATED TO THE MUSCULAR SYSTEM

Table 4.2 presents an overview of the abbreviations related to the terms introduced in this chapter. Note: To avoid errors or confusion, always be cautious when using abbreviations.

TABLE 4.2

ABBREVIATIONS RELATED TO THE MUSCULAR SYSTEM

carpal tunnel syndrome = CTS	**CTS** = carpal tunnel syndrome
electromyography = EMG	**EMG** = electromyography
fibromyalgia syndrome = FMS	**FMS** = fibromyalgia syndrome
hemiplegia = hemi	**hemi** = hemiplegia
impingement syndrome = IS	**IS** = impingement syndrome
intermittent claudication = IC	**IC** = intermittent claudication
muscular dystrophy = MD	**MD** = muscular dystrophy
myasthenia gravis = MG	**MG** = myasthenia gravis
polymyositis = PM	**PM** = polymyositis
quadriplegia, quadriplegic = quad	**quad** = quadriplegia, quadriplegic
repetitive stress disorder = RSD	**RSD** = repetitive stress disorder

Career Opportunities

In addition to the medical specialties already discussed, some of the health occupations involving the treatment of the muscular system include:

- **Physical therapist (PT):** plan, implement, and evaluate programs for their patients to aid postoperative recovery, improve mobility, and prevent or limit permanent disability of patients with injuries or diseases. Some PT specialties are:

    Cardiopulmonary physical therapy

    Geriatric physical therapy

    Neurological physical therapy

    Sports physical therapy

- **Physical therapy assistant (PTA):** works under the supervision of a PT to carry out treatment plans prescribed by the physician or physical therapist.
- **Massage therapist:** uses bodywork or therapeutic touch to provide pain relief and encourage healing.
- **Athletic trainer (AT):** works to prevent and treat athletic injuries and to provide rehabilitative services to athletes who have been injured. ATs can provide massage, corrective exercises, diet supervision, and equipment fittings.
- **Exercise physiologist:** in order to improve and maintain health and fitness, help in rehabilitation, or improve the performance of athletes, the exercise physiologist identifies and treats the physiological mechanisms underlying different types of physical activities.
- **Occupational therapist (OT):** by providing training and practice in the activities of daily living (ADL) skills, the OT enables those with physical, developmental, mental, and emotional disabilities to regain or improve their quality of life.
- **Occupational therapist assistant** or **aid:** works under the supervision of an OT to help patients with prescribed exercises and activities.

Health Occupation Profile

Physical Therapist

Barb Park is a physical therapist with many years of varied work experience. ***"I chose to study physical therapy because I liked science and working with people. I knew that PTs could find work in many settings, including hospitals, rehabilitation centers, schools, clinics, and institutions. I started out in a rehab setting helping patients who had suffered strokes, amputations, and spinal cord injuries. My work there included helping people increase mobility skills such as relearning how to walk. I then got a chance to work in hospitals with people with a wide variety of problems, including back pain, orthopedic problems, and burns. For the last 30 years, I've worked in an institution with severely developmentally disabled adults and children, making a real difference in their lives by helping them learn very basic skills such as head control and helping design wheelchairs for their comfort and optimal function."***

STUDY BREAK

Singultus, better known as the *hiccups*, are the result of an involuntary, spasmodic contraction of the diaphragm followed by the closing of the throat. Although hiccups usually eventually disappear on their own, an Iowa man is known to have hiccupped for over 60 years!

Thousands of folk "cures" for singultus have been proposed, including:

- **Drinking water from the far side of a glass with your head upside down**
- **Sucking on a lemon**
- **Blowing into and out of a paper bag**
- **Drinking water while pinching your nose closed**
- **Pulling on your forefingers**
- **Standing on your head**
- **Eating sugar**

However, a few unlucky, frequent hiccups sufferers require a physician's care because continuous hiccups are curtailing their work opportunities, sleep, and social life.

REVIEW TIME

Write the answers to the following questions on a separate piece of paper or in your notebook. In addition, be prepared to take part in the classroom discussion.

1. ***Written Assignment:*** Identify four ways in which **muscles can be named.**

   Discussion Assignment: Give an example of the muscles in each of the four categories.

2. ***Written Assignment:*** Use your own words to describe the difference between **intermittent claudication** and **nocturnal myoclonus.**

   Discussion Assignment: Describe which of these conditions occurs normally and which is caused by poor circulation.

3. Hilda has been a "wiz" on the computer keyboard for years. Recently, she has complained of pain and a burning sensation in her fingers.
   Written Assignment: Describe what happens within the wrist to cause **carpal tunnel syndrome.**

   Discussion Assignment: How would you explain this condition to Hilda?

4. In the ER, Dr. Woo performed a **myorrhaphy** on the gluteus maximus of a young stabbing victim.
   Written Assignment: Describe the procedure performed by Dr. Woo.

   Discussion Assignment: How do word parts work together to form this term, and is a combining vowel used?

5. Jennifer is the star of the track team; however, recently she has been experiencing pain when she runs. Dr. Hendrix performed several tests and established a diagnosis of **shin splints.**
   Written Assignment: Use terms a physician would understand to describe this condition and the muscles involved.

   Discussion Assignment: How would you present this diagnosis to Jennifer in terms she can understand?

continues

Optional Internet Activity

The goal of this activity is to help you learn more about medical terminology as it applies to the "real world." Select **one** *of these two options and follow the instructions.*

1. Search for information about the prevention of **carpal tunnel syndrome**. Write a brief (one- or two-paragraph) report on something new you learned here and include the address of the web site where you found this information.

2. Learn about **Achilles tendinitis** by finding one or more web sites that specialize in sports injuries, and describe this condition. Write a brief (one- or two-paragraph) report about how the injury happens, what the symptoms are, and what the treatments might be.

THE HUMAN TOUCH: CRITICAL THINKING ACTIVITY

The following story and questions are designed to stimulate critical thinking through class discussion or as a brief essay response. There are no right or wrong answers to these questions.

"Oh bummer! There's a 'no swimming' sign!"

"Let's just go ahead and take a dip—I trained as a lifeguard, you know. It'll be OK," ***his brother had responded. Now that Luke is confined to a wheelchair, that conversation runs through his head constantly. As do the events that followed it.***

Their family vacation had been going so well, and they were all feeling the freedom of being away from work and school. As he and his brother ran to dive into the crystal-blue lake, Luke was thinking of how much fun being captain of the swim team would be this year and of their chance of making it to the statewide competition. The events immediately after those thoughts were lost to him. The next thing he was aware of was waking up in the hospital and realizing that he couldn't feel or move his legs. His parents were sitting next to the bed, crying. He was paralyzed.

His father told Luke that when he hadn't come up from the dive, his brother had jumped in and dragged Luke out of the water. Their Mom ran screaming towards the shore and began to perform CPR on Luke while their Dad called 9-1-1. Soon the EMTs arrived, and they carefully immobilized Luke's neck before transporting him. Later, in the hospital, his parents' worst fears were confirmed: Luke had a spinal cord injury below the cervical vertebrae and would be a paraplegic for the rest of his life.

All of Luke's dreams about his senior year were shattered. Without the use of his legs, he would not be on the swim team, dance at the prom, or walk across the stage to receive his diploma. He would never forget the decision to dive that had changed his life.

continues

Suggested Discussion Topics

1. Discuss the poor decisions Luke made before he dove into the lake. If he and his brother could turn back the clock, what changes would they make on that fateful day?
2. Discuss Luke's current situation. As a paraplegic, which parts of his body can Luke move? What sorts of things can Luke do by himself?
3. Discuss what the damage would have been if Luke's injury had occurred higher on his spinal cord and had caused him to be a quadriplegic.
4. Luke is back in school now in a wheelchair. As one of his best friends, what should you do? Should you offer to push his chair, get his lunch, and run his errands? How can you help him and yet encourage him to find ways to be independent?

STUDENT WORKBOOK AND StudyWARE™ CD-ROM

1. Go to your **Student Workbook** and complete the Learning Exercises for this chapter.

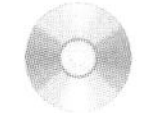

2. Go to the **StudyWARE™ CD-ROM** and have fun with the exercises and games for this chapter.

5

CHAPTER

THE CARDIOVASCULAR SYSTEM

OVERVIEW OF STRUCTURES, COMBINING FORMS, AND FUNCTIONS OF THE CARDIOVASCULAR SYSTEM

MAJOR STRUCTURES	RELATED COMBINING FORMS	PRIMARY FUNCTIONS
Heart	card/o, cardi/o	Pumps blood into the arteries.
Blood Vessels	angi/o, vas/o	Transport blood to and from all areas of the body.
Arteries	arteri/o	Transport blood away from the heart to all parts of the body.
Capillaries	capill/o	Permit the exchange of nutrients and waste products between the blood and the cells.
Veins	phleb/o, ven/o	Return blood from all body parts to the heart.
Blood	hem/o, hemat/o	Brings oxygen and nutrients to the cells and carries away waste.

Vocabulary Related to the Cardiovascular System

This list contains essential word parts and medical terms for this chapter. These terms are pronounced on the student StudyWARE™ CD-ROM and Audio CDs that are available for use with this text. These and the other important **primary terms** are shown in boldface throughout the chapter. *Secondary terms*, which appear in *orange* italics, clarify the meaning of primary terms.

Word Parts

- ☐ angi/o
- ☐ aort/o
- ☐ arteri/o
- ☐ ather/o
- ☐ brady-
- ☐ cardi/o
- ☐ -crasia
- ☐ -emia
- ☐ erythr/o
- ☐ hem/o, hemat/o
- ☐ leuk/o
- ☐ phleb/o
- ☐ tachy-
- ☐ thromb/o
- ☐ ven/o

Medical Terms

- ☐ **ACE inhibitor**
- ☐ **anemia** (ah-**NEE**-mee-ah)
- ☐ **aneurysm** (**AN**-you-rizm)
- ☐ **angina** (an-**JIH**-nuh)
- ☐ **angioplasty** (**AN**-jee-oh-**plas**-tee)
- ☐ **anticoagulant** (**an**-tih-koh-**AG**-you-lant)
- ☐ **aplastic anemia** (ay-**PLAS**-tick ah-**NEE**-mee-ah)
- ☐ **arrhythmia** (ah-**RITH**-mee-ah)
- ☐ **atherectomy** (**ath**-er-**ECK**-toh-mee)
- ☐ **atheroma** (**ath**-er-**OH**-mah)
- ☐ **atherosclerosis** (**ath**-er-**oh**-skleh-**ROH**-sis)
- ☐ **atrial fibrillation**
- ☐ **automated external defibrillator** (dee-**fih**-brih-**LAY**-ter)
- ☐ **beta-blocker**
- ☐ **blood dyscrasia** (dis-**KRAY**-zee-ah)
- ☐ **bradycardia** (**brad**-ee-**KAR**-dee-ah)
- ☐ **cardiac arrest**
- ☐ **cardiac catheterization** (**KAR**-dee-ack **kath**-eh-ter-eye-**ZAY**-shun)
- ☐ **cardiomyopathy** (**kar**-dee-oh-my-**OP**-pah-thee)
- ☐ **carotid endarterectomy** (kah-**ROT**-id **end**-ar-ter-**ECK**-toh-mee)
- ☐ **cholesterol** (koh-**LES**-ter-ol)
- ☐ **chronic venous insufficiency**
- ☐ **coronary thrombosis** (**KOR**-uh-**nerr**-ee throm-**BOH**-sis)
- ☐ **defibrillation** (dee-**fih**-brih-**LAY**-shun)
- ☐ **diuretic** (**dye**-you-**RET**-ick)
- ☐ **electrocardiogram** (ee-**leck**-troh-**KAR**-dee-oh-**gram**)
- ☐ **embolism** (**EM**-boh-lizm)
- ☐ **embolus** (**EM**-boh-lus)
- ☐ **endocarditis** (**en**-doh-kar-**DYE**-tis)
- ☐ **erythrocytes** (eh-**RITH**-roh-sights)
- ☐ **hemoglobin** (**hee**-moh-**GLOH**-bin)
- ☐ **hemolytic anemia** (**hee**-moh-**LIT**-ick ah-**NEE**-mee-ah)
- ☐ **hemostasis** (**hee**-moh-**STAY**-sis)
- ☐ **ischemic heart disease** (iss-**KEE**-mick)
- ☐ **leukemia** (loo-**KEE**-mee-ah)
- ☐ **leukocytes** (**LOO**-koh-sites)
- ☐ **leukopenia** (**loo**-koh-**PEE**-nee-ah)
- ☐ **megaloblastic anemia** (**MEG**-ah-loh-**blas**-tick ah-**NEE**-mee-ah)
- ☐ **myelodysplastic syndrome** (**my**-eh-loh-dis-**PLAS**-tick **SIN**-drohm)
- ☐ **myocardial infarction** (**my**-oh-**KAR**-dee-al in-**FARK**-shun)
- ☐ **orthostatic hypotension** (**or**-thoh-**STAT**-ick **high**-poh-**TEN**-shun)
- ☐ **paroxysmal atrial tachycardia** (**par**-ock-**SIZ**-mal **tack**-ee-**KAR**-dee-ah)
- ☐ **pericardium** (pehr-ih-**KAR**-dee-um)
- ☐ **pernicious anemia** (per-**NISH**-us ah-**NEE**-mee-ah)
- ☐ **phlebitis** (fleh-**BYE**-tis)
- ☐ **Raynaud's phenomenon** (ray-**NOHZ**)
- ☐ **septicemia** (**sep**-tih-**SEE**-mee-ah)
- ☐ **sickle cell anemia**
- ☐ **tachycardia** (**tack**-ee-**KAR**-dee-ah)
- ☐ **thallium stress test** (**THAL**-ee-um)
- ☐ **thrombocytopenia** (**throm**-boh-**sigh**-toh-**PEE**-nee-ah)
- ☐ **thrombolytic** (**throm**-boh-**LIT**-ick)
- ☐ **thrombosis** (throm-**BOH**-sis)
- ☐ **thrombotic occlusion** (throm-**BOT**-ick ah-**KLOO**-zhun)
- ☐ **thrombus** (**THROM**-bus)
- ☐ **transfusion reaction**
- ☐ **valvulitis** (**val**-view-**LYE**-tis)
- ☐ **varicose veins** (**VAR**-ih-kohs **VAYNS**)
- ☐ **ventricular fibrillation** (ven-**TRICK**-you-ler **fih**-brih-**LAY**-shun)
- ☐ **ventricular tachycardia** (ven-**TRICK**-you-ler **tack**-ee-**KAR**-dee-ah)

OBJECTIVES

On completion of this chapter, you should be able to:

1. Describe the heart in terms of chambers, valves, blood flow, heartbeat, and blood supply.
2. Differentiate among the three different types of blood vessels and describe the major function of each.
3. Identify the major components of blood and the major functions of each component.
4. State the difference between pulmonary and systemic circulation.
5. Recognize, define, spell, and pronounce the terms related to the pathology and the diagnostic and treatment procedures of the cardiovascular system.

FUNCTIONS OF THE CARDIOVASCULAR SYSTEM

The **cardiovascular system** consists of the heart, blood vessels, and blood. The term *cardiovascular* means pertaining to the heart and blood vessels (**cardi/o** means heart, **vascul** means blood vessels, and **-ar** means pertaining to).

These structures work together to efficiently pump blood to all body tissues.

- Blood is a fluid tissue that transports oxygen and nutrients to the other body tissues.
- Blood returns some waste products from these tissues to the kidneys and carries carbon dioxide back to the lungs.
- Blood cells also play important roles in the immune system, discussed in Chapter 6, and in the endocrine system, discussed in Chapter 13.

STRUCTURES OF THE CARDIOVASCULAR SYSTEM

The major structures of the cardiovascular system are the heart, blood vessels, and blood.

The Heart

The **heart** is a hollow, muscular organ located between the lungs. It is a very effective pump that furnishes the power to maintain the blood flow needed throughout the entire body (Figures 5.1 and 5.2). The pointed lower end of the heart is known as the *apex*.

The Pericardium

The **pericardium** (pehr-ih-**KAR**-dee-um), also known as the *pericardial sac*, is the double-walled membranous sac that encloses the heart (**peri-** means surrounding, **cardi** means heart, and **-um** is a singular noun ending). *Membranous* means pertaining to membrane, which is a thin layer of pliable tissue that covers or encloses a body part.

- The *parietal pericardium* is the tough outer layer that forms a fibrous sac that surrounds and protects the heart.
- The *visceral pericardium*, which is the inner layer of the pericardium, also forms the outer layer of the heart. When referred to as the outer layer of the heart, it is known as the epicardium (see Figure 5.3).
- *Pericardial fluid* is found between these two layers, where it acts as a lubricant to prevent friction when the heart beats.

The Walls of the Heart

The walls of the heart are made up of three layers: the epicardium, myocardium, and endocardium (Figure 5.3).

- The **epicardium** (**ep**-ih-**KAR**-dee-um) is the external layer of the heart and the inner layer of the pericardium (**epi-** means upon, **cardi** means heart, and **-um** is a singular noun ending).
- The **myocardium** (my-oh-**KAR**-dee-um), also known as *myocardial muscle*, is the middle and thickest of the heart's three layers and consists of specialized cardiac muscle tissue (**my/o** means muscle, **cardi** means heart, and **-um** is a singular noun ending). The constant contraction and relaxation of this muscle creates the pumping movement that maintains the flow of blood throughout the body. This muscle tissue is discussed in Chapter 4.
- The **endocardium** (**en**-doh-**KAR**-dee-um), which consists of epithelial tissue, is the inner lining of the heart (**endo-** means within, **cardi** means heart, and **-um** is a

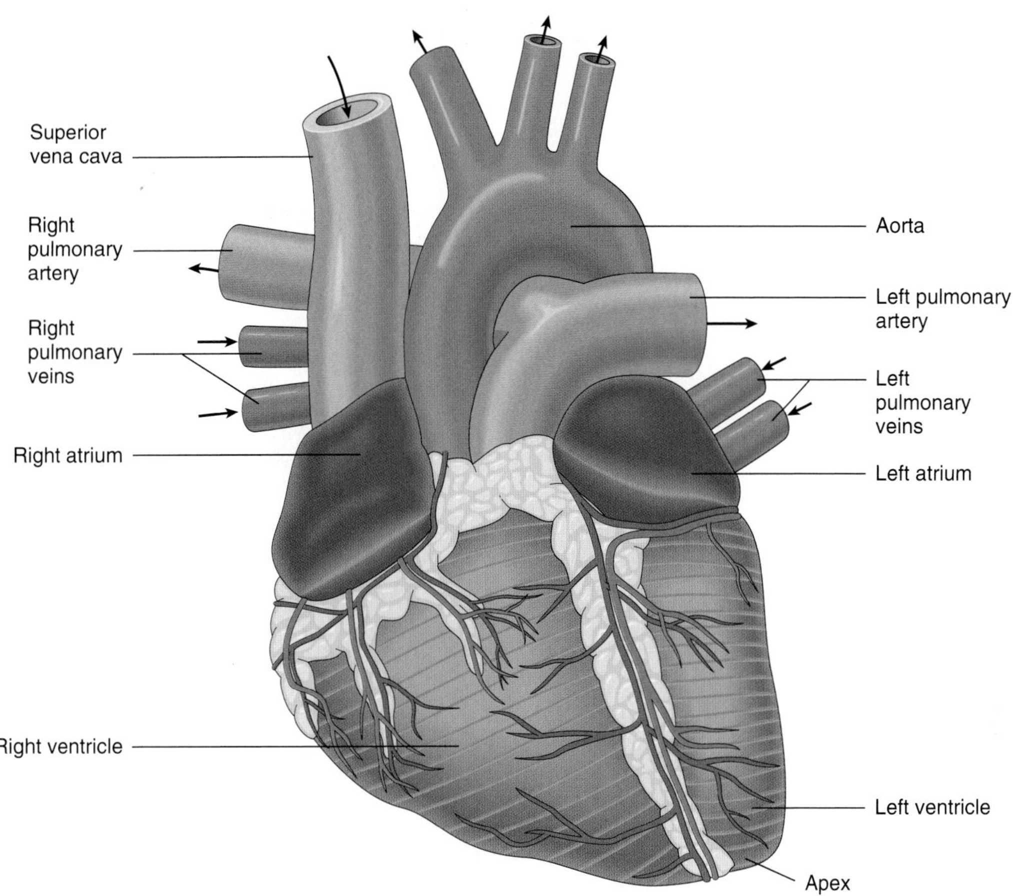

FIGURE 5.1 Anterior external view of the heart.

singular noun ending). This surface comes into direct contact with the blood as it is being pumped through the heart.

Blood Supply to the Myocardium

The myocardium, which beats constantly, must have a continuous supply of oxygen and nutrients plus prompt waste removal in order to survive. If for any reason this blood supply is disrupted, the myocardium in the affected area dies.

The **coronary arteries** (**KOR**-uh-**nerr**-ee), which supply oxygen-rich blood to the myocardium, are shown in red in Figure 5.4. The veins, which are shown here in blue, remove waste products from the myocardium.

The Chambers of the Heart

The heart is divided into left and right sides. Each side is subdivided to form the four chambers of the heart (see Figure 5.2).

- The **atria** (**AY**-tree-ah) are the two upper chambers of the heart. They are the receiving chambers, and all blood vessels coming into the heart enter here (singular, *atrium*).
- The atria are separated by the *interatrial septum*. A *septum* is a wall that separates two chambers.
- The **ventricles** (**VEN**-trih-kuhls) are the two lower chambers of the heart. They are the pumping chambers, and all blood vessels leaving the heart emerge from the ventricles. A *ventricle* is defined as a normal hollow chamber of the heart or the brain (see Chapter 10).
- The ventricles of the heart, which are separated by the *interventricular septum*, are the pumping chambers (**inter-** means between, **ventricul** means ventricle, and **-ar** means pertaining to). The walls of the ventricles are thicker than those of the atria because the ventricles must pump blood throughout the body.

The Valves of the Heart

The flow of blood through the heart is controlled by four valves: the tricuspid, pulmonary semilunar, mitral, and aortic semilunar valves. If any of these valves is not working correctly, blood does not flow properly through the heart

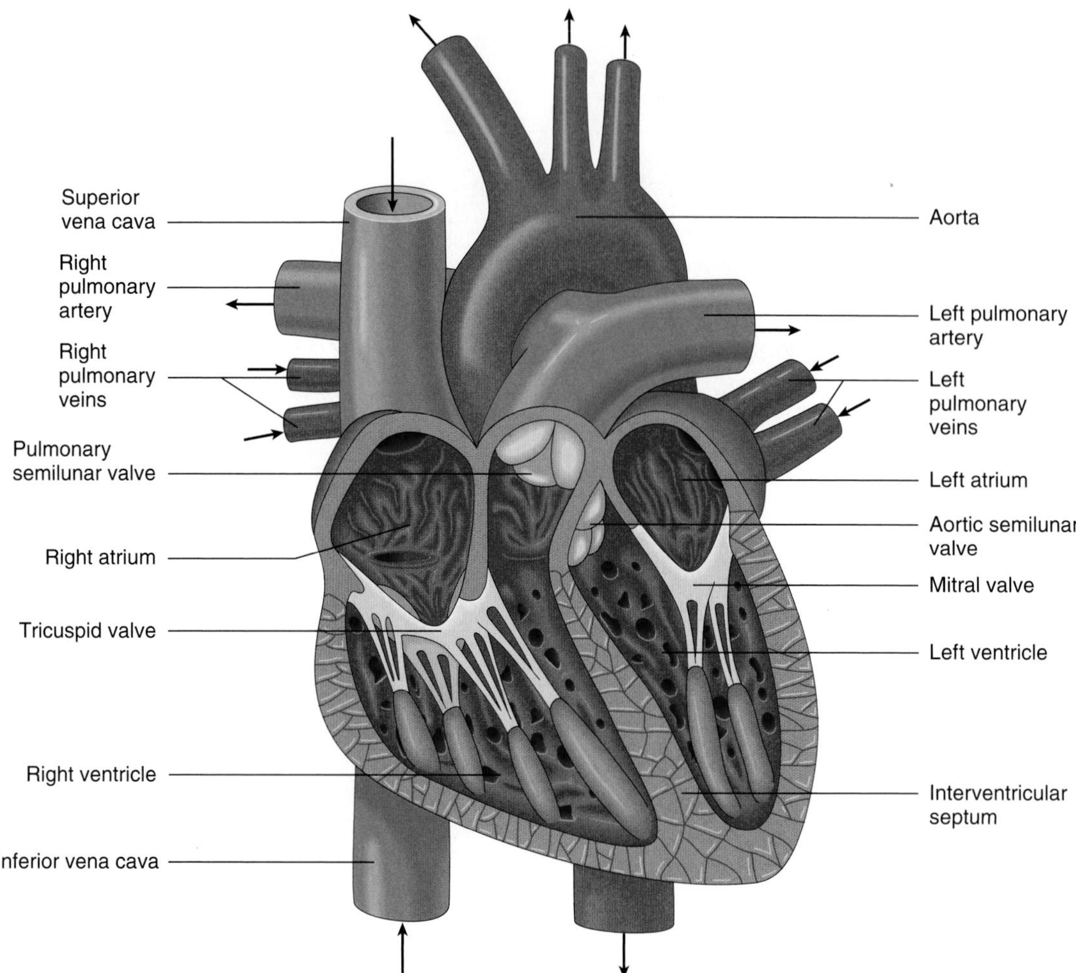

FIGURE 5.2 Anterior cross-section view of the heart.

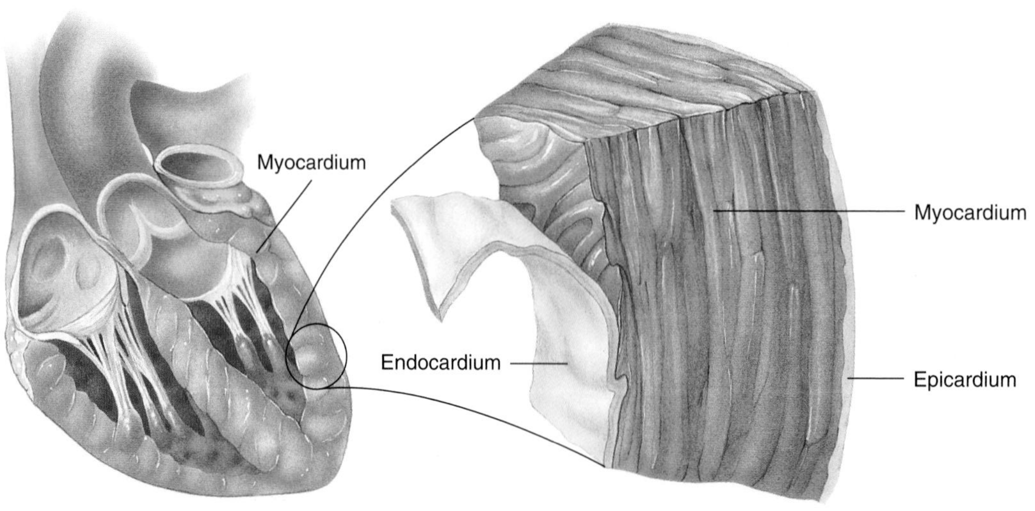

FIGURE 5.3 A simplified view of the tissues of the heart walls.

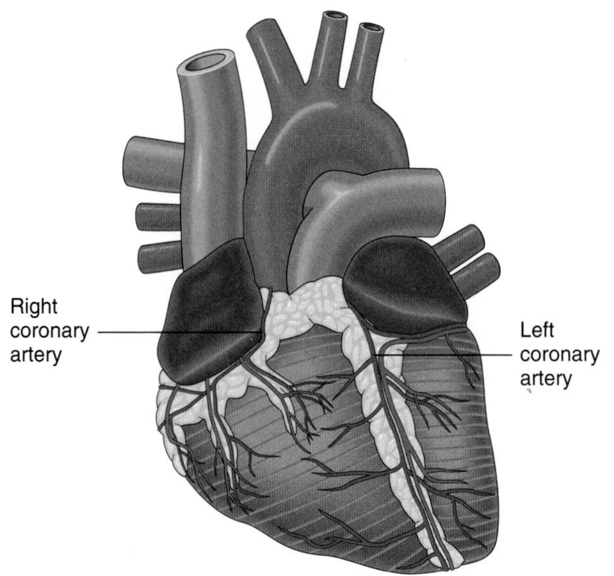

FIGURE 5.4 The coronary arteries supply blood to the myocardium.

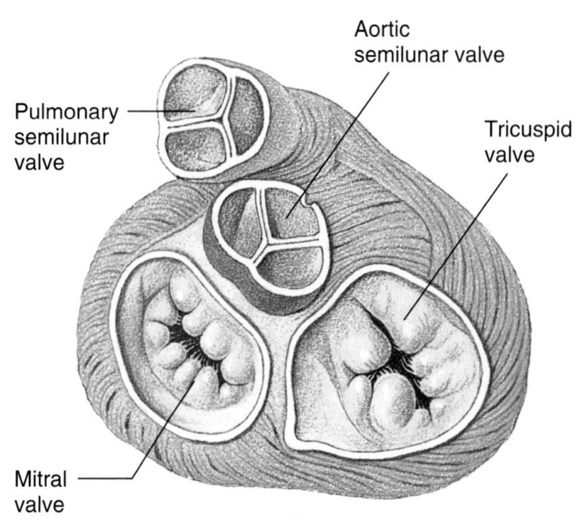

FIGURE 5.5 The valves of the heart. This is viewed from above with the atria removed.

and cannot be pumped effectively to all parts of the body (Figures 5.2 and 5.5).

- The **tricuspid valve** (try-**KUS**-pid) controls the opening between the right atrium and the right ventricle. *Tricuspid* means having three cusps (points), which describes the shape of this valve.
- The **pulmonary semilunar valve** (**sem**-ee-**LOO**-nar) is located between the right ventricle and the pulmonary artery. *Pulmonary* means pertaining to the lungs, and *semilunar* means half-moon; this valve is shaped like a half-moon.
- The **mitral valve** (**MY**-tral), also known as the *bicuspid valve*, is located between the left atrium and left ventricle. *Mitral* means shaped like a bishop's miter (hat). *Bicuspid* means having two cusps (points), which describes the shape of this valve.
- The **aortic semilunar valve** (ay-**OR**-tick **sem**-ee-**LOO**-nar) is located between the left ventricle and the aorta. *Aortic* means pertaining to the aorta, and *semilunar* means half-moon.
- The flow of blood through the heart is summarized in Table 5.1. The red arrows indicate oxygenated blood,

TABLE 5.1

Blood Flow Through the Heart

↓	The **right atrium** (RA) receives oxygen-poor blood from all tissues, except the lungs, through the superior and inferior venae cavae. Blood flows out of the RA through the tricuspid valve into the right ventricle.
↓	The **right ventricle** (RV) pumps the oxygen-poor blood through the pulmonary semilunar valve and into the pulmonary artery, which carries it to the lungs.
↓	The **left atrium** (LA) receives oxygen-rich blood from the lungs through the four pulmonary veins. The blood flows out of the LA, through the mitral valve, and into the left ventricle.
↓	**The left ventricle** (LV) receives oxygen-rich blood from the left atrium. Blood flows out of the LV through the aortic semilunar valve and into the aorta, which carries it to all parts of the body, except the lungs.
↓	Oxygen-poor blood is returned by the venae cavae to the right atrium and the cycle continues.

and blue arrows indicate deoxygenated blood. *Oxygenated* means oxygen-rich or containing an adequate supply of oxygen. *Deoxygenated* means oxygen-poor or not yet containing an adequate supply of oxygen.

Systemic and Pulmonary Circulation

Blood is pumped through the systemic and pulmonary circulation systems. Together these systems allow blood to bring oxygen to the cells and to remove waste products (Figure 5.6).

Pulmonary Circulation

Pulmonary circulation is the flow of blood only between the heart and lungs.

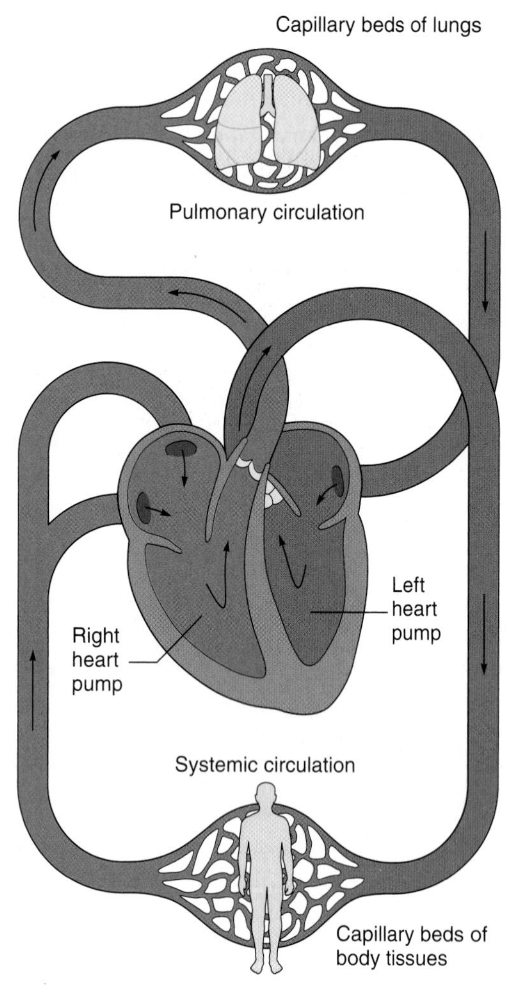

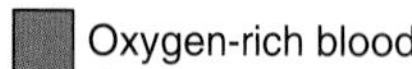

FIGURE 5.6 Systemic and pulmonary blood circulation.

- The **pulmonary arteries** carry deoxygenated blood out of the right ventricle and into the lungs. This is the only place in the body where deoxygenated blood is carried by arteries instead of veins.
- In the lungs, carbon dioxide from the body is exchanged for oxygen from the inhaled air.
- The **pulmonary veins** carry the oxygenated blood from the lungs into the left atrium of the heart. This is the only place in the body where veins carry oxygenated blood.

Systemic Circulation

Systemic circulation includes the flow of blood to all parts of the body *except* the lungs.

- Oxygenated blood flows out of the left ventricle and into arterial circulation.
- The veins carry deoxygenated blood into the right atrium.
- From here, the blood flows into the pulmonary circulation before being pumped out of the heart into the arteries again.

The Heartbeat

To pump blood effectively throughout the body, the contraction and relaxation (beating) of the heart must occur in exactly the correct sequence.

- The rate and regularity of the heart beat is determined by *electrical impulses* from nerves that stimulate the myocardium of the chambers of the heart.
- Also known as the *conduction system*, these electrical impulses are controlled by the sinoatrial (SA) node, atrioventricular (AV) node, and bundle of His (Figure 5.7).

The Sinoatrial Node

- The **sinoatrial node** (**sigh**-noh-**AY**-tree-ahl), which is often referred to as the *SA node*, is located in the posterior wall of the right atrium near the entrance of the superior vena cava (see Figure 5.7).
- The SA node establishes the basic rhythm and rate of the heartbeat. For this reason, it is known as the *natural pacemaker* of the heart.
- Electrical impulses from the SA node start each wave of muscle contraction in the heart.
- The impulse in the right atrium spreads over the muscles of both atria, causing them to contract simultaneously. This contraction forces blood into the ventricles.

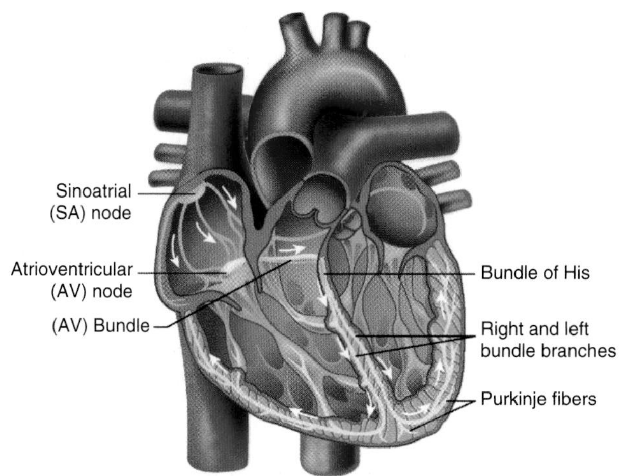

FIGURE 5.7 An electrical impulse from the SA node travels to the AV node and causes the ventricle to contract.

The Atrioventricular Node

- The impulses from the SA node also travel to the **atrioventricular node** (**ay**-tree-oh-ven-**TRICK**-you-lahr), which is also known as the *AV node*.
- The AV node is located on the floor of the right atrium near the interatrial septum (see Figure 5.7). From here, it transmits the electrical impulses onward to the bundle of His.

The Bundle of His

- The **bundle of His (HISS)** is a group of fibers located within the interventricular septum. These fibers carry an electrical impulse to ensure the sequence of the heart contractions (see Figure 5.7). These electrical impulses travel onward to the right and left ventricles and the Purkinje fibers.
- **Purkinje fibers** (per-**KIN**-jee) are specialized conductive fibers located within the walls of the ventricles. These fibers relay the electrical impulses to the cells of the ventricles, and it is this stimulation that causes the ventricles to contract. This contraction of the ventricles forces blood out of the heart and into the aorta and pulmonary arteries (see Figure 5.7).

Electrical Waves

The activities of the electrical conduction system of the heart can be visualized as wave movements on a monitor or an electrocardiogram (Figure 5.8).

- The *P wave* is due to the stimulation (contraction) of the atria.
- The *QRS complex* shows the stimulation (contraction) of the ventricles. The atria relax as the ventricles contract.

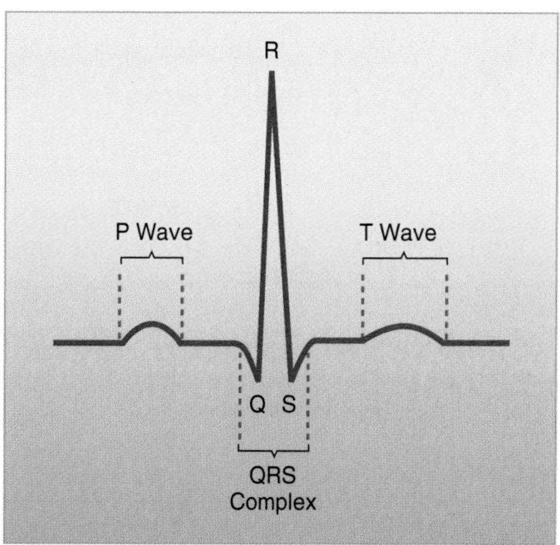

FIGURE 5.8 The waves of contraction and relaxation of the heart can be visualized on a monitor or as an electrocardiogram (EKG).

- The *T wave* is the recovery (relaxation) of the ventricles.

THE BLOOD VESSELS

There are three major types of blood vessels: arteries, capillaries, and veins. These vessels form the arterial and venous circulatory systems (Figures 5.9 and 5.10).

Arteries

- The **arteries** are large blood vessels that carry blood away from the heart to all regions of the body.
- The walls of the arteries are composed of three layers. This structure makes them muscular and elastic so they can expand and contract with the pumping beat of the heart. The term *endarterial* means pertaining to the inner portion of an artery or within an artery.
- *Arterial blood* is bright red in color because it is oxygen-rich. It is the pumping action of the heart that causes blood to spurt out when an artery is cut.
- The **aorta** (ay-**OR**-tah), which is the largest blood vessel in the body, is the main trunk of the arterial system and begins from the left ventricle of the heart (Figures 5.1 and 5.9).
- The **carotid arteries** (kah-**ROT**-id) are the major arteries that carry blood upward to the head. The *common carotid* located on each side of the neck divides into the *internal carotid*, which brings oxygen-rich blood to the brain, and the *external carotid*,

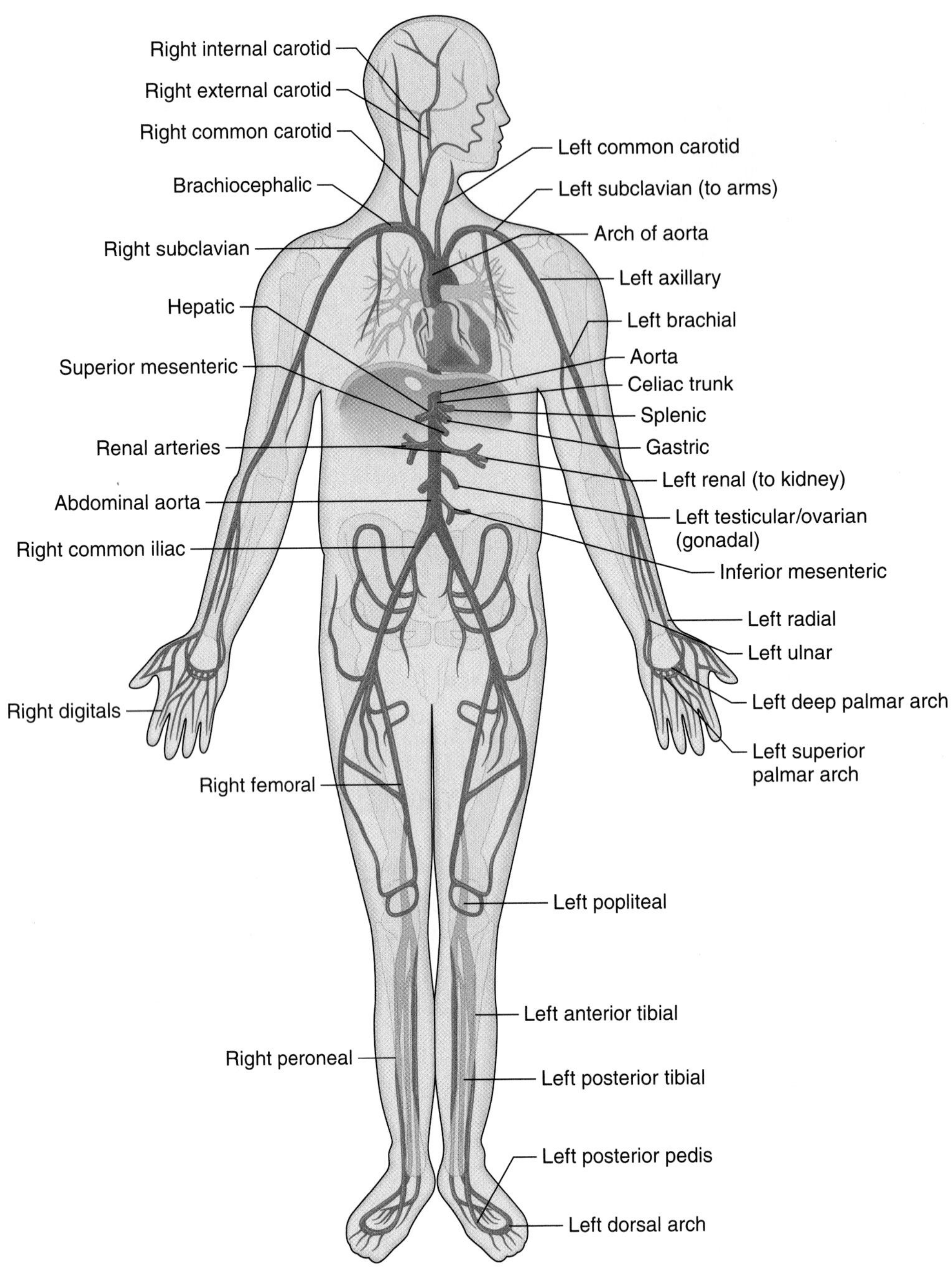

FIGURE 5.9 Anterior view of arterial circulation.

which brings blood to the face. Any disruption in this flow of blood can result in a stroke or other brain damage.

- The **arterioles** (ar-**TEE**-ree-ohlz) are the smaller, thinner branches of arteries that carry blood to the capillaries.

Veins

Veins form a low-pressure collecting system to return oxygen-poor blood to the heart (Figures 5.10 and 5.11).

- The walls of the veins are thinner and less elastic than those of the arteries.
- Veins have valves that enable blood to flow only toward the heart and prevent it from flowing away from the heart (see Figure 5.11).
- **Venules** (**VEN**-youls) are smallest veins that join to form the larger veins.
- *Superficial veins* are located near the body surface. *Deep veins* are located within the tissues and away from the body surface.

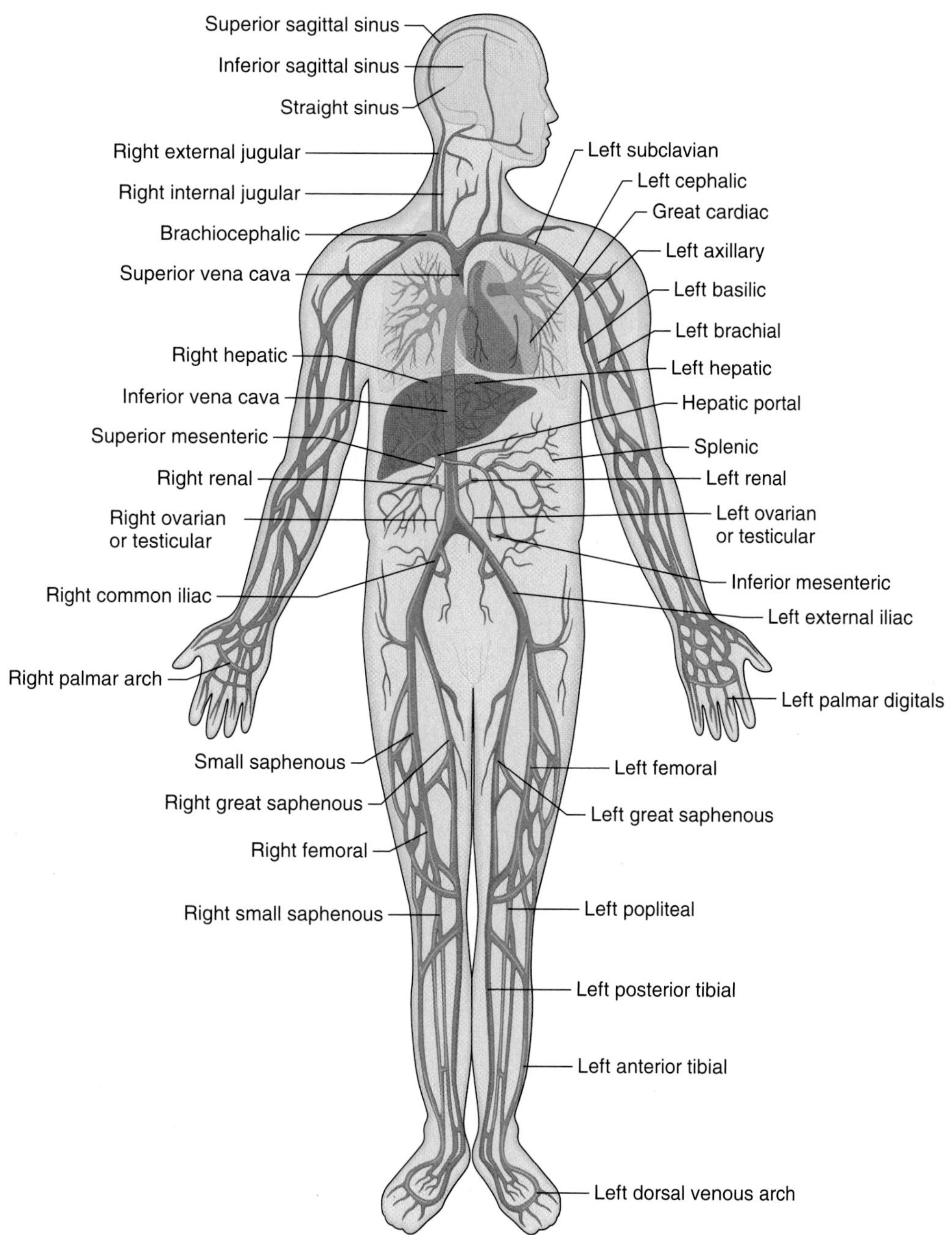

FIGURE 5.10 Anterior view of venous circulation.

The Venae Cavae

- The **venae cavae** (**VEE**-nee **KAY**-vee) are the two largest veins in the body. These are the veins that return blood into the heart (singular, *vena cava*).
- The *superior vena cava* transports blood from the upper portion of the body to the heart (Figures 5.1 and 5.2).
- The *inferior vena cava* transports blood from the lower portion of the body to the heart (Figure 5.2).

Capillaries

Capillaries, which are only one epithelial cell in thickness, are the smallest blood vessels in the body. The capillaries form networks of expanded vascular beds that have the important role of delivering oxygen and nutrients to the cells of the tissues (Figure 5.12). *Vascular* means pertaining to blood vessels.

- Arterioles deliver blood to the capillaries. Here the rate of flow of arterial blood slows as it enters one end of the bed.

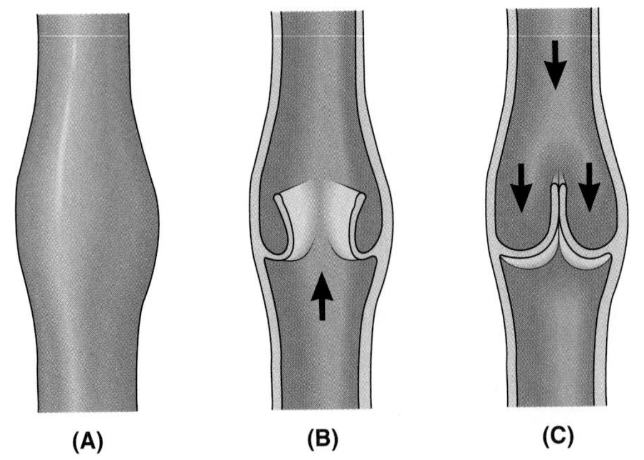

FIGURE 5.11 Veins contain valves to prevent the backward flow of blood. (A) External view of the vein shows wider area of valve. (B) Internal view with the valve open as blood flows through it toward the heart. (C) Internal view with the valve closed to prevent the back flow of blood.

- The capillaries further slow the flow of blood to allow plasma to flow into the tissues for the exchange of oxygen, nutrients, and waste materials with the surrounding cells.
- Ninety percent of this fluid, which is now oxygen-poor, leaves the opposite end of the capillary bed through the venules, and it continues to flow as venous blood that increases in speed as it begins its return journey to the heart. The remaining 10% of this fluid is left behind in the tissues and becomes lymph (see Chapter 6).

Pulse and Blood Pressure

- The **pulse** is the rhythmic pressure against the walls of an artery caused by the contraction of the heart. The *pulse rate* is discussed in Chapter 15.
- **Blood pressure** is the measurement of the amount of systolic and diastolic pressure exerted against the walls of the arteries. How to record blood pressure is discussed in Chapter 15.
- **Systolic pressure** (sis-**TOL**-ick), which occurs when the ventricles contract, is the highest pressure against the walls of an artery. The term *systole* means contraction of the heart, and *systolic* means pertaining to this contraction phase.
- **Diastolic pressure** (dye-ah-**STOL**-ick), which occurs when the ventricles are relaxed, is the lowest pressure against the walls of an artery. The term *diastole* means relaxation of the heart, and *diastolic* means pertaining to this relaxation phase.

BLOOD

Blood is the fluid tissue in the body. It is composed of 55% liquid plasma and 45% formed elements. As you study these elements, refer to Figure 5.13.

Plasma

Plasma (**PLAZ**-mah) is a straw-colored fluid that contains nutrients, hormones, and waste products. Plasma is 91% water. The remaining 9% consists mainly of proteins, including the clotting proteins.

- **Fibrinogen** (figh-**BRIN**-oh-jen) and **prothrombin** (proh-**THROM**-bin) are the clotting proteins found in plasma. They have an important role in clot formation to control bleeding.
- **Serum** (**SEER**-um) is plasma fluid after the blood cells and the clotting proteins have been removed.

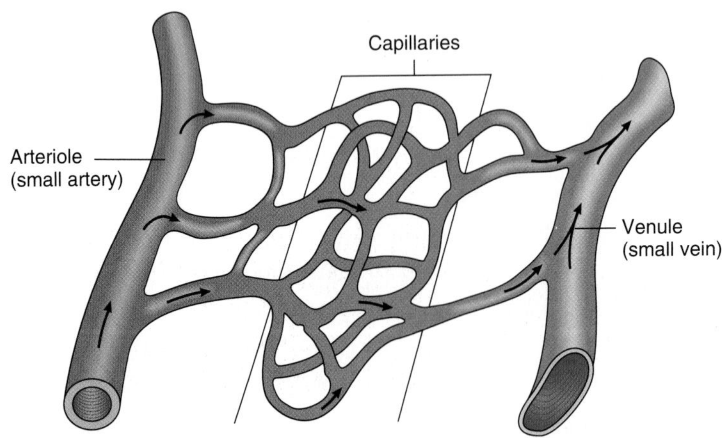

FIGURE 5.12 Oxygen-rich arterial blood is delivered by arterioles to the capillaries. After the oxygen has been extracted, the oxygen-poor blood is returned to circulation as venous blood.

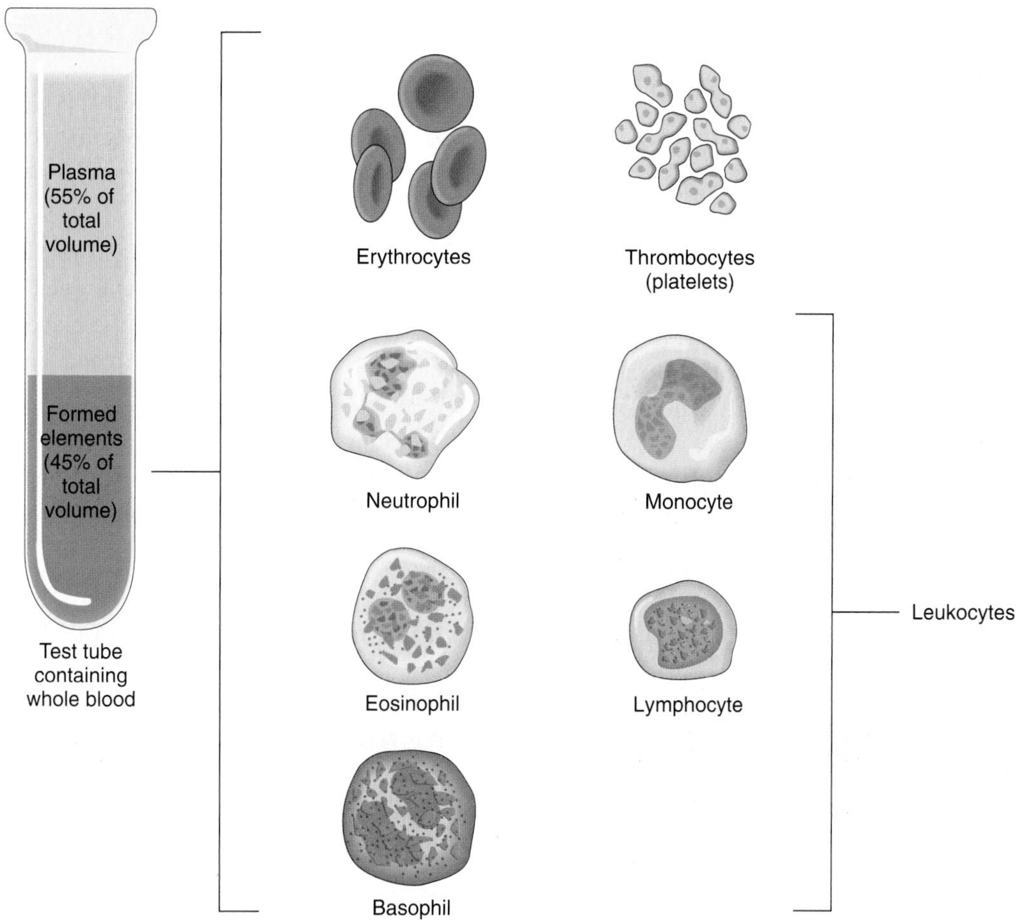

FIGURE 5.13 The major fluid and formed components of blood.

Formed Elements of the Blood

The formed elements of the blood include the erythrocytes, leukocytes, and thrombocytes.

Erythrocytes

Erythrocytes (eh-**RITH**-roh-sights), also known as *red blood cells* (RBC), are mature red blood cells produced by the red bone marrow (**erythr/o** means red, and **-cytes** means cells). The primary role of these cells is to transport oxygen to the tissues. This oxygen is transported by the **hemoglobin** (**hee**-moh-**GLOH**-bin), which is the iron-containing pigment of the erythrocytes.

Leukocytes

Leukocytes (**LOO**-koh-sites), also known as *white blood cells* (WBC), are the blood cells involved in defending the body against infective organisms and foreign substances (**leuk/o** means white, and **-cytes** means cells). The following are the major groups of leukocytes:

- **Neutrophils** (**NEW**-troh-fills), which are formed in red bone marrow, are the most common type of WBC. Through phagocytosis, neutrophils play a major role in the immune system's defense against pathogens including bacteria, viruses, and fungi. *Phagocytosis* is the process of destroying pathogens by surrounding and swallowing them.
- **Basophils** (**BAY**-soh-fills), which are formed in red bone marrow, are the least common type of WBC. Basophils are responsible for the symptoms of allergies.
- **Eosinophils** (**ee**-oh-**SIN**-oh-fills) are formed in red bone marrow and then migrate to tissues throughout the body. Eosinophils destroy parasitic organisms and play a major role in allergic reactions.
- **Lymphocytes** (**LIM**-foh-sights) are formed in red bone marrow, lymph nodes, and the spleen (**lymph/o** means lymph, and **-cytes** means cells). Lymphocytes identify foreign substances and germs (bacteria or viruses) in the body and produce antibodies that

specifically target them. Lymphocytes are discussed further in Chapter 6.

- **Monocytes** (**MON**-oh-sights) are formed in red bone marrow, lymph nodes, and the spleen. Through phagocytosis, monocytes provide immunological defenses against many infectious organisms.

Thrombocytes

Thrombocytes (**THROM**-boh-sights), also known as *platelets*, are the smallest formed elements of the blood (**thromb/o** means clot, and **-cytes** means cells). The throm-bocytes play an important role in the clotting of blood.

- When a blood vessel is damaged, the thrombocytes are activated and become sticky.
- This action causes the thrombocytes to clump together to form a clot that stops the bleeding.

Blood Types

Blood types are classified according to the presence, or absence, of certain antigens. An *antigen* is any substance that the body regards as being foreign.

The four major blood types are **A**, **AB**, **B**, and **O**. The A, AB, and B groups are based on the presence of the A and/or B antigens on the red blood cells. In type O blood, both antigens are absent.

The Rh Factor

The **Rh factor** refers to the presence, or absence of the Rh antigen on red blood cells. Because this antigen was first found in Rhesus monkeys, this factor was named for them.

- About 85% of Americans are *Rh positive* (Rh+). This means that these individuals *have* the Rh antigen.
- The remaining 15% are *Rh negative* (Rh–). This means that these individuals *do not have* the Rh antigen.
- The Rh factor is an important consideration in cross-matching blood for transfusions (see Chapter 15).
- The Rh factor can cause difficulties when an Rh-positive infant is born to an Rh-negative mother (see Chapter 14).

Blood Gases

Blood gases are gases that are normally dissolved in the liquid portion of blood. The major blood gases are *oxygen* (O_2), *carbon dioxide* (CO_2), and *nitrogen* (N_2).

MEDICAL SPECIALTIES RELATED TO THE CARDIOVASCULAR SYSTEM

- A **cardiologist** (**kar**-dee-**OL**-oh-jist) is a physician who specializes in diagnosing and treating abnormalities, diseases, and disorders of the heart (**cardi** means heart, and **-ologist** means specialist).
- A **hematologist** (**hee**-mah-**TOL**-oh-jist) is a physician who specializes in diagnosing and treating abnormalities, diseases, and disorders of the blood and blood-forming tissues (**hemat** means blood, and **-ologist** means specialist).
- A **vascular surgeon** is a physician who specializes in the diagnosis, medical management, and surgical treatment of disorders of the blood vessels.

PATHOLOGY OF THE CARDIOVASCULAR SYSTEM

Disorders of the heart can be present from before birth or develop at any time throughout life.

Congenital Heart Defects

Congenital heart defects are structural abnormalities caused by the failure of the heart to develop normally before birth (Figure 5.14). *Congenital* means present at birth. Some congenital heart defects are apparent at birth, whereas others may not be detected until later in life.

Coronary Artery Disease

Coronary artery disease is atherosclerosis of the coronary arteries that reduces the blood supply to the heart muscle. This creates an insufficient supply of oxygen that can cause angina (pain), a myocardial infarction (heart attack), or death. *End-stage coronary artery disease* is characterized by unrelenting angina pain and a severely limited lifestyle.

Atherosclerosis

Atherosclerosis (**ath**-er-**oh**-skleh-**ROH**-sis) is hardening and narrowing of the arteries caused by a buildup of cholesterol plaque on the interior walls of the arteries (**ather/o** means plaque or fatty substance, and **-sclerosis** means abnormal hardening) (Figures 5.14 and 5.15).

- This type of **plaque** (**PLACK**), which is found within the lumen of an artery, is a fatty deposit that is similar to the buildup of rust inside a pipe. (This substance is not the same as *dental plaque*, which is discussed in Chapter 8.)

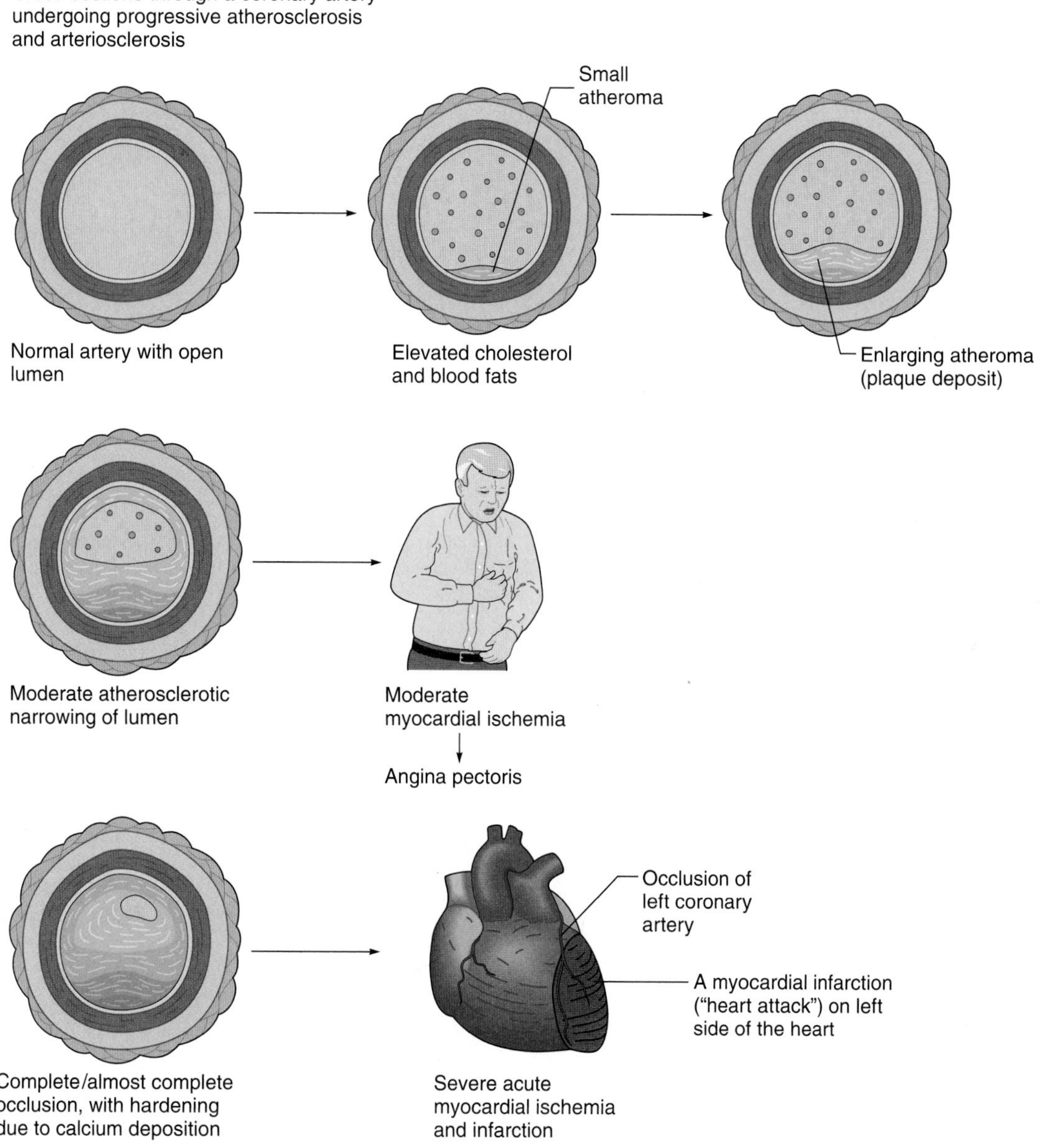

FIGURE 5.14 The progression of coronary heart disease resulting in a myocardial infarction.

- The plaque can protrude outward into the lumen of the vessel or protrude inward into the wall of the vessel. The *lumen* is the opening within these vessels through which the blood flows.
- An **atheroma** (**ath**-er-**OH**-mah), which is a characteristic of atherosclerosis, is a deposit of plaque on or within the arterial wall (**ather** means plaque, and **-oma** means tumor).

Ischemic Heart Disease

Ischemic heart disease (iss-**KEE**-mick) is a group of cardiac disabilities resulting from an insufficient supply of oxygenated blood to the heart. These diseases are usually associated with coronary artery disease. *Ischemic* means pertaining to the disruption of the blood supply.

- **Ischemia** (iss-**KEE**-mee-ah) is a condition in which there is an insufficient oxygen supply due to a restricted blood flow by to a part of the body (**isch** means to hold back, and **-emia** means blood). For example, *cardiac ischemia* is the lack of blood flow and oxygen to the heart muscle.

Angina

Angina (an-**JIH**-nuh), also known as *angina pectoris*, is a condition of episodes of severe chest pain due to inadequate blood flow to the myocardium. These episodes are due to ischemia of the heart muscle.

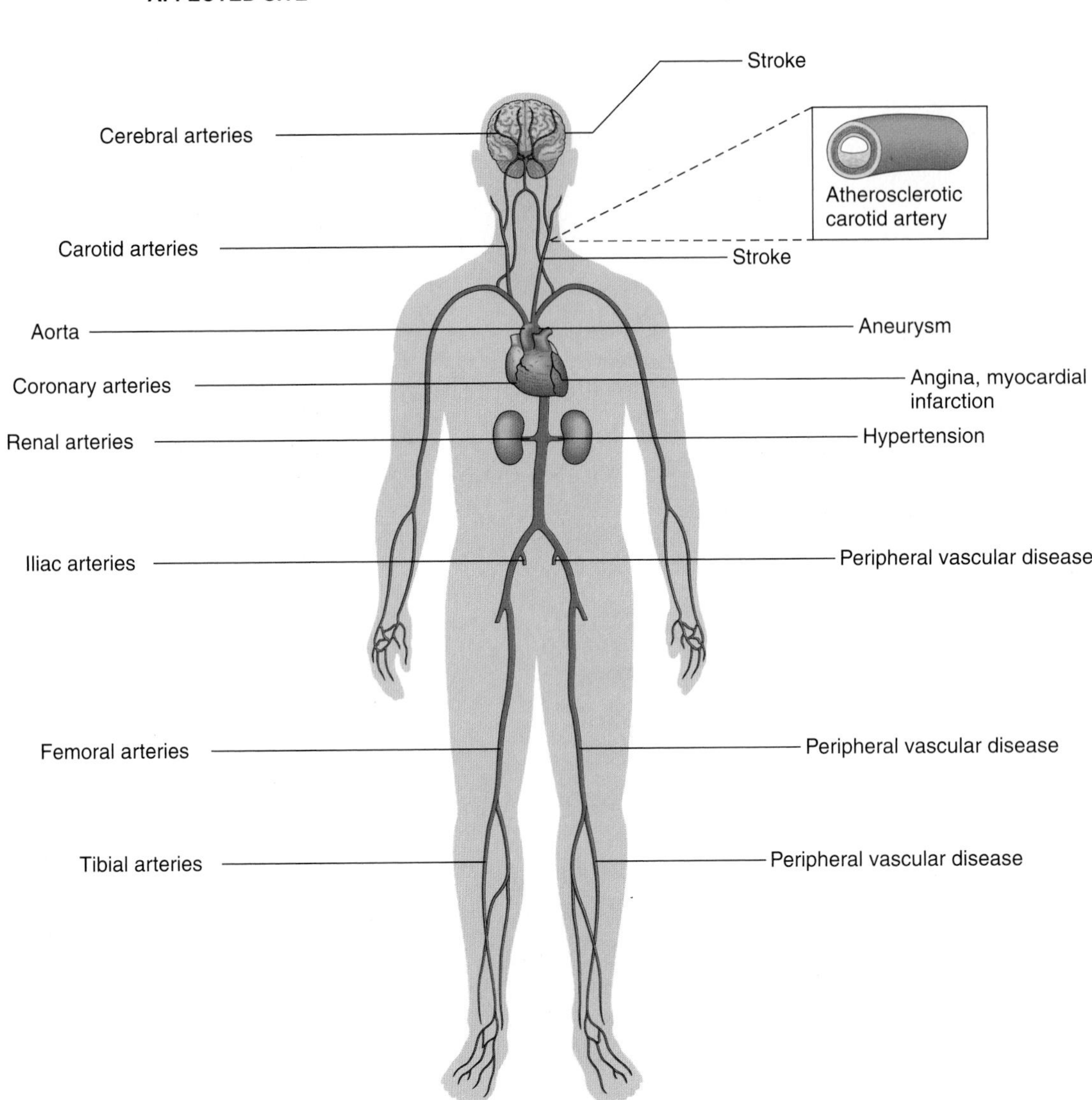

FIGURE 5.15 The sites affected by atherosclerosis (left column) and the potential complications of this condition (right column).

Myocardial Infarction

A **myocardial infarction** (**my**-oh-**KAR**-dee-al in-**FARK**-shun), also known as a *heart attack*, is the occlusion of one or more coronary arteries caused by plaque buildup. As used here, *occlusion* means total blockage.

- *Infarction* means a sudden insufficiency of blood. An *infarct* is a localized area of dead tissue caused by a lack of blood.
- This damage to the myocardium impairs the heart's ability to pump blood throughout the body (see Figure 5.14).
- The most frequently recognized symptoms of a myocardial infarction include pain in the middle of the chest that may spread to the back, jaw, or left arm. Many individuals having a heart attack have mild symptoms or none at all.

Heart Failure

Heart failure, which is also referred to as *congestive heart failure*, occurs most commonly in the elderly. This is a chronic condition in which the heart is unable to pump out all of the blood that it receives. The decreased pumping action causes congestion. *Congestion* means a fluid buildup (Figure 5.16).

- *Left-sided heart failure*, which is also known as *pulmonary edema*, causes an accumulation of fluid in

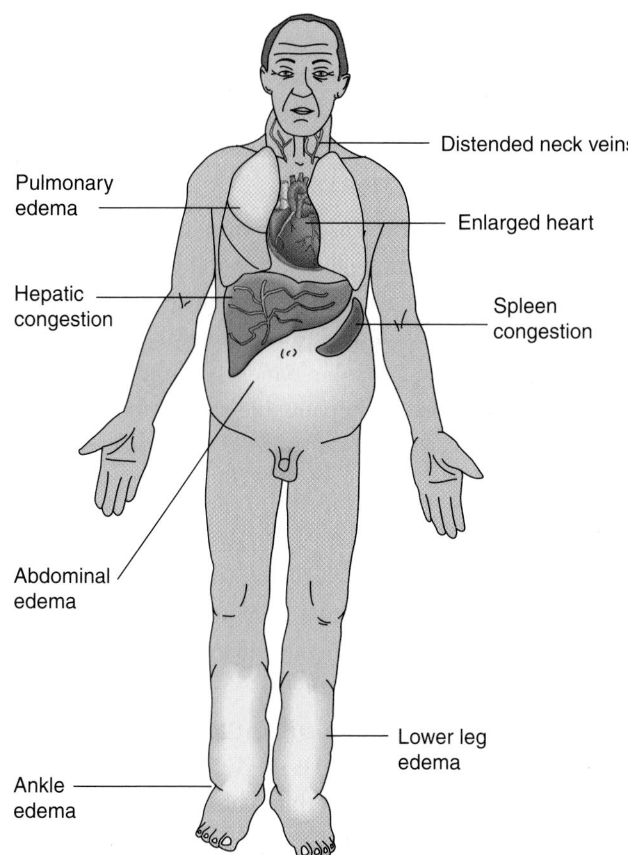

FIGURE 5.16 Signs of congestive heart failure.

the lungs. This occurs because the left side of the heart is not efficiently pumping blood to and from the lungs.

- *Right-sided heart failure* causes fluid buildup beginning with the feet and legs. This swelling can also affect the liver, gastrointestinal tract, or arms. This occurs because the right side of the heart is not efficiently pumping blood to and from the rest of the body, with the exception of the lungs.
- **Cardiomegaly** (**kar**-dee-oh-**MEG**-ah-lee) is the abnormal enlargement of the heart that is frequently associated with heart failure when the heart enlarges in an effort to compensate for the loss of its pumping ability (**cardi/o** means heart, and **-megaly** means abnormal enlargement).

Carditis

Carditis (kar-**DYE**-tis) is an inflammation of the heart (**card** means heart, and **-itis** means inflammation). Note the spelling of *carditis*: In this term, the word root (combining form) **card/o** is used to avoid having a double *i* when it is joined with the suffix **-itis**.

- **Endocarditis** (**en**-doh-kar-**DYE**-tis) is an inflammation of the inner lining of the heart (**endo-** means within, **card** means heart, and **-itis** means inflammation).
- **Bacterial endocarditis** is an inflammation of the lining or valves of the heart caused by the presence of bacteria in the bloodstream. One cause of this condition is bleeding during dental surgery because it allows bacteria from the mouth to enter the bloodstream.
- **Myocarditis** (**my**-oh-kar-**DYE**-tis) is an inflammation of the myocardium (**my/o** means muscle, **card** means heart, and **-itis** means inflammation). This uncommon condition can develop as a complication of a viral infection.
- **Pericarditis** (**pehr**-ih-kar-**DYE**-tis) is an inflammation of the pericardium that causes an accumulation of fluid within the pericardial sac (**peri-** means surrounding, **card** means heart, and **-itis** means inflammation). This fluid restricts the beating of the heart and reduces the ability of the heart to pump blood throughout the body.

Diseases of the Myocardium

- **Cardiomyopathy** (**kar**-dee-oh-my-**OP**-pah-thee) is the term used to describe all diseases of the heart muscle (**cardi/o** means heart, **my/o** means muscle, and **-pathy** means disease).
- *Dilated cardiomyopathy* is a disease of the heart muscle that causes the heart to become enlarged, and to pump less strongly. The progression of this condition is usually slow and only presents with symptoms when quite advanced. *Dilated* means the expansion of a hollow structure.

Heart Valves

- A **heart murmur** is an abnormal sound heard when listening to the heart or neighboring large blood vessels. Heart murmurs are most often caused by defective heart valves.
- **Valvulitis** (**val**-view-**LYE**-tis) is an inflammation of a heart valve (**valvul** means valve, and **-itis** means inflammation).
- **Valvular prolapse** (**VAL**-voo-lar proh-**LAPS**) is the abnormal protrusion of a heart valve that results in the inability of the valve to close completely (**valvul** means valve, and **-ar** means pertaining to). *Prolapse* means the falling or dropping down of an organ or internal

part. This condition is named for the affected valve, such as a *mitral valve prolapse*.

- **Valvular stenosis** (steh-**NOH**-sis) is a condition in which there is narrowing, stiffening, thickening, or blockage of one or more valves of the heart. *Stenosis* is the abnormal narrowing of an opening. These conditions are named for the affected valve, such as *aortic valve stenosis*.

Cardiac Arrest and Arrhythmias

Cardiac arrest is an event in which the heart abruptly stops or develops a very abnormal arrhythmia that prevents it from pumping blood. **Sudden cardiac death** results if treatment is not provided within a few minutes.

The term **arrhythmia** (ah-**RITH**-mee-ah) describes an abnormality, or the loss of the normal rhythm, of the heartbeat.

- **Bradycardia** (**brad**-ee-**KAR**-dee-ah) is an abnormally slow resting heart rate (**brady-** means slow, **card** means heart, and **-ia** means abnormal condition). This term is usually applied to rates less than 60 beats per minute. Bradycardia is the opposite of *tachycardia*.
- **Tachycardia** (**tack**-ee-**KAR**-dee-ah) is an abnormally rapid resting heart rate (**tachy-** means rapid, **card** means heart, and **-ia** means abnormal condition). This term is usually applied to rates greater than 100 beats per minute. Tachycardia is the opposite of *bradycardia*.
- **Palpitation** (**pal**-pih-**TAY**-shun) is a pounding or racing heart with or without irregularity in rhythm. This is associated with certain heart disorders; however, it also occur as part of a panic attack (see Chapter 10).

Atrial and Ventricular Fibrillation

- **Atrial fibrillation**, also known as *A fib*, occurs when the normal rhythmic contractions of the atria are replaced by rapid irregular twitching of the muscular heart wall. This condition causes an irregular and quivering action of the atria (Figure 5.17A). The term *fibrillation* means a fast, uncontrolled heart beat.
- **Paroxysmal atrial tachycardia** (**par**-ock-**SIZ**-mal **tack**-ee-**KAR**-dee-ah), also known as *PAT*, is an episode that begins and ends abruptly during which there are very rapid and regular heartbeats that originate in the atrium (Figure 5.17B). PAT is caused by an abnormality in the body's electrical system. *Paroxysmal* means pertaining to sudden occurrence. Compare with *ventricular tachycardia.*
- **Ventricular fibrillation** (ven-**TRICK**-you-ler **fih**-brih-**LAY**-shun), also known as *V fib*, is the rapid, irregular, and useless contractions of the ventricles. Instead of pumping strongly, the heart muscle quivers ineffectively. This condition is the cause of many sudden cardiac deaths (Figure 5.17C).
- **Ventricular tachycardia**, also known as *V tach*, a very rapid heart beat that begins within the ventricles. This condition is potentially fatal because the heart is beating so rapidly that it is unable to adequately pump blood through the body. For some patients, this condition can be controlled with an implantable cardioverter defibrillator. Compare with *paroxysmal atrial tachycardia.*

Blood Vessels

- **Angiitis** (**an**-jee-**EYE**-tis), also known as *vasculitis*, is the inflammation of a blood or lymph vessel (**angi** means vessel, and **-itis** means inflammation). Note: This term is also spelled *angitis.*
- **Angiostenosis** (**AN**-jee-oh-steh-**NOH**-sis) is the abnormal narrowing of a blood vessel (**angi/o** means vessel, and **-stenosis** means abnormal narrowing).
- A **hemangioma** (hee-**man**-jee-**OH**-mah) is a benign tumor made up of newly formed blood vessels (**hem** means blood, **angi** means blood or lymph vessel, and **-oma** means tumor) (see birthmarks in Chapter 12).
- **Hypoperfusion** (**high**-poh-per-**FYOU**-zhun) is a deficiency of blood passing through an organ or body part. *Perfusion* is the flow of blood through the vessels of an organ.
- **Polyarteritis** (**pol**-ee-**ar**-teh-**RYE**-tis), also known as *polyarteritis nodosa*, is a form of angiitis involving several medium and small arteries at the same time (**poly-** means many, **arter** means artery, and **-itis** mean inflammation). Polyarteritis is a serious blood vessel disease that occurs when certain immune cells attack the affected arteries.

Peripheral Vascular Disease

The term **peripheral vascular disease** refers to disorders of the blood vessels located outside the heart and brain. These disorders usually involve narrowing of the vessels that carry blood to the legs, arms, stomach, or kidneys.

- **Peripheral arterial occlusive disease**, also known as *peripheral artery disease*, is an example of a peripheral vascular disease caused by atherosclerosis. It is a common, and serious, problem affecting more than

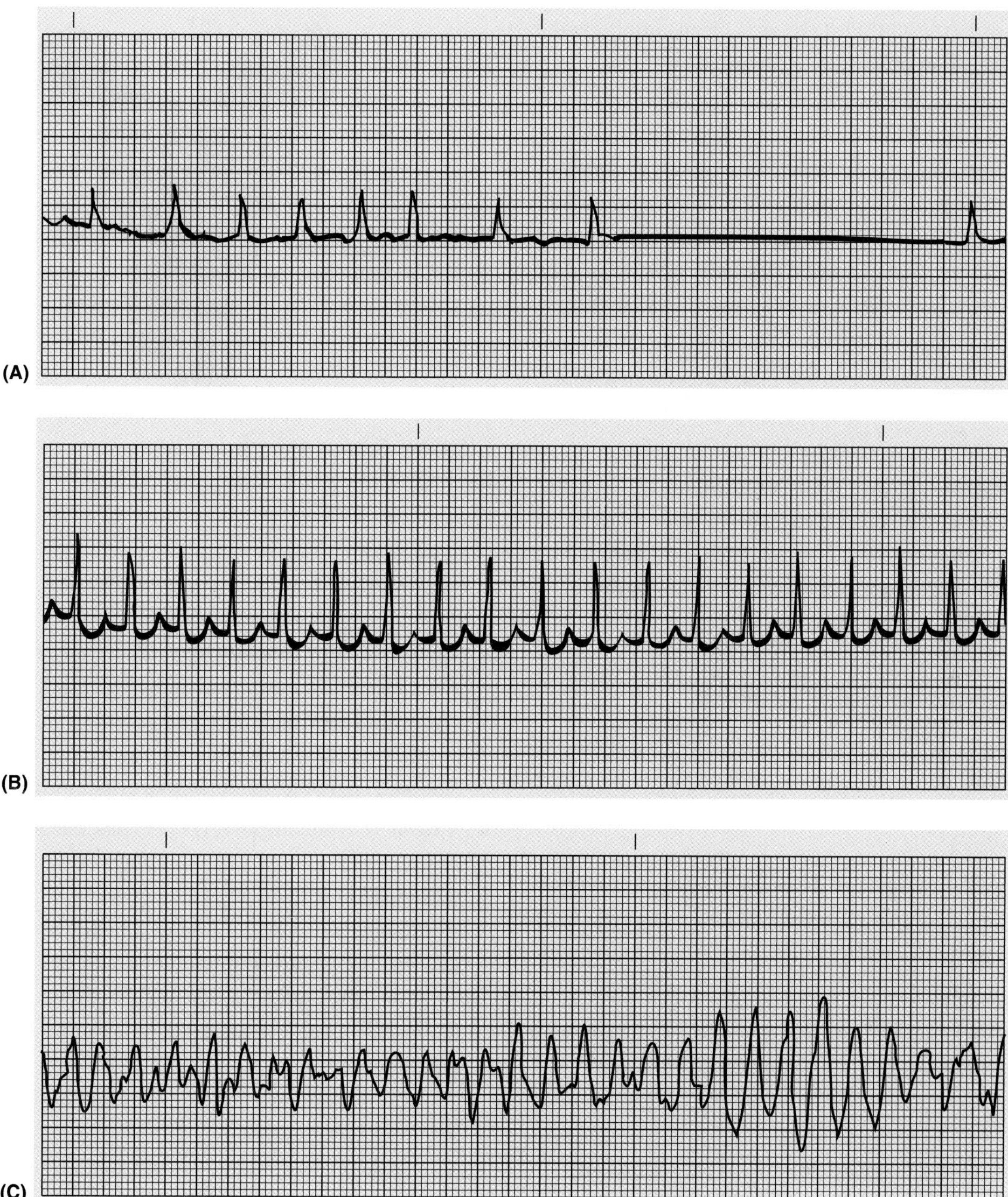

FIGURE 5.17 Electrocardiograms showing disruptions of heart rhythms. (A) Atrial fibrillation. (B) Paroxysmal atrial tachycardia. (C) Ventricular fibrillation.

20% of patients over 70 years of age. Impaired circulation to the extremities and vital organs causes changes in the skin color and temperature, plus intermittent claudication (see Chapter 4).

- **Raynaud's phenomenon** (ray-**NOHZ**) is a peripheral arterial occlusive disease in which intermittent attacks are triggered by cold or stress. The symptoms, which are due to constricted circulation, include pallor (paleness), cyanosis (blue color), and then redness of the fingers and toes.

Arteries

- An **aneurysm** (**AN**-you-rizm) is a localized weak spot, or balloon-like enlargement, of the wall of an artery. The rupture of an aneurysm can be fatal because of the rapid loss of blood. Aneurysms are named for the artery involved such as *aortic aneurysms*, *abdominal aortic aneurysms*, and *popliteal aneurysms*.
- **Arteriosclerosis** (ar-**tee**-ree-oh-skleh-**ROH**-sis), also known as *hardening of the arteries*, is any of a group of

diseases characterized by thickening and the loss of elasticity of arterial walls (**arteri/o** means artery, and **-sclerosis** mean abnormal hardening).

Veins

- **Chronic venous insufficiency**, also known as *venous insufficiency*, is a condition in which venous circulation is inadequate due to partial vein blockage or leakage of venous valves. This condition primarily affects the feet and ankles, and the leakage of venous blood into the tissues causes discoloration of the skin.
- **Phlebitis** (fleh-**BYE**-tis) is the inflammation of a vein (**phleb** means vein, and **-itis** mean inflammation). This usually occurs in a superficial vein (Figure 5.18).
- **Varicose veins** (**VAR**-ih-kohs **VAYNS**) are abnormally swollen veins, usually occurring in the superficial veins of the legs. Varicose veins occur when the valves in the veins malfunction and allow blood to pool in these veins, causing them to enlarge.

Thromboses and Embolisms

Thromboses and embolisms are both serious conditions that can result in the blockage of a blood vessel.

Thrombosis

A **thrombosis** (throm-**BOH**-sis) is the abnormal condition of having a thrombus (**thromb** means clot, and **-osis** means abnormal condition or disease) (plural, *thromboses*) (Figure 5.19).

- A **thrombus** (**THROM**-bus) is a blood clot attached to the interior wall of an artery or vein (**thromb** means clot, and **-us** is a singular noun ending) (plural, *thrombi*).
- A **thrombotic occlusion** (throm-**BOT**-ick ah-**KLOO**-zhun) is the blocking of an artery by a thrombus.

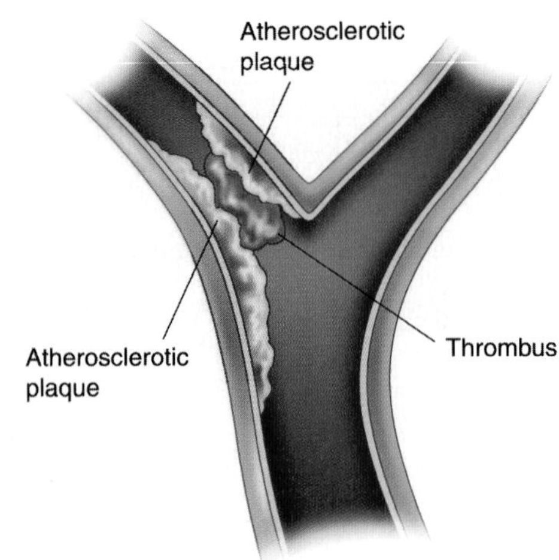

FIGURE 5.19 A thrombus is a blood clot attached to the interior wall of an artery or vein.

Thrombotic means caused by a thrombus. As used here, *occlusion* means blockage.

- A **coronary thrombosis** (**KOR**-uh-**nerr**-ee throm-**BOH**-sis) is damage to the heart muscle caused by a thrombus blocking a coronary artery (**coron** means crown, and **-ary** means pertaining to; **thromb** means clot, and **-osis** means abnormal condition).
- A **deep vein thrombosis** (DVT), also known as a *deep venous thrombosis*, is the condition of having a thrombus attached to the wall of a deep vein. Sometimes such a blockage forms in the legs of a bedridden patient or in someone who has remained seated too long on an airplane. The danger is that the thrombus will break loose and travel to a lung where it can be fatal (see Figure 5.18).

Embolism

An **embolism** (**EM**-boh-lizm) is the sudden blockage of a blood vessel by an embolus (**embol** means something

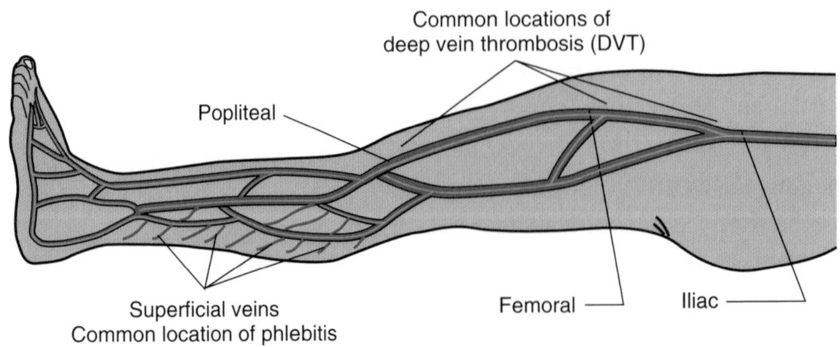

FIGURE 5.18 Common sites for the development of phlebitis and deep vein thrombosis.

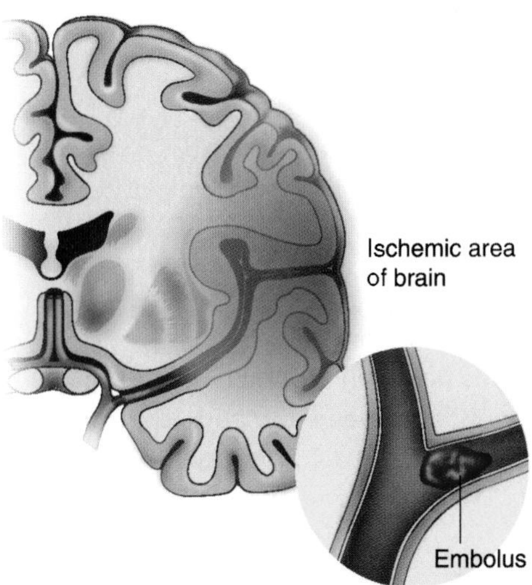

FIGURE 5.20 An embolus is a foreign object circulating in the blood.

inserted, and **-ism** means condition). The embolism is often named for the causative factor, such as an *air embolism* or a *fat embolism* (Figure 5.20).

- An **embolus** (**EM**-boh-lus) is a foreign object, such as a blood clot, quantity of air or gas, or a bit of tissue or tumor that is circulating in the blood (**embol** means something inserted, and **-us** is a singular noun ending) (plural, *emboli*).

Blood Disorders

- **Blood dyscrasia** (dis-**KRAY**-zee-ah) is any pathologic condition of the cellular elements of the blood (**dys-** means bad, and **-crasia** means a mixture or blending).
- **Hemochromatosis** (**hee**-moh-**kroh**-mah-**TOH**-sis), also known as *iron overload disease*, is a genetic disorder in which the intestines absorb too much iron (**hem/o** means blood, **chromat** means color, and **-osis** means abnormal condition or disease). The excess iron that is absorbed enters the bloodstream and accumulates in organs where it causes damage.
- The term **leukopenia** (**loo**-koh-**PEE**-nee-ah) describes any situation in which the total number of leukocytes in the circulating blood is less than normal (**leuk/o** means white, and **-penia** means deficiency). Since these cells combat infection, this condition can place patients at an increased of risk.
- **Polycythemia** (**pol**-ee-sy-**THEE**-mee-ah) is an abnormal increase in the number of red cells in the blood due to excess production of these cells by the bone marrow.
- **Septicemia** (**sep**-tih-**SEE**-mee-ah), formerly known as *blood poisoning*, is a systemic condition caused by the spread of microorganisms and their toxins via the circulating blood.
- **Thrombocytopenia** (**throm**-boh-**sigh**-toh-**PEE**-nee-ah) is a condition in which there is an abnormally small number of platelets circulating in the blood (**thromb/o** means thrombus, **cyt/o** means cell and **-penia** means deficiency). Because these cells help the blood to clot, this condition is sometimes associated with abnormal bleeding.
- **Thrombocytosis** (**throm**-boh-sigh-**TOH**-sis) is an abnormal increase in the number of platelets in the circulating blood (**thromb/o** means thrombus, **cyt** means cell, and **-osis** means abnormal condition).
- A **hemorrhage** (**HEM**-or-idj) is the loss of a large amount of blood in a short time. This term also means to bleed.
- A **transfusion reaction** is a serious, and potentially fatal, complication of a blood transfusion in which a severe immune response occurs because the patient's blood and the donated blood do not match.

Cholesterol

- **Cholesterol** (koh-**LES**-ter-ol) is a fatty substance that travels through the blood and is found in all parts of the body. It aids in the production of cell membranes, some hormones, and vitamin D. Some cholesterol comes from dietary sources, and some is created by the liver. Excessively high levels of certain types of cholesterol can lead to heart disease (see Table 5.2).
- **Hyperlipidemia** (**high**-per-**lip**-ih-**DEE**-mee-ah), also known as *hyperlipemia*, is the general term used to described elevated levels of cholesterol and other fatty substances in the blood (**hyper-** means excessive, **lipid** means fat, and **-emia** means blood condition).

Leukemia

- **Myelodysplastic syndrome** (**my**-eh-loh-dis-**PLAS**-tick), previously known as *preleukemia*, is a group of bone marrow disorders that are characterized by the insufficient production of one or more types of blood cells due to dysfunction of the bone marrow.
- **Leukemia** (loo-**KEE**-mee-ah) is a type of cancer characterized by a progressive increase in the number of abnormal leukocytes (white blood cells) found in blood forming tissues, other organs, and in the circulating blood (**leuk** means white, and **-emia** means blood condition).

TABLE 5.2

INTERPRETING CHOLESTEROL LEVELS

Total cholesterol is measured in terms of milligrams (mg) per deciliter (dL) of blood. A *milligram* is equal to one thousandth of a gram. A *deciliter* is equal to one tenth of a liter.	*Desirable levels* are below 200 mg/dL. *Borderline high levels* are 200–239 mg/dL. *High levels* are 240 mg/dL and above.
Low-density lipoprotein cholesterol (LDL) is referred to as *bad cholesterol* because excess quantities of LDL contribute to plaque buildup in the arteries.	*Optimal levels* are below 100 mg/dL. *Near optimal* is between 100 and 129 mg/dL. *Borderline high* is between 130 and 159 mg/dL. *High* is between 160 and 189 mg/dL. *Very high* is 190 mg/dL and above.
High-density lipoprotein cholesterol (HDL) is referred to as *good cholesterol* because it carries unneeded cholesterol back to the liver for processing and does not contribute to plaque buildup.	*Bad levels* are below 40 mg/dL. *Better levels* are between 40 and 59 mg/dL. *Best levels* are 60 mg/dL and above.
Triglycerides (try-**GLIS**-er-eyeds) are combinations of fatty acids attached to glycerol that are also found normally in the blood in limited quantities.	*Desirable levels* are below 150 mg/dL. *Borderline high levels* are between 150 and 199 mg/dL. *High levels* are between 200 and 499 mg/dL. *Very high levels* are 500 or above.

Source: National Heart, Lung, and Blood Institute, 2006.

Anemias

Anemia (ah-**NEE**-mee-ah) is a lower than normal number of erythrocytes (red blood cells) in the blood (**an-** means without or less than, and **-emia** means blood condition). The severity of this condition is usually measured by a decrease in the amount of hemoglobin in the blood. When inadequate hemoglobin is present, all parts of the body receive less oxygen and have less energy than is needed to function properly.

- **Aplastic anemia** (ay-**PLAS**-tick ah-**NEE**-mee-ah) is characterized by an absence of *all* formed blood elements caused by the failure of blood cell production in the bone marrow (**a-** means without, **plast** means growth, and **-ic** means pertaining to). Anemia, a low red blood cell count, leads to fatigue and weakness. Leukopenia, a low white blood cell count, causes an increased risk of infection. Thrombocytopenia, a low platelet count, results in bleeding especially from mucus membranes and skin.
- **Hemolytic anemia** (**hee**-moh-**LIT**-ick ah-**NEE**-mee-ah) is a condition of an inadequate number of circulating red blood cells due to the premature destruction of red blood cells by the spleen (**hem/o** means relating to blood, and **-lytic** means to destroy). *Hemolytic* means pertaining to breaking down of red blood cells.
- **Iron-deficiency anemia** is the most common form of anemia. Iron, an essential component of hemoglobin, is normally obtained through food diet and by recycling iron from old red blood cells. Without sufficient iron to help create hemoglobin, blood cannot carry oxygen effectively.
- **Megaloblastic anemia** (**MEG**-ah-loh-**blas**-tick ah-**NEE**-mee-ah) is a blood disorder characterized by anemia in which the red blood cells are larger than normal. This condition usually results from a deficiency of folic acid or of vitamin B_{12}.
- **Pernicious anemia** (per-**NISH**-us ah-**NEE**-mee-ah) is caused by a lack of the protein *intrinsic factor* (IF) that helps the body absorb vitamin B_{12} from the gastrointestinal tract. Vitamin B_{12} is necessary for the formation of red blood cells.
- **Sickle cell anemia** is a genetic disorder that causes abnormal hemoglobin, resulting in some red blood cells assuming an abnormal sickle shape (Figure 5.21). This sickle shape interferes with normal blood flow, resulting in damage to most of the body systems. The

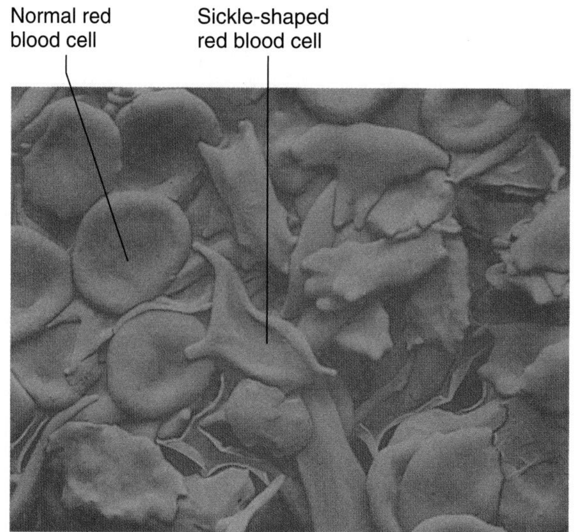

FIGURE 5.21 Normal and sickle-shaped red blood cells magnified through a scanning electron microscope. (Courtesy of Philips Electronic Instruments Company.)

genetic transmission of sickle cell anemia is discussed in Chapter 2.

- **Thalassemia** (thal-ah-**SEE**-mee-ah) is an inherited blood disorder that causes mild or severe anemia due to reduced hemoglobin and fewer red blood cells than normal. *Cooley's anemia* is the name that is sometimes is used to refer to any type of thalassemia that requires treatment with regular blood transfusions.

Hypertension

Hypertension, commonly known as *high blood pressure*, is the elevation of arterial blood pressure to a level that is likely to cause damage to the cardiovascular system. Hypertension is the opposite of *hypotension*.

- *Essential hypertension*, also known as *primary* or *idiopathic hypertension*, is consistently elevated blood pressure of unknown cause. *Idiopathic* means a disease of unknown cause. The classifications of blood pressure for adults with this condition are summarized in Table 5.3.
- *Secondary hypertension* is caused by a different medical problem, such as a kidney disorder or a tumor on the adrenal glands. When the other problem is cured, the secondary hypertension is usually resolved.
- *Malignant hypertension* is characterized by very high blood pressure. This condition, which can be fatal, is usually accompanied by damage to the organs, the brain, and optic nerves, or failure of the heart and kidneys.

Hypotension

Hypotension (**high**-poh-**TEN**-shun) is lower than normal arterial blood pressure. Symptoms can include dizziness, lightheadedness, or fainting. Hypotension is the opposite of *hypertension*.

- **Orthostatic hypotension** (**or**-thoh-**STAT**-ick **high**-poh-**TEN**-shun), also known as *postural hypotension*, is low blood pressure that occurs upon standing up. *Orthostatic* means relating to an upright or standing position.

DIAGNOSTIC PROCEDURES OF THE CARDIOVASCULAR SYSTEM

- **Blood tests** and **ultrasonic diagnostic procedures** are discussed in Chapter 15.
- **Angiography** (**an**-jee-**OG**-rah-fee) is a radiographic (x-ray) study of the blood vessels after the injection of a contrast medium (**angi/o** means blood vessel, and **-graphy** means the process of recording). The resulting film is an *angiogram* (Figure 5.22).
- **Cardiac catheterization** (**KAR**-dee-ack **kath**-eh-ter-eye-**ZAY**-shun) is a diagnostic procedure in which a catheter is passed into a vein or artery and then guided into the heart (Figure 5.23). When the catheter is in

TABLE 5.3

BLOOD PRESSURE CLASSIFICATIONS FOR ADULTS

Category	Systolic (mm Hg)	Diastolic (mm Hg)
Normal blood pressure	less than 120	less than 80
Prehypertension	120–139	80–89
Stage 1 Hypertension	140–159	90–99
Stage 2 Hypertension	160 and higher	100 and higher

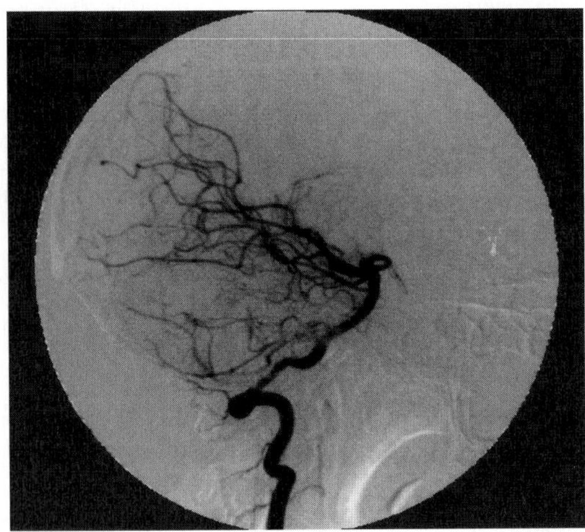

FIGURE 5.22 In an angiogram, the blood vessels (in black) are made visible through the use of a contrast medium.

place, a contrast medium is introduced to produce an angiogram to determine how well the heart is working. This procedure is also used during treatment. See the section on clearing blocked arteries later in this chapter.

- **Digital subtraction angiography** (DSA) combines angiography with computerized components to clarify the view of the area of interest by removing the soft tissue and bones from the images.
- **Duplex ultrasound** is a diagnostic procedure to image the structures of the blood vessels and the flow of blood through these vessels. This is a combination of *diagnostic ultrasound* to shows the structure of the blood vessels and *Doppler ultrasound* to show the movement of the red blood cells through these vessels. Diagnostic and Doppler ultrasound are discussed in Chapter 15.
- **Phlebography** (fleh-**BOG**-rah-fee), also known as *venography*, is a radiographic test that provides an image of the leg veins after a contrast dye is injected into a vein in the patient's foot (**phleb/o** means vein, and **-graphy** means the process of recording). The resulting film is a *phlebogram*. This is a very accurate test for detecting deep vein thrombosis.

Electrocardiography

Electrocardiography (ee-**leck**-troh-kar-dee-**OG**-rah-fee) is the noninvasive process of recording the electrical activity of the myocardium (**electr/o** means electric, **cardi/o** means heart, and **graphy** means the process of recording a picture or record). A *noninvasive* procedure does not require the insertion of an instrument or device through the skin or a body opening for diagnosis or treatment.

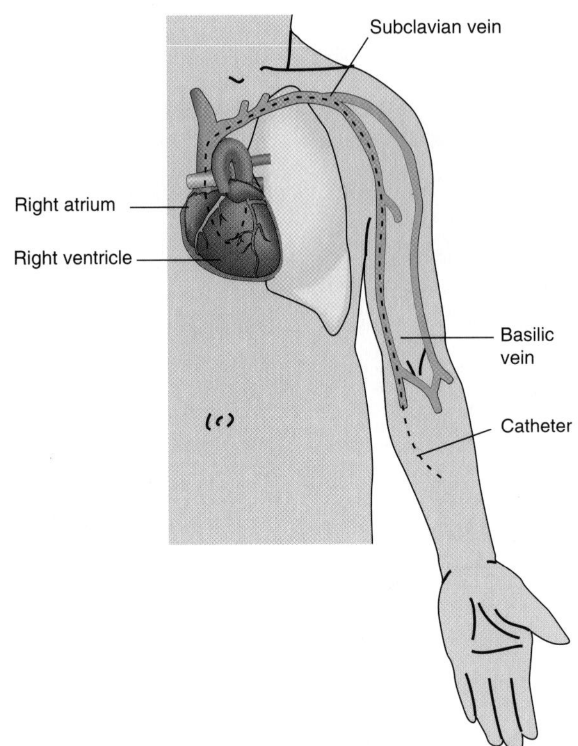

FIGURE 5.23 Cardiac catheterization is a diagnostic procedure in which a catheter is passed into a vein or artery and then guided into the heart.

- An **electrocardiogram** (ee-**leck**-troh-**KAR**-dee-oh-**gram**) is a record of the electrical activity of the myocardium (**electr/o** means electric, **cardi/o** means heart, and **-gram** means picture or record). See Figure 5.17.
- A **Holter monitor** is a portable electrocardiograph that is worn by an ambulatory patient to continuously monitor the heart rates and rhythms over a 24-hour period.
- A **stress test** is performed to assess cardiovascular health and function during and after stress. This involves monitoring with an electrocardiogram while the patient exercises on a treadmill.
- A **thallium stress test** (**THAL**-ee-um) is performed to evaluate how well blood flows through the coronary arteries of the heart muscle during exercise.

TREATMENT PROCEDURES OF THE CARDIOVASCULAR SYSTEM

Medications

Many heart conditions are controlled with medications; however, successful treatment depends on patient compliance. *Compliance* is the accuracy and consistency with which the patient follows the physician's instructions.

Antihypertensives

An **antihypertensive** (**an**-tih-**high**-per-**TEN**-siv) is a medication administered to lower blood pressure. Some of these drugs are also used to treat other heart conditions.

- An **ACE inhibitor** (*Angiotensin-Converting Enzyme*) blocks the action of the enzyme that causes the blood vessels to contract resulting in hypertension. When this enzyme is blocked, the blood vessels are able to dilate (enlarge), and this reduces the blood pressure. These medications are used primarily to treat hypertension and heart failure.
- A **beta-blocker** reduces the workload of the heart by slowing the rate of the heart beat. They are commonly prescribed to lower blood pressure, relieve angina, or to treat heart failure.
- **Calcium channel blocker agents** cause the heart and blood vessels to relax by decreasing the movement of calcium into the cells of these structures. This relaxation reduces the workload of the heart by increasing the supply of blood and oxygen. Some calcium channel blocking agents are used to treat hypertension or to relieve and control angina.
- A **diuretic** (**dye**-you-**RET**-ick) is administered to stimulate the kidneys to increase the secretion of urine to rid the body of excess sodium and water. These medications are administered to treat hypertension and heart failure by reducing the amount of fluid circulating in the blood.

Additional Medications

- An **antiarrhythmic** (**an**-tih-ah-**RITH**-mick) is a medication administered to control irregularities of the heartbeat.
- An **anticoagulant** (**an**-tih-koh-**AG**-you-lant) slows coagulation and prevents new clots from forming. *Coagulation* is the process of clotting blood (see Coumadin).
- **Aspirin** in very small daily dose, such as an 81 mg *baby aspirin*, may be recommended to reduce the risk of a heart attack or stroke by slightly reducing the ability of the blood to clot.
- **Cholesterol-lowering drugs**, such as *statins*, are used to combat hyperlipidemia by reducing the undesirable cholesterol levels in the blood.
- **Coumadin**, which is the brand name for *warfarin*, is an anticoagulant administered to prevent blood clots from forming or growing larger. This medication is often prescribed for patients with clotting difficulties, certain types of heartbeat irregularities, or after a heart attack or after heart valve replacement surgery.
- **Digitalis** (**dij**-ih-**TAL**-is), also known as *digoxin*, strengthens the contraction of the heart muscle, slows the heart rate, and helps eliminate fluid from body tissues. It is often used to treat heart failure or certain types of arrhythmias.
- A **thrombolytic** (**throm**-boh-**LIT**-ick), also known as a *clot-busting drug*, dissolves or causes a thrombus to break up (**thromb/o** means clot, **and -lytic** means to destroy).
- **Tissue plasminogen activator** (plaz-**MIN**-oh-jen) is a thrombolytic that is administered to some patients having a heart attack or stroke. If administered within a few hours after symptoms begin, this medication can dissolve the damaging blood clots.
- A **vasoconstrictor** (**vas**-oh-kon-**STRICK**-tor) causes blood vessels to narrow. Examples of uses of these medications include antihistamines and decongestants. A vasoconstrictor is the opposite of a *vasodilator*.
- A **vasodilator** (**vas**-oh-dye-**LAYT**-or) causes blood vessels to expand. A vasodilator is the opposite of a *vasoconstrictor*.
- **Nitroglycerin** is a vasodilator that is prescribed to prevent or relieve the pain of angina by dilating the blood vessels to the heart. This increases the blood flow and oxygen supply to the heart. Nitroglycerin can be administered sublingually (under the tongue), transdermally (through the skin), or orally as a spray.

Clearing Blocked Arteries

- **Percutaneous transluminal coronary angioplasty** (PTCA), commonly referred to simply as **angioplasty** (**AN**-jee-oh-**plas**-tee), is also known as a *balloon angioplasty*. This is a procedure in which a small balloon on the end of a catheter is used to open a partially blocked coronary artery by flattening the plaque deposit and stretching the lumen (see Figure 5.24).
- A **stent** is a wire-mesh tube that is commonly placed after the artery has been opened. This provides support to the arterial wall, keeps the plaque from expanding again, and prevents restenosis (Figure 5.25).
- **Restenosis** describes the condition when an artery that has been opened by angioplasty closes again (**re-** means again, and **-stenosis** means narrowing).

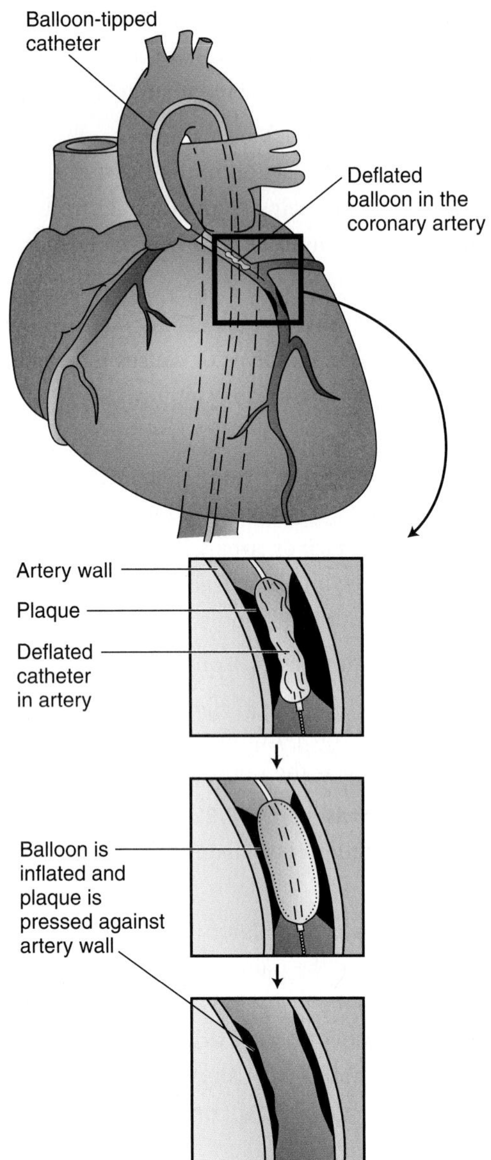

FIGURE 5.24 Balloon angioplasty is performed to reopen a blocked coronary artery.

- An **atherectomy** (**ath**-er-**ECK**-toh-mee) is the surgical removal of plaque buildup from the interior of an artery (**ather** means plaque, and **-ectomy** means surgical removal). A stent may be put in place after the atherectomy to prevent the artery from becoming blocked again.
- A **carotid endarterectomy** (kah-**ROT**-id **end**-ar-ter-**ECK**-toh-mee) is the surgical removal of the lining of a portion of a clogged carotid artery leading to the brain. This procedure is performed to reduce the risk of a stroke caused by a disruption of the blood flow to the brain. Strokes are discussed in Chapter 10.

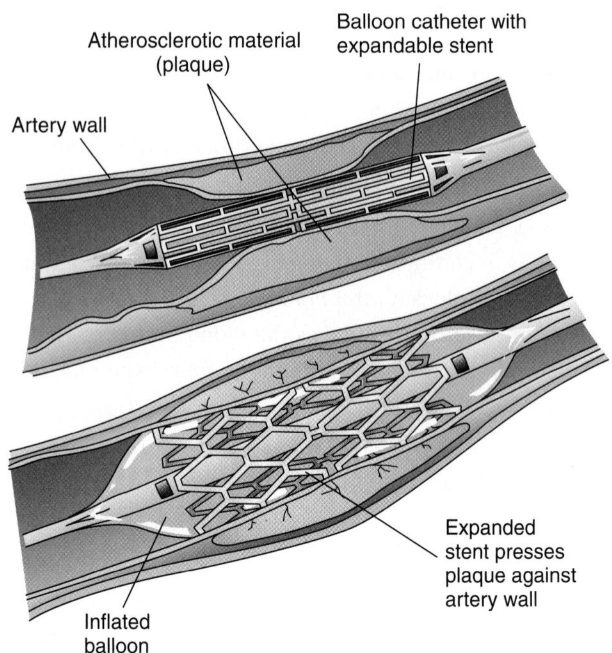

FIGURE 5.25 A stent is placed to prevent restenosis of a treated artery.

Coronary Artery Bypass Graft

Coronary artery bypass graft (CABG) is also known as *bypass surgery* (Figure 5.26). In this surgery, which requires opening the chest, a piece of vein from the leg or chest is implanted on the heart to replace a blocked coronary artery and to improve the flow of blood to the heart.

- A **minimally invasive coronary artery bypass**, also known as a *keyhole bypass* or a *buttonhole bypass*, is an alternative technique for some bypass patients. This procedure is performed with the aid of a fiber optic camera through small openings between the ribs.

Treatment of Cardiac Arrhythmias

- **Defibrillation** (dee-**fih**-brih-**LAY**-shun), also known as *cardioversion*, is the use of electrical shock to restore the heart's normal rhythm. This shock is provided by a device known as a *defibrillator*.
- An **automated external defibrillator** (AED) is designed for use by nonprofessionals in emergency situations when defibrillation is required. This piece of equipment automatically samples the electrical rhythms of the heart and, if necessary, externally shocks the heart to restore a normal cardiac rhythm (Figure 5.27).
- An **artificial pacemaker** is used primarily as treatment for bradycardia or atrial fibrillation. This electronic

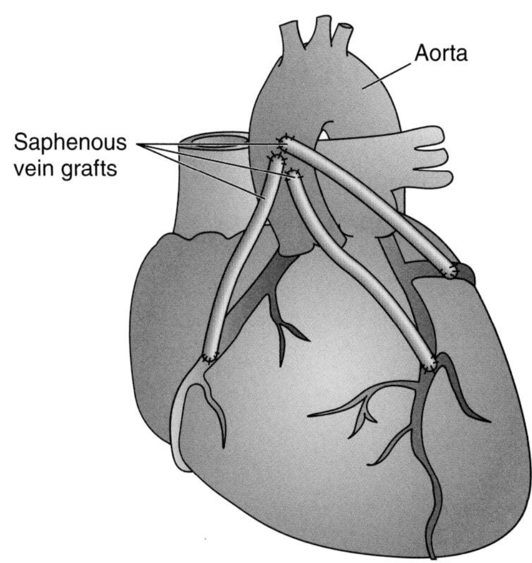

FIGURE 5.26 Coronary artery bypass surgery is performed to allow the flow of blood by placing vein grafts to bypass blocked arteries.

device can be attached externally or implanted under the skin with connections leading into the heart to regulate the heartbeat.

- An **implantable cardioverter defibrillator** (**KAR**-dee-oh-**ver**-ter dee-**fib**-rih-**LAY**-ter) is a double-action pacemaker. (1) It constantly regulates the heartbeat to ensure that the heart does not beat too slowly. (2) If a dangerous disruption of the heart's rhythm occurs, it acts as an automatic defibrillator (Figure 5.28).
- **Valvoplasty** (**VAL**-voh-**plas**-tee), also known as *valvuloplasty*, is the surgical repair or replacement of a heart valve (**valv/o** means valve, and **-plasty** means surgical repair).

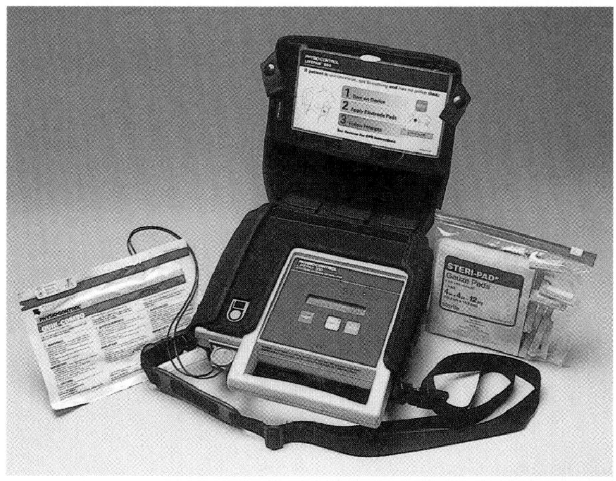

FIGURE 5.27 An automated external defibrillator (AED) is designed for use by nonprofessionals in emergency situations when defibrillation is required.

- **Cardiopulmonary resuscitation**, commonly known as *CPR*, is an emergency procedure for life support consisting of artificial respiration and manual external cardiac compression. *Cardiopulmonary* means pertaining to the heart and lungs.

Blood Vessels, Blood, and Bleeding

- An **aneurysmectomy** (**an**-you-riz-**MECK**-toh-mee) is the surgical removal of an aneurysm (**aneurysm** means aneurysm, and **-ectomy** means surgical removal).
- An **aneurysmorrhaphy** (**an**-you-riz-**MOR**-ah-fee), also known as *aneurysmoplasty*, is the surgical suturing of an aneurysm (**aneurysm/o** means aneurysm, and **-rrhaphy** means surgical suturing).
- An **arteriectomy** (**ar**-teh-ree-**ECK**-toh-mee) is the surgical removal of part of an artery (**arteri** means artery, and **-ectomy** means surgical removal).
- **Hemostasis** (**hee**-moh-**STAY**-sis) means to stop or control bleeding (**hem/o** means blood, and **-stasis** means stopping or controlling). This could be accomplished by the formation of a blood clot by the body or

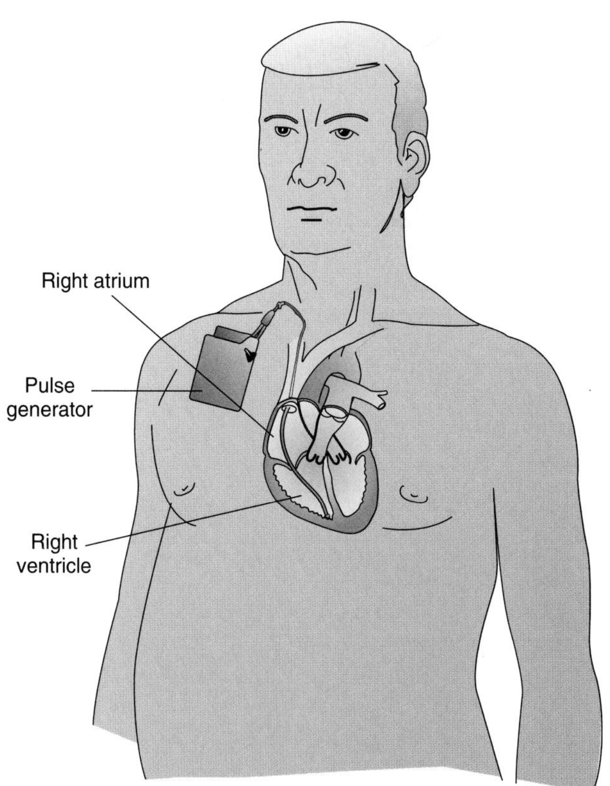

FIGURE 5.28 An implantable cardioverter defibrillator constantly regulates the heartbeat and, if necessary, acts as an automatic defibrillator.

through the external application of pressure to block the flow of blood.

- **Plasmapheresis** (**plaz**-mah-feh-**REE**-sis) is the removal of whole blood from the body and separation of the blood's cellular elements. The red blood cells and platelets are suspended in saline or a plasma substitute and returned to the circulatory system. For blood donors, this makes more frequent donations possible. Patients with certain autoimmune disorders receive their own red blood cells and platelets back cleansed of antibodies.

ABBREVIATIONS RELATED TO THE CARDIOVASCULAR SYSTEM

Table 5.4 presents an overview of the abbreviations related to the terms introduced in this chapter. Note: To avoid errors or confusion, always be cautious when using abbreviations.

TABLE 5.4
Abbreviations Related to the Cardiovascular System

anticoagulant = AC	**AC** = anticoagulant
atrial fibrillation = AF	**AF** = atrial fibrillation
cardiac catheterization = card cath, CC	**card cath, CC** = cardiac catheterization
cholesterol = C	**C** = cholesterol
chronic venous insufficiency = CVI	**CVI** = chronic venous insufficiency
coronary artery disease = CAD	**CAD** = coronary artery disease
electrocardiogram = EKG, ECG	**EKG, ECG** = electrocardiogram
ischemic heart disease = IHD	**IHD** = ischemic heart disease
minimally invasive direct coronary artery bypass = MIDCAB	**MIDCAB** = minimally invasive direct coronary artery bypass
myocardial infarction = MI	**MI** = myocardial infarction
peripheral artery disease = PAD	**PAD** = Peripheral artery disease
peripheral vascular disease = PVD	**PVD** = peripheral vascular disease
thallium stress test = TST	**TST** = thallium stress test
tissue plasminogen activator = tPA	**tPA** = tissue plasminogen activator
ventricular fibrillation = VF	**VF** = ventricular fibrillation

CAREER OPPORTUNITIES

In addition to the medical specialties already discussed, some of the health occupations involving the treatment of the cardiovascular system include:

- **Phlebotomist**, or **venipuncture technician:** takes patient blood samples and prepares them for testing
- **Perfusionist:** operates a heart-lung machine during coronary bypass surgery
- **Cardiovascular technologist:** assists with cardiac catheterization procedures and angioplasty, monitors patients during open-heart surgery and the implantation of pacemakers, and performs tests to check circulation
- **Electrocardiograph (ECG** or **EKG) technician:** a cardiovascular technologist who operates electrocardiograph machines and Holter monitors, and performs other specialized cardiac tests
- **Vascular nurse:** RN who treats patients with coronary heart disease and those who have had heart surgery, providing services such as postoperative rehabilitation

HEALTH OCCUPATION PROFILE

CARDIAC SONOGRAPHER

Michael C. Foster is a cardiac sonographer. ***"I take pictures (still and moving) of people's hearts using ultrasound. As a runner, I've always been fascinated by the heart and how it works, how it acquires disease, and how it is repaired. I completed the 2-year cardiovascular technology program at our local community college and now have a great job at Duke University Medical Center. It's my job to make a 'movie' that will inform the doctor about the patient's heart function. I do this by using a handheld probe placed on the patient's chest. The study usually takes about 30 minutes, and I see eight to ten patients a day. Since my skills center on diagnosis, I'm often the first person to have an idea of what might be wrong with a patient's heart.***

"I work closely with doctors to identify the cardiac problem. My work helps the medical team to plan the patient's care. I like my job because my specialized skills help solve important medical problems and often make people's quality of life significantly better."

Study Break

Have you ever taken a big bite of a Popsicle or a mouthful of an ice-cold drink and felt a sudden pain in your head? The not-very-scientific term "ice cream headache" is sometimes used to describe this phenomenon, as are as the alarming (and inaccurate) terms "brain freeze" or "frozen brain syndrome." An ice cream headache occurs when a really cold food or beverage comes into contact with the roof of the mouth; the pain usually lasts only about 30 seconds.

The cause of the pain is the dilation of blood vessels in the head. This dilation is probably caused by a reaction in the nerve center located above the roof of your mouth. When this nerve center gets cold, it seems to overreact and tries to heat your brain with warm blood. The *carotid arteries*, which carry blood to the brain, send a sudden surge of blood to all the blood vessels in the forehead and face, causing a temporary, but painful, buildup of pressure.

About one out of every three people experience ice cream headaches from time to time. The best way to avoid them is to keep icy cold foods and beverages away from the roof of the mouth, or to cool the mouth down gradually by taking small bites or sips if you are really hot.

Review Time

Write the answers to the following questions on a separate piece of paper or in your notebook. In addition, be prepared to take part in the classroom discussion.

1. ***Written Assignment:*** Describe how **pulmonary arteries** and **pulmonary veins** differ from all other arteries and veins.

   Discussion Assignment: Which heart chambers pump deoxygenated blood to the lungs, and which chambers received oxygenated blood from the lungs? Include in your discussion the names of the vessels that carry this blood as it travels between the heart and lungs.

2. ***Written Assignment:*** Explain the meaning of the abbreviation **CAD**. Include with your explanation some of the symptoms a patient with this condition experiences.

   Discussion Assignment: This condition includes atherosclerosis of the coronary arteries. How would you explain it in terms that a patient's family can understand?

3. Mike Muldoon's **blood pressure** is 160/90.
   Written Assignment: What condition does the patient have? Describe what each of these numbers indicates.

   Discussion Assignment: How would you explain to Mr. Muldoon the risks of not controlling his blood pressure?

4. James Macintosh has been diagnosed with **high cholesterol**, and he is confused about the difference between LDL and HDL.
   Written Assignment: Describe the differences between LDL and HDL.

   Discussion Assignment: How would you explain to Mr. Macintosh why one is considered good and the other is considered bad?

continues

5. Mrs. Warren requires an **artificial pacemaker**.

   Written Assignment: Identify which structure is known as the natural pacemaker, and list two conditions that might make this surgery necessary.

   Discussion Assignment: Mrs. Warren's children are concerned that an artificial pacemaker might fail. How would you explain to them how Mrs. Warren's artificial pacemaker will work in her body?

Optional Internet Activity

The goal of this activity is to help you learn more about medical terminology as it applies to the "real world." Select **one** *of these two options and follow the instructions.*

1. Search for information about **myelodysplastic syndrome** and **leukemia**. Write a brief (one- or two-paragraph) report on something new you learned here and include the address of the web site where you found this information.

2. To learn more about **heart attack symptoms**, go to the web site of the American Heart Association. Write a brief (one- or two-paragraph) report on something new you learned here.

THE HUMAN TOUCH: CRITICAL THINKING ACTIVITY

The following story and questions are designed to stimulate critical thinking through class discussion or as a brief essay response. There are no right or wrong answers to these questions.

When she heard the TV turn off downstairs in the middle of her Grandma Julia's favorite show, 14-year-old Jenny Duvitsky assumed that Grandma Julia was tired from another long day at her job. Continuing with her math homework, Jenny finished the row of problems and then headed downstairs to grab a soda from the fridge. Passing by the living room, she was surprised to see her grandmother sitting bent over at the waist and breathing shallowly. **"Something wrong, Grandma?"**

Her grandmother looked up at Jenny and grimaced in pain. She pressed her hand over her heart to ease the pain that radiated upward to her chin and down along her abdomen. **"It must be that angina again, Jenny. Be a good girl and run and get me more of my nitroglycerin pills. Those I took already just didn't help."**

Jenny remembered the family discussion about her grandmother's recent doctor's visit. The doctor was worried about grandmother's weight, cholesterol, blood pressure, and increasingly frequent angina attacks. The doctor had warned that if the nitroglycerin didn't ease the pain of an angina attack quickly, the pain might be a heart attack.

Jenny gave Grandma another nitroglycerin pill and looked at her watch. Ten minutes passed and the pills didn't seem to be helping. Grandma Julia looked worse. She was pale and sweating with pain.

Jenny was scared. Her dad wouldn't be home from work for hours and Jenny knew she had to do something now. **"Okay, Grandma, I think you need to go to the hospital, and I'm going to call an ambulance."** ***Jenny's hands were shaking as she dialed 9-1-1.*** **"Hello? Yes ... it's an emergency. I need an ambulance, please. I think my Grandma is having a heart attack."**

continues

Help arrived quickly, and within minutes, the EMTs had evaluated Grandma Julia's condition and conveyed her to the ambulance. In the hospital, additional tests revealed that Grandma Julia had two blocked coronary arteries.

Suggested Discussion Topics

1. Discuss whether heart attack symptoms are the same in men and in women. What made Jenny decide her grandmother might be having a heart attack?
2. Discuss the risk factors mentioned in the story that indicate Grandma Julia might be having a heart attack.
3. Jenny responded appropriately to her grandmother's situation. But is there training available that would help her feel more capable in an emergency?
4. Should Grandma Julia have asked Jenny to call 9-1-1 instead of asking for more nitroglycerin pills? Why do you think she didn't do that?

STUDENT WORKBOOK AND StudyWARE™ CD-ROM

1. Go to your **Student Workbook** and complete the Learning Exercises for this chapter.

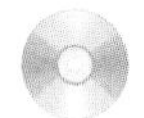

2. Go to the **StudyWARE™ CD-ROM** and have fun with the exercises and games for this chapter.

CHAPTER 6

THE LYMPHATIC AND IMMUNE SYSTEMS

OVERVIEW OF STRUCTURES, COMBINING FORMS, AND FUNCTIONS OF THE LYMPHATIC AND IMMUNE SYSTEMS

MAJOR STRUCTURES	RELATED COMBINING FORMS	PRIMARY FUNCTIONS
Lymph	lymph/o	The fluid that removes cellular waste products, pathogens, and dead blood cells from the tissues.
Lymphatic Vessels and Ducts	lymphangi/o	Returns lymph from the tissue to the circulatory system.
Lymph Nodes	lymphaden/o	Filter pathogens and harmful substances from the lymph.
Tonsils and Adenoids	tonsill/o, adenoid/o	Protect the entry into the respiratory system.
Spleen	splen/o (Notice that this combining form is spelled with only one *e*.)	Filters foreign materials from the blood. Maintains the appropriate balance between cells and plasma in the blood. Destroys worn-out blood cells, releases hemoglobin, acts as a blood reservoir, and stores platelets.
Bone Marrow	myel/o	Produces blood cells (see Chapter 3). This word part also refers to the spinal cord.
Lymphocytes	lymphocyt/o	The specialized white blood cells that play an important role in immune reactions.
Thymus	thym/o	Secretes the endocrine thymosin that aids in the maturation of T lymphocytes for use by the immune system.
Immune System	immun/o	Defends the body against harmful substances, such as pathogenic microorganisms, allergens, toxins, and malignant cells.

Vocabulary Related to the Lymphatic and Immune Systems

This list contains essential word parts and medical terms for this chapter. These terms are pronounced on the student StudyWARE™ CD-ROM and Audio CDs that are available for use with this text. These and the other important **primary terms** are shown in boldface throughout the chapter. *Secondary terms*, which appear in *orange* italics, clarify the meaning of primary terms.

Word Parts

- ☐ **anti-**
- ☐ **carcin/o**
- ☐ **immun/o**
- ☐ **lymph/o**
- ☐ **lymphaden/o**
- ☐ **lymphangi/o**
- ☐ **neo-, ne/o**
- ☐ **-oma**
- ☐ **onc/o**
- ☐ **phag/o**
- ☐ **-plasm**
- ☐ **sarc/o**
- ☐ **splen/o**
- ☐ **-tic**
- ☐ **tox/o**

Medical Terms

- ☐ **acquired immunodeficiency syndrome** (**im**-you-noh-deh-**FISH**-en-see)
- ☐ **allergen** (**AL**-er-jen)
- ☐ **anaphylaxis** (**an**-ah-fih-**LACK**-sis)
- ☐ **antibiotic**
- ☐ **antibody** (**AN**-tih-**bod**-ee)
- ☐ **antifungal** (**an**-tih-**FUNG**-gul)
- ☐ **antigen** (**AN**-tih-jen)
- ☐ **antigen-antibody reaction**
- ☐ **autoimmune disorder** (**aw**-toh-ih-**MYOUN**)
- ☐ **bacilli** (bah-**SILL**-eye)
- ☐ **bacteria** (back-**TEER**-ree-ah)
- ☐ **carcinoma** (**kar**-sih-**NOH**-mah)
- ☐ **carcinoma in situ** (**kar**-sih-**NOH**-mah in **SIGH**-too)
- ☐ **complement** (**KOM**-pleh-ment)
- ☐ **cytomegalovirus** (**sigh**-toh-**meg**-ah-loh-**VYE**-rus)
- ☐ **cytotoxic drug** (**sigh**-toh-**TOK**-sick)
- ☐ **ductal carcinoma in situ**
- ☐ **hemolytic** (**hee**-moh-**LIT**-ick)
- ☐ **herpes zoster** (**HER**-peez **ZOS**-ter)
- ☐ **Hodgkin's lymphoma** (**HODJ**-kinz lim-**FOH**-mah)
- ☐ **human immunodeficiency virus** (**im**-you-noh-deh-**FISH**-en-see)
- ☐ **immunodeficiency disorder** (**im**-you-noh-deh-**FISH**-en-see)
- ☐ **immunoglobulins** (**im**-you-noh-**GLOB**-you-lins)
- ☐ **immunosuppressant** (**im**-you-noh-soo-**PRES**-ant)
- ☐ **immunotherapy** (ih-**myou**-noh-**THER**-ah-pee)
- ☐ **infectious mononucleosis** (**mon**-oh-**new**-klee-**OH**-sis)
- ☐ **infiltrating ductal carcinoma** (in-**FILL**-trate-ng **DUK**-tal kar-sih-**NOH**-mah)
- ☐ **interferon** (**in**-ter-**FEAR**-on)
- ☐ **lymphadenitis** (lim-**fad**-eh-**NIGH**-tis)
- ☐ **lymphadenopathy** (lim-**fad**-eh-**NOP**-ah-thee)
- ☐ **lymphangioma** (lim-**fan**-jee-**OH**-mah)
- ☐ **lymphedema** (**lim**-feh-**DEE**-mah)
- ☐ **lymphocytes** (**LIM**-foh-sights)
- ☐ **lymphokines** (**LIM**-foh-kyens)
- ☐ **lymphoma** (lim-**FOH**-mah)
- ☐ **lymphoscintigraphy** (**lim**-foh-sin-**TIH**-grah-fee)
- ☐ **macrophage** (**MACK**-roh-fayj)
- ☐ **malaria** (mah-**LAY**-ree-ah)
- ☐ **mammography** (mam-**OG**-rah-fee)
- ☐ **metastasis** (meh-**TAS**-tah-sis)
- ☐ **metastasize** (meh-**TAS**-tah-sighz)
- ☐ **myoma** (my-**OH**-mah)
- ☐ **myosarcoma** (**my**-oh-sahr-**KOH**-mah)
- ☐ **non-Hodgkin's lymphoma** (non-**HODJ**-kinz lim-**FOH**-mah)
- ☐ **opportunistic infection** (**op**-ur-too-**NIHS**-tick)
- ☐ **osteosarcoma** (**oss**-tee-oh-sar-**KOH**-mah)
- ☐ **parasite** (**PAR**-ah-sight)
- ☐ **pathogen** (**PATH**-oh-jen)
- ☐ **rabies** (**RAY**-beez)
- ☐ **rickettsia** (rih-**KET**-see-ah)
- ☐ **rubella** (roo-**BELL**-ah)
- ☐ **sarcoma** (sar-**KOH**-mah)
- ☐ **spirochetes** (**SPY**-roh-keets)
- ☐ **splenomegaly** (**splee**-noh-**MEG**-ah-lee)
- ☐ **staphylococci** (**staf**-ih-loh-**KOCK**-sigh)
- ☐ **streptococci** (**strep**-toh-**KOCK**-sigh)
- ☐ **teletherapy** (**tel**-eh-**THER**-ah-pee)
- ☐ **tetanus** (**TET**-ah-nus)
- ☐ **toxoplasmosis** (**tock**-soh plaz-**MOH**-sis)
- ☐ **varicella** (**var**-ih-**SEL**-ah)

OBJECTIVES

On completion of this chapter, you should be able to:

1. Identify the medical specialists who treat disorders of the lymphatic and immune systems.
2. Describe the major functions and structures of the lymphatic and immune systems.
3. Recognize, define, spell, and pronounce the major terms related to the pathology, diagnostic, and treatment procedures of the lymphatic and immune systems.
4. Recognize, define, spell, and pronounce terms related to oncology.

INTRODUCTION

The lymphatic and immune systems work in close cooperation to protect and maintain the health of the body. Some functions and structures of these systems are performed by specialized structures or shared structures. Additional roles are performed by other body systems.

MEDICAL SPECIALTIES RELATED TO THE LYMPHATIC AND IMMUNE SYSTEMS

- An **allergist** (**AL**-er-jist) specializes in diagnosing and treating conditions of altered immunologic reactivity, such as allergic reactions.
- An **immunologist** (**im**-you-**NOL**-oh-jist) specializes in diagnosing and treating disorders of the immune system (**immun** means protected, and **-ologist** means specialist).
- An **oncologist** (ong-**KOL**-oh-jist) is a physician who specializes in diagnosing and treating malignant disorders such as tumors and cancer (**onc** means tumor, and **-ologist** means specialist).

FUNCTIONS OF THE LYMPHATIC SYSTEM

The lymphatic system performs three primary functions in cooperation with other body systems. These are:

- Absorbing fats and fat-soluble vitamins from the small intestine.
- Removing waste from the tissues.
- Providing aid to the immune system.

Absorption of Fats and Fat-Soluble Vitamins

Food is digested in the small intestine. From here, the nutrients, fats, and fat-soluble vitamins are absorbed for use throughout the body.

- The *villi* are small finger-like projections that line the small intestine. These structures contain blood vessels and **lacteals** (**LACK**-tee-ahls), which are specialized structures of the lymphatic system.
- The blood vessels in the villi absorb most of the nutrients from the digested food directly into the bloodstream. This is discussed further in Chapter 8.
- Fats and fat-soluble vitamins that cannot be absorbed directly into the bloodstream are absorbed and transported by the lacteals of the lymphatic system.

Waste Removal from the Tissues

The lymphatic system removes waste products and excess fluids created by the cells. It also destroys pathogens and takes away foreign substances that are present in the tissues.

Cooperating with the Immune System

The lymph nodes play an active role in cooperation with the immune system to protect the body against invading microorganisms and diseases. These functions are described in the discussion of the immune system.

STRUCTURES OF THE LYMPHATIC SYSTEM

The major structures of the lymphatic system are lymph, lymphatic vessels and ducts, and lymph nodes. Additional structures include the tonsils, thymus, spleen, lacteals, Peyer's patches, the vermiform appendix, and lymphocytes (Figure 6.1). Lymphocytes, which are specialized white blood cells, have roles in both the lymphatic and immune systems and are discussed under the heading of "Specialized Cells of the Antigen-Antibody Reaction."

Lymphatic Circulation

Lymphatic circulation transports lymph from tissues throughout the body and eventually returns this fluid to

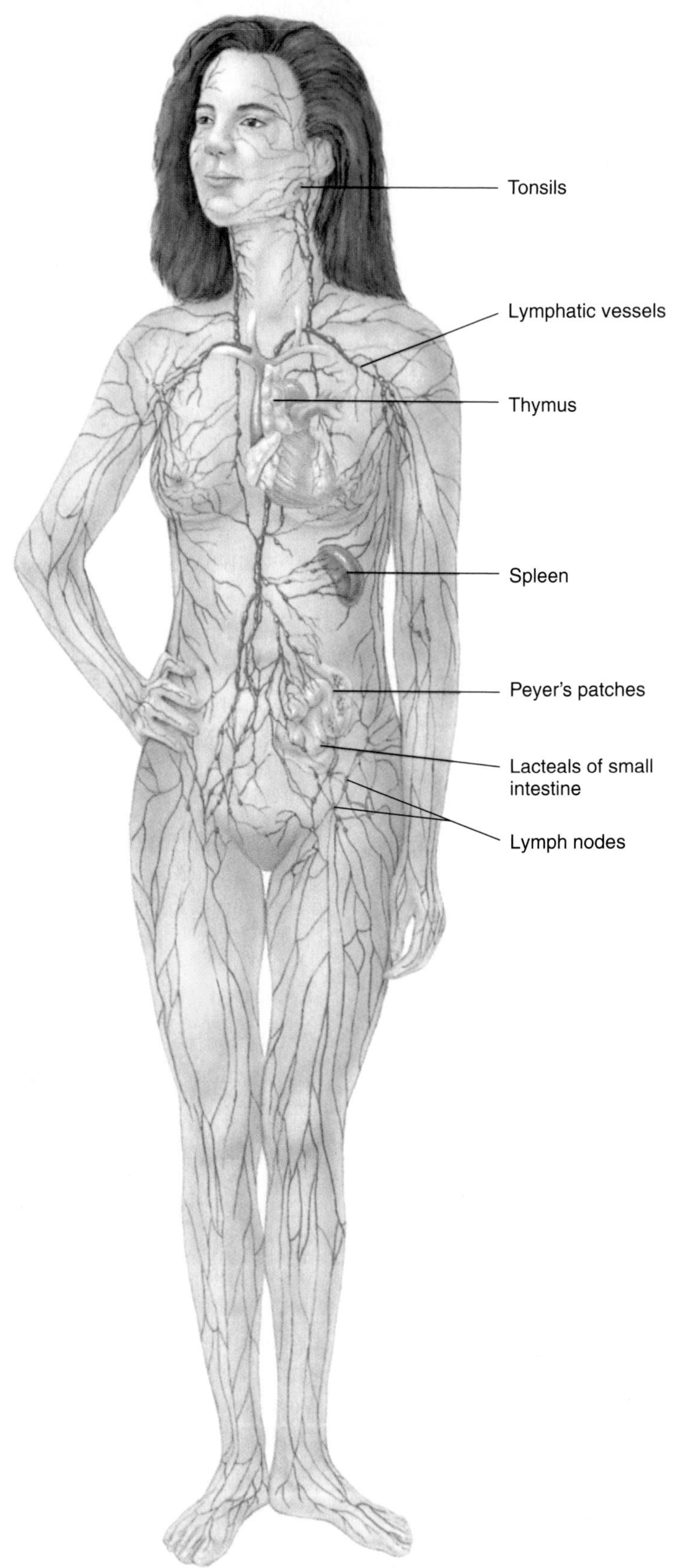

FIGURE 6.1 The vessels and organs of the lymphatic system.

the venous circulation. **Lymph** is a clear, watery fluid that transports waste products and proteins out of the spaces between the cells of the body tissues. It also destroys bacteria or other pathogens that are present in the tissues.

Because the lymphatic vessels are closely aligned with those of the cardiovascular system, the lymphatic system is sometimes referred to as the *secondary circulatory system*. Despite the similarities, there are major differences between these two circulatory systems. While studying this section, compare Figures 6.1 and 5.9.

- Blood circulates throughout the entire body. Lymph flows in only one direction, from its point of origin until its return to the venous circulation in the region of the neck.
- Blood flows in an open system in which it leaves, and re-enters, the blood vessels through the capillaries. Lymphatic circulation is a closed system. From the time lymph enters the lymphatic capillaries, it does not leave the lymphatic vessels again until it returns to the venous circulation.
- Blood is pumped throughout the body by the heart. The lymphatic system does not have a pump-like organ. Instead, lymph must depend on help from the movements of nearby muscles and blood vessels to aid in its flow.
- The color of blood makes the arteries and veins readily visible. Lymph is a clear fluid, and the lymphatic vessels are not readily visible.
- Blood is filtered by the kidneys, and waste products are excreted by the urinary system. Lymph is filtered by lymph nodes located along the lymphatic vessels throughout the body.

Interstitial Fluid and Lymph Creation

Interstitial fluid (**in**-ter-**STISH**-al), also known as *intercellular* or *tissue fluid*, is plasma from arterial blood that flows out of the capillaries and into the spaces between the cells. This interstitial fluid transports food, oxygen, and hormones to the cells.

- About 90% of this fluid is reabsorbed by the capillaries and returned to the venous circulation. *Reabsorbed* means to be taken up again by the body.
- The remaining 10% of the interstitial fluid that was not reabsorbed becomes lymph. It is transported by the lymphatic vessels and is filtered by lymph nodes located along these vessels.

Lymphatic Capillaries

Lymphatic capillaries are microscopic, blind-ended tubes located near the surface of the body. The capillary walls are only one cell in thickness. These cells separate briefly to allow lymph to enter the capillary, and the action of the cells as they close forces the lymph to flow forward (Figure 6.2).

Lymphatic Vessels and Ducts

Lymph flows from the lymphatic capillaries into the progressively larger **lymphatic vessels**, which are located deeper within the tissues. Like veins, lymphatic vessels have valves to prevent the backward flow of lymph.

The larger lymphatic vessels eventually join together to form two ducts. Each duct drains a specific part of the body and returns the lymph to the venous circulation (see Figure 6.1).

- The **right lymphatic duct** collects lymph from the right side of the head and neck, the upper right quadrant of the body and the right arm. The right lymphatic duct empties into the right subclavian vein.
- The **thoracic duct**, which is the largest lymphatic vessel in the body, collects lymph from the left side of the head and neck, the upper left quadrant of the trunk, the left arm, and the entire lower portion of the trunk and both legs. The thoracic duct empties into the left subclavian vein.

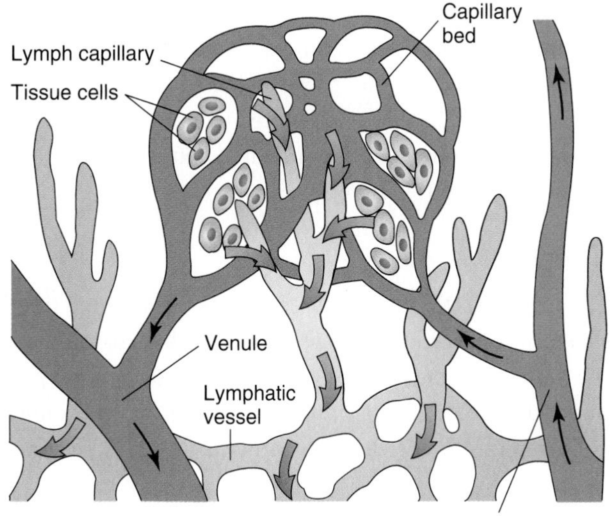

FIGURE 6.2 Lymph capillaries begin as blind-ended tubes. Lymph enters between the cells of the capillary wall and flows into progressively larger lymphatic vessels.

Lymph Nodes

Each small, bean-shaped **lymph node** contains specialized lymphocytes that are capable of destroying pathogens. Unfiltered lymph flows into the nodes, and here the lymphocytes destroy harmful substances such as bacteria, viruses, and malignant cells. Additional structures within the node filter the lymph to remove additional impurities. After these processes are complete, the lymph leaves the node and continues its journey to again become part of the venous circulation.

There are between 400 and 700 lymph nodes located along the larger lymphatic vessels, and approximately half of these nodes are in the abdomen. Most of the others nodes are positioned on the branches of the larger lymphatic vessels throughout the body. The exceptions are the three major groups of lymph nodes that are named for their locations (see Figure 6.1).

- **Cervical lymph nodes** (**SER**-vih-kal) are located along the sides of the neck (**cervic** means neck, and **-al** means pertaining to).
- **Axillary lymph nodes** (**AK**-sih-**lar**-ee) are located under the arms in the area known as the armpits (**axill** means armpit, and **-ary** means pertaining to).
- **Inguinal lymph nodes** (**ING**-gwih-nal) are located in the inguinal (groin) area of the lower abdomen (**inguin** means groin, and **-al** means pertaining to).

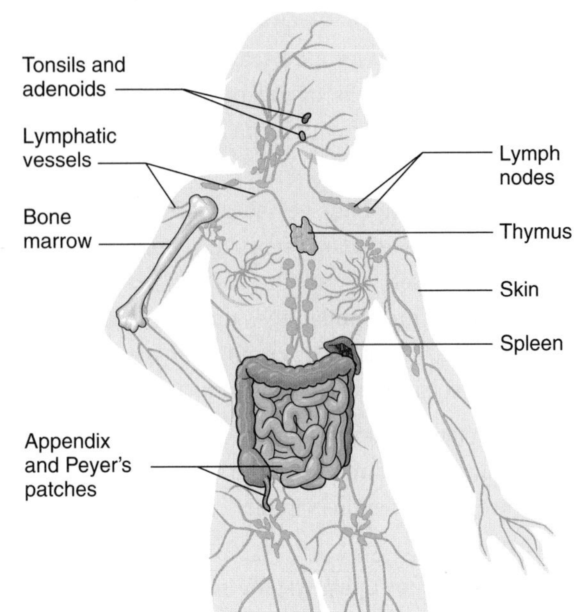

FIGURE 6.3 Many important roles in the immune system are filled by structures consisting of lymphoid tissues.

Additional Structures of the Lymphatic System

The remaining structures of this body system are made up of lymphoid tissue. The term *lymphoid* means pertaining to the lymphatic system or resembling lymph or lymphatic tissue. Although these structures consist of lymphoid tissue, their primary roles are in conjunction with the immune system (Figure 6.3).

The Tonsils

The **tonsils** (**TON**-sils) are three masses of lymphoid tissue that form a protective ring around the back of the nose and the upper throat (Figure 6.4). These structures play an important role in the immune system by preventing pathogens from entering the body through the nose and mouth.

- The **adenoids** (**AD**-eh-noids), also known as the *nasopharyngeal tonsils*, are located in the nasopharynx, which is described in Chapter 7.

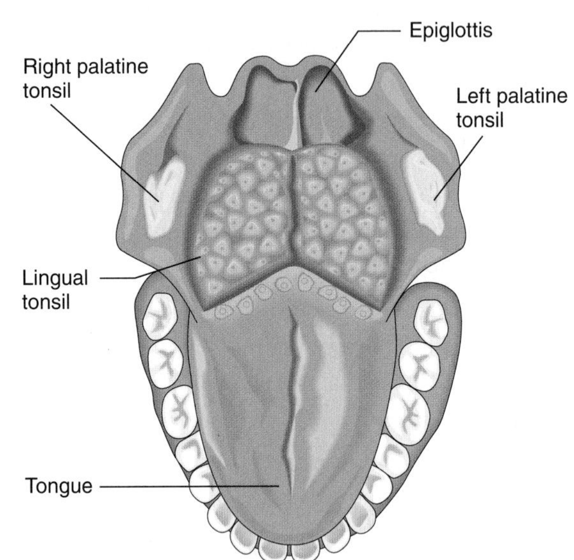

FIGURE 6.4 The tonsils form a protective ring around the entrance to the respiratory system.

- The **palatine tonsils** (**PAL**-ah-tine) are located on the left and right sides of the throat in the area that is visible through the mouth. *Palatine* means referring to the hard and soft palates.
- The **lingual tonsils** (**LING**-gwal) are located at the base of the tongue. *Lingual* means pertaining to the tongue.

The Thymus

The **thymus** (**THIGH**-mus) is located superior to (above) the heart (see Figure 6.3). Although it is composed largely of lymphoid tissue, the thymus is an endocrine gland that assists the immune system (see Chapter 13).

Peyer's Patches and the Vermiform Appendix

These structures, which consist of lymphoid tissue, work with the immune system to protect against the entry of pathogens through the digestive system (see Figure 6.3).

- **Peyer's patches** (**PIE**-erz) are located on the walls of the ileum. The *ileum* is last section of the small intestine.
- The **vermiform appendix** hangs from the lower portion of the cecum. The *cecum* is the first section of the large intestine. Recent research indicates that the appendix plays an important role in the immune system.

The Spleen

The **spleen** is a saclike mass of lymphoid tissue located in the left upper quadrant of the abdomen, just inferior to (below) the diaphragm and posterior to (behind) the stomach (Figure 6.5).

- The spleen filters microorganisms and other foreign material from the blood.
- The spleen forms lymphocytes and monocytes, which are specialized white blood cells with roles in the immune system.
- The spleen has the **hemolytic** (**hee**-moh-**LIT**-ick) function of destroying worn-out red blood cells and releasing their hemoglobin for reuse (**hem/o** means blood, and **-lytic** means to destroy).
- The spleen also stores extra erythrocytes (red blood cells) and maintains the appropriate balance between these cells and the plasma of the blood.

Pathology and Diagnostic Procedures of the Lymphatic System

- **Lymphadenitis** (lim-**fad**-eh-**NIGH**-tis), also known as *swollen glands*, is an inflammation of the lymph nodes (**lymphaden** means lymph node, and **-itis** means inflammation). The terms lymph nodes and lymph glands are sometimes used interchangeably. Swelling of the lymph nodes is frequently an indication of the presence of an infection.
- **Lymphadenopathy** (lim-**fad**-eh-**NOP**-ah-thee) is any disease process affecting a lymph node or nodes (**lymphaden/o** means lymph node, and **-pathy** means disease).
- A **lymphangioma** (lim-**fan**-jee-**OH**-mah) is a benign tumor formed by an abnormal collection of lymphatic

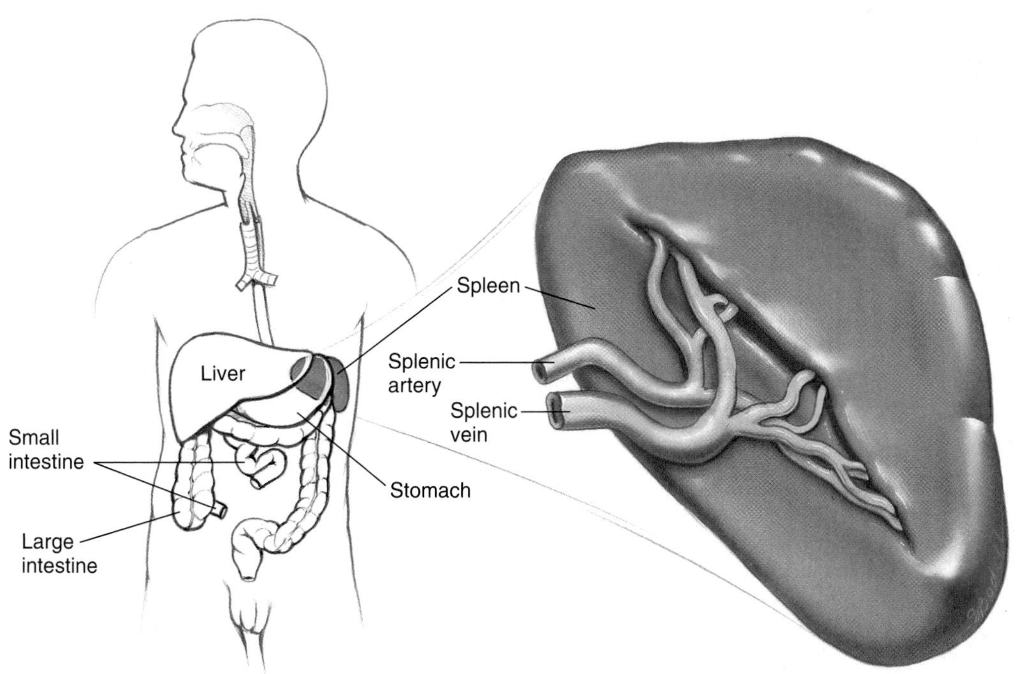

FIGURE 6.5 The spleen performs important functions related to both the immune and cardiovascular systems.

vessels due to a congenital malformation of the lymphatic system (**lymphangi** means lymph vessel, and **-oma** means tumor).

- **Splenomegaly** (**splee**-noh-**MEG**-ah-lee) is an abnormal enlargement of the spleen (**splen/o** means spleen, and **-megaly** means abnormal enlargement). This condition can be due to bleeding caused by an injury, an infectious disease such as mononucleosis, or abnormal functioning of the immune system.
- **Splenorrhagia** (**splee**-noh-**RAY**-jee-ah) is bleeding from the spleen (**splen/o** means spleen, and **-rrhagia** means bleeding).
- *Tonsillitis* and *tonsillectomy* are discussed in Chapter 1.
- **Lymphoscintigraphy** (**lim**-foh-sin-**TIH**-grah-fee) is a diagnostic test that is performed to detect damage or malformations of the lymphatic vessels.

Lymphedema

Lymphedema (**lim**-feh-**DEE**-mah) is swelling due to an abnormal accumulation of lymph fluid within the tissues (**lymph** means lymph, and **-edema** means swelling).

- **Primary lymphedema** is a hereditary disorder due to malformation of the lymphatic system. This condition, which can appear at any time in life, most commonly produces swelling in the feet and legs.
- **Secondary lymphedema** is caused by damage to the lymphatic system that most commonly produces swelling in the limb nearest to the damaged lymphatic vessels. Cancer treatment (surgery, chemotherapy, and/or radiation) and trauma (burns, injuries, and scarring) are the most frequent causes of this condition.

FUNCTIONS AND STRUCTURES OF THE IMMUNE SYSTEM

Functions of the Immune System

The primary function of the immune system is to maintain good health and to protect the body from harmful substances including:

- *Pathogens*, which are disease-producing microorganisms.
- *Allergens*, which are substances that produce allergic reactions.
- *Toxins*, which are poisonous or harmful substances.
- *Malignant cells*, which are potentially life-threatening cancer cells.

The immune system first attempts to prevent the entry of these harmful substances into the body. If they do gain entry, the immune system immediately begins working to destroy them.

Structures of the Immune System

Unlike other body systems, the immune system is not contained within a single set of organs or vessels. Instead, its functions depend on structures from several other body systems.

The First Lines of Defense

- **Intact skin** wraps the body in a physical barrier that prevents invading organisms from entering the body. *Intact* means there are no cuts, scrapes, open sores, or breaks in the skin.
- The **respiratory system** traps breathed-in foreign matter with nose hairs and the moist mucous membrane lining of the respiratory system. The tonsils form a protective ring around the entrance to the throat. If foreign matter gets past these barriers, coughing and sneezing help to expel it from the respiratory system.
- The **digestive system** uses the acids and enzymes produced by the stomach to destroy invaders that are swallowed or consumed with food.
- The structures of the **lymphatic system**, and specialized white blood cells, work together in specific ways to attack and destroy pathogens that have succeeded in entering the body.

The Antigen-Antibody Reaction

An **antigen-antibody reaction**, also known as the *immune reaction*, involves binding antigens to antibodies. This reaction labels a potentially dangerous antigen so it can be recognized, and destroyed, by other cells of the immune system.

- An **antigen** (**AN**-tih-jen) is any substance that the body regards as being foreign, and includes viruses, bacteria, toxins, and transplanted tissues. The immune system immediately responds to the presence of any antigen.
- An **allergen** (**AL**-er-jen) is a substance that produces an allergic reaction in an individual.
- An **antibody** (**AN**-tih-**bod**-ee) is a disease-fighting protein created by the immune system in response to the presence of a specific antigen (the prefix **anti-** means against). The terms *antibody* and *immunoglobulin* are often used interchangeably.

Immunoglobulins

Immunoglobulins (**im**-you-noh-**GLOB**-you-lins) bind with specific antigens in the antigen-antibody response. The five primary types of immunoglobulins, which are secreted by plasma cells, are also known as antibodies (see Table 6.1). **Plasma cells** are specialized white blood cells that produce antibodies coded to destroy specific antigens.

Specialized Cells of the Antigen-Antibody Reaction

The immune response requires the actions of many specialized cells.

Lymphocytes

Lymphocytes (**LIM**-foh-sights) are white blood cells that are formed in bone marrow as stem cells (**lymph/o** means lymph, and **-cytes** means cells). These cells undergo further maturation and differentiation in lymphoid tissues throughout the body.

These changes enable these lymphocytes to act as specialized antibodies that are capable of attacking specific antigens. *Maturation* means the process of becoming mature. *Differentiation* means to be modified to perform a specific function.

B Cells

B cells, also known as *B lymphocytes*, are specialized lymphocytes that produce and secrete antibodies. Each lymphocyte makes a specific antibody that is capable of destroying a specific antigen.

- B cells are most effective against viruses and bacteria circulating in the blood.
- When a B cell is confronted with the antigen that it is coded to destroy, that B cell is transformed into a *plasma B cell*. These cells are capable of producing and secreting antibodies that are coded to destroy a specific antigen.

Dendritic Cells

Dendritic cells (den-**DRIT**-ic) are specialized white blood cells that patrol the body searching for antigens that produce infections. When such a cell is found the dendritic cells grab, swallow, and internally break apart the captured antigen.

Fragments of the destroyed antigen are then moved to the surface of the cell where these fragments are displayed on tentacle-like extensions of the dendritic cell. The purpose of this display is to alert, and activate, T cells to protect against this specific antigen.

T Cells

T cells, also known as *T lymphocytes*, are small lymphocytes that mature in the thymus as a result of exposure to the hormone *thymosin*, which is secreted by the thymus.

- T cells contribute to the immune defense by coordinating immune defenses and by killing infected cells on contact.

TABLE 6.1
IMMUNOGLOBULINS AND THEIR ROLES

Immunoglobulin G (IgG) is the most abundant class of antibodies, and they are found in blood serum and lymph. These antibodies are active against bacteria, fungi, viruses, and foreign particles.
Immunoglobulin A (IgA) is the class of antibodies produced predominantly against ingested antigens. These antibodies are found in body secretions such as saliva, sweat, or tears, and function to prevent the attachment of viruses and bacteria to the epithelial surfaces that line most organs.
Immunoglobulin M (IgM) is the class of antibodies that are found in circulating body fluids. These are the first antibodies to appear in response to an initial exposure to an antigen.
Immunoglobulin D (IgD) is the class of antibodies found only on the surface of B cells. These antibodies are important in B cell activation which is discussed later in this chapter.
Immunoglobulin E (IgE) is the class of antibodies produced in the lungs, skin, and mucous membranes. These antibodies are responsible for allergic reactions.
Note: Synthetic immunoglobulins, which are used as medications, are discussed later in this chapter.

- **Interferon** (**in**-ter-**FEAR**-on) is a family of proteins produced by the T cells whose specialty is fighting viruses by slowing or stopping their multiplication.
- **Lymphokines** (**LIM**-foh-kyens), which are produced by the T cells, direct the antigen-antibody response by signaling between the cells of the immune system. Lymphokines attract macrophages to the infected site and prepare them to attack the invaders.
- A **macrophage** (**MACK**-roh-fayj) is a type of white blood cell that surrounds and kills invading cells (**macro-** means large, and **-phage** means a cell that eats). Macrophages also remove dead cells and stimulate the action of other immune cells.
- A **phagocyte** (**FAG**-oh-sight) is a large white blood cell that can destroy substances such as cell debris, dust, pollen, and pathogens by the process of phagocytosis (**phag/o** means to eat or swallow, and **-cyte** means cell). *Phagocytosis* is the process of destroying pathogens by surrounding and swallowing them.

Complement

Complement (**KOM**-pleh-ment) is a group of proteins that normally circulate in the blood in an inactive form and are activated by contact with nonspecific antigens such as foreign blood cells or bacteria. Complement then marks these foreign invaders and attracts phagocytes to destroy these antigens.

Immunity

Immunity is the state of being resistant to a specific disease.

- *Natural immunity* is passed from the mother to her fetus (developing child) before birth. This immunity lasts only a short time.
- *Passive immunity* is passed from the mother to her child after birth through breast milk.
- *Acquired immunity*, also known as *active immunity*, is the production of antibodies against a specific antigen by the immune system either by contracting an infectious disease such as chickenpox, or by vaccination against a disease such as poliomyelitis (polio).
- *Vaccination*, also known as *immunization*, is providing protection for susceptible individuals from communicable diseases by the administration of a vaccine to provide acquired immunity against a specific disease. A *vaccine* is a preparation containing an antigen, consisting of whole or partial disease-causing organisms, which have been killed or weakened.

Pathology and Diagnostic Procedures of the Immune System

The effectiveness of the immune system depends upon the individual's

- *General health*. If the immune system is compromised by poor health, it cannot be fully effective.
- *Age*. Older individuals usually have more acquired immunity; however, their immune systems tend to respond less quickly and effectively to new challenges. Babies and very young children do not yet have as much acquired immunity, and their bodies sometimes have difficulty resisting challenges to the immune system.
- *Heredity*. Genes and genetic disorders affect the individual's general health and the functioning of his or her immune system.

Allergic Reactions

- An **allergic reaction** occurs when the body's immune system reacts to a harmless allergen such as pollen, food, or animal dander as if it were a dangerous invader.
- An **allergy**, also known as *hypersensitivity*, is an overreaction by the body to a particular antigen.
- A **localized allergic response**, also known as a *cellular response*, includes redness, itching, and burning where the skin has come into contact with an allergen. For example, contact with poison ivy can cause a localized allergic response in the form of an itchy rash (see Chapter 12). Although the body reacts mildly the first time it is exposed to the allergen, sensitivity is established, and future contacts can cause much more-severe symptoms.
- A **systemic reaction**, which is also described as **anaphylaxis** (**an**-ah-fih-**LACK**-sis) or as *anaphylactic shock*, is a severe response to an allergen. As shown in Figure 6.6, the symptoms of this response develop quickly. Without medical aid, the patient can die within a few minutes.
- A **scratch test** is a diagnostic test to identify commonly troublesome allergens such as tree pollen and ragweed. Swelling and itching indicate an allergic reaction (see Figure 6.7).
- **Antihistamines** are medications administered to relieve or prevent the symptoms of hay fever, which is a common allergy to wind-borne pollens, and other types of allergies. Antihistamines work by preventing the

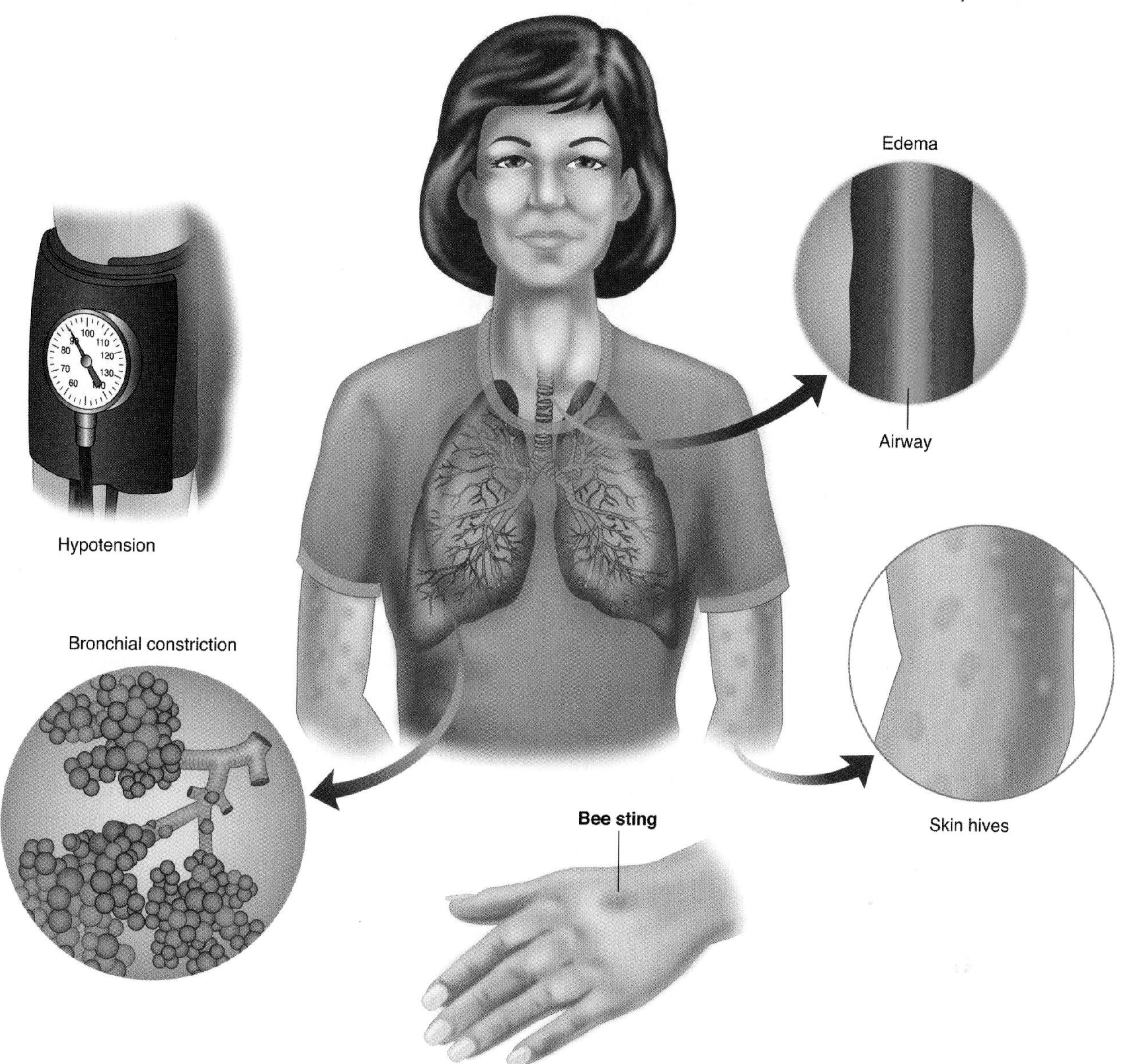

FIGURE 6.6 A severe anaphylactic allergic reaction involves several body systems and requires prompt treatment. Shown here are the many systems that may respond to a bee sting.

effects of *histamine*, which is a substance produced by the body that causes the itching, sneezing, runny nose, and watery eyes of an allergic reaction.

Autoimmune Disorders

An **autoimmune disorder** (**aw**-toh-ih-**MYOUN**), also known as an *autoimmune disease*, is any of a large group of diseases characterized by a condition in which the immune system produces antibodies against its own tissues. This abnormal functioning of the immune system appears to be genetically transmitted and predominantly occurs in women during the childbearing years. Autoimmune disorders affect most body systems. For examples, see Table 6.2.

Immunodeficiency Disorders

An **immunodeficiency disorder** (**im**-you-noh-deh-**FISH**-en-see) occurs when the immune response is compromised. *Compromised* means weakened, reduced, absent, or not functioning properly.

The Human Immunodeficiency Virus

The **human immunodeficiency virus** (**im**-you-noh-deh-**FISH**-en-see), commonly known as *HIV*, is a bloodborne

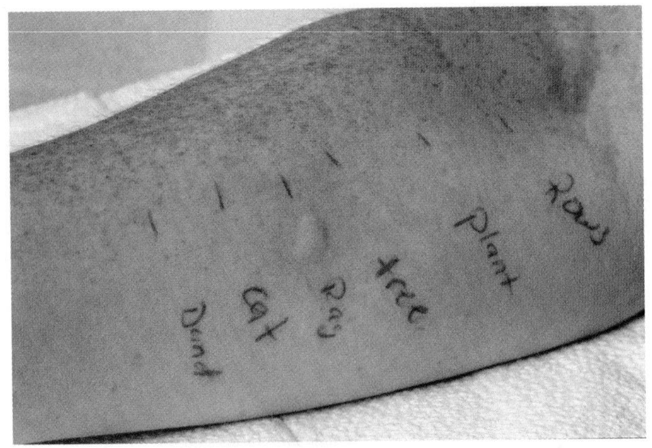

FIGURE 6.7 In scratch tests, allergens are placed on the skin, the skin is scratched, and the allergen is labeled. Reactions usually occur within 20 minutes. Pictured is a reaction to ragweed.

infection in which the virus damages or kills the cells of the immune system, causing it to progressively fail, thus leaving the body at risk of developing many life-threatening opportunistic infections (Figure 6.8). In the early stages of HIV, medical intervention can prolong the patient's life.

- An **opportunistic infection** (**op**-ur-too-**NIHS**-tick) is caused by a pathogen that does not normally produce an illness in healthy humans. However, when the host is debilitated, these pathogens are able to cause an infection. *Debilitated* means weakened by another condition. Because the immune systems of patients with HIV or AIDS are weakened, many opportunistic infections can develop.
- **Acquired immunodeficiency syndrome**, commonly known as *AIDS*, is the most advanced, and fatal, stage of an HIV infection.
- **Kaposi's sarcoma** (**KAP**-oh-seez sar-**KOH**-mah) is an example of an opportunistic infection that is frequently associated with HIV. This cancer causes patches of abnormal tissue to grow under the skin, in the lining of the mouth, nose, and throat, or in other organs.
- **ELISA**, which is the acronym for *enzyme-linked immunosorbent assay*, is a blood test used to screen for the presence of HIV antibodies.
- A **Western blot test** is a blood test that produces more accurate results than the ELISA test. The Western blot test is performed to confirm the diagnosis when the results of the ELISA test are positive. This is necessary because the ELISA test sometimes produces a *false positive* result in which the test erroneously indicates the presence of HIV.

Treatment of the Immune System

A variety of treatment procedures are used to correct or control the symptoms of disorders of the immune system.

Immunotherapy

Immunotherapy (ih-**myou**-noh-**THER**-ah-pee) is a disease treatment that involves either stimulating or repressing the immune response (**immun/o** means immune, and **-therapy** means treatment).

- In the treatment of cancers, immunotherapy is used to stimulate the immune response to fight the malignancy. *Stimulate* means to cause greater activity.
- In the treatment of allergies, immunotherapy is used to repress the body's sensitivity to a particular allergen.

TABLE 6.2
EXAMPLES OF AUTOIMMUNE DISORDERS AND THE AFFECTED BODY SYSTEMS

Body System	Autoimmune Disorder
Skeletal System	*Rheumatoid arthritis* affects joints and connective tissue.
Muscular System	*Myasthenia gravis* affects nerve and muscle synapses.
Cardiovascular System	*Pernicious anemia* affects the red blood cells.
Digestive System	*Crohn's disease* affects the intestines, ileum, or the colon.
Nervous System	*Multiple sclerosis* affects the brain and spinal cord.
Integumentary System	*Scleroderma* affects the skin and connective tissues.
Endocrine System	*Graves' disease* affects the thyroid gland.

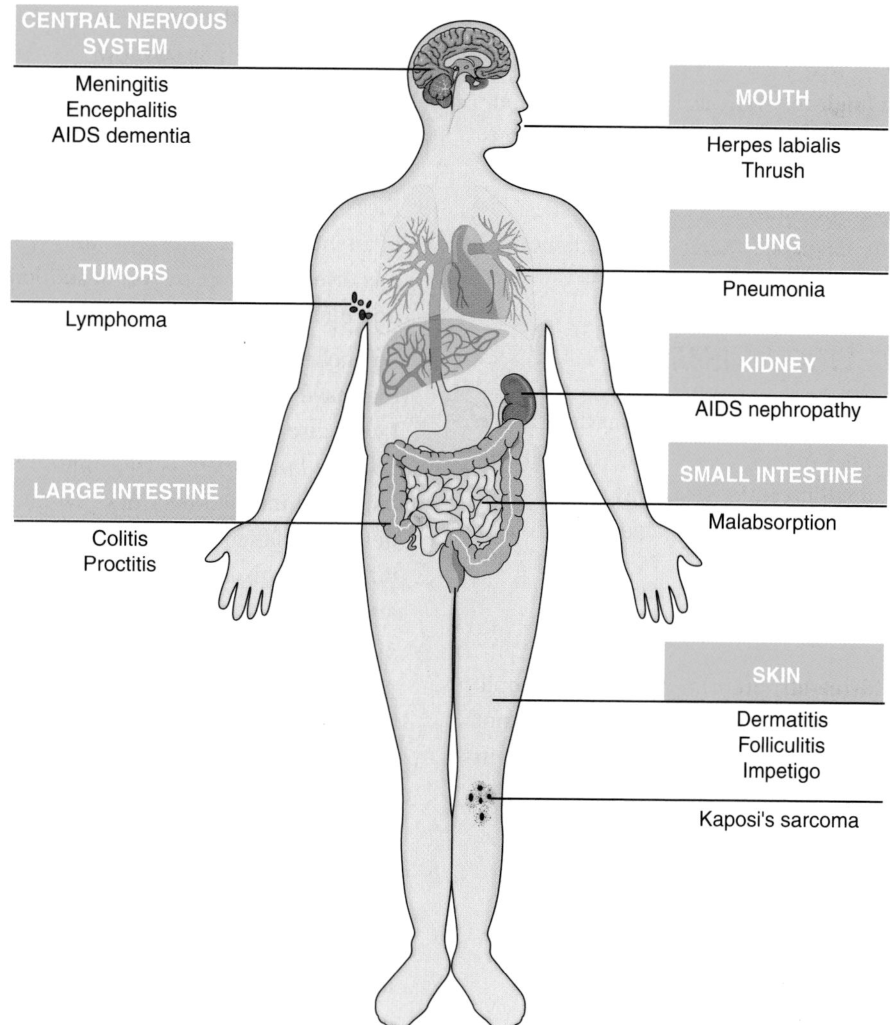

FIGURE 6.8 Pathologies associated with AIDS. (Each condition is discussed in the appropriate body system chapter.)

Repress means to decrease, slow, or stop a normal response. This treatment is also known as *allergy desensitization*.

Antibody Therapy

- **Synthetic immunoglobulins**, also known as *immune serum*, are used as a postexposure preventive measure against certain viruses, including rabies and some types of hepatitis. *Postexposure* means that the patient has been exposed to the virus, for example, has been bitten by an animal with rabies. The goal of this treatment is to prevent the disease from developing.
- **Synthetic interferon** is used in the treatment of multiple sclerosis, hepatitis C, and some cancers.
- **Monoclonal antibodies** are any of a class of antibodies produced in the laboratory by identical offspring of a clone of specific cells. These artificially produced antibodies are used to enhance the patient's immune response to certain malignancies, including some non-Hodgkin's lymphoma, melanoma, breast cancer and colon cancer. *Monoclonal* means pertains to a single clone of cells. As used here, a *clone* is an exact replica of a group of bacteria.

Immunosuppression

Immunosuppression (**im**-you-noh-sup-**PRESH**-un) is treatment to repress or interfere with the ability of the immune system to respond to stimulation by antigens.

- An **immunosuppressant** (**im**-you-noh-soo-**PRES**-ant) is a substance that prevents or reduces the body's normal immune response. This medication is administered to prevent the rejection of donor tissue and to depress autoimmune disorders.
- A **corticosteroid drug** (**kor**-tih-koh-**STEHR**-oid) is a hormone-like preparation administered primarily as an anti-inflammatory and as an immunosuppressant. The

natural production of corticosteroids by the endocrine system is discussed in Chapter 13.

- A **cytotoxic drug** (**sigh**-toh-**TOK**-sick) is a medication that kills or damages cells (**cyt/o** means cell, **tox** means poison, and **-ic** means pertaining to). These drugs are used as immunosuppressants or as antineoplastics. Antineoplastics are discussed under "Chemotherapy" later in this chapter.

PATHOGENIC ORGANISMS

A **pathogen** (**PATH**-oh-jen) is a microorganism that causes a disease in humans. A *microorganism* is a living organism that is so small it can be seen only with the aid of a microscope. *Pathogenic* means capable of producing disease (Figure 6.9).

Bacteria

Bacteria (back-**TEER**-ree-ah) are one-celled microscopic organisms (singular, *bacterium*). Most bacteria are not harmful to humans. Bacteria that are pathogenic in humans include bacilli, rickettsia, spirochetes, staphylococci, and streptococci.

- **Bacilli** (bah-**SILL**-eye) are rod-shaped spore-forming bacteria (singular, *bacillus*). **Tetanus** (**TET**-ah-nus) is caused by the bacillus *Clostridium tetani*, and is transmitted through a cut or wound. Tetanus is commonly known as *lockjaw* because it produces muscle spasms that are so severe a patient cannot open his or her mouth or swallow.
- A **rickettsia** (rih-**KET**-see-ah) is a small bacterium that lives in lice, fleas, ticks, and mites (plural, *rickettsiae*). **Rocky Mountain spotted fever**, which is caused by *Rickettsia rickettsii*, is transmitted to humans by the bite of an infected tick. The signs and symptoms of this serious disease include a fever of sudden onset, headache, and muscle pain followed by the development of a rash.
- **Spirochetes** (**SPY**-roh-keets) are spiral-shaped bacteria that have flexible walls and are capable of movement. **Lyme disease**, which is caused by the spirochete *Borrelia burgdorferi*, is transmitted to humans by the bite of an infected deer tick. Symptoms include fever, headache, fatigue, and a characteristic skin rash. If left untreated, this infection can spread to the joints, heart, and nervous system.
- **Staphylococci** (**staf**-ih-loh-**KOCK**-sigh) are a group of about 30 species of bacteria that form irregular groups or clusters resembling grapes (singular, *staphylococcus*). Most staphylococci are harmless and reside normally on the skin and mucous membranes of humans and other organisms; however, others are capable of producing very serious infections.
- **Staphylococcus aureus** (**staf**-ih-loh-**KOCK**-us **OR**-ee-us), also known as *staph aureus*, is a form of staphylococci that commonly infects wounds and causes serious problems such as toxic shock syndrome or

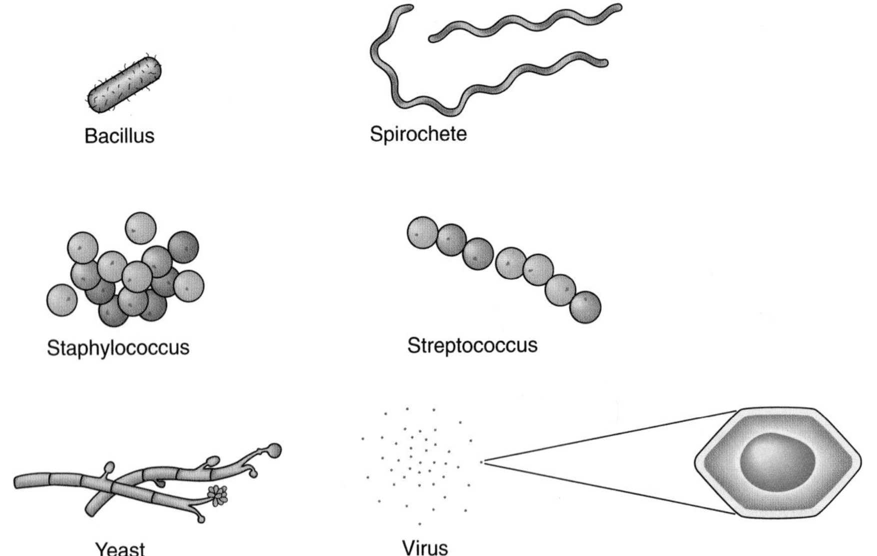

FIGURE 6.9 Shown here are examples of types of pathogens. The single virus shown at the right is magnified to illustrate details of its structure.

produces food poisoning. *Toxic shock syndrome* is a rare but potentially fatal disease caused by bacterial toxins.

- **Streptococci** (**strep**-toh-***KOCK***-sigh) are bacteria that form a chain (singular, *streptococcus*). Many streptococcal species are harmless; however, other members of this group are responsible for illnesses including *strep throat*, *meningitis* (see Chapter 10), *endocarditis* (see Chapter 5), and *necrotizing fasciitis* (see Chapter 12).

Septic Shock

Septic shock is a serious condition that occurs when an overwhelming bacterial infection affects the body. Toxins released by these pathogens can produce direct tissue damage resulting in low blood pressure. This damage causes vital organs (the brain, heart, kidneys, and liver) to not function properly or to fail completely. Septic shock occurs most often in the very old and the very young. It also occurs in those with underlying or debilitating illnesses.

Antibiotic Resistant Bacteria

- **Antibiotic resistant bacteria**, also known as *superbugs*, develop when an antibiotic fails to kill all of the bacteria it targets. When this occurs the surviving bacteria become resistant to that particular drug. When more and more bacteria become resistant to first-line treatments, the consequences are severe, as illnesses last longer, and the risks of complications and death increase.
- **Methicillin-resistant *Staphylococcus aureus***, commonly known as *MRSA*, is resistant to most antibiotics. The first symptom of MRSA looks like small, red bumps with a black top. These bumps soon become red-hot abscesses that require immediate care. MRSA infections are serious, difficult to treat, and can be fatal. Originally these infections were nosocomial (hospital acquired); however, MRSA infections are increasingly present in the general population.

Fungus, Yeast, and Parasites

- A **fungus** (**FUNG**-gus) is a simple parasitic organism (plural, *fungi*). Some of these fungi are harmless to humans, others are pathogenic. **Tinea pedis**, commonly known as *athlete's foot*, is a fungal infection that commonly develops between the toes and on the feet.
- **Yeast** is a type of fungus. **Candidiasis** (**kan**-dih-**DYE**-ah-sis), formerly known as *moniliasis*, is now also known as a *yeast infection* or *thrush*. These infections, which are caused by the pathogenic yeast *Candida albicans*, occur on the skin or mucous membranes in the warm, moist areas such as the vagina or the mouth.
- A **parasite** (**PAR**-ah-sight) is a plant or animal that lives on, or within, another living organism at the expense of that organism. For example, **malaria** (mah-**LAY**-ree-ah) is a disease caused by a parasite that lives in certain mosquitoes that is transferred to humans by the bite of an infected mosquito. Symptoms develop from 7 days to 4 weeks after being infected and include fever, shaking chills, headache, muscle aches, and tiredness.
- Another parasite is **toxoplasmosis** (**tock**-soh-plaz-**MOH**-sis) which is most commonly transmitted from animals (pets) to humans by contact with contaminated feces. If a woman contracts this condition during pregnancy, it can result in abnormalities in the developing child such as microcephalus or hydrocephalus. *Microcephalus* is an abnormally small head and underdeveloped brain. *Hydrocephalus* is a condition in which excess cerebrospinal fluid accumulates in the ventricles of the brain. For this reason, it is recommended that pregnant women not perform tasks such as cleaning a kitty-litter box.

Viruses

Viruses (**VYE**-rus-ez) are very small infectious agents that live only by invading other cells (singular, *virus*). After invading the cell, the virus reproduces and then breaks the cell wall to release the newly formed viruses. These viruses spread to other cells and repeat the process.

Viral Infections

- **Herpes zoster** (**HER**-peez **ZOS**-ter), which is also known as *shingles*, is an acute viral infection characterized by painful skin eruptions that follow the underlying route of an inflamed nerve. This inflammation occurs when the dormant varicella (chickenpox) virus is reactivated later in life. A vaccine is available to prevent such a reoccurance.
- **Infectious mononucleosis** (**mon**-oh-**new**-klee-**OH**-sis), also known as *mono*, is caused by the *Epstein-Barr virus* (EBV). This condition is characterized by fever, a sore throat, and enlarged lymph nodes. Swelling of the spleen or liver involvement can also develop.

- **Measles** is an acute, highly contagious infection caused by the *rubeola virus* and transmitted by respiratory droplets. Symptoms include a high fever, a runny nose, coughing, photophobia, and a red, itchy rash over the entire body. *Photophobia* means sensitivity to light. Complications of measles can be serious.
- **Mumps** is an acute viral disease characterized by the swelling of the parotid glands, which are the salivary glands located just in front of the ears. In adults, mumps can also cause painful swelling of the ovaries or testicles.
- **Rubella** (roo-**BELL**-ah), also known as *German measles* or *3-day measles*, is a viral infection characterized by a low-grade fever, swollen glands, inflamed eyes, and a fine, pink rash. Although not usually severe or long lasting, rubella is serious in a woman during early pregnancy because of its ability to cause defects in a developing fetus. Measles and rubella share similar symptoms, and in fact the term "German" measles comes from the Latin word "*germanus*," meaning similar.
- The **measles, mumps, and rubella vaccination** (MMR) can prevent these three viral conditions.
- **Rabies** (**RAY**-beez) is an acute viral infection that is most commonly transmitted to humans by the bite or saliva of an infected animal. In humans, signs and symptoms of rabies usually occur 30–90 days after the bite. Once symptoms develop, rabies is almost always fatal. If at risk, it is necessary to undergo testing immediately so that postexposure treatment can be started as quickly as possible.
- **Varicella** (**var**-ih-**SEL**-ah), also known as *chickenpox*, is caused by the herpes virus *Varicella zoster* and is highly contagious. This condition is characterized by a fever and a rash consisting of hundreds of itchy, fluid-filled blisters that burst and form crusts.
- **West Nile virus** is spread to humans by the bite of an infected mosquito. A mild form of this condition has flu-like symptoms. A more severe variety spreads to the spinal cord and brain.

Cytomegalovirus

Cytomegalovirus (**sigh**-toh-**meg**-ah-loh-**VYE**-rus) (CMV) is a member of the herpesvirus family that cause a variety of diseases (**cyt/o** means cell, **megal/o** means large, **vir** means virus, and **-us** is a singular noun ending).

- CMV is found in most body fluids and can be present as a *silent infection* in which the individual has no signs or symptoms of the infection.
- CMV can potentially cause a serious illness when the individual has a weakened immune system.
- CMV can be transmitted from the mother to her unborn child. This transmission can cause serious congenital disabilities in the child.

Medications to Control Infections

- **Antibiotics** are medications that are capable of inhibiting growth, or killing pathogenic bacterial microorganisms (**anti-** means against, **bio** means life, and **-tic** means pertaining to). *Inhibit* means to slow the growth or development. Antibiotics are not effective against viral infections.
- A *bactericide* is a substance that causes the death of bacteria (**bacteri** means bacteria, and **-cide** means causing death). This group of antibiotics includes penicillins and cephalosporins. A *bacteriostatic* is an agent that slows or stops the growth of bacteria (**bacteri** means bacteria, and **-static** means causing control). This group of antibiotics includes tetracycline, sulfonamide, and erythromycin.
- An **antifungal** (**an**-tih-**FUNG**-gul) is an agent that destroys or inhibits the growth of fungi (**anti-** means against, **fung** means fungus, and **-al** means pertaining to). Lotrimin is an example of a topical antifungal that is applied to treat, or prevent, athlete's foot. This type of medication is also known as an *antimycotic*.
- An **antiviral drug** (**an**-tih-**VYE**-ral), such as acyclovir, is used to treat viral infections or to provide temporary immunity (**anti-** means against, **vir** means virus, and **-al** means pertaining to).

ONCOLOGY

Oncology (ong-**KOL**-oh-jee) is the study of the prevention, causes, and treatment of tumors and cancer (**onc** means tumor, and **-ology** means study of). Most cancers are named for the part of the body where the cancer originated. Cancer can attack all body systems and is the second leading cause of death in the United States after heart conditions.

Tumors

A **tumor**, which is also known as a *neoplasm*, is a growth of tissue that forms an abnormal mass. Within this mass, the multiplication of cells is uncontrolled, abnormally rapid, and progressive (**neo-** means new or strange, and **-plasm** means formation).

- A tumor can be *benign* (not life-threatening) or *malignant* (harmful, capable of spreading, and potentially life-threatening).
- A **benign tumor** is a noncancerous growth; however, these tumors can cause problems by placing pressure on adjacent structures. For example, a **myoma** (my-**OH**-mah) is a benign tumor made up of muscle tissue (**my** means muscle, and **-oma** means tumor).
- A **malignant tumor** is harmful, capable of spreading to distant body sites including other body system, can become progressively worse, and is progressively life-threatening. For example, a **myosarcoma** (**my**-oh-sahr-**KOH**-mah) is a malignant tumor derived from muscle tissue (**myo** means muscle, **sarc** means flesh, and **-oma** means tumor).
- **Angiogenesis** (**an**-jee-oh-**JEN**-eh-sis) is the process through which the tumor supports its growth by creating its own blood supply (**angi/o** means vessel, and **-genesis** means reproduction). Angiogenesis is the opposite of *antiangiogenesis.*
- **Antiangiogenesis** is a form of treatment that disrupts this blood supply to the tumor (**anti-** means against, **angi/o** means vessel, and **-genesis** means reproduction). Antiangiogenesis is the opposite of *angiogenesis.*

Cancer

Cancer is a class of diseases characterized by the uncontrolled division of cells and the ability of these cells to invade other tissues, either by invasion through direct growth into adjacent tissue or by spreading into distant sites by metastasizing.

- To **metastasize** (meh-**TAS**-tah-sighz) is the process by which cancer spreads from one place to another. The cancer moves from the primary site and metastasizes (spreads) to a secondary site.
- A **metastasis** (meh-**TAS**-tah-sis) is a new cancer site that results from the spreading process (**meta-** means beyond, and **-stasis** means stopping). The metastasis can be within the same body system or within another body system at a distance from the primary site (plural, *metastases*).

Carcinomas

A **carcinoma** (**kar**-sih-**NOH**-mah) is a malignant tumor that occurs in epithelial tissue (**carcin** means cancer, and **-oma** means tumor). Epithelial tissue forms the protective covering for all of the internal and external surfaces of the body (Figure 6.10).

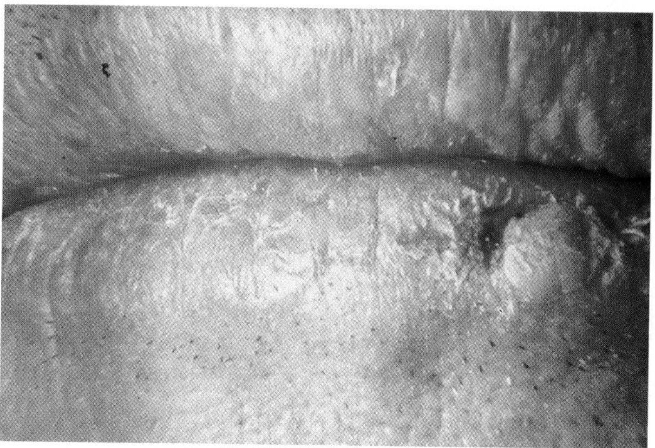

FIGURE 6.10 Carcinoma of the lip. (Courtesy of Dr. Joseph Konzelman, School of Dentistry, Medical College of Georgia.)

- Carcinomas tend to infiltrate and produce metastases that can affect any organ or part of the body.
- **Carcinoma in situ** (**kar**-sih-**NOH**-mah in **SIGH**-too) describes a malignant tumor in its original position that has not yet disturbed or invaded the surrounding tissues. *In situ* means in the place where the cancer first occurred.
- For example, an **adenocarcinoma** (**ad**-eh-noh-**kar**-sih-**NOH**-mah) is any one of a large group of carcinomas derived from glandular tissue (**aden/o** means gland, **carcin** means cancer, and **-oma** means tumor).

Sarcomas

A **sarcoma** (sar-**KOH**-mah) is a malignant tumor that arises from connective tissues, including hard tissues, soft tissues, and liquid tissues (**sarc** means flesh, and **-oma** means tumor) (plural, *sarcomas* or *sarcomata*).

- *Hard tissue sarcomas* arise from bone or cartilage (see Chapter 3). For example, an **osteosarcoma** (**oss**-tee-oh-sar-**KOH**-mah) is a malignant tumor usually involving the upper shaft of long bones, the pelvis, or knee (**oste/o** means bone, **sarc** means flesh, and **-oma** means tumor).
- *Soft tissue sarcomas* arise from tissues such as muscle, connective tissues such as tendons, blood and lymphatic vessels, nerves, and fat. For example, a **synovial sarcoma** (sih-**NOH**-vee-al sar-**KOH**-mah) is a malignant tumor of the tissue surrounding a synovial joint. The most common locations are the knee, ankle, shoulder, and hip.
- *Liquid tissue sarcomas* arise from blood and lymph. One example is **leukemia** (loo-**KEE**-mee-ah), which affects the blood, and is discussed in Chapter 5.

Staging

Staging is the process of classifying tumors with respect to how far the disease has progressed, the potential for its responding to therapy, and the patient's prognosis. Specific staging systems are used for different types of cancer (see Figure 6.11).

Lymphomas

Lymphoma (lim-**FOH**-mah) is a general term applied to malignancies affecting lymphoid tissues (**lymph** means lymph, and **-oma** means tumor). This includes lymph nodes, the spleen, liver, and bone marrow. The two most common types of lymphomas are Hodgkin's lymphoma and non-Hodgkin's lymphoma.

- **Hodgkin's lymphoma** (**HODJ**-kinz lim-**FOH**-mah), also known as *Hodgkin's disease*, is distinguished from other lymphomas by the presence of large, cancerous lymphocytes known as *Reed-Sternberg cells*.

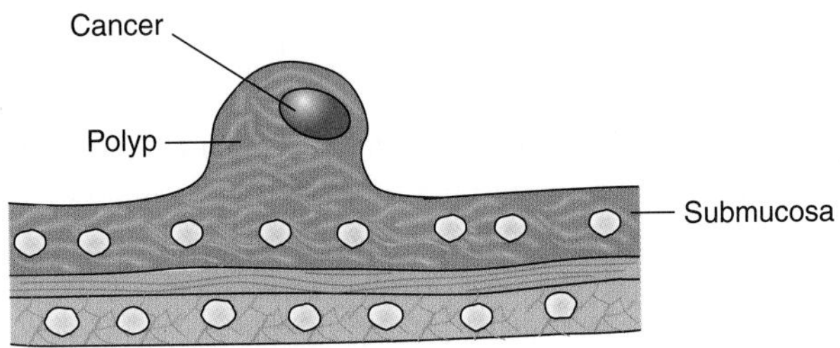

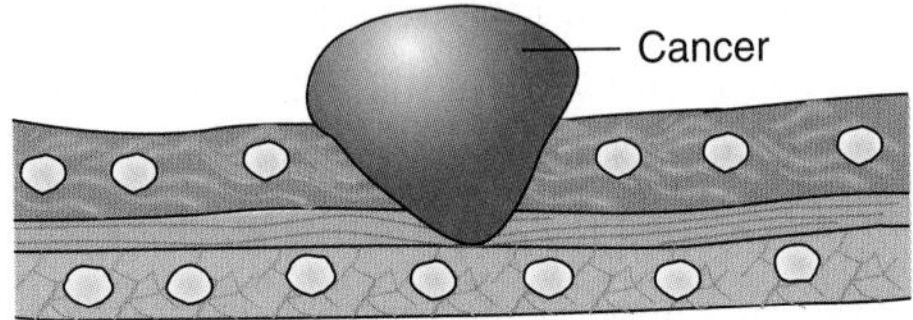

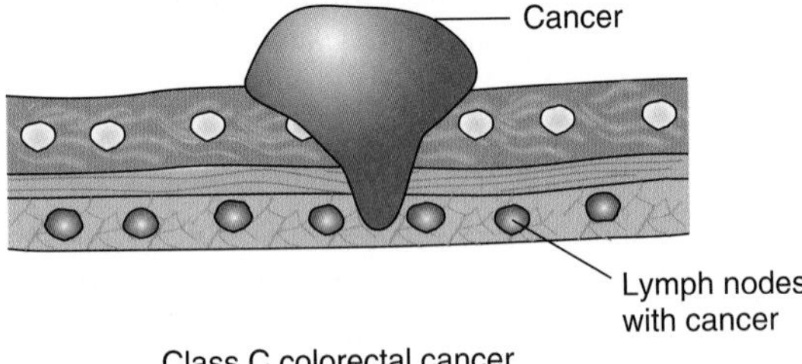

FIGURE 6.11 Stages of colorectal cancer. *Class A:* The cancerous tumor has formed within a polyp inside the colon, but has not yet invaded the surrounding tissue. *Class B:* The cancer has invaded the underlying tissue. *Class C:* The cancer has spread to the underlying tissues and nearby lymph nodes.

- **Non-Hodgkin's lymphoma** is the term used to describe all lymphomas *other than* Hodgkin's lymphoma. There are many different types of non-Hodgkin's lymphoma, some aggressive (fast-growing) and some indolent (slow-growing).

Breast Cancer

Breast cancer is a carcinoma that develops from the cells of the breast and can spread to adjacent lymph nodes and other body sites (Figure 6.12). There are several types of breast cancer named for their location or amount of spreading.

- **Ductal carcinoma in situ** is breast cancer at its earliest stage before the cancer has broken through the wall of the milk duct. At this stage, the cure rate is nearly 100%.
- **Infiltrating ductal carcinoma** (in-**FILL**-trate-ng **DUK**-tal kar-sih-**NOH**-mah), also known as *invasive ductal carcinoma*, starts in the milk duct, breaks through the wall of that duct, and invades the fatty breast tissue. This form of cancer accounts for the majority of all breast cancers. *Infiltrating* and *invasive* are terms used to describe cancer that has spread beyond the layer of tissue in which it developed and the cancer is now growing into surrounding, healthy tissues.
- **Infiltrating lobular carcinoma**, also known as *invasive lobular carcinoma*, is cancer that starts in the milk glands (lobules), breaks through the wall of the gland, and invades the fatty tissue of the breast. Once this cancer reaches the lymph nodes, it can rapidly spread to distant parts of the body.
- **Inflammatory breast cancer** (IBC) is the most aggressive and least common form of breast cancer. IBC grows rapidly, and symptoms include pain, rapid increase in the breast size, redness or a rash on the breast, and the

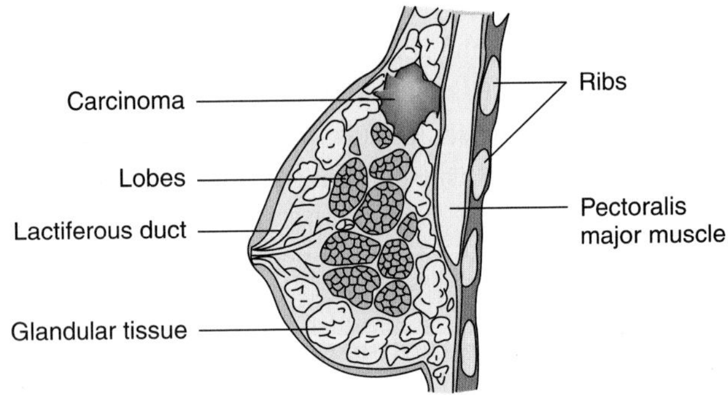

FIGURE 6.12 Most breast cancers are initially detected as a lump. When this lump is malignant, it is a form of carcinoma.

swelling of nearby lymph nodes. IBC can be detected by magnetic resonance imaging (MRI); however, it is not detected by mammography or ultrasound.

- **Male breast cancer** can occur in the small amount of breast tissue that is normally present in men. The types of cancers are similar to those occurring in women.

Detection of Breast Cancer

Early detection of breast cancer is very important and utilizes the following techniques.

- **Breast self-examination** is an essential self-care procedure for the early detection of breast cancer. The focus of this self-examination is checking for a new lump or for changes in an existing lump, shape of the nipple, or the skin covering the breast.
- **Professional palpation of the breast** is performed to feel the texture, size, and consistency of the breast. *Palpation* is explained in Chapter 15.
- **Mammography** (mam-**OG**-rah-fee) is a radiographic examination of the breasts to detect the presence of tumors or precancerous cells (**mammo/o** means breast, and **-graphy** means the process of producing a picture or record) (Figure 6.13). The resulting record is a *mammogram* (Figure 6.14).

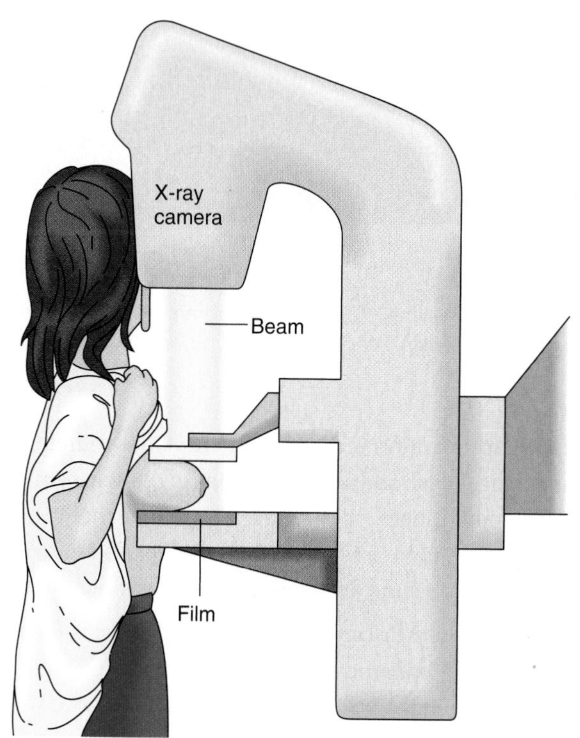

FIGURE 6.13 In mammography, the breast is gently flattened and radiographed from various angles.

- Ultrasound is used as an initial follow-up test when an abnormality is found by mammography. (Ultrasound is discussed further in Chapter 15.)
- A **surgical biopsy** (**BYE**-op-see) is the removal of a small piece of tissue for examination to confirm or establish a diagnosis (**bi-** means pertaining to life, and **-opsy** means view of). After a diagnosis has been established, treatment is then based on the stage of the cancer.
- A **needle breast biopsy** is a technique in which an x-ray-guided needle is used to remove small samples of tissue from the breast. It is less painful and disfiguring than a surgical biopsy.
- In a **sentinel-node biopsy**, after the sentinel lymph node has been identified, only this and the other affected nodes are removed for biopsy. If the cancer has not spread, this spares the remaining nodes in that group. The *sentinel node* is the first lymph node to come into contact with cancer cells as they leave the organ of origination and start spreading into the rest of the body.
- **Lymph node dissection** is a surgical procedure in which all of the lymph nodes in a major group are removed to determine or slow the spread of cancer. For example, an *axillary lymph node dissection* (ALND) is sometimes performed as part of the surgical treatment of the breast.

Surgical Treatment of Breast Cancer

- A **lumpectomy** is the surgical removal of only the cancerous tissue and a surrounding margin of normal tissue (Figure 6.15).
- A **mastectomy** (mas-**TECK**-toh-mee) is the surgical removal of the entire breast and nipple (**mast** means breast, and **-ectomy** means surgical removal). Although simply described as a mastectomy, this procedure often includes the removal of axillary lymph nodes under the adjacent arm.
- A **modified radical mastectomy** is the surgical removal of the entire breast and all of the axillary lymph nodes under the adjacent arm (Figure 6.16).
- A **radical mastectomy** is the surgical removal of an entire breast and many of the surrounding tissues.

Cancer Treatments

The most common forms of cancer treatments are surgery, chemotherapy, and radiation therapy.

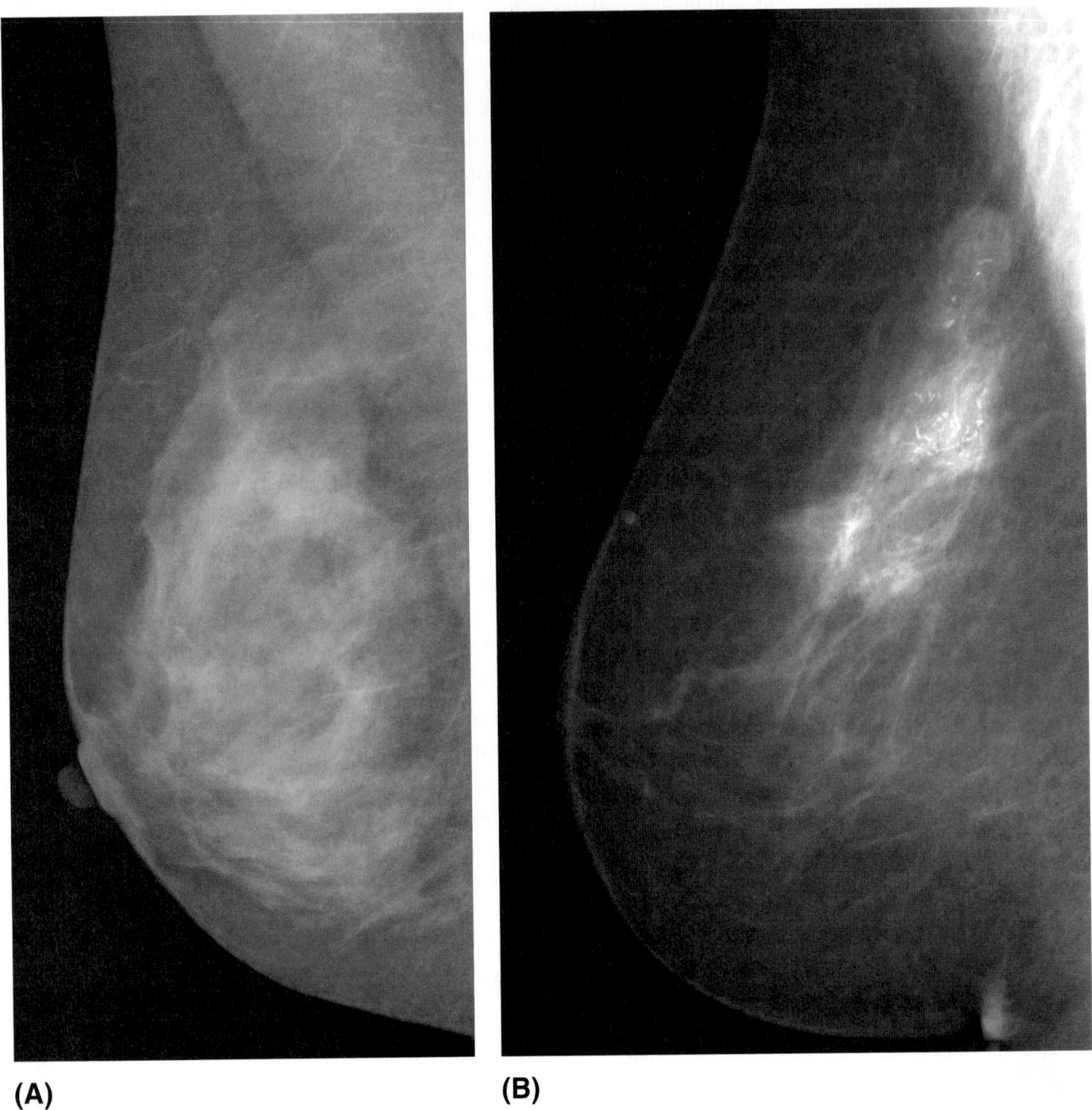

FIGURE 6.14 (A) A normal mammogram in which no abnormal mass is visible. (B) A mammogram in which breast cancer is visible. (Films courtesy of Lonie R. Salkoski, M.D., University of Wisconsin School of Medicine and Public Health, Madison, WI.)

Surgery

Most commonly cancer surgery involves removing the malignancy plus a margin of normal surrounding tissue. It may also involve the removal of one or more nearby lymph nodes to detect whether the cancer has stated to spread.

Chemotherapy

Chemotherapy is the use of chemical agents and drugs in combinations selected to destroy malignant cells and tissues.

- **Chemoprevention** is the use of natural or synthetic substances such as drugs or vitamins to reduce the risk of developing cancer, or to reduce the chance that cancer will recur. Chemoprevention may also be used to reduce the size or slow the development of an existing tumor.
- An **antineoplastic** (**an**-tih-nee-oh-**PLAS**-tick) is medication that blocks the development, growth, or proliferation of malignant cells (**anti-** means against, **ne/o** means new, **plast** means growth or formation, and **-ic** means pertaining to). *Proliferation* means to increase rapidly.

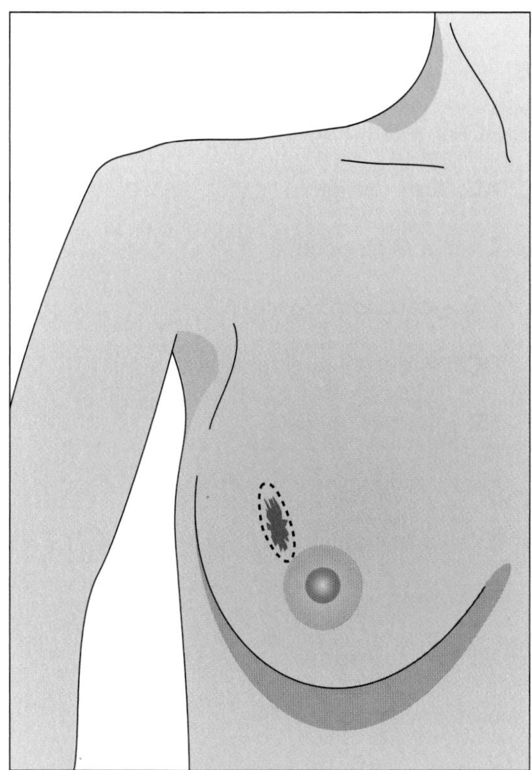

FIGURE 6.15 A lumpectomy is the removal of the cancerous tissue plus a margin of healthy tissue.

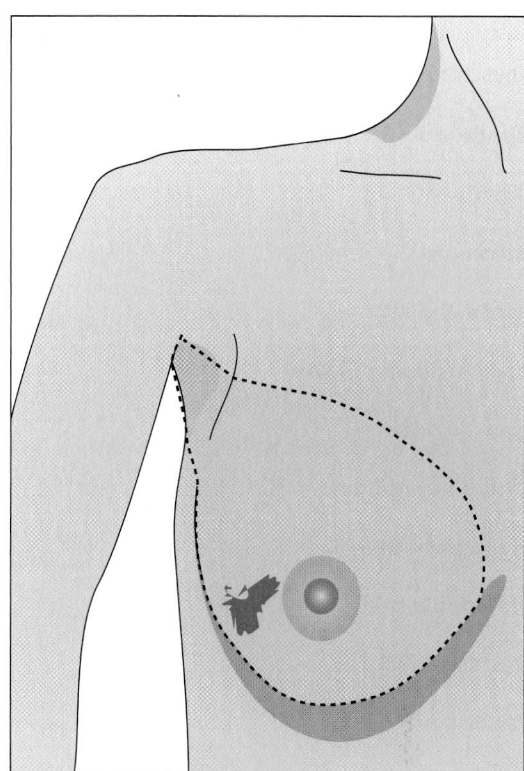

FIGURE 6.16 A modified radical mastectomy is the removal of the entire breast and the adjacent lymph nodes.

- Cytotoxic drugs, which are also used for both immunosuppression and chemotherapy, are discussed earlier in this chapter.

Radiation Therapy

Radiation therapy is used in the treatment of some cancers, with the goal of destroying the cancer while sparing healthy tissues.

- **Brachytherapy** (**brack**-ee-**THER**-ah-pee) is the use of radioactive materials in contact with, or implanted into, the tissues to be treated (**brachy-** means short, and **-therapy** means treatment).
- **Teletherapy** (**tel**-eh-**THER**-ah-pee) is radiation therapy administered at a distance from the body (**tele-** means distant, and **-therapy** means treatment). With the assistance of three-dimensional computer imaging, it is possible to aim doses more precisely.

Additional Therapies

- **Adjuvant therapy** (**AD**-jeh-vant) is used after the primary treatments have been completed to decrease the chance that a cancer will recur. The term *adjuvant* refers to an agent intended to increase the effectiveness of a drug; however, adjuvant treatments for cancer can also include chemotherapy, hormone therapy, radiation, immunotherapy, or targeted therapy.
- **Targeted therapy** is a developing form of anti-cancer drug therapy that uses drugs or other substances to identify and attack specific cancer cells without harming normal cells. A monoclonal antibody is a type of targeted therapy.

ABBREVIATIONS RELATED TO THE LYMPHATIC AND IMMUNE SYSTEMS

Table 6.3 presents an overview of the abbreviations related to the terms introduced in this chapter. Note: To avoid errors or confusion, always be cautious when using abbreviations.

TABLE 6.3

Abbreviations Related to the Lymphatic and Immune Systems

antibody = A, Ab	**A, Ab** = antibody
antigen = AG, Ag	**AG, Ag** = antigen
carcinoma = CA, Ca	**CA, Ca** = carcinoma
carcinoma in situ = CIS	**CIS** = carcinoma in situ
ductal carcinoma in situ = DCIS	**DCIS** = ductal carcinoma in situ
herpes zoster = HZ	**HZ** = herpes zoster
Hodgkin's lymphoma = HL	**HL** = Hodgkin's lymphoma
immunoglobulin = IG	**IG** = immunoglobulin
lymphedema = LE	**LE** = lymphedema
metastasis = MET	**MET** = metastasis
metastasize = met	**met** = metastasize
non-Hodgkin's lymphoma = NHL	**NHL** = non-Hodgkin's lymphoma
rickettsia = Rick	**Rick** = rickettsia
varicella = VSZ	**VSZ** = varicella

CAREER OPPORTUNITIES

In addition to the medical specialties already discussed, some of the health occupations involving the treatment of the lymphatic and immune systems include:

- **Cytotechnologist:** a clinical laboratory technologist who prepares slides of body cells and examines these cells microscopically for abnormalities that can signal the beginning of a cancerous growth
- **Immunology technologist:** a laboratory technician who examines elements of the human immune system and its response to foreign bodies
- **Lymphedema therapist:** an occupational or physical therapist with specialized postgraduate training to provide treatment for lymphedema patients
- **Mammographer:** a radiographer who specializes in performing mammograms

HEALTH OCCUPATION PROFILE

LYMPHEDEMA THERAPIST

Early in her career as a lymphedema therapist, Doris Laing, LMBT, CLT-LANA, worked in a hospital in "the snow belt." There, she was the only therapist qualified to provide the manual lymph drainage (MLD) and other treatment modalities recommended for lymphedema patients.

Several years ago, Doris moved south to join a group practice where several qualified lymphedema therapists are treating lymphedema patients with challenging, severe cases of this condition. As Doris describes it, *"The therapists, and our patients, benefit from our being able to discuss difficult situations and find innovative solutions to provide the patients with the highest quality of care in the management of this chronic condition. And yes, I do miss the snow—but that is what ski vacations are for!"*

STUDY BREAK

Very few scientists are lucky enough to be immortalized by having a body part carry their name. It's obvious that Peyer's patches is an eponym (named after a person), so you're probably wondering who Dr. Peyer was—and why the small areas of lymphatic tissue on the walls of the large intestine are named after him.

Johann Conrad Peyer was a Swiss anatomist who lived from 1653 to 1712. He was born into a wealthy family and studied medicine in Switzerland and Paris. In addition to working as a physician, he taught rhetoric, logic, and medicine, and conducted scientific experiments. In 1682, he was the first person to describe the lymphatic nodules on the walls of the ileum that now bear his name.

Humans are not the only species with lymphatic tissue called Peyer's patches. Johann Conrad Peyer also lives on in veterinary studies, where all students learning about the intestines of cows, dogs, rats, and other mammals must remember his name.

Review Time

Write the answers to the following questions on a separate piece of paper or in your notebook. In addition, be prepared to take part in the classroom discussion.

1. ***Written Assignment:*** Describe the primary characteristic that differentiates **Hodgkin's lymphoma** from **non-Hodgkin's lymphoma**.

   Discussion Assignment: Define the term **lymphoma** in terms that a layperson could understand.

2. ***Written Assignment:*** Identify **autoimmune disorders** of at least four body systems.

   Discussion Assignment: Be prepared to describe the four autoimmune disorders you identified in the written assignment. (The conditions listed in Table 6.2 are described in other chapters of the text.)

3. ***Written Assignment:*** Identify three major functions of the **lymphatic system**.

   Discussion Assignment: Describe how the lymphatic system absorbs fats and fat-soluble vitamins.

4. ***Written Assignment:*** Identify the four body systems that make up the first lines of defense of the **immune system**.

   Discussion Assignment: Describe how each of these defenses assists the immune system.

5. ***Written Assignment:*** Use terms a patient would understand to describe the role of **immunosuppression**.

   Discussion Assignment: **Cytotoxic drugs** can be used as immunosuppressants or as antineoplastics. Discuss what antineoplastics are used for.

Optional Internet Activity

The goal of this activity is to help you learn more about medical terminology as it applies to the "real world." Select **one** *of these two options and follow the instructions.*

1. Search for information about **Lyme disease** or **Rocky Mountain spotted fever**. Write a brief (one- or two-paragraph) report on something new you learned here and include the address of the web site where you found this information.

2. To learn more about **acquired immunodeficiency syndrome** (AIDS), go to the Medline Plus web site sponsored by the National Institutes of Health. Explore the site and then write a brief (one- or two-paragraph) report on something new you learned here.

THE HUMAN TOUCH: CRITICAL THINKING ACTIVITY

The following story and questions are designed to stimulate critical thinking through class discussion or as a brief essay response. There are no right or wrong answers to these questions.

"Man, summer seems so long ago. Remember everything that we had to do to prepare for college life?" ***Jackie asked.*** **"Buy extra-long sheets for the dorm bed, say good-bye to high school friends—and then there was a trip to the clinic for that bacterial meningitis vaccine. Why'd we need to get that anyway? Are dorms cesspools for disease or something?"**

"My mom's a nurse, and while she was giving me the vaccination, she explained it to me," ***Crystal rolled her eyes and put on her best "mom" voice.*** **"If there is an outbreak of meningitis in the dormitory, everyone who had come in contact with the patient and had not been vaccinated would be required to take antibiotics. Otherwise, they might catch it, and meningitis can be fatal. So she said I had to get the shot. That's my mom for you. Tough love."**

"Listen, I didn't get one and you don't see me getting sick. It's no big deal, they just blow it way out of proportion," ***Sara added casually.***

Crystal and Jackie gave each other a look. The medical form for entry to college had said that all freshmen living in the dorms had to be vaccinated against bacterial meningitis. It said that some schools had recently had outbreaks of it and a few students had died. The three of them were living in such a small dorm room together, Jackie couldn't imagine what would happen if one of them got seriously sick. Why hadn't Sara gotten the shot?

Sara sat biting her lip, hoping that the conversation would go no further. Sure, she had gotten the medical form and filled it out, but the meningitis shot was over $50. Her mom was working two jobs to pay for the tuition that the scholarship didn't cover. Neither of the jobs offered health coverage, so how could Sara ask her mom to pay for an expensive shot when she wasn't even sick?

Suggested Discussion Topics

1. Discuss whether or not you think that the college has a responsibility to provide required vaccinations for students who cannot afford to get them on their own.
2. Talk about whether there is anything that Crystal and Jackie could do to change Sara's mind about getting vaccinated.
3. Should Crystal or Jackie report the fact that Sara was not vaccinated to their dorm advisor?
4. Discuss why a student living in a dorm, rather than at home, would be more likely to contract meningitis.

STUDENT WORKBOOK AND StudyWARE™ CD-ROM

1. Go to your **Student Workbook** and complete the Learning Exercises for this chapter.

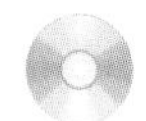

2. Go to the **StudyWARE™ CD-ROM** and have fun with the exercises and games for this chapter.

7

CHAPTER

THE RESPIRATORY SYSTEM

OVERVIEW OF STRUCTURES, COMBINING FORMS, AND FUNCTIONS OF THE RESPIRATORY SYSTEM

MAJOR STRUCTURES	RELATED COMBINING FORMS	PRIMARY FUNCTIONS
Nose	**nas/o**	Exchanges air during inhaling and exhaling; warms, moisturizes, and filters inhaled air.
Sinuses	**sinus/o**	Produce mucus for the nasal cavities, make bones of the skull lighter, aid in sound production.
Pharynx	**pharyng/o**	Transports air back and forth between the nose and the trachea.
Larynx	**laryng/o**	Makes speech possible.
Epiglottis	**epiglott/o**	Closes off the trachea during swallowing.
Trachea	**trache/o**	Transports air back and forth between the pharynx and the bronchi.
Bronchi	**bronch/o, bronchi/o**	Transports air from the trachea into the lungs.
Alveoli	**alveol/o**	Air sacs that exchange gases with the pulmonary capillary blood.
Lungs	**pneum/o, pneumon/o, pulmon/o**	Bring oxygen into the body and remove carbon dioxide and some water waste from the body.

VOCABULARY RELATED TO THE RESPIRATORY SYSTEM

This list contains essential word parts and medical terms for this chapter. These terms are pronounced on the student StudyWARE™ CD-ROM and Audio CDs that are available for use with this text. These and the other important **primary terms** are shown in boldface throughout the chapter. *Secondary terms*, which appear in *orange* italics, clarify the meaning of primary terms.

Word Parts

- ☐ **bronch/o, bronchi/o**
- ☐ **cyan/o**
- ☐ **laryng/o**
- ☐ **ox/i, ox/o, ox/y**
- ☐ **pharyng/o**
- ☐ **phon/o**
- ☐ **pleur/o**
- ☐ **-pnea**
- ☐ **pneum/o, pneumon/o, pneu-**
- ☐ **pulm/o, pulmon/o**
- ☐ **somn/o**
- ☐ **spir/o**
- ☐ **tachy-**
- ☐ **thorac/o, -thorax**
- ☐ **trache/o**

Medical Terms

- ☐ **anoxia** (ah-**NOCK**-see-ah)
- ☐ **anthracosis** (**an**-thrah-**KOH**-sis)
- ☐ **antitussive** (**an**-tih-**TUSS**-iv)
- ☐ **aphonia** (ah-**FOH**-nee-ah)
- ☐ **apnea** (**AP**-nee-ah)
- ☐ **asbestosis** (**ass**-beh-**STOH**-sis)
- ☐ **asphyxia** (ass-**FICK**-see-ah)
- ☐ **asphyxiation** (ass-**fick**-see-**AY**-shun)
- ☐ **aspiration pneumonia** (**ass**-pih-**RAY**-shun)
- ☐ **asthma** (**AZ**-mah)
- ☐ **atelectasis** (**at**-ee-**LEK**-tah-sis)
- ☐ **bradypnea** (**brad**-ihp-**NEE**-ah)
- ☐ **bronchodilator** (**brong**-koh-dye-**LAY**-tor)
- ☐ **bronchorrhea** (**brong**-koh-**REE**-ah)
- ☐ **bronchoscopy** (brong-**KOS**-koh-pee)
- ☐ **bronchospasm** (**brong**-koh-spazm)
- ☐ **Cheyne-Stokes respiration** (**CHAYN-STOHKS**)
- ☐ **croup** (**KROOP**)
- ☐ **cystic fibrosis** (**SIS**-tick figh-**BROH**-sis)
- ☐ **diphtheria** (dif-**THEE**-ree-ah)
- ☐ **dysphonia** (dis-**FOH**-nee-ah)
- ☐ **dyspnea** (**DISP**-nee-ah)
- ☐ **emphysema** (**em**-fih-**SEE**-mah)
- ☐ **empyema** (**em**-pye-**EE**-mah)
- ☐ **endotracheal intubation** (**en**-doh-**TRAY**-kee-al **in**-too-**BAY**-shun)
- ☐ **epistaxis** (**ep**-ih-**STACK**-sis)
- ☐ **hemoptysis** (hee-**MOP**-tih-sis)
- ☐ **hemothorax** (**hee**-moh-**THOH**-racks)
- ☐ **hypercapnia** (**high**-per-**KAP**-nee-ah)
- ☐ **hyperpnea** (**high**-perp-**NEE**-ah)
- ☐ **hypopnea** (**high**-poh-**NEE**-ah)
- ☐ **hypoxemia** (**high**-pock-**SEE**-mee-ah)
- ☐ **hypoxia** (high-**POCK**-see-ah)
- ☐ **laryngectomy** (**lar**-in-**JECK**-toh-mee)
- ☐ **laryngitis** (**lar**-in-**JIGH**-tis)
- ☐ **laryngoplegia** (**lar**-ing-goh-**PLEE**-jee-ah)
- ☐ **laryngoscopy** (**lar**-ing-**GOS**-koh-pee)
- ☐ **mediastinum** (**mee**-dee-as-**TYE**-num)
- ☐ **nebulizer** (**NEB**-you-lye-zer)
- ☐ **otolaryngologist** (**oh**-toh-**lar**-in-**GOL**-oh-jist)
- ☐ **pertussis** (per-**TUS**-is)
- ☐ **pharyngitis** (**fah**-rin-**JIGH**-tis)
- ☐ **pharyngoplasty** (fah-**RING**-goh-**plas**-tee)
- ☐ **pleurectomy** (ploor-**ECK**-toh-mee)
- ☐ **pleurisy** (**PLOOR**-ih-see)
- ☐ **pleurodynia** (**ploor**-oh-**DIN**-ee-ah)
- ☐ **pneumoconiosis** (**new**-moh-**koh**-nee-**OH**-sis)
- ☐ **pneumonectomy** (**new**-moh-**NECK**-toh-mee)
- ☐ **pneumothorax** (**new**-moh-**THOR**-racks)
- ☐ **polysomnography** (**pol**-ee-som-**NOG**-rah-fee)
- ☐ **pulmonologist** (**pull**-mah-**NOL**-oh-jist)
- ☐ **pulse oximeter** (ock-**SIM**-eh-ter)
- ☐ **pyothorax** (**pye**-oh-**THOH**-racks)
- ☐ **sinusitis** (**sigh**-nuh-**SIGH**-tis)
- ☐ **tachypnea** (**tack**-ihp-**NEE**-ah)
- ☐ **thoracentesis** (**thoh**-rah-sen-**TEE**-sis)
- ☐ **thoracostomy** (**thoh**-rah-**KOS**-toh-mee)
- ☐ **tracheostomy** (**tray**-kee-**OS**-toh-mee)
- ☐ **tracheotomy** (**tray**-kee-**OT**-oh-mee)
- ☐ **tuberculosis** (too-**ber**-kew-**LOH**-sis)

OBJECTIVES

On completion of this chapter, you should be able to:

1. Identify and describe the major structures and functions of the respiratory system.
2. Recognize, define, spell, and pronounce terms related to the pathology and the diagnostic and treatment procedures of the respiratory system.

FUNCTIONS OF THE RESPIRATORY SYSTEM

The functions of the respiratory system are to

- Bring oxygen from the inhaled air into the blood for delivery to the body cells.
- Expel waste products (carbon dioxide and some water waste) returned to the lungs by the blood.
- Produce the airflow through the larynx that makes speech possible.

STRUCTURES OF THE RESPIRATORY SYSTEM

The **respiratory system** brings oxygen into the body for transportation to the cells. It also removes carbon dioxide and some water waste from the body. For descriptive purposes, the respiratory system is divided into upper and lower respiratory tracts (Figures 7.1 and 7.2).

- The **upper respiratory tract** consists of the nose, mouth, pharynx, epiglottis, larynx, and trachea.

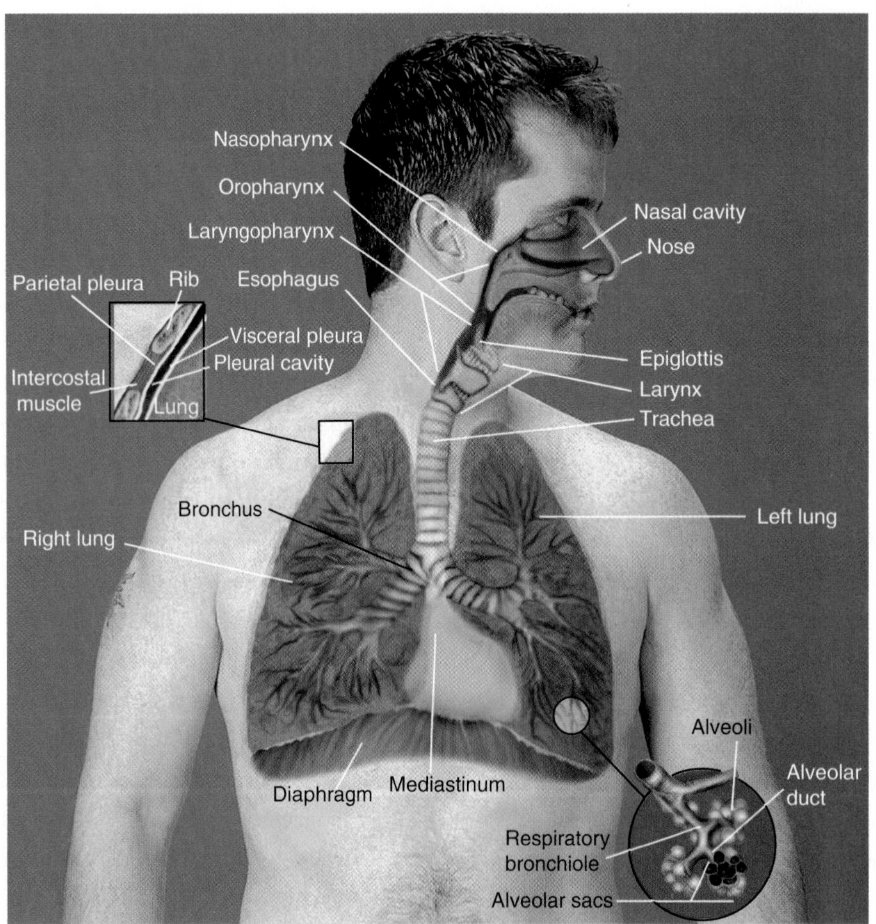

FIGURE 7.1 Structures of the respiratory system.

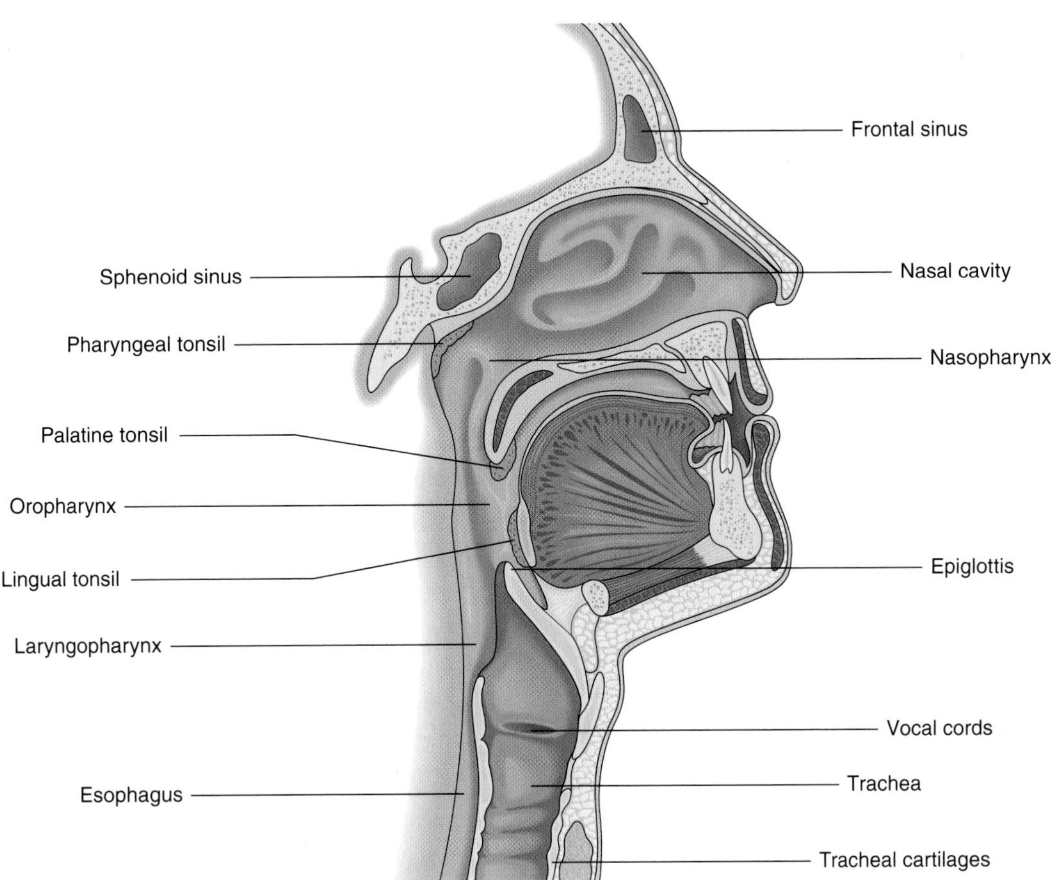

FIGURE 7.2 Structures of the upper respiratory tract.

- The **lower respiratory tract** consists of the bronchial tree and lungs. These structures are located within, and protected by, the **thoracic cavity** which is also known as the *rib cage*.

The Nose

Air enters the body through the **nose** and passes through the *nasal cavity*, which is the interior portion of the nose.

- The **nasal septum** (**NAY**-zal **SEP**-tum) is a wall of cartilage that divides the nose into two equal sections. A *septum* is a wall that separates two chambers.
- **Cilia** (**SIL**-ee-ah), the thin hairs located just inside the nostrils, filter incoming air to remove debris.
- **Mucous membranes** (**MYOU**-kus) are the specialized tissues that line the respiratory, digestive, reproductive, and urinary systems.
- **Mucus** (**MYOU**-kus), which is secreted by the mucous membranes, protects and lubricates these tissues. In the nose mucus helps to moisten, warm, and filter the air as it enters. Notice the different spellings; however, they have the same pronunciation. Muc*o*us is the name of the tissue; mucus is the secretion that flows from the tissue.
- The **olfactory receptors** (ol-**FACK**-toh-ree) are nerve endings that act as the receptors for the sense of smell. They are also important to the sense of taste. These receptors are located in the mucous membrane in the upper part of the nasal cavity.

The Tonsils

The **tonsils** form a protective circle of lymphatic tissue around the entrance to the respiratory system and are discussed in Chapter 6.

The Paranasal Sinuses

The **paranasal sinuses**, which are air-filled cavities lined with mucous membrane, are located in the bones of the skull. These sinuses are connected to the nasal cavity via short ducts (**para-** means near, **nas** means nose, and **-al** means pertaining to).

The functions of these sinuses are (1) to make the bones of the skull lighter, (2) to help produce sound by giving resonance to the voice, and (3) to produce mucus to provide lubrication for the tissues of the nasal cavity. The four paired sinuses are located on either side of the nose and are named for the bones in which they are located.

- The **frontal sinuses** are located in the frontal bone just above the eyebrows. An infection here can cause severe pain in this area.
- The **sphenoid sinuses**, which are located in the sphenoid bone, are close to the optic nerves and an infection here can damage vision.
- The **maxillary sinuses**, which are the largest of the paranasal sinuses, are located in the maxillary bones. An infection in these sinuses can cause pain in the posterior maxillary teeth.
- The **ethmoid sinuses**, which are located in the ethmoid bones, are irregularly shaped air cells that are separated from the orbital (eye) cavity by only a thin layer of bone.

The Pharynx

The **pharynx** (**FAR**-inks), which is commonly known as the *throat*, receives the air after it passes through the nose. The pharynx is made up of three divisions (see Figure 7.2).

- The **nasopharynx** (**nay**-zoh-**FAR**-inks), which is the first division, is posterior to the nasal cavity and continues downward to behind the mouth (**nas/o** means nose, and **-pharynx** means throat). This portion of the pharynx is used only by the respiratory system for the transport of air and opens into the oropharynx.
- The **oropharynx** (**oh**-roh-**FAR**-inks), which is the second division, is the portion that is visible when looking into the mouth (**or/o** means mouth, and **-pharynx** means throat). The oropharynx is shared by the respiratory and digestive systems and transports air, food, and fluids downward to the laryngopharynx (see Figure 7.2).
- The **laryngopharynx** (lah-**ring**-goh-**FAR**-inks), which is the third division, is also shared by both the respiratory and digestive systems (**laryng/o** means larynx, and **-pharynx** means throat). Air, food, and fluids continue downward to the openings of the esophagus and trachea where air enters the trachea and food and fluids flow into the esophagus. See Protective Swallowing Mechanisms below.

The Larynx

The **larynx** (**LAR**-inks), also known as the *voice box*, is a triangular chamber located between the pharynx and the trachea (Figure 7.3).

- The larynx is protected and supported by a series of nine separate cartilages. The *thyroid cartilage* is the largest, and when enlarged, it is commonly known as the *Adam's apple*.
- The larynx contains the *vocal cords*. During breathing, the cords are separated to let air pass. During speech, they close together, and sound is produced as air is expelled from the lungs, causing the cords to vibrate against each other.

Protective Swallowing Mechanisms

The respiratory and digestive systems share part of the pharynx. During swallowing, there is the risk of a blocked airway or pneumonia caused by food or water going into the trachea and entering the lungs instead of traveling into the esophagus. Two protective mechanisms act automatically during swallowing to ensure that *only* air goes into the lungs.

- During swallowing, the soft palate, which is the muscular posterior portion of the roof of the mouth, moves up and backward to close off the nasopharynx. This movement prevents food or liquid from going up into the nose. Structures of the mouth are discussed further in Chapter 8.
- At the same time, the **epiglottis** (**ep**-ih-**GLOT**-is), which is a lid-like structure located at the base of the tongue, swings downward and closes off the laryngopharynx so that food does not enter the trachea and the lungs.

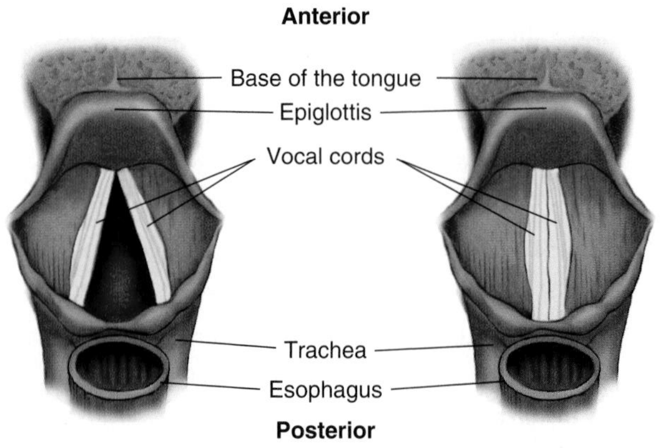

Anterior

Base of the tongue

Epiglottis

Vocal cords

Trachea

Esophagus

Posterior

FIGURE 7.3 View of the larynx and vocal cords from above. Shown on the left, the vocal cords are open during breathing. On the right, the vocal cords vibrate together during speech.

The Trachea

The **trachea** (**TRAY**-kee-ah), commonly known as the *windpipe*, is the tube located directly in front of the esophagus that extends from the neck to the chest. Its role is to transport air to, and from, the lungs (Figure 7.4).

- The trachea is held open by a series of C-shaped cartilage rings. The wall between these rings is flexible, and this feature makes it possible for the trachea to adjust to different body positions.

The Bronchi

The **bronchi** (**BRONG**-kye) are formed where the trachea divides into two branches known as the *primary bronchi* (singular, *bronchus*). Because of the similarity of these branching structures to an inverted tree, this is referred to as the *bronchial tree* with one branch going into each lung.

- Within the lung, each primary bronchus divides and subdivides into increasingly smaller **bronchioles** (**BRONG**-kee-ohlz), which are the smallest branches of the bronchi.

The Alveoli

Alveoli (al-**VEE**-oh-lye), also known as *air sacs*, are the very small grape-like clusters found at the end of each bronchiole (singular, *alveolus*). Each lung contains millions of alveoli that are filled with air from the bronchioles (Figures 7.1 and 7.4).

- A network of microscopic pulmonary capillaries surrounds the thin, elastic walls of the alveoli.
- During respiration, the exchange of oxygen and carbon dioxide between the alveolar air and the pulmonary capillary blood occurs through the walls of the alveoli.

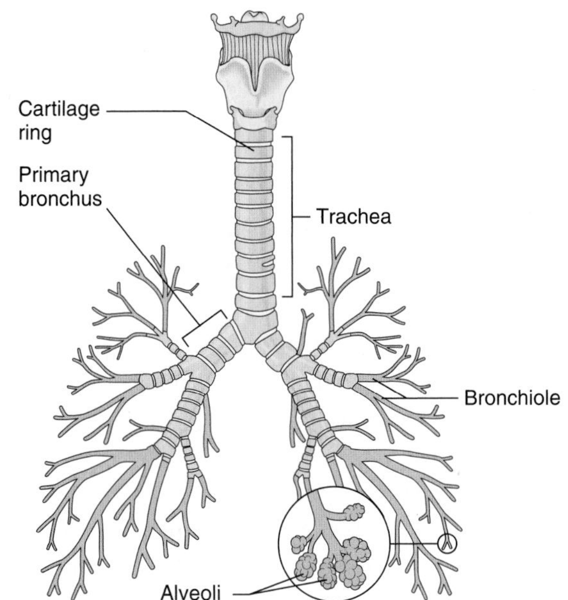

FIGURE 7.4 The trachea, bronchial tree, and alveoli.

The Lungs

The **lungs**, which are the organs of respiration, are divided into lobes (Figure 7.5). A *lobe* is a subdivision or part of an organ.

- The **right lung** has three lobes: the superior, middle, and inferior.
- The **left lung** has only two lobes: the superior and inferior. It is slightly smaller than the right lung because of the space taken up by the heart.

The lungs produce a detergent-like substance, known as a *surfactant*, which reduces the surface tension of the lungs. This allows air to flow over the lungs and be absorbed more easily.

The Mediastinum

The **mediastinum** (**mee**-dee-as-**TYE**-num) is the cavity located between the lungs. This cavity contains connective tissue and organs, including the heart and its veins and arteries, the esophagus, trachea, bronchi, the thymus gland, and lymph nodes (see Figure 7.1).

The Pleura

The **pleura** (**PLOOR**-ah) is a thin, moist, and slippery membrane that covers the outer surface of the lungs and lines the inner surface of the rib cage (Figure 7.6).

- The **parietal pleura** (pah-**RYE**-eh-tal) is the outer layer of the pleura that lines the walls of the thoracic cavity, covers the diaphragm, and forms the sac containing each lung. *Parietal* means relating to the walls of a cavity.
- The **visceral pleura** (**VIS**-er-al) is the inner layer of pleura that surrounds each lung. *Visceral* means relating to the internal organs.
- The **pleural cavity**, also known as the *pleural space*, is the airtight area between the layers of the pleural membranes. This space contains a thin layer of fluid that allows the membranes to slide easily during breathing.

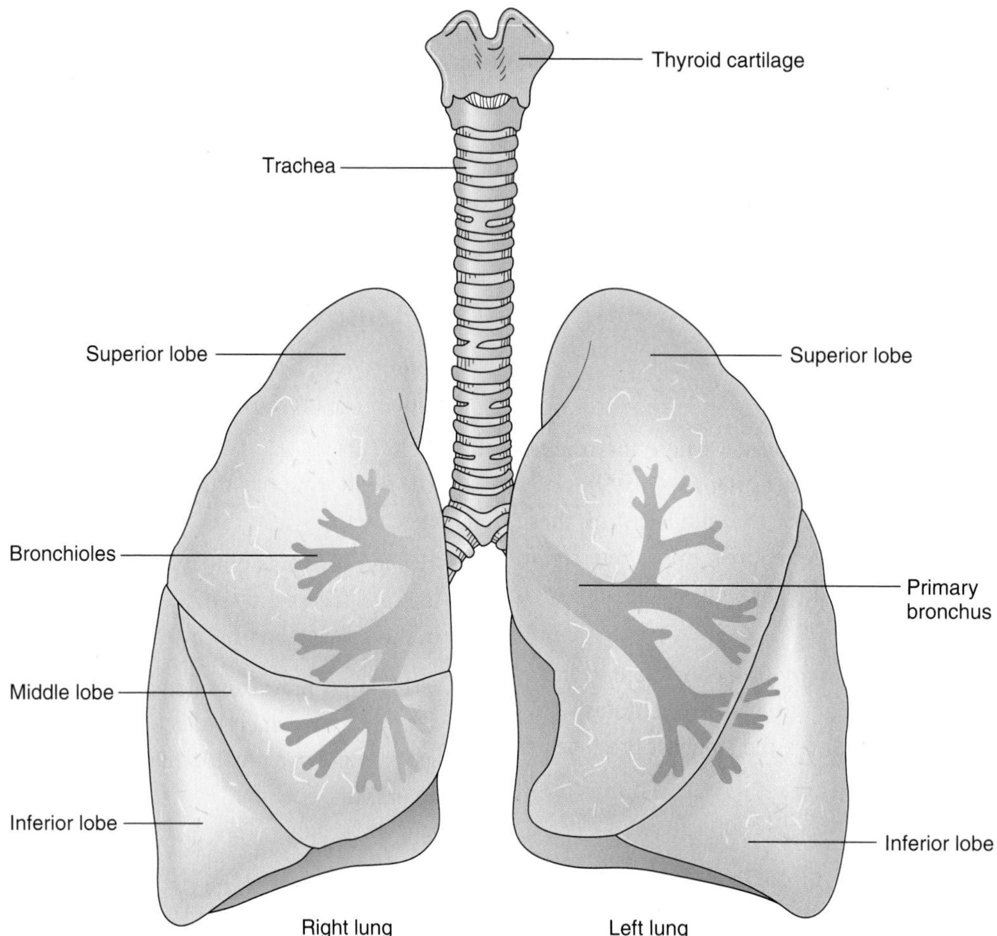

FIGURE 7.5 External view of the lungs. Note the three lobes of the right lung and the two lobes of the left lung.

The Diaphragm

The **diaphragm** (**DYE**-ah-fram) is the muscle that separates the thoracic cavity from the abdomen. It is the contraction and relaxation of this muscle that makes breathing possible. The **phrenic nerves** (**FREN**-ick) stimulate the diaphragm and cause it to contract (Figure 7.7).

RESPIRATION

Respiration is the exchange of oxygen and carbon dioxide that is essential to life. A single respiration consists of one inhalation and one exhalation (Figure 7.8).

Inhalation and Exhalation

Inhalation (**in**-hah-**LAY**-shun) is the act of taking in air as the diaphragm contracts and pulls downward (Figure 7.8 left). This action causes the thoracic cavity to expand. This produces a vacuum within the thoracic cavity that draws air into the lungs.

Exhalation (**ecks**-hah-**LAY**-shun) is the act of breathing out. As the diaphragm relaxes, it moves upward, causing the thoracic cavity to become narrower. This action forces air out of the lungs (Figure 7.8 right).

External Respiration

External respiration is the act of bringing air into and out of the lungs and exchanging gases from this air (Figure 7.9A).

- As air is *inhaled* into the alveoli, oxygen immediately passes into the surrounding capillaries and is carried by the erythrocytes (red blood cells) to all body cells.
- At the same time, the waste product carbon dioxide that has passed into the bloodstream is transported into the airspaces of the lungs to be *exhaled*.

Internal Respiration

Internal respiration is the exchange of gases within the cells of the body organs, cells, and tissues (see Figure 7.9B).

- In this process, oxygen passes from the bloodstream into the cells.

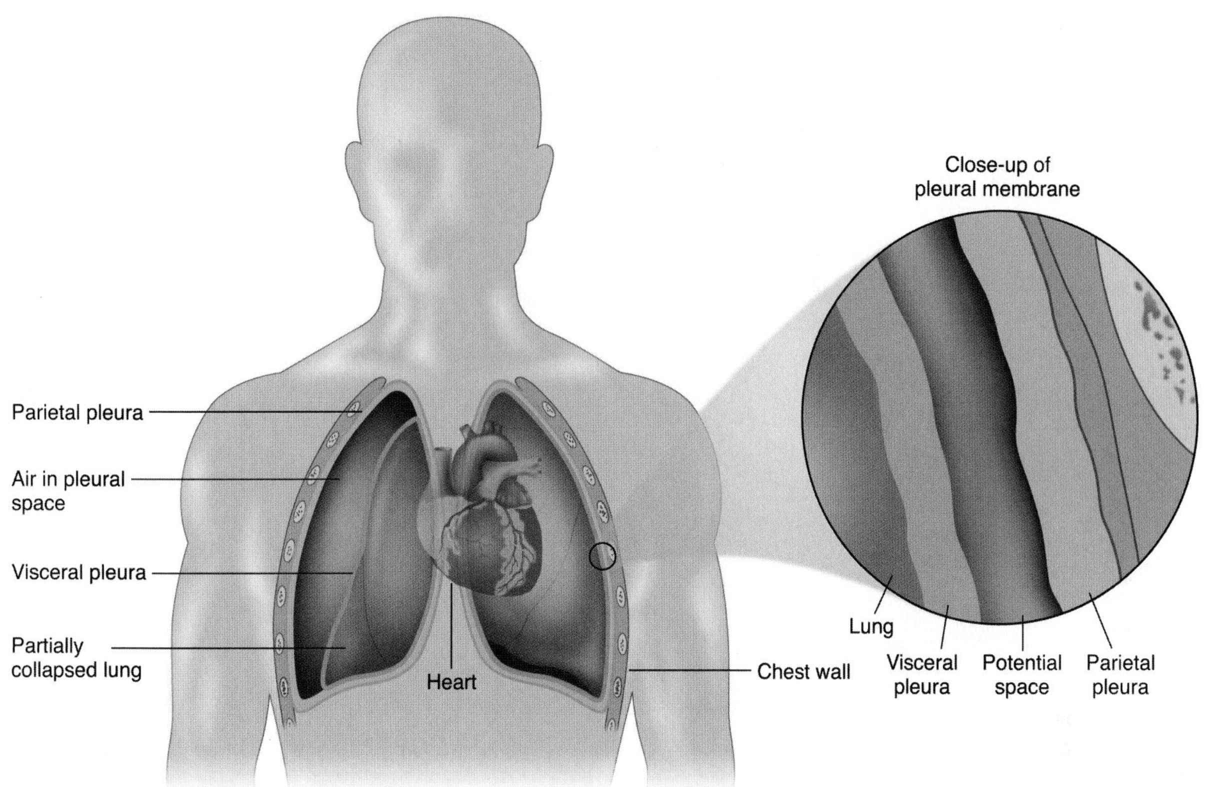

FIGURE 7.6 The pleura allows the lungs to move smoothly within the chest.

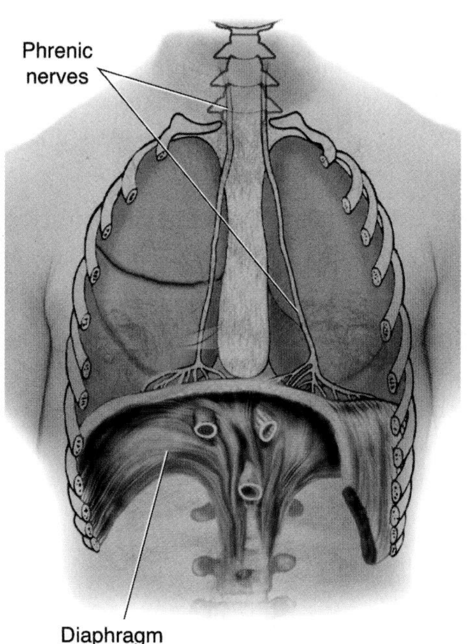

FIGURE 7.7 The diaphragm is controlled by the phrenic nerves.

- The cells give off the waste product carbon dioxide, and this passes into the bloodstream.
- The bloodstream transports the carbon dioxide to the lungs where it is expelled during exhalation.

MEDICAL SPECIALTIES RELATED TO THE RESPIRATORY SYSTEM

- An **otolaryngologist** (**oh**-toh-**lar**-in-**GOL**-oh-jist), also known as an ENT, is a physician with specialized training in the diagnosis and treatment of diseases and disorders of the ears, nose, throat, and related structures of the head and neck (**ot/o** means ear, **laryng/o** means larynx, and **-ologist** means specialist).
- A **pulmonologist** (**pull**-mah-**NOL**-oh-jist) is a physician who specializes in diagnosing and treating diseases and disorders of the lungs and associated tissues (**pulmon** means lung, and **-ologist** means specialist).

PATHOLOGY OF THE RESPIRATORY SYSTEM

Chronic Obstructive Pulmonary Diseases

Chronic obstructive pulmonary disease, also known as *COPD*, is a lung disease in which it is hard to breathe. In this condition, damage to the bronchi partially obstructs them, making it difficult to get air in and out. Most people with COPD, who are usually smokers or former smokers, also have both chronic bronchitis and emphysema.

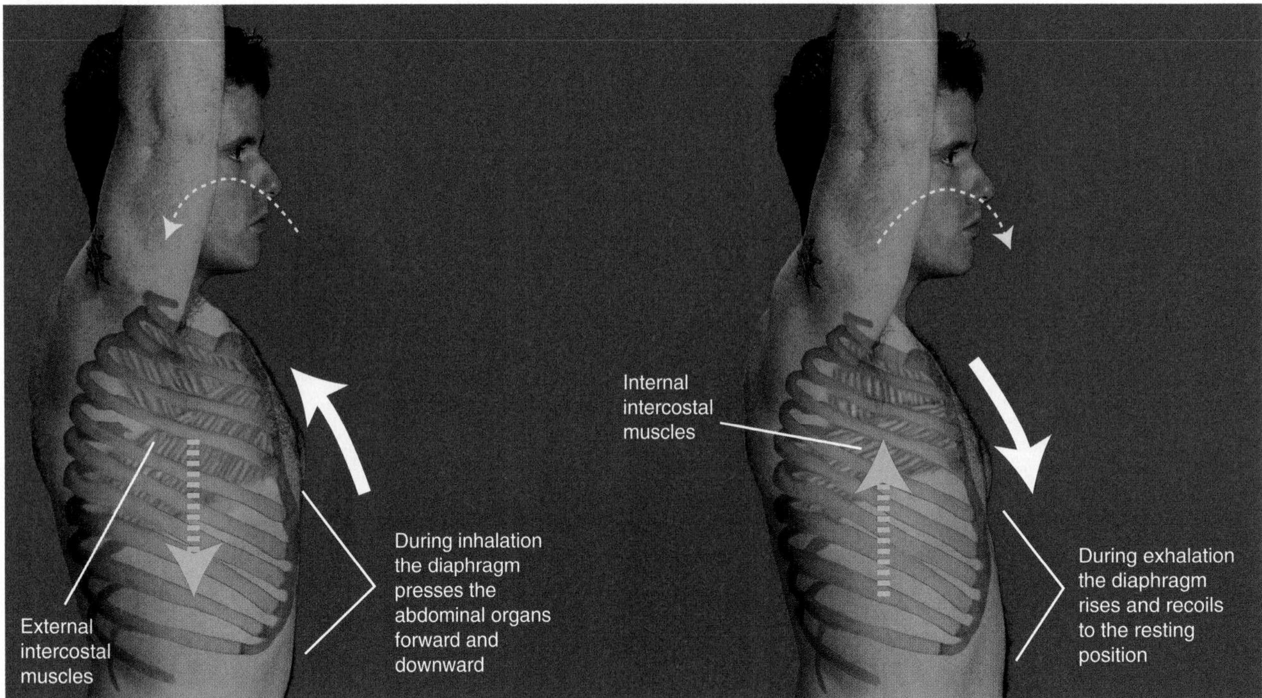

FIGURE 7.8 Movements of the diaphragm and thoracic cavity produce inhalation (left) and exhalation (right).

Chronic Bronchitis

In **chronic bronchitis** (brong-**KYE**-tis), the airways have become inflamed and thickened, and there is an increase in the number and size of mucus-producing cells (**bronch** means bronchus, and **-itis** means inflammation). This results in excessive mucus production, which in turn causes coughing and difficulty getting air in and out of the lungs.

Emphysema

Emphysema (**em**-fih-**SEE**-mah) is the progressive loss of lung function that is characterized by (1) a decrease in the total number of alveoli, (2) the enlargement of the remaining alveoli, and (3) the progressive destruction of the walls of the remaining alveoli.

As the alveoli are destroyed, breathing becomes increasingly rapid, shallow, and difficult. In an effort to compensate for the loss of capacity, the lungs expand, and the chest sometimes assumes an enlarged barrel shape (Figure 7.10).

Asthma

Asthma (**AZ**-mah) is a chronic allergic disorder characterized by episodes of severe breathing difficulty, coughing, and wheezing. These episodes are known as *asthmatic attacks*. *Wheezing* is a breathing sound caused by a partially obstructed airway. The frequency and severity of asthmatic attacks is influenced by a variety of factors including allergens, environmental agents, exercise, or infection.

- Figure 7.11A shows the exterior of the airway before an attack. Figure 7.11B shows the factors within and surrounding the airway that cause breathing difficulty during an attack.
- **Airway inflammation** is the swelling and clogging of the airways with mucus. This usually occurs after the airway has been exposed to inhaled allergens.
- A **bronchospasm** (**brong**-koh-spazm) is a contraction of the smooth muscle in the walls of the bronchi and bronchioles that tighten and squeeze the airway shut (**bronch/o** means bronchi, and **-spasm** means involuntary contraction).
- *Exercise-induced bronchospasms* (EIB) are the narrowing of the airways that develops after 5–15 minutes of physical exertion. This also can be due to cold weather or allergies.

Asthma Treatment

Most asthmatics take two kinds of medicines. *Controller medicines*, such as inhaled corticosteroids, are taken daily to prevent attacks. These medications help to control inflammation and to stop the airways from reacting to the factors that trigger the asthma.

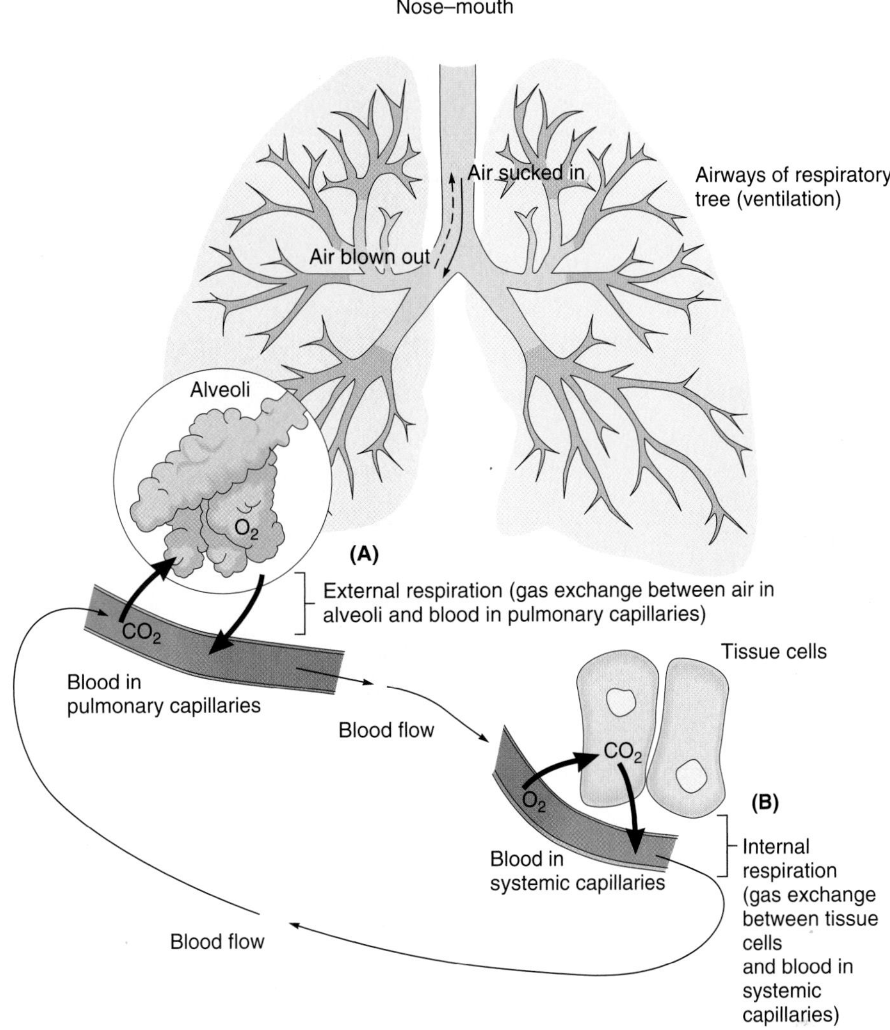

FIGURE 7.9 External and internal respiration compared. (A) External respiration occurs in the lungs. (B) Internal respiration occurs within the cells and tissues.

Quick-relief, or *rescue medicines*, are taken at the first sign of an attack to dilate the airways and make breathing easier. These medications are known as bronchodilators and are discussed later in this chapter under medications.

Upper Respiratory Diseases

- **Upper respiratory infections** and *acute nasopharyngitis* are among the terms used to describe the *common cold*. An upper respiratory infection can be caused by any one of 200 different viruses.
- **Allergic rhinitis** (rye-**NIGH**-tis), commonly referred to as an *allergy*, is an allergic reaction to airborne allergens that causes an increased flow of mucus (**rhin** means nose, and **-itis** means inflammation). Allergies are discussed in Chapter 6.
- **Croup** (**KROOP**) is an acute respiratory syndrome in children and infants characterized by obstruction of the larynx, hoarseness, and a barking cough.
- **Diphtheria** (dif-**THEE**-ree-ah), now largely prevented through immunization, is an acute bacterial infection of the throat and upper respiratory tract. The diphtheria bacteria produce toxins that can damage the heart muscle and peripheral nerves.
- **Epistaxis** (**ep**-ih-**STACK**-sis), also known as a *nosebleed*, is bleeding from the nose that is usually caused by an injury, excessive use of blood thinners, or bleeding disorders.
- **Influenza** (**in**-flew-**EN**-zah), also known as the *flu*, is an acute, highly contagious viral respiratory infection that is spread by respiratory droplets and occurs most commonly in epidemics during the colder months.

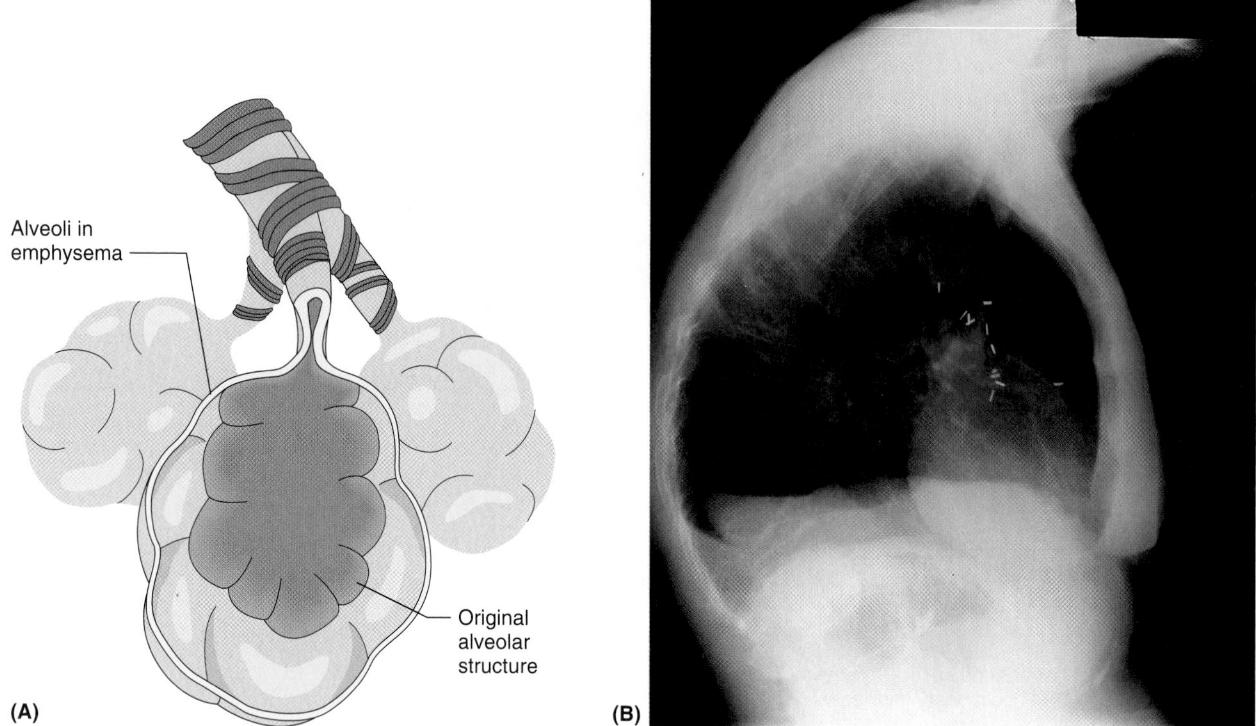

FIGURE 7.10 Emphysema. (A) Changes in the alveoli as the disease progresses. (B) Lateral x-ray showing lung enlargement and abnormal barrel chest in emphysema.

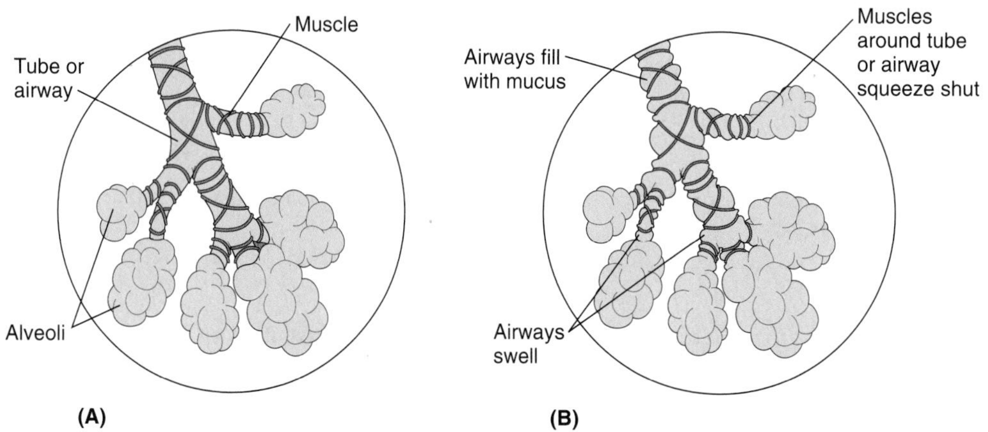

FIGURE 7.11 Changes in the airways during an asthma episode. (A) Before the episode, the muscles are relaxed and the airways are open. (B) During the episode, the muscles tighten and the airways fill with mucus.

There are many strains of the influenza virus. Some strains can be prevented by annual immunization.

- **Pertussis** (per-**TUS**-is), also known as *whooping cough*, is a contagious bacterial infection of the upper respiratory tract that is characterized by recurrent bouts of a paroxysmal cough, followed by breathlessness, and a noisy inspiration. *Paroxysmal* means sudden or spasm-like.
- **Rhinorrhea** (**rye**-noh-**REE**-ah), also known as a *runny nose*, is the watery flow of mucus from the nose (**rhin/o** means nose, and **-rrhea** means abnormal discharge).
- **Sinusitis** (**sigh**-nuh-**SIGH**-tis) is an inflammation of the sinuses (**sinus** means sinus, and **-itis** means inflammation).

Pharynx and Larynx

- **Pharyngitis** (**fah**-rin-**JIGH**-tis), also known as a *sore throat*, is an inflammation of the pharynx (**pharyng** means pharynx, and **-itis** means inflammation).

- **Laryngoplegia** (**lar**-ing-goh-**PLEE**-jee-ah) is paralysis of the larynx (**laryng/o** means larynx, and **-plegia** means paralysis).
- A **laryngospasm** (lah-**RING**-goh-spazm) is the sudden spasmodic closure of the larynx (**laryng/o** means larynx, and **-spasm** means a sudden involuntary contraction).

Voice Disorders

- **Aphonia** (ah-**FOH**-nee-ah) is the loss of the ability of the larynx to produce normal speech sounds (**a-** means without, **phon** means voice or sound, and **-ia** means abnormal condition).
- **Dysphonia** (dis-**FOH**-nee-ah) is any change in vocal quality, including hoarseness, weakness, or the cracking of a boy's voice during puberty (**dys-** means bad, **phon** means voice or sound, and **-ia** means abnormal condition).
- **Laryngitis** (**lar**-in-**JIGH**-tis) is an inflammation of the larynx (**laryng** means larynx, and **-itis** means inflammation). This term is also commonly used to describe voice loss that is caused by this inflammation.

Trachea and Bronchi

- **Tracheorrhagia** (**tray**-kee-oh-**RAY**-jee-ah) is bleeding from the mucous membranes of the trachea (**trache/o** means trachea, and **-rrhagia** means bleeding).
- **Bronchorrhea** (**brong**-koh-**REE**-ah) is an excessive discharge of mucus from the bronchi (**bronch/o** means bronchus, and **-rrhea** means abnormal flow).

Pleural Cavity

- **Pleurisy** (**PLOOR**-ih-see), also known as *pleuritis*, is an inflammation of the pleura that produces sharp chest pain with each breath. Pleurisy can be caused by influenza or by damage to the lung beneath the pleura (**pleur** means pleura, and **-isy** is a noun ending).
- **Pleurodynia** (**ploor**-oh-**DIN**-ee-ah) is pain in the pleura that occurs in relation to breathing movements (**pleur/o** means pleura, and **-dynia** means pain).
- A **pneumothorax** (**new**-moh-**THOR**-racks) is the accumulation of air in the pleural space causing a pressure imbalance that prevents the lung from fully expanding or can cause it to collapse (**pneum/o** means lung or air, and **-thorax** means chest). This can have an external cause such as a stab wound through the chest wall. It can be caused internally by a rupture in the pleura that allows air to leak into the pleural space (Figure 7.12).
- **Pleural effusion** (eh-**FEW**-zhun) is the abnormal accumulation of fluid in the pleural space. This produces a feeling of breathlessness because it prevents the lung from fully expanding. *Effusion* is the escape of fluid from blood or lymphatic vessels into the tissues or into a body cavity (Figure 7.13).
- **Hemothorax** (**hee**-moh-**THOH**-racks) is a collection of blood in the pleural cavity (**hem/o** means blood, and

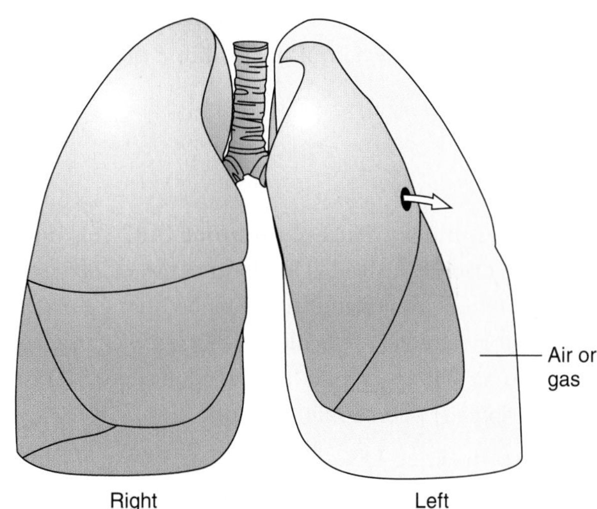

FIGURE 7.12 Pneumothorax is an accumulation of air or gas in the pleural space that causes the lung to collapse. In the left lung, a perforation in the pleura allowed air to escape into the pleural space.

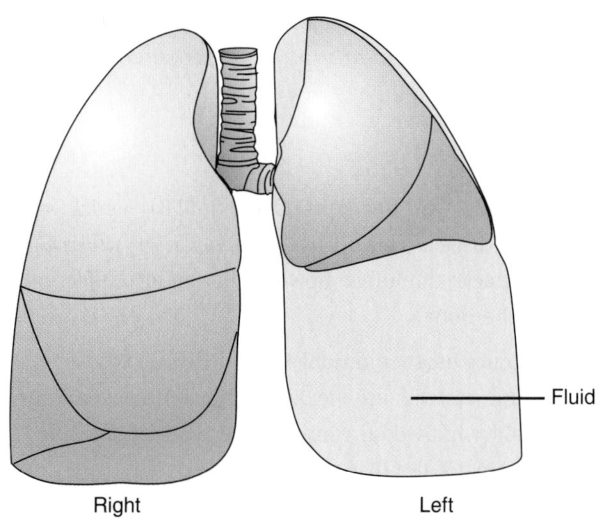

FIGURE 7.13 In pleural effusion, fluid in the pleural cavity prevents the lung from fully expanding.

-**thorax** means chest). This condition often results from chest trauma, such as a stab wound, or it can be caused by disease or surgery.

- **Hemoptysis** (hee-**MOP**-tih-sis) is coughing up of blood or bloodstained sputum derived from the lungs or bronchial tubes as the result of a pulmonary or bronchial hemorrhage (**hem/o** means blood, and -**ptysis** means spitting).
- **Pyothorax** (**pye**-oh-**THOH**-racks) is the presence of pus in the pleural cavity between the layers of the pleural membrane (**py/o** means pus, and -**thorax** means chest). This condition is also known as *empyema of the pleural cavity*. An **empyema** (**em**-pye-**EE**-mah) is a collection of pus within a body cavity.

Lungs

- **Acute respiratory distress syndrome** (ARDS) is not a specific disease. Instead, it is a form of the sudden onset of severe lung dysfunction affecting both lungs, making breathing extremely difficult. This syndrome is caused by trauma (injury), sepsis (systemic infection), diffuse (wide spread) pneumonia, or shock.
- **Atelectasis** (**at**-ee-**LEK**-tah-sis) is the collapse of part or all of a lung by blockage of the air passages or by very shallow breathing (**atel** means incomplete, and -**ectasis** means stretching or enlargement).
- A **collapsed lung** is unable to expand to receive air due to a pneumothorax or atelectasis.
- **Pulmonary edema** (eh-**DEE**-mah) is an accumulation of fluid in lung tissues. *Edema* means swelling.
- **Pneumorrhagia** (**new**-moh-**RAY**-jee-ah) is bleeding from the lungs (**pneum/o** means lungs, and -**rrhagia** means bleeding).

Tuberculosis

Tuberculosis (too-**ber**-kew-**LOH**-sis) (TB), which is an infectious disease caused by *Mycobacterium tuberculosis*, usually attacks the lungs; however, it can also affect other parts of the body.

- TB occurs most commonly in individuals whose immune systems are weakened by another condition. A healthy individual can carry TB without showing symptoms of the disease.
- *Multidrug-resistant tuberculosis* is a dangerous form of tuberculosis because the germs have become resistant to the effect of the primary TB drugs.

Pneumonia Named for the Affected Lung Tissue

Pneumonia (new-**MOH**-nee-ah) is a serious infection or inflammation of the lungs in which the smallest bronchioles and alveoli fill with pus and other liquid (**pneumon** means lung, and -**ia** means abnormal condition). There are two types of pneumonia named for the parts of the lungs affected (Figure 7.14). These are:

- **Bronchopneumonia** (**brong**-koh-new-**MOH**-nee-ah) is a localized form of pneumonia that often affects the bronchioles and surrounding alveoli (**bronch/o** means bronchial tubes, **pneumon** means lung, and -**ia** means abnormal condition).
- **Lobar pneumonia** affects larger areas of the lungs, often including one or more sections, or lobes, of a lung. *Double pneumonia* is lobar pneumonia involving both lungs, and is usually a form of bacterial pneumonia.

Pneumonia Named for the Causative Agent

As many as 30 causes of pneumonia have been identified; however, the most common causative agents are inhaled substances, bacteria, fungi, and viruses.

- **Aspiration pneumonia** (**ass**-pih-**RAY**-shun) can occur when a foreign substance, such as vomit, is inhaled into the lungs. As used here, *aspiration* means inhaling or drawing a foreign substance into the upper respiratory tract.
- **Bacterial pneumonia**, which is often caused by *Streptococcus pneumoniae*, is the only form of pneumonia that can be prevented through vaccination.
- **Mycoplasma pneumonia** (**my**-koh-**PLAZ**-mah new-**MOH**-nee-ah) is a milder but longer lasting form of the disease caused by the bacteria *Mycoplasma*

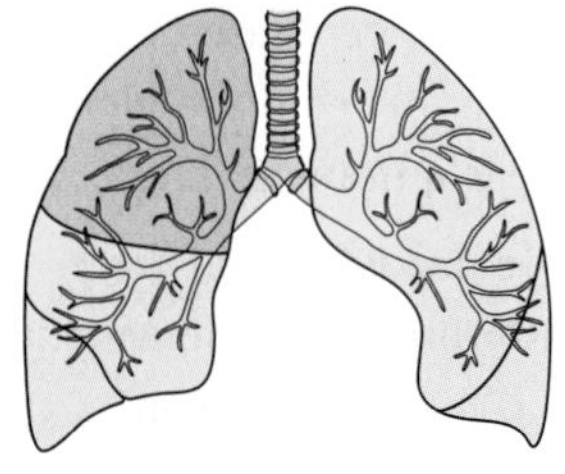

(A) Lobar pneumonia

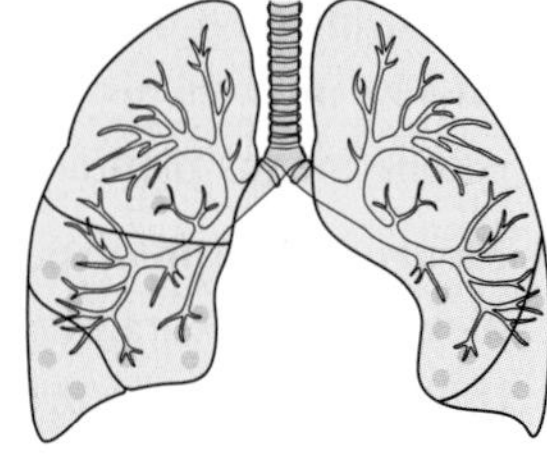

(B) Bronchopneumonia

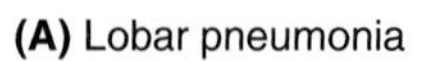

FIGURE 7.14 Types of pneumonia are usually named for the causative agent or for the area of the lung that is involved. (A) Lobar pneumonia affects larger areas of the lungs. (B) Bronchopneumonia affects the bronchioles and surrounding alveoli.

pneumoniae. It is sometimes referred to as *walking pneumonia* because often the patient is not bedridden.

- **Pneumocystis carinii pneumonia** (**new**-moh-**SIS**-tis kah-**RYE**-nee-eye new-**MOH**-nee-ah) is an opportunistic infection caused by the fungus *Pneumocystis carinii*. Opportunistic infections are discussed in Chapter 6.
- **Viral pneumonia**, which is caused by several different types of viruses, accounts for approximately half of all pneumonias.

Interstitial Lung Diseases

Interstitial lung diseases (**in**-ter-**STISH**-al) are a group of almost 200 diseases that cause inflammation and scarring of the alveoli and their supporting structures. *Interstitial* means pertaining to between, but not within, the parts of a tissue. These lung conditions lead to a reduction of oxygen being transferred to the blood.

- **Interstitial fibrosis** is another name for the inflammation and thickening of the walls of the alveoli. *Fibrosis* is a condition in which normal tissue is replaced by fibrotic (hardened) tissue.
- Many connective tissue diseases such as rheumatoid arthritis, scleroderma, and lupus can cause interstitial lung disease. These conditions are also caused by environmental and occupational toxins that are inhaled.

Environmental and Occupational Lung Diseases

- **Pneumoconiosis** (**new**-moh-**koh**-nee-**OH**-sis) is fibrosis of the lung tissues caused by dust in the lungs that usually develops after prolonged environmental or occupational contact (**pneum/o** means lung, **coni** means dust, and **-osis** means abnormal condition or disease).
- **Anthracosis** (**an**-thrah-**KOH**-sis), also known as *coal miner's pneumoconiosis* or *black lung disease*, is caused by coal dust in the lungs (**anthrac** means coal dust, and **-osis** means abnormal condition or disease).
- **Asbestosis** (**ass**-beh-**STOH**-sis) is caused by asbestos particles in the lungs and usually occurs after working with asbestos (**asbest** means asbestos, and **-osis** means abnormal condition or disease).
- **Byssinosis** (**biss**-ih-**NOH**-sis), also known as *brown lung disease*, is caused by inhaling cotton dust into the lungs and usually occurs after working in a textile factory (**byssin** means cotton dust, and **-osis** means abnormal condition or disease).
- **Silicosis** (**sill**-ih-**KOH**-sis) is caused by inhaling silica dust in the lungs and usually occurs after working in occupations including foundry work, quarrying, ceramics, glass work, and sandblasting (**silic** means glass, and **-osis** means abnormal condition or disease).

Pulmonary Fibrosis

Pulmonary fibrosis (figh-**BROH**-sis) is the formation of scar tissue in the lung, resulting in decreased lung capacity and increased difficulty in breathing. This condition can be caused by autoimmune disorders, infections, dust, gases, toxins, and some drugs.

Cystic Fibrosis

Cystic fibrosis (**SIS**-tick figh-**BROH**-sis) is a genetic disorder in which the lungs and pancreas are clogged with large quantities of abnormally thick mucus. Treatment for cystic fibrosis includes:

- Digestive enzymes are administered to aid the digestive system.
- Antibiotics are administered to control lung infections.
- *Postural drainage* is performed with the patient positioned at various angles to allow gravity to help drain secretions from the lungs.
- *Chest percussion* is also performed to remove excess mucus from the lungs. Percussion is described in Chapter 15.

Lung Cancer

Lung cancer, which is the leading cause of cancer death in the United States, is a condition in which cancer cells form in the tissues of the lung. Important risk factors for lung cancer are tobacco smoking and inhaling second-hand smoke (Figure 7.15).

The two tests most commonly used to diagnose lung cancer are chest x-rays and sputum cytology. *Sputum cytology* is a procedure in which a sample of mucus is coughed up from the lungs and then examined under a microscope to detect cancer cells.

Breathing Disorders

The general term *breathing disorders* describes abnormal changes in the rate or depth of breathing. Specific terms describe in greater detail the changes that are occurring (Figure 7.16).

- **Eupnea** (youp-**NEE**-ah) is easy or normal breathing (**eu-** means good, and **-pnea** means breathing).

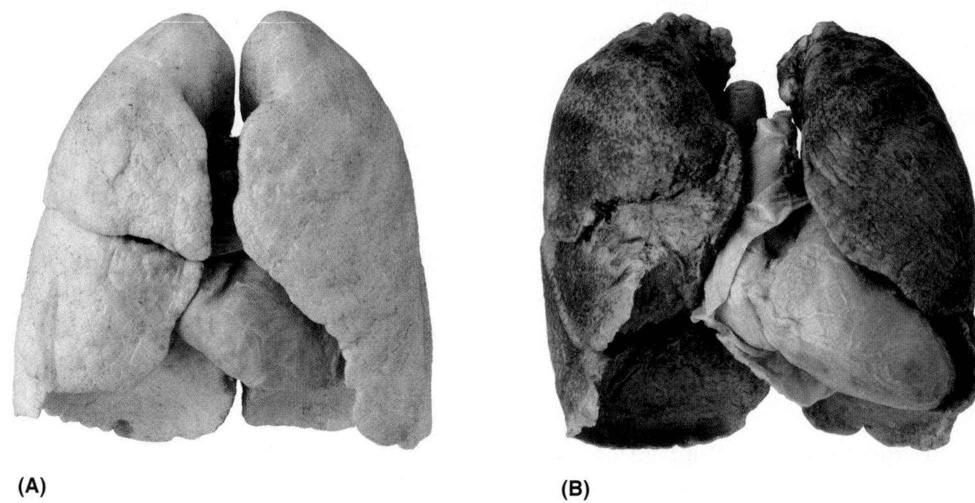

FIGURE 7.15 Photographs of actual lung and heart specimens. (A) Healthy lungs of a nonsmoker. (B) Damaged lungs from a smoker. (Copyright Gunther von Hagens, Institute for Plastination, Heidelburg, Germany)

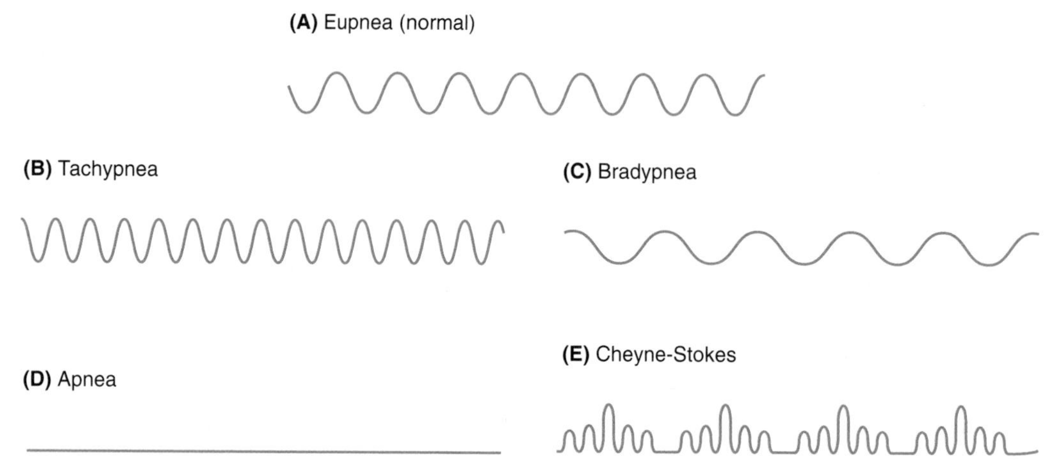

FIGURE 7.16 Respiratory patterns. (A) Eupnea is normal breathing. (B) Tachypnea is abnormally rapid breathing. (C) Bradypnea is abnormally slow breathing. (D) Apnea is the absence of breathing. (E) Cheyne-Stokes is an alternating series of abnormal patterns.

This is the baseline for judging some breathing disorders (Figure 7.16A). Eupnea is the opposite of *apnea*.

- **Apnea** (**AP**-nee-ah) is the absence of spontaneous respiration (**a-** means without and **-pnea** means breathing) (Figure 7.16D). Apnea is the opposite of *eupnea*.
- **Sleep apnea syndromes** are a group of potentially fatal disorders in which breathing repeatedly stops during sleep for long-enough periods to cause a measurable decrease in blood oxygen levels. *Snoring*, which can be a symptom of sleep apnea, is noisy breathing caused by vibration of the soft palate during sleep.
- **Bradypnea** (**brad**-ihp-**NEE**-ah) is an abnormally slow rate of respiration usually of less than 10 breaths per minute (**brady-** means slow, and **-pnea** means breathing) (Figure 7.16C). Bradypnea is the opposite of *tachypnea*.
- **Tachypnea** (**tack**-ihp-**NEE**-ah) is an abnormally rapid rate of respiration usually of more than 20 breaths per minute (**tachy-** means rapid, and **-pnea** means breathing) (Figure 7.16B). Tachypnea is the opposite of *bradypnea*.
- **Cheyne-Stokes respiration** (**CHAYN-STOHKS**) is a pattern of alternating periods of hypopnea or apnea, followed by hyperpnea (Figure 7.16E).

- **Dyspnea** (**DISP**-nee-ah), also known as *shortness of breath* (SOB), is difficult or labored breathing (**dys-** means painful, and **-pnea** means breathing). Shortness of breath is frequently one of the first symptoms of heart failure. It can also be caused by strenuous physical exertion or can be due to lung damage that produces dyspnea even at rest.
- **Hyperpnea** (**high**-perp-**NEE**-ah), which is commonly associated with exertion, is breathing that is deeper and more rapid than is normal at rest (**hyper-** means excessive, and **-pnea** means breathing). Hyperpnea is the opposite of *hypopnea.*
- **Hypopnea** (**high**-poh-**NEE**-ah) is shallow or slow respiration (**hypo-** means decreased, and **-pnea** means breathing). Hypopnea is the opposite of *hyperpnea.*
- **Hyperventilation** (**high**-per-**ven**-tih-**LAY**-shun) is an abnormally rapid rate of deep respiration that is usually associated with anxiety (**hyper-** means excessive, and **-ventilation** means breathing). This causes changes in the blood gas levels due to a decrease in carbon dioxide at the cellular level.

Lack of Oxygen

- **Airway obstruction**, commonly known as *choking*, occurs when food or a foreign object blocks the airway and prevents air from entering or leaving the lungs. This is a life-threatening emergency requiring immediate action by performing the *abdominal thrust maneuver*. This is also known as the *Heimlich maneuver*.
- **Anoxia** (ah-**NOCK**-see-ah) is the absence of oxygen from the body's gases, blood, or tissues (**an-** means without, **ox** means oxygen, and **-ia** means abnormal condition). If anoxia continues for more than 4–6 minutes, irreversible brain damage can occur.
- **Asphyxia** (ass-**FICK**-see-ah) is the condition that occurs when the body cannot get the air it needs to function. In this life-threatening condition, oxygen levels in the blood drop quickly, carbon dioxide levels rise, and unless the patient's breathing is restored within a few minutes, death or serious brain damage follows.
- **Asphyxiation** (ass-**fick**-see-**AY**-shun), also known as *suffocation*, is any interruption of normal breathing resulting in asphyxia. Asphyxiation can be caused by an airway obstruction, drowning, smothering, choking, or inhaling gases such as carbon monoxide instead of air.
- **Cyanosis** (**sigh**-ah-**NOH**-sis) is a bluish discoloration of the skin caused by a lack of adequate oxygen (**cyan** means blue, and **-osis** means abnormal condition or disease).
- **Hypercapnia** (**high**-per-**KAP**-nee-ah) is the abnormal buildup of carbon dioxide in the blood (**hyper-** means excessive, **capn** means carbon dioxide, and **-ia** means abnormal condition).
- **Hypoxemia** (**high**-pock-**SEE**-mee-ah) is a condition of having below-normal oxygen level in the blood (**hyp-** means deficient, **ox** means oxygen, and **-emia** means blood). This condition is less severe than anoxia. Compare with *hypoxia.*
- **Hypoxia** (high-**POCK**-see-ah) is the condition of having below-normal oxygen levels in the body tissues and cells; however, it is less severe than anoxia (**hyp-** means deficient, **ox** means oxygen, and **-ia** means abnormal condition). Compare with *hypoxemia.*
- *Altitude hypoxia*, also known as *altitude sickness*, is a condition that can be brought on by the decreased oxygen in the air at higher altitudes, usually above 8,000 feet.
- **Respiratory failure** (RF), also known as *respiratory acidosis*, is a condition in which the level of oxygen in the blood becomes dangerously low or the level of carbon dioxide becomes dangerously high.
- **Smoke inhalation** is damage to the lungs in which particles from a fire coat the alveoli and prevent the normal exchange of gases.

Sudden Infant Death Syndrome

Sudden infant death syndrome, also known as *SIDS* or *crib death*, is the sudden and unexplainable death of an apparently healthy sleeping infant between the ages of 2 weeks and 1 year. This happens more often among babies who sleep on their stomach. For this reason, it is recommended that infants be put down to sleep on their back or side.

DIAGNOSTIC PROCEDURES OF THE RESPIRATORY SYSTEM

- The *respiratory rate*, which is an important vital sign, is discussed in Chapter 15.
- **Bronchoscopy** (brong-**KOS**-koh-pee) is the visual examination of the bronchi using a bronchoscope (**bronch/o** means bronchus, and **-scopy** means direct visual examination). A *bronchoscope* is a flexible, fiber optic device that is passed through the nose and down the airways. It can also be used for operative

procedures, such as tissue repair, or the removal of a foreign object.

- **Chest imaging**, also known as a *chest x-ray*, is a valuable tool for diagnosing pneumonia, lung tumors, pneumothorax, pleural effusion, tuberculosis, and emphysema (see Figure 7.10B).
- **Laryngoscopy** (**lar**-ing-**GOS**-koh-pee) is the visual examination of the larynx using a laryngoscope inserted through the mouth and placed into the pharynx to examine the larynx (**laryng/o** means larynx, and **-scopy** means a direct visual examination). *Mirror laryngoscopy* is a simpler version of this test in which the larynx is viewed by shining a light on an angled mirror held at the back of the soft palate.
- A **peak flow meter** is a handheld device often used to test those with asthma to measure how quickly the patient can expel air (Figure 7.17).
- **Polysomnography** (**pol**-ee-som-**NOG**-rah-fee), also known as a *sleep apnea study*, measures physiological activity during sleep and is most often performed to detect nocturnal defects in breathing associated with sleep apnea (**poly-** means many, **somn/o** means sleep, and **-graphy** means the process of recording).
- **Pulmonary function tests** (PFT) are a group of tests that measure volume and flow of air by utilizing a spirometer. These tests are measured against a norm for the individual's age, height, and sex.
- A **spirometer** (spih-**ROM**-eh-ter) is a recording device that measures the amount of air inhaled or exhaled (volume) and the length of time required for each breath (**spir/o** means to breathe, and **-meter** means to measure).
- A **pulse oximeter** (ock-**SIM**-eh-ter) is an external monitor placed on the patient's finger or earlobe to measure the oxygen saturation level in the blood (**ox/i** means oxygen, and **-meter** means to measure). In a normal reading, 95%–100% of the blood is saturated by oxygen (Figure 7.18).
- **Sputum** (**SPYOU**-tum) is phlegm ejected through the mouth that can be examined for diagnostic purposes. **Phlegm** (**FLEM**) is thick mucus secreted by the tissues lining the respiratory passages.

Tuberculosis Testing

- **Tuberculin skin testing** is a screening test for tuberculosis in which the skin of the arm is injected with a harmless antigen extracted from TB bacteria. The *tuberculin tine test* is performed using an instrument with several small prongs called tines. A positive result indicates the possibility of exposure to the disease, and this response warrants further testing.
- The **Mantoux PPD skin test** is considered a more accurate skin test for diagnosing tuberculosis. A very small amount of PPD tuberculin (a purified protein derivative) is injected just under the top layer of the skin on the forearm. The site is checked for a reaction 48–72 hours later.

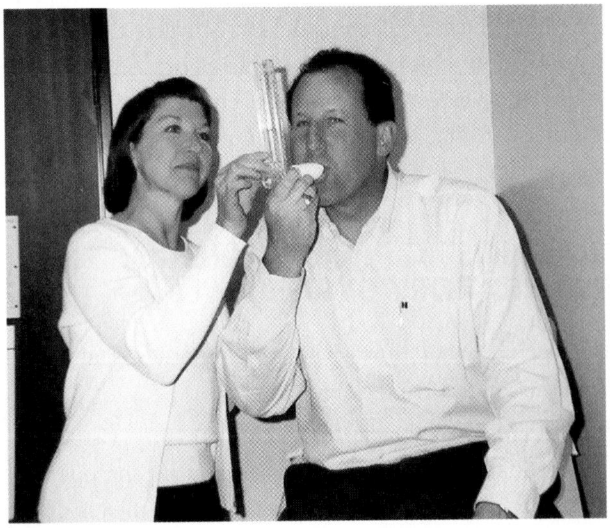

FIGURE 7.17 A peak flow meter is often used to test those with asthma to measure how quickly the patient can expel air.

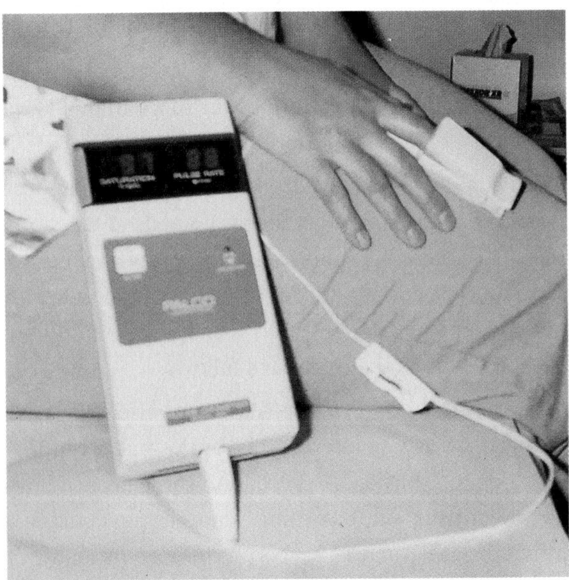

FIGURE 7.18 A pulse oximeter is applied to a finger to provide continuous reassessment of the patient's levels of oxygenation.

TREATMENT PROCEDURES OF THE RESPIRATORY SYSTEM

Medications and Their Administration

- An **antitussive** (**an**-tih-**TUSS**-iv), commonly known as *cough medicine*, is administered to prevent or relieve coughing (**anti-** means against, **tuss** means cough, and **-ive** means performs).
- A **bronchodilator** (**brong**-koh-dye-**LAY**-tor) is a medication that expands the opening of the passages into the lungs. At the first sign of an asthma attack, the patient uses a metered-dose inhaler to self-administer the bronchodilator.
- A **metered-dose inhaler** mixes a single dose of the medication with a puff of air and pushes it into the mouth via a chemical propellant (Figure 7.19).
- A **nebulizer** (**NEB**-you-lye-zer), also known as an *atomizer*, pumps air or oxygen through a liquid medicine to turn it into a vapor, which is then inhaled by the patient via a face mask or mouth piece.

The Nose, Throat, and Larynx

- **Endotracheal intubation** (**en**-doh-**TRAY**-kee-al **in**-too-**BAY**-shun) is the passage of a tube through the nose or mouth into the trachea to establish or maintain an open airway (**endo-** means within, **trache** means trachea, and **-al** means pertaining to). *Intubation* is the insertion of a tube, usually for the passage of air or fluids.

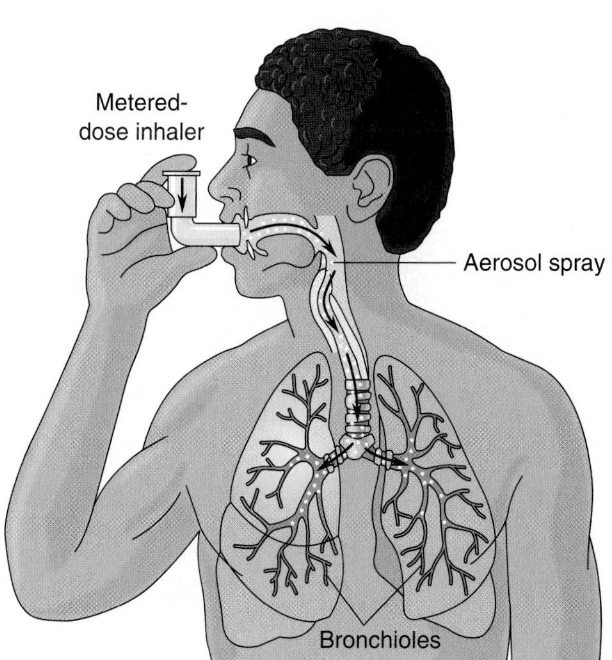

FIGURE 7.19 The metered-dose inhaler delivers medication for inhalation directly into the airways.

- **Functional endoscopic sinus surgery** (FESS) is a procedure performed using an endoscope in which chronic sinusitis is treated by enlarging the opening between the nose and sinus.
- A **laryngectomy** (**lar**-in-**JECK**-toh-mee) is the surgical removal of the larynx (**laryng** means larynx, and **-ectomy** means surgical removal).
- A **laryngoplasty** (lah-**RING**-goh-**plas**-tee) is the surgical repair of the larynx (**laryng** means larynx, and **-plasty** means surgical repair).
- **Pharyngoplasty** (fah-**RING**-goh-**plas**-tee) is the surgical repair of the pharynx (**pharyng/o** means pharynx, and **-plasty** means surgical repair).
- A **pharyngotomy** (**far**-ing-**GOT**-oh-mee) is a surgical incision of the pharynx (**pharyng** means pharynx and **-otomy** means a surgical incision).
- **Septoplasty** (**SEP**-toh-**plas**-tee) is the surgical repair or alteration of parts of the nasal septum (**sept/o** means septum, and **-plasty** means surgical repair).

The Trachea

- **Tracheoplasty** (**TRAY**-kee-oh-**plas**-tee) is the surgical repair of the trachea (**trache/o** means trachea, and **-plasty** means surgical repair).
- A **tracheostomy** (**tray**-kee-**OS**-toh-mee) is the creation of a stoma into the trachea and inserting a tube to facilitate the passage of air or the removal of secretions (**trache** means trachea, and **-ostomy** means surgically creating an opening). Placement of this tube can be temporary or permanent. As used here, a *stoma* means a surgically created opening on a body surface (Figure 7.20).
- A **tracheotomy** (**tray**-kee-**OT**-oh-mee) is usually an emergency procedure in which an incision is made into the trachea to gain access to the airway below a blockage (**trache** means trachea, and **-otomy** means surgical incision).

The Lungs, Pleura, and Thorax

- A **lobectomy** (loh-**BECK**-toh-mee) is the surgical removal of a lobe of the lung (**lob** means lobe, and **-ectomy** means surgical removal). This term is also used to describe the removal of a lobe of the liver, brain, or thyroid gland.

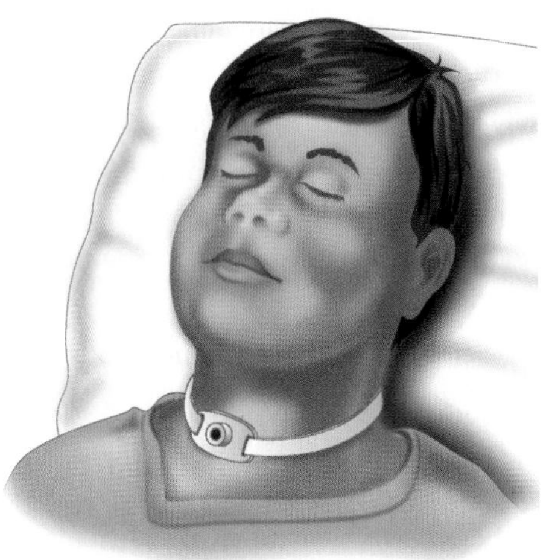

FIGURE 7.20 A tracheostomy tube creates an open airway for a patient who is unable to maintain his own airway.

- A **pleurectomy** (ploor-**ECK**-toh-mee) is the surgical removal of part of the pleura (**pleur** means pleura, and **-ectomy** means surgical removal).
- A **pneumonectomy** (**new**-moh-**NECK**-toh-mee) is the surgical removal of all or part of a lung (**pneumon** means lung, and **-ectomy** means surgical removal).
- **Thoracentesis** (**thoh**-rah-sen-**TEE**-sis) is the surgical puncture of the chest wall with a needle to obtain fluid from the pleural cavity (**thor/a** means chest, and **-centesis** means surgical puncture to remove fluid). This procedure is performed for diagnostic purposes or to drain excess fluid from severe pleural effusion.
- A **thoracostomy** (**thoh**-rah-**KOS**-toh-mee) is the surgical creation of an opening into the chest cavity (**thorac** means thorax or chest, and **-ostomy** means the surgical creation of an opening). This procedure is performed to establish drainage of empyema, which is pus in the pleural space.
- A **thoracotomy** (**thoh**-rah-**KOT**-toh-mee) is a surgical treatment of lung cancer by removing all or part of a lung (**thorac** means chest, and **-otomy** means surgical incision).This surgery involves cutting between the ribs on one side of the thorax and then removing the affected portion of the lung. A thoracotomy is also used for the visual examination of internal organs and the procurement of tissue specimens from the thorax.
- **Video-assisted thoracic surgery** (VATS) is the use of a video-assisted thoracoscope to view the inside of the chest cavity through very small incisions. A *thoracoscope* is a specialized endoscope used for treating the thorax. This procedure is used to obtain biopsy specimens to diagnose certain types of pneumonia, infections, or tumors of the chest wall. It is also used to treat repeatedly collapsing lungs.

Respiratory Therapy

- **Diaphragmatic breathing**, also known as *abdominal breathing*, is a relaxation technique used to relieve anxiety.
- A **CPAP device** (*continuous positive airway pressure*) is also known as a **positive pressure ventilation device**. This is treatment for sleep apnea that includes a mask, tubes, and a fan to create air pressure that pushes the tongue forward to maintain an open airway. Although this does not cure sleep apnea, it does reduce snoring and prevents dangerous apnea disturbances.
- A **respirator** is an apparatus for administering artificial respiration in cases of respiratory failure. For example, when a spinal cord injury destroys the natural breathing mechanism, the patient can continue to breathe through the use of a respirator. The term *respirator* also refers to any device that controls the quality of the air a person inhales. For example, it can also be a disposable dust mask or a piece of scuba diving equipment.
- A **ventilator** is a mechanical device for artificial ventilation of the lungs that is used to replace or supplement the patient's natural breathing function (Figure 7.21). The ventilator forces air into the lungs; exhalation takes place passively as the lungs contract.

Supplemental Oxygen

Supplemental oxygen is administered when the patient is unable to maintain an adequate oxygen saturation level in

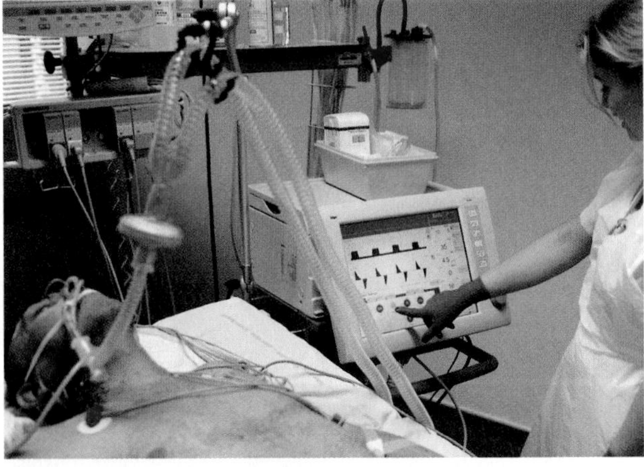

FIGURE 7.21 A ventilator forces air into and out of the lungs of a patient who is unable to breathe on his own. (Courtesy Draeger Medical, Inc., Telford, PA.)

the blood. This oxygen is administered by the following methods.

- A *nasal cannula* is a small tube that divides into two nasal prongs (Figure 7.22).
- A *rebreather mask* allows the exhaled breath to be partially reused, delivering up to 60% oxygen.
- A *non-rebreather mask* allows higher levels of oxygen to be added to the air taken in by the patient.

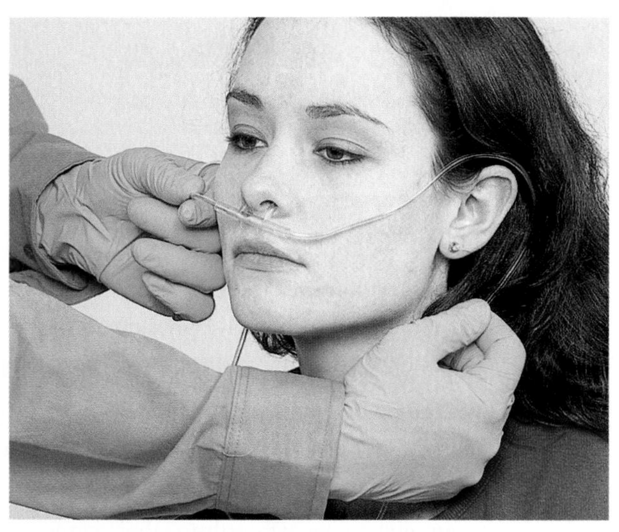

FIGURE 7.22 One method of delivering supplemental oxygen is through a nasal cannula.

ABBREVIATIONS RELATED TO THE RESPIRATORY SYSTEM

Table 7.1 presents an overview of the abbreviations related to the terms introduced in this chapter. Note: To avoid errors or confusion, always be cautious when using abbreviations.

TABLE 7.1

ABBREVIATIONS RELATED TO THE RESPIRATORY SYSTEM

bronchitis = BR, Br	**BR, Br** = bronchitis
bronchoscopy = BRO, bronch	**BRO, bronch** = bronchoscopy
Cheyne-Stokes breathing = CSB	**CSB** = Cheyne-Stokes breathing
cystic fibrosis = CF	**CF** = cystic fibrosis
diphtheria = diph	**diph** = diphtheria
***Pneumocystis carinii* pneumonia** = PCP	**PCP** = *Pneumocystis carinii* pneumonia
pneumothorax = Pno	**Pno** = pneumothorax
positive pressure ventilation = PPV	**PPV** = positive pressure ventilation
sleep apnea syndromes = SAS	**SAS** = sleep apnea syndromes
upper respiratory infection = URI	**URI** = upper respiratory infection

Career Opportunities

In addition to the medical specialties already discussed, some of the health occupations involving the treatment of the respiratory system include:

- **Respiratory therapist (RT):** treats patients with heart or lung problems by administering oxygen, gases, or aerosol medications under a physician's orders. RTs also perform diagnostic tests, connect and monitor patients on ventilators, and use exercises to improve patient breathing
- **Respiratory therapy technician (RTT):** works under the supervision of an RT to administer respiratory treatment, perform basic diagnostic tests, clean and maintain equipment, and keep records
- **Asthma educator:** a health professional who promotes optimal asthma management and quality of life among individuals with asthma, their families, and communities

Health Occupation Profile

Respiratory Therapist

Karen Zilles Hickel is a registered respiratory therapist (RT). She specializes in pediatrics, which means she helps children with breathing problems such as asthma and cystic fibrosis. *"My job involves giving a variety of treatments, including breathing medicines, oxygen, and using small machines to treat diseases of the lung. As a respiratory therapist, I also work in the intensive care unit where I see children who have had surgery, been in accidents, or have severe medical problems. When these patients are very sick, they often require a mechanical ventilator or respirator to breathe for them, which is run by an RT.*

"Respiratory therapists are an important part of the hospital's resuscitation team, keeping the patient's airway open and providing oxygen during CPR. I work in a pulmonary clinic, too. Here, I teach patients and their families how to use devices such as inhalers or nebulizers to treat asthma, and encourage adults and teens to avoid smoking to keep their lungs healthy. It is very rewarding to help people, particularly children, breathe more easily!"

STUDY BREAK

We do it when we're bored. We do it when we're sleepy. We sometimes do it because we see someone else do it. We may try not to, but can't help ourselves. What is it? A yawn. (The word *yawn* doesn't sound like most other medical terms because it comes from the Anglo-Saxon word *geonian* rather than Latin or Greek.)

A yawn is an involuntary *inhalation* of breath, accompanied by an opened mouth. Why do we yawn? Scientists are not entirely sure, but it seems to be a way for the body to get a sudden surge of oxygen into the lungs and to equalize the pressure in the ear. A spasm in the throat muscles opens the mouth so that we try to take in a deep breath.

We may yawn because:

- We are drowsy and not breathing deeply enough
- The body's vital functions are depressed, for example, after a *hemorrhage*
- The pressure in the ear needs to be equalized, such as during a plane landing
- We see someone else yawn (try this on a group of friends and see how many can resist)!

REVIEW TIME

Write the answers to the following questions on a separate piece of paper or in your notebook. In addition, be prepared to take part in the classroom discussion.

1. ***Written Assignment:*** Identify the four types of **paranasal sinuses** and state the location of each.

   Discussion Assignment: What is the role of the sinuses? What is the term used to describe the condition when they become infected or inflamed?

2. ***Written Assignment:*** Use your own words to describe what occurs within the lungs and chest as **emphysema** progresses.

   Discussion Assignment: How would you explain the progressive nature of emphysema to a patient's family?

3. ***Written Assignment:*** Using terms a physician would understand, describe at least two different kinds of **pneumonia**.

   Discussion Assignment: What type of pathogen causes **mycoplasma pneumonia** and **bacterial pneumonia**?

4. ***Written Assignment:*** Using terms the family could understand, describe each of the four forms of **cystic fibrosis** treatment and explain why each type of treatment is important.

   Discussion Assignment: How is cystic fibrosis transmitted?

5. ***Written Assignment:*** Describe **endotracheal intubation** and state why this procedure is performed.

   Discussion Assignment: State the primary differences between endotracheal intubation and bronchoscopy.

continues

Optional Internet Activity

The goal of this activity is to help you learn more about medical terminology as it applies to the "real world." Select **one** *of these two options and follow the instructions.*

1. Search for information about **sudden infant death syndrome** (SIDS). Write a brief (one- or two-paragraph) report on why it is recommended that infants be placed on their backs to sleep. Include the address of the web site where you found this information.

2. To learn more about **asthma**, go to the web site of the American Lung Association. Write a brief (one- or two-paragraph) report on something new you learned here.

THE HUMAN TOUCH: CRITICAL THINKING ACTIVITY

The following story and questions are designed to stimulate critical thinking through class discussion or as a brief essay response. There are no right or wrong answers to these questions.

BEEP! BEEP! BEEP! Chris Falke, 15, lifted his head groggily and turned off his alarm clock, staring in disbelief at the time. Late again! He must've hit the snooze button without realizing it. Rushing to get ready, he ran to the bus stop, only to see the school bus leaving as he arrived. Sighing, he started to walk to school instead. At least he had a warm coat on, he thought to himself, since it was snowing lightly.

By the time he reached school, he was wheezing with each breath, his asthma flaring up from the cold air and exertion. Sitting down at his desk, he reached into his backpack for his inhaler, only to realize that he'd left it at home. He didn't want to miss any more class time by going to the office to call his Dad and have him bring the inhaler from home. Hopefully, if he sat still in class and bent forward to make breathing easier, the warm air would make his asthma recede.

Wheezing noisily with each indrawn breath, it wasn't until he started feeling light-headed that he realized that this asthma attack was more serious than he had realized. The teacher glanced over at him and frowned. **"Chris, do you have your inhaler with you?"** ***Chris shook his head, concentrating on breathing, and his teacher nodded to one of the other students.*** **"Judy, take Chris's backpack and walk with him to the secretary's office."**

It wasn't the first time that Chris had forgotten his inhaler and suffered an asthma attack at school. The only thing that the school could do was to call his father to bring the inhaler to him, or to call an ambulance if the asthma attack was serious enough to be life-threatening. Judy left Chris in the secretary's office and returned to class as the secretary called his father. Thankfully, Chris's father worked at home, and it wasn't long before he arrived at school muttering a bit about Chris needing to be more responsible. It was almost 20 minutes before the medication had enough effect to let Chris breathe normally, but soon after that, Chris was back in class.

continues

Suggested Discussion Topics

1. Chris is a junior this year and plans to go away to college after he graduates from high school. Discuss Chris's responsibility now in learning how to manage his asthma.
2. Discuss why you think the school nurse did not have a spare inhaler with her supplies and use it to administer medicine to Chris when he came in. Could Chris, or his parents, have given the nurse an inhaler to keep on hand for him in case he forgot his?
3. Why would Chris have been reluctant to go to the nurses' office as soon as he realized that he'd forgotten his inhaler?
4. Is there any way that Chris could avoid having asthma attacks?

STUDENT WORKBOOK AND StudyWARE™ CD-ROM

1. Go to your **Student Workbook** and complete the Learning Exercises for this chapter.

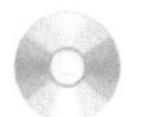

2. Go to the **StudyWARE™ CD-ROM** and have fun with the exercises and games for this chapter.

8

CHAPTER

THE DIGESTIVE SYSTEM

OVERVIEW OF STRUCTURES, COMBINING FORMS, AND FUNCTIONS OF THE DIGESTIVE SYSTEM

MAJOR STRUCTURES	RELATED COMBINING FORMS	PRIMARY FUNCTIONS
Mouth	or/o, stomat/o	Begins preparation of food for digestion.
Pharynx	pharyng/o	Transports food from the mouth to the esophagus.
Esophagus	esophag/o	Transports food from the pharynx to the stomach.
Stomach	gastr/o	Breaks down food and mixes it with digestive juices.
Small intestine	enter/o	Completes digestion and absorption of most nutrients.
Large intestine	col/o, colon/o	Absorbs excess water and prepares solid waste for elimination.
Rectum and anus	an/o, proct/o, rect/o	Control the excretion of solid waste.
Liver	hepat/o	Secretes bile and enzymes to aid in the digestion of fats.
Gallbladder	cholecyst/o	Stores bile and releases it to the small intestine as needed.
Pancreas	pancreat/o	Secretes digestive juices and enzymes into small intestine as needed.

VOCABULARY RELATED TO THE DIGESTIVE SYSTEM

This list contains essential word parts and medical terms for this chapter. These terms are pronounced on the student StudyWARE™ CD-ROM and Audio CDs that are available for use with this text. These and the other important **primary terms** are shown in boldface throughout the chapter. *Secondary terms*, which appear in *orange* italics, clarify the meaning of primary terms.

Word Parts

- ☐ an/o
- ☐ chol/e
- ☐ cholecyst/o
- ☐ col/o, colon/o
- ☐ -emesis
- ☐ enter/o
- ☐ esophag/o
- ☐ gastr/o
- ☐ hepat/o
- ☐ -lithiasis
- ☐ -pepsia
- ☐ -phagia
- ☐ proct/o
- ☐ rect/o
- ☐ sigmoid/o

Medical Terms

- ☐ **aerophagia** (**ay**-er-oh-**FAY**-jee-ah)
- ☐ **amebic dysentery** (ah-**MEE**-bik **DIS**-en-**ter**-ee)
- ☐ **anastomosis** (ah-**nas**-toh-**MOH**-sis)
- ☐ **anorexia nervosa** (**an**-oh-**RECK**-see-ah ner-**VOH**-sah)
- ☐ **antiemetic** (**an**-tih-ee-**MET**-ick)
- ☐ **aphthous ulcers** (**AF**-thus **UL**-serz)
- ☐ **ascites** (ah-**SIGH**-teez)
- ☐ **bariatrics** (**bayr**-ee-**AT**-ricks)
- ☐ **borborygmus** (**bor**-boh-**RIG**-mus)
- ☐ **botulism** (**BOT**-you-lizm)
- ☐ **bulimia nervosa** (byou-**LIM**-ee-ah ner-**VOH**-sah)
- ☐ **cachexia** (kah-**KEKS**-eeh-ah)
- ☐ **cheilosis** (kee-**LOH**-sis)
- ☐ **cholangiography** (koh-**LAN**-jee-**og**-rah-fee)
- ☐ **cholangitis** (**koh**-lan-**JIGH**-tis)
- ☐ **cholecystalgia** (**koh**-lee-sis-**TAL**-jee-ah)
- ☐ **cholecystectomy** (**koh**-lee-sis-**TECK**-toh-mee)
- ☐ **cholecystitis** (**koh**-lee-sis-**TYE**-tis)
- ☐ **choledocholithotomy** (koh-**led**-oh-koh-lih-**THOT**-oh-mee)
- ☐ **cholelithiasis** (**koh**-lee-lih-**THIGH**-ah-sis)
- ☐ **cholera** (**KOL**-er-ah)
- ☐ **cirrhosis** (sih-**ROH**-sis)
- ☐ **colonoscopy** (**koh**-lun-**OSS**-koh-pee)
- ☐ **Crohn's disease**
- ☐ **diverticulitis** (**dye**-ver-tick-you-**LYE**-tis)
- ☐ **diverticulosis** (**dye**-ver-**tick**-you-**LOH**-sis)
- ☐ **dyspepsia** (dis-**PEP**-see-ah)
- ☐ **dysphagia** (dis-**FAY**-jee-ah)
- ☐ **emesis** (**EM**-eh-sis)
- ☐ **enteritis** (**en**-ter-**EYE**-tis)
- ☐ **eructation** (eh-ruk-**TAY**-shun)
- ☐ **esophageal varices** (eh-**sof**-ah-**JEE**-al **VAYR**-ih-seez)
- ☐ **esophagogastroduodenoscopy** (eh-**sof**-ah-goh-**gas**-troh-**dew**-oh-deh-**NOS**-koh-pee)
- ☐ **gastroduodenostomy** (**gas**-troh-**dew**-oh-deh-**NOS**-toh-mee)
- ☐ **gastroesophageal reflux disease** (gas-troh-eh-**sof**-ah-**JEE**-al **REE** flucks)
- ☐ **gastrostomy tube** (gas-**TROS**-toh-mee)
- ☐ **hematemesis** (**hee**-mah-**TEM**-eh-sis)
- ☐ **Hemoccult test** (**HEE**-moh-kult)
- ☐ **hepatitis** (**hep**-ah-**TYE**-tis)
- ☐ **herpes labialis** (**HER**-peez **lay**-bee-**AL**-iss)
- ☐ **hiatal hernia** (high-**AY**-tal **HER**-nee-ah)
- ☐ **hyperemesis** (**high**-per-**EM**-eh-sis)
- ☐ **ileus** (**ILL**-ee-us)
- ☐ **inguinal hernia** (**ING**-gwih-nal **HER**-nee-ah)
- ☐ **jaundice** (**JAWN**-dis)
- ☐ **melena** (meh-**LEE**-nah)
- ☐ **morbid obesity** (**MOR**-bid oh-**BEE**-sih-tee)
- ☐ **nasogastric intubation** (**nay**-zoh-**GAS**-trick **in**-too-**BAY**-shun)
- ☐ **obesity** (oh-**BEE**-sih-tee)
- ☐ **periodontium** (**pehr**-ee-oh-**DON**-shee-um)
- ☐ **peristalsis** (**pehr**-ih-**STAL**-sis)
- ☐ **proctopexy** (**PROCK**-toh-**peck**-see)
- ☐ **regurgitation** (ree-**gur**-jih-**TAY**-shun)
- ☐ **salmonellosis** (**sal**-moh-nel-**LOH**-sis)
- ☐ **sigmoidoscopy** (**sig**-moi-**DOS**-koh-pee)
- ☐ **stomatorrhagia** (**stoh**-mah-toh-**RAY**-jee-ah)
- ☐ **trismus** (**TRIZ**-mus)
- ☐ **ulcerative colitis** (**UL**-ser-**ay**-tiv koh-**LYE**-tis)
- ☐ **volvulus** (**VOL**-view-lus)
- ☐ **xerostomia** (**zeer**-oh-**STOH**-mee-ah)

OBJECTIVES

On completion of this chapter, you should be able to:

1. Identify and describe the major structures and functions of the digestive system.
2. Describe the processes of digestion, absorption, and metabolism.
3. Recognize, define, spell, and pronounce terms related to the pathology and the diagnostic and treatment procedures of the digestive system.

STRUCTURES OF THE DIGESTIVE SYSTEM

The major structures of the digestive system include the oral cavity (mouth), pharynx (throat), esophagus, stomach, small intestine, large intestine, rectum, and anus.

The *accessory organs* of the digestive system aid with digestion, but are not part of the digestive system. These organs include the liver, gallbladder, and pancreas (Figure 8.1).

The Gastrointestinal Tract

The structures of the digestive system are also described as the **gastrointestinal tract** or *GI tract* (**gastr/o** means stomach, **intestin** means intestine, and **-al** means pertaining to).

- The *upper GI tract* consists of the mouth, esophagus, and stomach.
- The *lower GI tract* is made up of the small and large intestines (sometimes referred to as the *bowels*), plus the rectum, and anus.

The Oral Cavity

The major structures of the **oral cavity**, also known as the *mouth*, are the lips, hard and soft palates, salivary glands, tongue, teeth, and the periodontium (Figure 8.2).

The Lips

The **lips**, also known as *labia*, form the opening to the oral cavity (singular, *labium*). The term *labia* is also used to describe parts of the female genitalia (see Chapter 14).

During eating, the lips hold food in the mouth and aid the tongue and cheeks in guiding food between the teeth for chewing. The lips also have important roles in breathing, speaking, and the expression of emotions.

The upper and lower *labial frenum* are narrow bands of tissue that attach the lips to the jaws (see Figure 8.2).

The Palate

The **palate** (**PAL**-at) forms the roof of the mouth (see Figure 8.2).

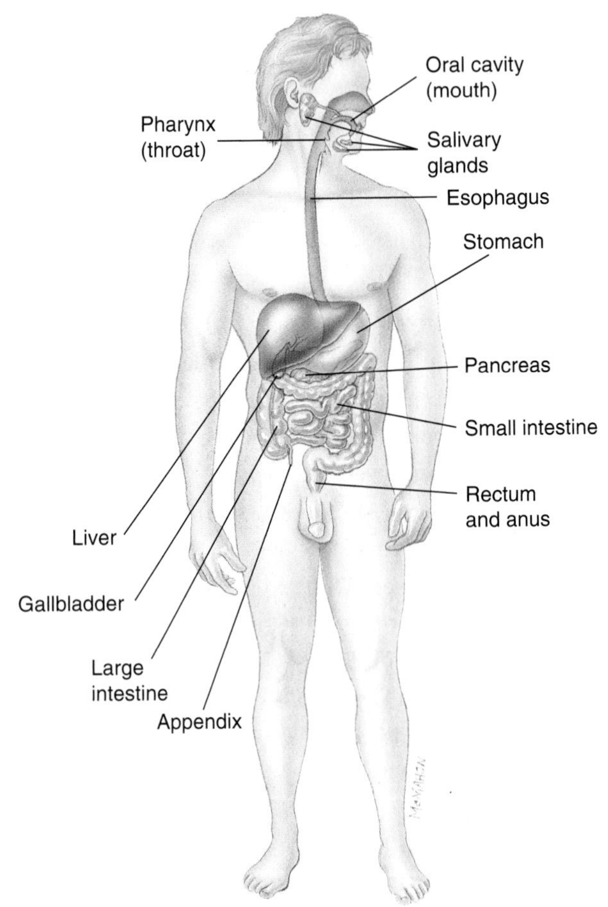

FIGURE 8.1 Major structures and accessory organs of the digestive system.

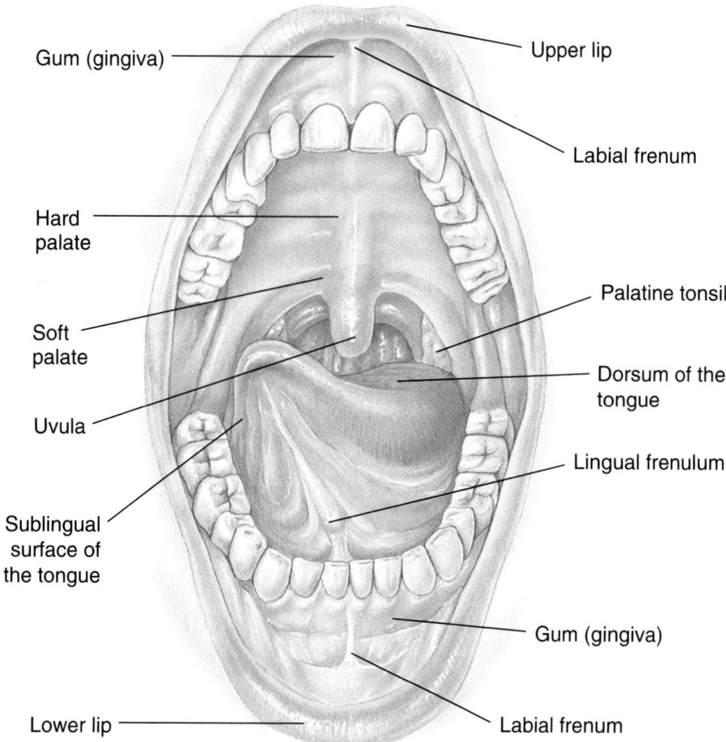

FIGURE 8.2 Structures of the tongue and oral cavity.

- The **hard palate** is the bony anterior portion of the palate that is covered with specialized mucous membrane. *Rugae* are irregular ridges or folds in this mucous membrane (singular, *ruga).*
- The **soft palate** is the flexible posterior portion of the palate. It has the important role of closing off the nasal passage during swallowing to prevent food and liquid from moving upward into the nasal cavity.
- The **uvula** (**YOU**-view-lah) hangs from the free edge of the soft palate. During swallowing, it moves upward with the soft palate. It also plays an important role in snoring and in the formation of some speech sounds.

The Tongue

The **tongue** is very strong, flexible, and muscular. It aids in speech and moves food during chewing and swallowing (see Figure 8.2).

- The upper surface of the tongue is the *dorsum*. This surface has a tough protective covering and, in some areas, small bumps known as **papillae** (pah-**PILL**-ee) (singular, *papilla*). These papillae contain *taste buds*, which are the sensory receptors for the sense of taste.
- The *sublingual surface* of the tongue, and the tissues that lie under the tongue, are covered with delicate highly vascular tissues. *Sublingual* means under the tongue. *Highly vascular* means containing many blood vessels.
- It is the presence of this rich blood supply under the tongue that makes it suitable for administering certain medications by placing them sublingually where they are quickly absorbed into the bloodstream.
- The *lingual frenum* attaches the tongue to the floor of the mouth and limits its motion.

Soft Tissues of the Oral Cavity

- The **periodontium** (**pehr**-ee-oh-**DON**-shee-um) consists of the bone and soft tissues that surround and support the teeth (**peri-** means surrounding, **odonti** means the teeth, and **-um** is the noun ending).
- The **gingiva** (**JIN**-jih-vah), commonly known as the *gums*, is the specialized mucous membrane that surrounds the teeth, covers the bone of the dental arches, and lines the cheeks.

The Dental Arches

The boney structures of the oral cavity consist of the *maxillary* and *mandibular arches*. These structures, which are commonly referred to as the *upper and lower jaws*, firmly hold the teeth in position to facilitate chewing and speaking.

The **temporomandibular joint** (**tem**-poh-roh-man-**DIB**-you-lar), commonly known as the *TMJ*, is formed at the back of the mouth where the maxillary and mandibular arches come together. The maxillary arch, which is part of the skull, does not move. The mandibular arch, which is a separate bone, is the moveable component of this joint.

The Teeth

The term **dentition** (den-**TISH**-un) refers to the natural teeth arranged in the upper and lower jaws.

- The human dentition includes four types of teeth: *incisors* and *canines* (also known as *cuspids*) that are used for biting and tearing, plus *premolars* (also known as *bicuspids*) and *molars* that are used for chewing and grinding.
- The **primary dentition**, also known as the *deciduous dentition* or *baby teeth*, consists of 20 teeth that are normally lost during childhood and are replaced by the permanent teeth. These teeth include: 8 incisors, 4 canines, 8 molars, and no premolars.
- The **permanent dentition** consists of 32 teeth that are designed to last a lifetime. These teeth include: 8 incisors, 4 canines, 8 premolars, and 12 molars.
- **Edentulous** (ee-**DEN**-too-lus) means without teeth. This term describes the situation after the natural permanent teeth have been lost.
- As used in dentistry, **occlusion** (ah-**KLOO**-zhun) describes any contact between the chewing surfaces of the upper and lower teeth.
- **Malocclusion** (**mal**-oh-**KLOO**-zhun) is any deviation from the normal positioning of the upper teeth against the lower teeth.

Structures and Tissues of the Teeth

The *crown* is the portion of a tooth that is visible in the mouth. It is covered with *enamel*, which is the hardest substance in the body (Figure 8.3).

- The *roots* of the tooth hold it securely in place within the dental arch. The roots are protected by *cementum*, which is strong, but not as hard as enamel.
- The *cervix* (neck) of the tooth is where the crown and root meet.
- *Dentin* makes up the bulk of the tooth structure and is protected on the outer surfaces by the enamel and cementum.

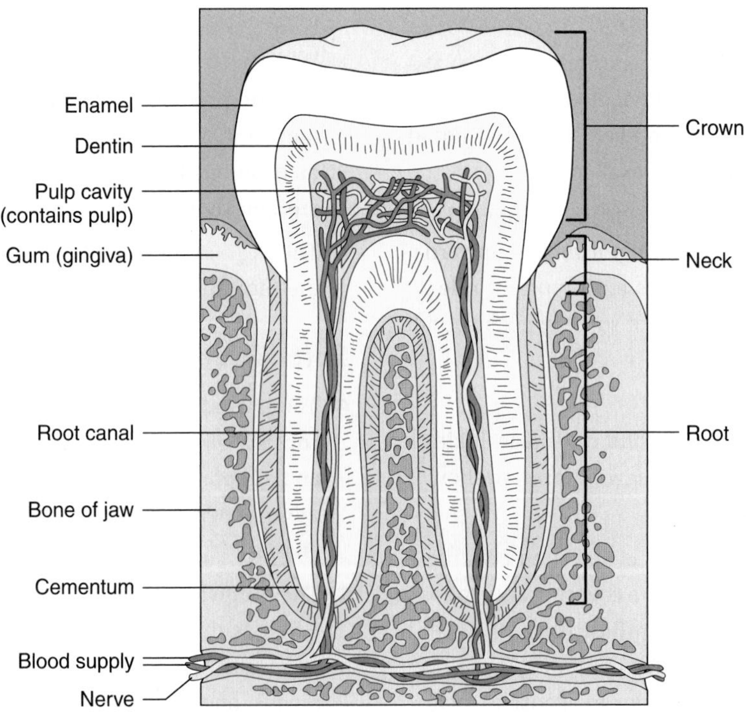

FIGURE 8.3 Structures and tissues of the tooth.

- The *pulp* consists of a rich supply of blood vessels and nerves that provide nutrients and innervation to the tooth. In the crown, the pulp is located in the *pulp cavity*. In the roots, the pulp continues through the *root canals*.

Saliva and Salivary Glands

Saliva is a colorless liquid that moistens the mouth, begins the digestive process, and lubricates food during chewing and swallowing. The three pairs of **salivary glands** (**SAL**-ih-ver-ee) secrete saliva that is carried by ducts into the mouth (Figure 8.4).

- The *parotid glands* are located on the face in front of and slightly lower than each ear. The ducts for these glands are on the inside of the cheek near the upper molars.
- The *sublingual glands* and their ducts are located on the floor of the mouth under the tongue.
- The *submandibular glands* and their ducts are located on the floor of the mouth near the mandible.

The Pharynx

The **pharynx** (**FAR**-inks), which is the common passageway for both respiration and digestion, is discussed in Chapter 7.

- The **epiglottis** (**ep**-ih-**GLOT**-is) is a lid-like structure that closes off the entrance to the trachea (windpipe) to prevent food and liquids from moving from the pharynx during swallowing. This is discussed further in Chapter 7.

The Esophagus

The **esophagus** (eh-**SOF**-ah-gus) is the muscular tube through which ingested food passes from the pharynx to the stomach (see Figure 8.1).

- The **lower esophageal sphincter**, also known as the *cardiac sphincter* or the *gastroesophageal sphincter*, is a muscular ring controls the flow between the esophagus and stomach (see Figure 8.5). This sphincter normally opens to allow the flow of food into the stomach and closes to prevent the stomach contents from regurgitating into the esophagus. *Regurgitating* means to flow backward.

The Stomach

The **stomach** is a sac-like organ composed of the *fundus* (upper, rounded part), *body* (main portion), and *antrum* (lower part) (Figure 8.5).

- **Rugae** (**ROO**-gay) are the folds in the mucosa lining the stomach. Glands located within these folds produce gastric juices that aid in digestion and mucus to create a protective coating on the lining of the stomach.
- The **pylorus** (pye-**LOR**-us) is the narrow passage that connects the stomach with the small intestine.

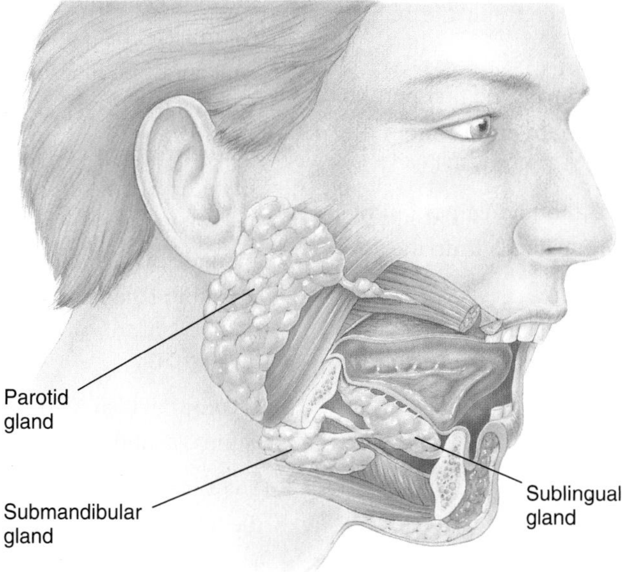

FIGURE 8.4 The salivary glands.

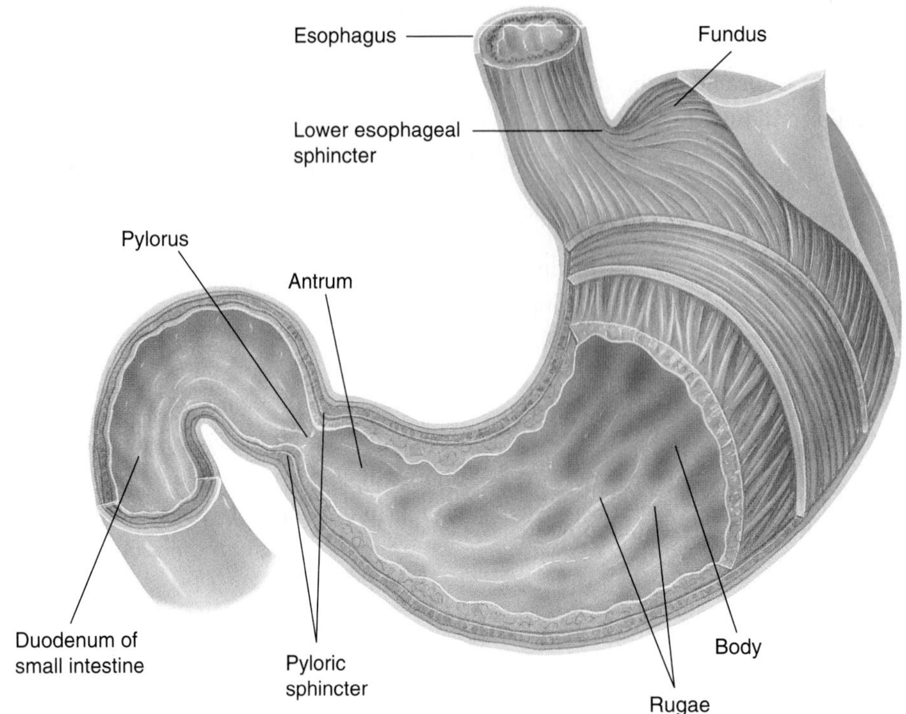

FIGURE 8.5 Structures of the stomach.

- The **pyloric sphincter** (pye-**LOR**-ick) is the ring-like muscle that controls the flow from the stomach to the duodenum of the small intestine.

The Small Intestine

The **small intestine** extends from the pyloric sphincter to the first part of the large intestine. The small intestine is a coiled organ up to 20 feet in length (see Figure 8.1). The small intestine consists of three sections where food is digested and the nutrients are absorbed into the bloodstream.

- The **duodenum** (**dew**-oh-**DEE**-num) is the first portion of the small intestine. The duodenum extends from the pylorus to the jejunum.
- The **jejunum** (jeh-**JOO**-num) is the middle portion of the small intestine. The jejunum extends from the duodenum to the ileum.
- The **ileum** (**ILL**-ee-um), which is the last and longest portion of the small intestine, extends from the jejunum to the cecum of the large intestine.

The Large Intestine

The **large intestine** extends from the end of the small intestine to the anus. It is about twice as wide as the small intestine, but only one-fourth as long. It is here that the waste products of digestion are processed in preparation for excretion through the anus. The major parts of the large intestine are the cecum, colon, rectum, and anus (Figure 8.6).

The Cecum

The **cecum** (**SEE**-kum) is a pouch that lies on the right side of the abdomen. It extends from the end of the ileum to the beginning of the colon.

- The **ileocecal sphincter** (**ill**-ee-oh-**SEE**-kull) is the ring-like muscle that controls the flow from the ileum of the small intestine into the cecum of the large intestine (see Figure 8.6).
- The **vermiform appendix**, commonly called the *appendix*, hangs from the lower portion of the cecum. The term *vermiform* refers to a worm-like shape. The appendix, which consists of lymphoid tissue, is discussed in Chapter 6.

The Colon

The **colon**, which is the longest portion of the large intestine, is subdivided into four parts (see Figure 8.6):

- The **ascending colon** travels upward from the cecum to the undersurface of the liver. *Ascending* means upward.
- The **transverse colon** passes horizontally from right to left toward the spleen. *Transverse* means across.

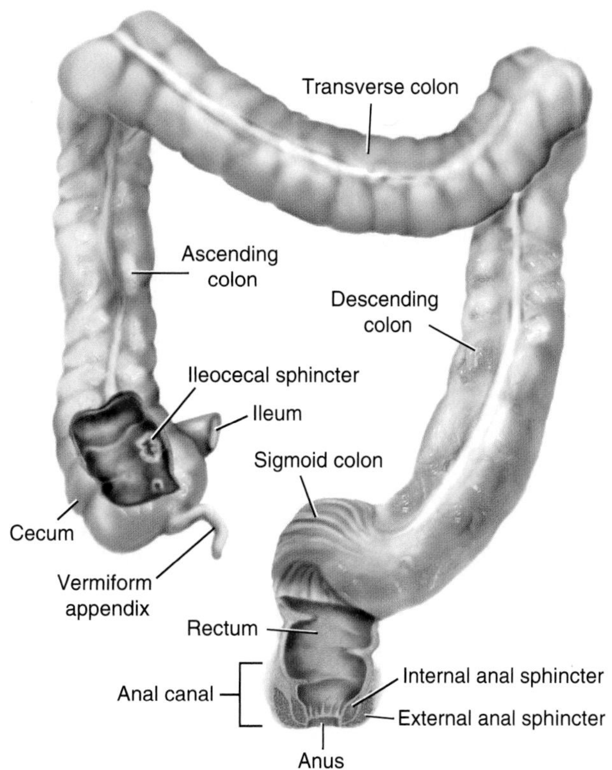

FIGURE 8.6 Structures of the large intestine.

- The **descending colon** travels down the left side of the abdominal cavity to the sigmoid colon. *Descending* means downward.
- The **sigmoid colon** (**SIG**-moid) is an S-shaped structure that continues from the descending colon above and joins with the rectum below. *Sigmoid* means curved like the letter *S*.

The Rectum and Anus

- The **rectum**, which is the widest division of the large intestine, makes up the last 4 inches of the large intestine and ends at the anus.
- The **anus** is the lower opening of the digestive tract. The flow of waste through the anus is controlled by the *internal anal sphincter* and the *external anal sphincter*.
- The term *anorectal* refers to the anus and rectum as a single unit (**an/o** means anus, **rect** means rectum, and **-al** means pertaining to).

Accessory Digestive Organs

The accessory organs of the digestive system are so named because they play a key role in the digestive process, but are not part of the gastrointestinal tract (Figure 8.7).

The Liver

The **liver** is a large organ located in the right upper quadrant of the abdomen (see Figures 8.7 and 8.8). It has several important functions related to removing toxins from the blood and turning food into the fuel and nutrients the body needs. The term *hepatic* means pertaining to the liver (**hepat** means liver, and **-ic** means pertaining to).

- The liver removes excess *glucose*, commonly known as blood sugar from the bloodstream and stores it as *glycogen*, which is a form of starch. When the blood sugar level is low, the liver converts glycogen back into glucose and releases it for use by the body.
- The liver also destroys old erythrocytes (red blood cells), removes toxins from the blood, and manufactures some blood proteins. **Bilirubin** (bill-ih-**ROO**-bin), which is the pigment produced from the destruction of hemoglobin, is released by the liver in bile.
- **Bile**, which aids in the digestion of fats, is a digestive juice secreted by the liver. Bile travels from the liver to the gallbladder, where it is concentrated and stored.

The Biliary Tree

The **biliary tree** (**BILL**-ee-air-ee) provides the channels through which bile is transported from the liver to the small intestine. *Biliary* means pertaining to bile.

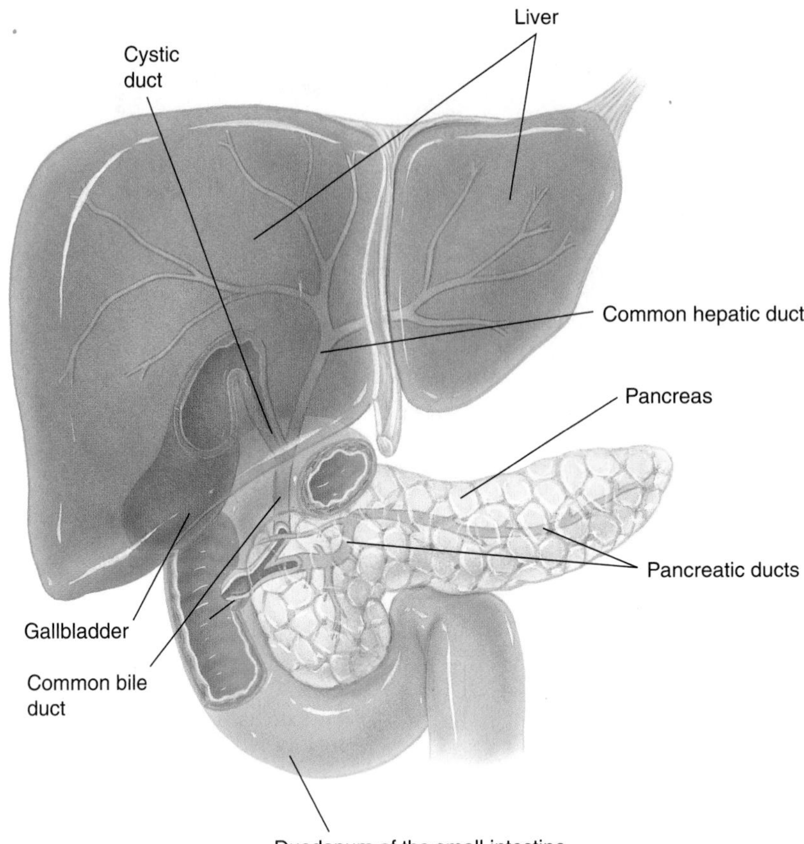

FIGURE 8.7 Accessory digestive organs: the liver, gallbladder, and pancreas.

- Small ducts in the liver join together like branches to form the biliary tree. The trunk, which is just outside the liver, is known as the *common hepatic duct*.
- The bile travels from the liver through the common hepatic duct to the gallbladder where it enters and exits through the narrow *cystic duct*.
- The cystic duct leaving the gallbladder rejoins the common hepatic duct to form the *common bile duct*. The common bile duct joins the *pancreatic duct*, and together they enter the duodenum of the small intestine.

The Gallbladder

The **gallbladder** is a pear-shaped organ about the size of an egg located under the liver. It stores and concentrates the bile for later use (see Figures 8.7 and 8.8).

- The term **cholecystic** means pertaining to the gallbladder (**cholecyst** means gallbladder, and **-ic** means pertaining to).
- When bile is needed, the gallbladder contracts, forcing the bile out through the biliary tree.

The Pancreas

The **pancreas** (**PAN**-kree-as) is a soft, 6 inch long oblong gland that is located behind the stomach (see Figures 8.7 and 8.8). This gland has important roles in both the digestive and endocrine systems. The digestive functions are discussed here. The endocrine functions, plus the pathology and procedures related to the pancreas, are discussed in Chapter 13.

- The pancreas produces and secretes *pancreatic juices* that aid in digestion and contain sodium bicarbonate to help neutralize stomach acids and digestive enzymes. *Pancreatic* means pertaining to the pancreas (**pancreat** means pancreas, and **-tic** means pertaining to.)
- The pancreatic juices leave the pancreas through the *pancreatic duct* that joins the *common bile duct* just before the entrance into the duodenum.

DIGESTION

Digestion is the process by which complex foods are broken down into nutrients in a form the body can use. The flow of food through the digestive system is shown in Figure 8.8.

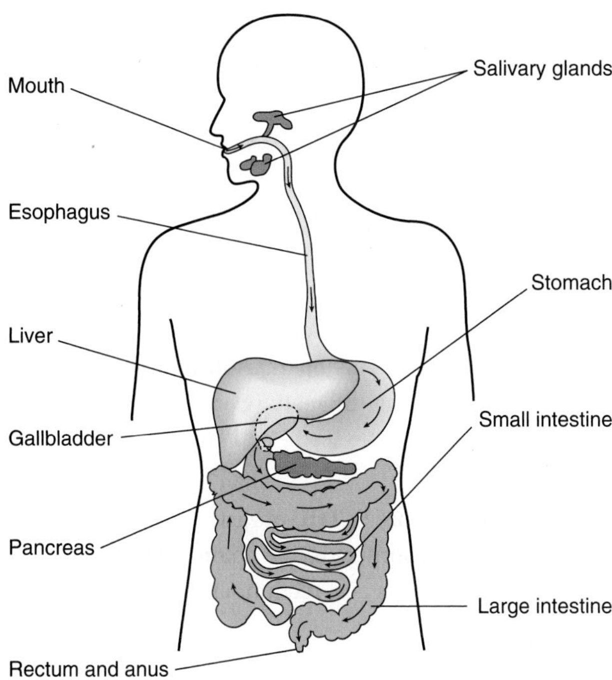

FIGURE 8.8 A schematic diagram showing the pathway of food through the digestive system.

- *Digestive enzymes* are responsible for the chemical changes that break foods down into simpler forms of nutrients for use by the body.
- A *nutrient* is a substance, usually from food, that is necessary for normal functioning of the body. The primary nutrients are *carbohydrates*, *fats*, and *proteins*. *Vitamins* and *minerals* are essential nutrients, which are required only in small amounts.

Metabolism

The term **metabolism** (meh-**TAB**-oh-lizm) includes all of the processes involved in the body's use of nutrients (**metabol** means change, and **-ism** means condition). It consists of two parts: anabolism and catabolism.

- **Anabolism** (an-**NAB**-oh-lizm) is the building up of body cells and substances from nutrients. Anabolism is the opposite of *catabolism*.
- **Catabolism** (kah-**TAB**-oh-lizm) is the breaking down of body cells or substances, releasing energy and carbon dioxide. Catabolism is the opposite of *anabolism*.

Absorption

Absorption (ab-**SORP**-shun) is the process by which completely digested nutrients are transported to the cells throughout the body.

- The mucosa that lines the small intestine is covered with finger-like projections called **villi** (**VILL**-eye) (singular, *villus*). Each villus contains blood vessels and lacteals.
- The blood vessels absorb nutrients directly from the digestive system into the bloodstream for delivery to the cells of the body.
- Fats and fat-soluble vitamins cannot be transported directly by the bloodstream. Instead the *lacteals*, which are specialized structures of the lymphatic system, absorb these nutrients and transport them via lymphatic vessels. As these nutrients are being transported, they are filtered by the lymph nodes in preparation for their delivery to the bloodstream. (Lacteals are discussed in Chapter 6.)

The Role of the Mouth, Salivary Glands, and Esophagus

- **Mastication** (**mass**-tih-**KAY**-shun), also known as *chewing*, breaks food down into smaller pieces, mixes it with saliva, and prepares it to be swallowed.
- A **bolus** (**BOH**-lus) is a mass of food that has been chewed and is ready to be swallowed. The term bolus is also used in relation to the administration of medication and is discussed in Chapter 15.
- During swallowing, food travels from the mouth into the pharynx and on into the esophagus.
- In the esophagus, food moves downward through the action of gravity and peristalsis. **Peristalsis** (**pehr**-ih-**STAL**-sis) is a series of wave-like contractions of the smooth muscles in a single direction.

The Role of the Stomach

- The *gastric juices* of the stomach contain hydrochloric acid and digestive enzymes to begin the digestive process. Few nutrients enter the bloodstream through the walls of the stomach.
- The churning action of the stomach works with the gastric juices by converting the food into chyme. **Chyme** (**KYM**) is the semifluid mass of partly digested food that passes out of the stomach, through the pyloric sphincter, and into the small intestine.

The Role of the Small Intestine

The conversion of food into usable nutrients is completed as the chyme is moved through the small intestine by peristaltic action.

- In the duodenum, chyme is mixed with pancreatic juice and bile. The bile breaks apart large fat globules so enzymes in the pancreatic juices can digest the fats. This action is called *emulsification* and must be completed before the nutrients can be absorbed into the body.
- The jejunum secretes large amounts of digestive enzymes and continues the process of digestion.
- The primary function of the ileum is the absorption of nutrients from the digested food.

The Role of the Large Intestine

The role of the entire large intestine is to receive the waste products of digestion and store them until they are eliminated from the body.

- Food waste enters the large intestine in liquid form. Excess water is reabsorbed into the body through the walls of the large intestine, helping to maintain the body's fluid balance, and the remaining waste forms into feces. **Feces** (**FEE**-seez), also known as *stools*, are solid body wastes expelled through the rectum and anus.
- **Defecation** (**def**-eh-**KAY**-shun), also known as a *bowel movement*, is the evacuation or emptying of the large intestine.
- The large intestine contains billions of bacteria, most of them harmless, which help break down organic waste material. This process produces gas. **Borborygmus** (**bor**-boh-**RIG**-mus) is the rumbling noise caused by the movement of gas in the intestine.
- **Flatulence** (**FLAT**-you-lens), also known as *flatus*, is the passage of gas out of the body through the rectum.

MEDICAL SPECIALTIES RELATED TO THE DIGESTIVE SYSTEM

- **Bariatrics** (**bayr**-ee-**AT**-ricks) is the branch of medicine concerned with the prevention and control of obesity and associated diseases.
- A **dentist** holds a Doctor of Dental Surgery (DDS) or Doctor of Medical Dentistry (DMD) degree and specializes in diagnosing and treating diseases and disorders of teeth and tissues of the oral cavity.
- A **gastroenterologist** (**gas**-troh-**en**-ter-**OL**-oh-jist) is a physician who specializes in diagnosing and treating diseases and disorders of the stomach and intestines (**gastr/o** means stomach, **enter** means small intestine, and **-ologist** means specialist).
- An **internist** is a physician who specializes in diagnosing and treating diseases and disorders of the internal organs and related body systems.
- An **orthodontist** (**or**-thoh-**DON**-tist) is a dental specialist who prevents or corrects malocclusion of the teeth and related facial structures (**orth** means straight or normal, **odont** means the teeth, and **-ist** means specialist).
- A **periodontist** (**pehr**-ee-oh-**DON**-tist) is a dental specialist who prevents or treats disorders of the tissues surrounding the teeth (**peri-** means surrounding, **odont** means the teeth, and **-ist** means specialist).
- A **proctologist** (prock-**TOL**-oh-jist) is a physician who specializes in disorders of the colon, rectum, and anus (**proct** means anus and rectum, and **-ologist** means specialist).

PATHOLOGY OF THE DIGESTIVE SYSTEM

Tissues of the Oral Cavity

- **Aphthous ulcers** (**AF**-thus **UL**-serz), also known as *canker sores* or *mouth ulcers*, are grey-white pits with a red border in the soft tissues lining the mouth. Although the exact cause is unknown, the appearance of these very common sores is associated with stress, certain foods, or fever.
- **Cheilosis** (kee-**LOH**-sis), also known as *cheilitis*, is a disorder of the lips characterized by crack-like sores at the corners of the mouth (**cheil** means lips, and **-osis** means abnormal condition or disease).
- **Herpes labialis** (**HER**-peez **lay**-bee-**AL**-iss), also known as *cold sores* or *fever blisters*, are blister-like sores on the lips and adjacent facial tissue that are caused by the *oral herpes simplex virus type 1* (HSV-1). Most adults have been infected by this extremely common virus, and in some, it becomes re-activated periodically, causing cold sores.
- **Oral thrush** develops when the fungus *Candida albicans* grows out of control. The symptoms are creamy white lesions on the tongue or inner cheeks, and this condition occurs most often in infants, older adults with weakened immune systems, or individuals who have been taking antibiotics.
- **Stomatomycosis** (**stoh**-mah-toh-my-**KOH**-sis) is any disease of the mouth due to a fungus (**stomat/o**

means mouth or oral cavity, **myc** means fungus, and **-osis** means abnormal condition or disease). See oral thrush.

- **Stomatorrhagia** (**stoh**-mah-toh-**RAY**-jee-ah) describes bleeding from any part of the mouth (**stomat/o** means mouth or oral cavity, and **-rrhagia** means bursting forth of blood).
- The term **trismus** (**TRIZ**-mus) describes any restriction to the opening of the mouth caused by trauma, surgery, or radiation associated with the treatment of oral cancer. This condition causes difficulty in speaking and affects the patient's nutrition due to impaired ability to chew and swallow.
- **Xerostomia** (**zeer**-oh-**STOH**-mee-ah), also known as *dry mouth*, is the lack of adequate saliva due to diminished secretions by the salivary glands (**xer/o** means dry, **stom** means mouth, and **-ia** means pertaining to). This condition can be due to medications or radiation of the salivary glands, and can cause discomfort, difficulty in swallowing, changes in the taste of food, and dental decay.

Cleft Lip and Cleft Palate

- A **cleft lip**, also known as a *harelip*, is a birth defect in which there is a deep groove of the lip running upward to the nose as a result of the failure of this portion of the lip to close during prenatal development.
- A **cleft palate** is the failure of the palate to close during the early development of the fetus. This opening can involve the upper lip, hard palate, and/or soft palate. If not corrected, this opening between the nose and mouth makes it difficult for the child to eat and speak. Cleft lip and cleft palate can occur singly or together and usually can be corrected surgically (Figure 8.9).

Dental Diseases

- **Acute necrotizing ulcerative gingivitis** (ANUG), also known as *trench mouth*, is caused by the abnormal growth of bacteria in the mouth. As this condition progresses, the inflammation, bleeding, deep ulceration, and the death of gum tissue become more severe. *Necrotizing* means causing ongoing tissue death.
- **Bruxism** (**BRUCK**-sizm) is the involuntary grinding or clenching of the teeth that usually occurs during sleep and is associated with tension or stress. Bruxism wears away tooth structure, damages periodontal tissues, and injures the temporomandibular joint.
- **Dental calculus** (**KAL**-kyou-luhs), also known as *tartar*, is dental plaque that has calcified (hardened) on the teeth. These deposits irritate the surrounding tissues and cause increasingly serious periodontal diseases. The term *calculus* is also used to describe hard deposits, such as gallstones or kidney stones, which form in other parts of the body.
- **Dental caries** (**KAYR**-eez), also known as *tooth decay* or a *cavity*, is an infectious disease caused by bacteria that destroy the enamel and dentin of the tooth. If the decay process is not arrested, the pulp can be exposed and become infected.

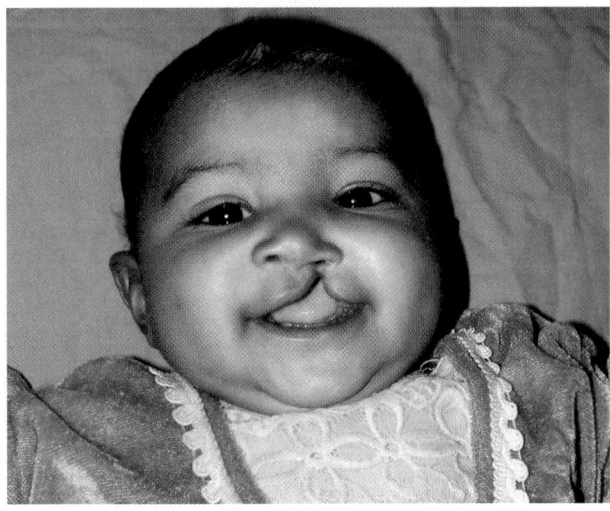

(A)

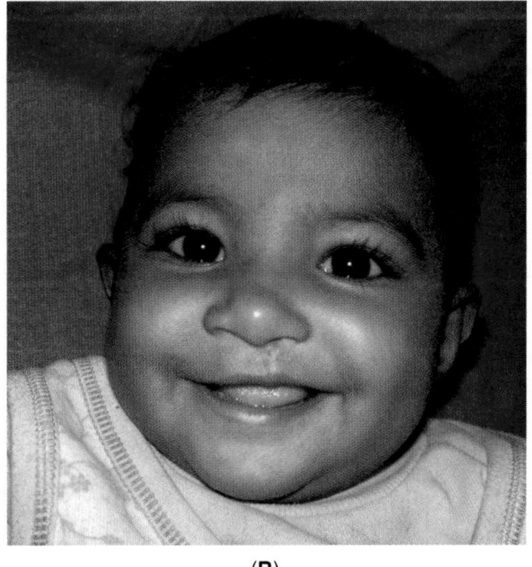

(B)

FIGURE 8.9 A child with a cleft palate before and after treatment. (A) Before treatment. (B) After treatment. (Photos courtesy of The Smile Train: www.smiletrain.org.)

- **Dental plaque** (**PLACK**), which is a major cause of dental caries and periodontal disease, forms as soft deposits in sheltered areas near the gums and between the teeth. Dental plaque consists of bacteria and bacterial by-products. In contrast, the *plaque* associated with heart conditions consists of deposits of cholesterol that form within blood vessels.
- **Gingivitis** (**jin**-jih-**VYE**-tis) is the earliest stage of periodontal disease, and the inflammation affects only the gums (**gingiv** means gums, and **-itis** means inflammation).
- **Halitosis** (hal-ih-**TOH**-sis), also known as *bad breath*, is an unpleasant odor coming from the mouth that can be caused by dental diseases or respiratory or gastric disorders (**halit** means breath, and **-osis** means abnormal condition or disease).
- **Periodontal disease**, also known as *periodontitis*, is an inflammation of the tissues that surround and support the teeth (**peri-** means surrounding, **odont** means tooth or teeth, and **-al** means pertaining to). This progressive disease is classified according to the degree of tissue involvement. In severe cases, the gums and bone surrounding the teeth are involved.
- A **temporomandibular disorder** (**tem**-poh-roh-man-**DIB**-you-lar) part of the group of complex symptoms that include pain, headache, or difficulty in chewing that are related to the functioning of the temporomandibular joint.

The Esophagus

- **Dysphagia** (dis-**FAY**-jee-ah) is difficulty in swallowing (**dys-** means difficult, and **-phagia** means swallowing).
- **Gastroesophageal reflux disease** (**gas**-troh-eh-**sof**-ah-**JEE**-al **REE**-flucks), also known as *GERD*, is the upward flow of acid from the stomach into the esophagus (**gastr/o** means stomach, **esophag** means esophagus, and **-eal** means pertaining to). *Reflux* means a backward or return flow. When this occurs, the stomach acid irritates and damages the delicate lining of the esophagus.
- **Pyrosis** (pye-**ROH**-sis), also known as *heartburn*, is the burning sensation caused by the return of acidic stomach contents into the esophagus (**pyr** means fever or fire, and **-osis** means abnormal condition or disease).
- **Esophageal varices** (eh-**sof**-ah-**JEE**-al **VAYR**-ih-seez) are enlarged and swollen veins at the lower end of the esophagus (singular, *varix*). Severe bleeding occurs if one of these veins ruptures.
- A **hiatal hernia** (high-**AY**-tal **HER**-nee-ah) is a condition in which a portion of the stomach protrudes upward into the chest, through an opening in the diaphragm (**hiat** means opening, and **-al** means pertaining to). A *hernia* is the protrusion of a part or structure through the tissues that normally contain it. This condition can cause esophageal reflux and pyrosis (Figure 8.10).

The Stomach

- **Gastritis** (gas-**TRY**-tis) is a common inflammation of the stomach lining that is often caused by the bacterium *Helicobacter pylori* (**gastr** means stomach, and **-itis** means inflammation).
- **Gastroenteritis** (**gas**-troh-en-ter-**EYE**-tis) is an inflammation of the mucous membrane lining the stomach and intestines (**gastr/o** means stomach, **enter** means small intestine, and **-itis** means inflammation).
- **Gastrorrhea** (**gas**-troh-**REE**-ah) is the excessive secretion of gastric juice or mucus in the stomach (**gastr/o** is stomach, and **-rrhea** means flow or discharge).

Peptic Ulcers

Peptic ulcers (**UL**-serz) are sores that affect the mucous membranes of the digestive system (**pept** means

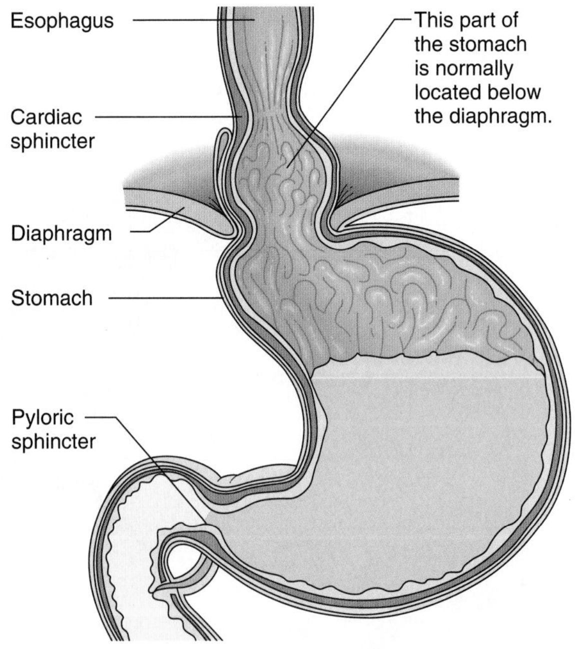

FIGURE 8.10 In a hiatal hernia, part of the stomach protrudes through the esophageal opening in the diaphragm.

digestion, and -ic means pertaining to). An *ulcer* is an erosion of the skin or mucous membrane. Peptic ulcers are caused by the bacterium *Helicobacter pylori* or by medications, such as aspirin, that irritate the mucous membranes (Figure 8.11).

- *Gastric ulcers* are peptic ulcers that occur in the stomach.
- *Duodenal ulcers* are peptic ulcers that occur in the upper part of the small intestine.
- A *perforating ulcer* is a complication of a peptic ulcer in which the ulcer erodes through the entire thickness of the organ wall.

Eating Disorders

- **Anorexia** (**an**-oh-**RECK**-see-ah) is the loss of appetite for food, especially when caused by disease.
- **Anorexia nervosa** (**an**-oh-**RECK**-see-ah ner-**VOH**-sah) is an eating disorder characterized by a false perception of body appearance. This leads to an intense fear of gaining weight and refusal to maintain a normal body weight. Voluntary starvation and excessive exercising often cause the patient to become emaciated. *Emaciated* means abnormally thin.
- **Bulimia nervosa** (byou-**LIM**-ee-ah ner-**VOH**-sah) is an eating disorder characterized by frequent episodes of binge eating followed by compensatory behaviors such as self-induced vomiting or the misuse of laxatives, diuretics, or other medications. The term *bulimia* means continuous, excessive hunger.

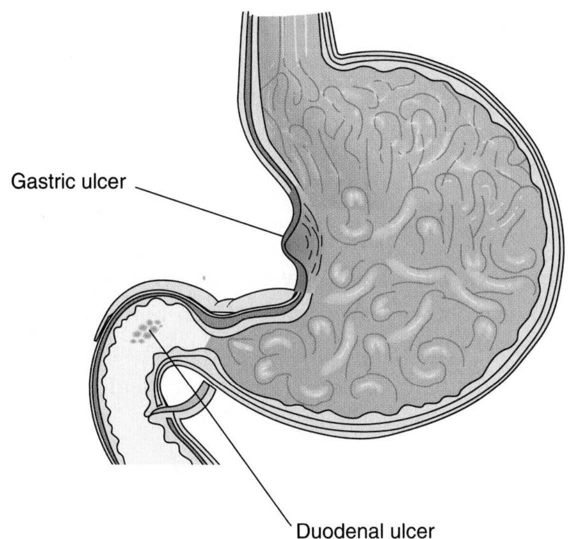

FIGURE 8.11 The locations of gastric and duodenal ulcers.

- **Cachexia** (kah-**KEKS**-eeh-ah) is a condition of physical wasting away due to the loss of weight and muscle mass that occurs in patients with diseases such as advanced cancer or AIDS. Although these patients are eating enough, the wasting happens because their bodies are unable to absorb the nutrients.
- **Pica** (**PYE**-kah) is an abnormal craving or appetite for nonfood substances, such as dirt, paint, or clay that lasts for at least 1 month. Pica is not the same as the short-lasting abnormal food cravings that are sometimes associated with pregnancy.

Nutritional Conditions

- **Dehydration** is a condition in which fluid loss exceeds fluid intake and disrupts the body's normal electrolyte balance.
- **Malnutrition** is a lack of proper food or nutrients in the body due to a shortage of food, poor eating habits, or the inability of the body to digest, absorb, and distribute these nutrients.
- **Malabsorption** (**mal**-ab-**SORP**-shun) is a condition in which the small intestine cannot absorb nutrients from food that passes through it.

Obesity

Obesity (oh-**BEE**-sih-tee) is an excessive accumulation of fat in the body. The term *obese* is usually used to refer to individuals who are more than 20%–30% over the established weight standards for their height, age, and gender. The term *gender* refers to the differences between men and women.

- **Morbid obesity** (**MOR**-bid oh-**BEE**-sih-tee) is the condition of weighing two to three times, or more, than the ideal weight or having a body mass index value greater than 39. As used here, the term *morbid* means a diseased state.
- The **body mass index** (BMI) is a number that shows body weight adjusted for height. The results fall into one of these categories: underweight, normal, overweight, or obese. A high BMI is one of many factors related to developing chronic diseases such as heart disease, cancer, or diabetes.
- Obesity is frequently present as a comorbidity with conditions such as hypertension (Chapter 5) and diabetes (Chapter 13). *Comorbidity* means the presence of more than one disease or health condition in an individual at a given time.

Indigestion and Vomiting

- **Aerophagia** (**ay**-er-oh-**FAY**-jee-ah) is the excessive swallowing of air while eating or drinking, and is a common cause of gas in the stomach (**aer/o** means air, and **-phagia** means swallowing).
- **Dyspepsia** (dis-**PEP**-see-ah), also known as *indigestion*, is pain or discomfort in digestion (**dys-** means painful, and **-pepsia** means digestion).
- **Emesis** (**EM**-eh-sis), also known as *vomiting*, is the reflex ejection of the stomach contents through the mouth. Note that emesis is used both as a stand alone term and as a suffix.
- **Eructation** (eh-ruk-**TAY**-shun) is the act of belching or raising gas orally from the stomach.
- **Hematemesis** (**hee**-mah-**TEM**-eh-sis) is the vomiting of blood (**hemat** means blood, and **-emesis** means vomiting).
- **Hyperemesis** (**high**-per-**EM**-eh-sis) is extreme, persistent vomiting that can cause dehydration (**hyper-** means excessive, and **-emesis** means vomiting). During the early stages of pregnancy, this is known as *morning sickness*.
- **Nausea** (**NAW**-see-ah) is the urge to vomit.
- **Regurgitation** (ree-**gur**-jih-**TAY**-shun) is the return of swallowed food into the mouth.

Intestinal Disorders

- **Colorectal carcinoma**, also known as colon cancer, often first manifests itself in polyps in the colon (see Figure 6.11).
- **Diverticulosis** (**dye**-ver-**tick**-you-**LOH**-sis) is the presence of a number of diverticula in the colon (**diverticul** means diverticulum, and **-osis** means abnormal condition or disease). A **diverticulum** (**dye**-ver-**TICK**-you-lum) is a small pouch or sac occurring in the lining or wall of a tubular organ such as the colon (plural, *diverticula*).
- **Diverticulitis** (**dye**-ver-tick-you-**LYE**-tis) is the inflammation of one or more diverticula in the colon (**diverticul** means diverticulum, and **-itis** means inflammation).
- **Enteritis** (**en**-ter-**EYE**-tis) is an inflammation of the small intestine caused by eating or drinking substances contaminated with viral and bacterial pathogens (**enter** means small intestine, and **-itis** means inflammation).

Ileus

Ileus (**ILL**-ee-us) is the partial or complete blockage of the small and/or large intestine. It is caused by the cessation (stopping) of intestinal peristalsis. Symptoms of ileus can include severe pain, cramping, abdominal distention, vomiting, and the failure to pass gas or stools.

Postoperative ileus is a temporary impairment of bowel motility that is considered to be a normal response to abdominal surgery. It is often present for 24–72 hours depending on what part of the digestive system was treated.

Irritable Bowel Syndrome

Irritable bowel syndrome (IBS), also known as *spastic colon*, is a common condition of unknown cause with symptoms that can include intermittent cramping, abdominal pain, bloating, constipation, and/or diarrhea. This condition, which is usually aggravated by stress, is *not* caused by pathogens (bacteria or viruses) or by structural changes.

Inflammatory Bowel Diseases

Inflammatory bowel disease (IBD) is the general name for diseases that cause inflammation in the intestines. The two most common inflammatory bowel diseases are ulcerative colitis and Crohn's disease.

- These conditions are grouped together because both are chronic, incurable, and can affect the large and small intestines. They also have similar symptoms, which include abdominal pain, weight loss, fatigue, fever, rectal bleeding, and diarrhea.
- These conditions tend to occur at intervals of active disease known as *flares* alternating with periods of remission. These disorders are treated with medication and surgery to remove diseased portions of the intestine.

Ulcerative colitis

Ulcerative colitis (**UL**-ser-**ay**-tiv koh-**LYE**-tis) is a chronic condition of unknown cause in which repeated episodes of inflammation in the rectum and large intestine cause ulcers and irritation (**col** means colon, and **-itis** means inflammation) (Figure 8.12).

- Ulcerative colitis usually starts in the rectum and progresses upward to the lower part of the colon; however, it can affect the entire large intestine.
- Ulcerative colitis affects only the innermost lining and not the deep tissues of the colon.

Crohn's disease

Crohn's disease (CD) is a chronic autoimmune disorder that can occur anywhere in the digestive tract; however, it is most often found in the ileum and in the colon.

- In contrast to ulcerative colitis, CD generally penetrates every layer of tissue in the affected area. This commonly results in scarring and thickening of the walls of the affected structures.
- The term *regional ileitis* is used to describe CD that affects the ileum. Ileitis is an inflammation of the ileum.
- The term *Crohn's colitis* is used to describe CD that affects the colon. Colitis is an inflammation of the colon. Note: This term is not the same as the condition ulcerative colitis.

Intestinal Obstructions

An **intestinal obstruction** is the partial or complete blockage of the small and/or large intestine caused by a physical obstruction. This blockage can result from many causes such as scar tissue or a tumor.

- *Intestinal adhesions* abnormally hold together parts of the intestine that normally should be separate. This condition, which is caused by inflammation or trauma, can lead to intestinal obstruction.
- In a *strangulating obstruction*, the blood flow to a segment of the intestine is cut off. This can lead to gangrene and perforation. *Gangrene* is tissue death that is usually associated with a loss of circulation. As used here, a *perforation* is a hole through the wall of a structure.
- **Volvulus** (**VOL**-view-lus) is the twisting of the intestine on itself that causes an obstruction (see Figure 8.13). Volvulus is a condition that usually occurs in infancy.
- **Intussusception** (**in**-tus-sus-**SEP**-shun) is the telescoping of one part of the small intestine into the opening of an immediately adjacent part. This is a rare condition sometimes found in infants and young children (see Figure 8.14).
- An **inguinal hernia** (**ING**-gwih-nal **HER**-nee-ah) is the protrusion of a small loop of bowel through a weak place in the lower abdominal wall or groin. This condition can be caused by obesity, pregnancy, heavy lifting, or straining to pass a stool.
- A **strangulated hernia** occurs when a portion of the intestine is constricted inside the hernia and its blood supply is cut off.

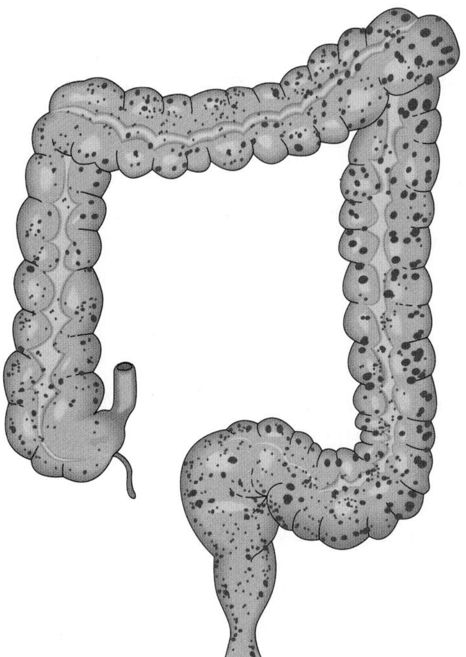

FIGURE 8.12 Ulcerative colitis causes ulcers and irritation in the rectum and large intestine.

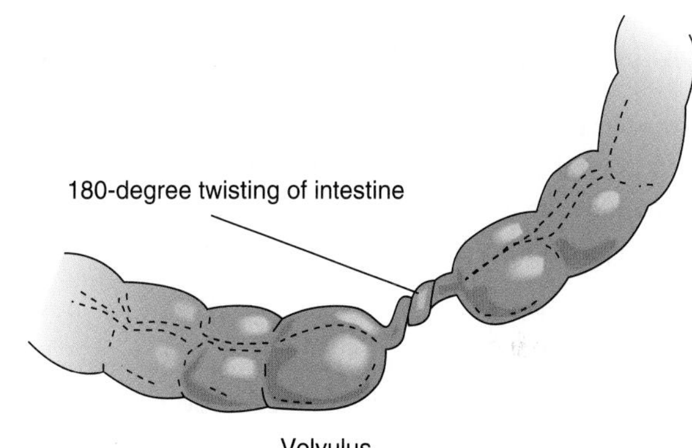

FIGURE 8.13 Volvulus is the twisting of the bowel on itself.

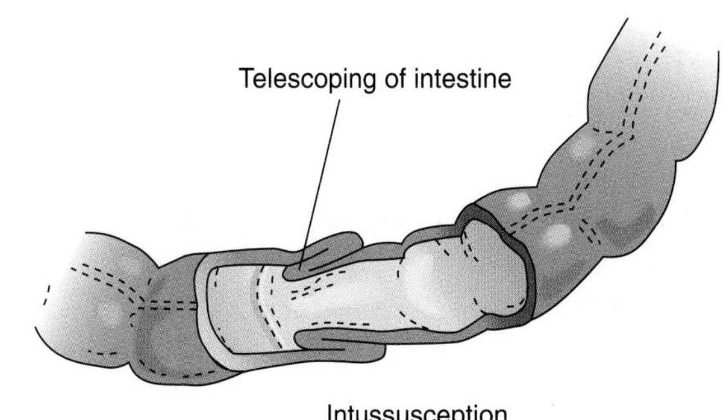

FIGURE 8.14 Intussusception is the telescoping of the bowel on itself.

Infectious Diseases of the Intestines

Infectious diseases of the intestines can be transmitted through contaminated food and water or through poor sanitation practices. The more common of these diseases are described in Table 8.1.

Anorectal Disorders

- An **anal fissure** is a small crack-like sore in the skin of the anus that can cause severe pain during a bowel movement. As used here, a *fissure* is a groove or crack-like sore of the skin.
- **Bowel incontinence** (in-**KON**-tih-nents) is the inability to control the excretion of feces. (Urinary incontinence is discussed in Chapter 9.)
- **Constipation** is defined as having a bowel movement fewer than three times per week. With constipation, stools are usually hard, dry, small in size, and difficult to eliminate.
- **Diarrhea** (**dye**-ah-**REE**-ah) is an abnormal frequent flow of loose or watery stools that can lead to dehydration (**dia-** means through, and **-rrhea** means flow or discharge).
- **Hemorrhoids** (**HEM**-oh-roids), also known as *piles*, occur when a cluster of veins, muscles, and tissues slip near or through the anal opening. The veins can become inflamed, resulting in pain, fecal leakage, and bleeding.
- **Melena** (meh-**LEE**-nah) is the passage of black, tarry, and foul-smelling stools (**melan** means black or dark, and **-a** is a noun ending). This appearance of the stools is caused by the presence of digested blood and often indicates an injury or disorder in the upper part of the gastrointestinal tract. In contrast, *bright red blood in the stool* usually indicates that the blood is coming from the lower part of the gastrointestinal tract.

TABLE 8.1

INFECTIOUS DISEASES OF THE INTESTINES

Disease and Mode of Transmission	Causative Agent and Symptoms
Amebic dysentery (ah-**MEE**-bik **DIS**-en-**ter**-ee), also known as *amebiasis*, is transmitted by food or water that is contaminated due to poor sanitary conditions.	*Caused by:* The one-celled parasite *Entamoeba histolytica.* *Symptoms:* In the mild form, symptoms include loose stools, stomach pain, and stomach cramping. In the severe form, there can be bloody stools and fever.
Botulism (**BOT**-you-lizm), also known as *food poisoning*, is a rare, but very serious, condition transmitted through contaminated food or an infected wound.	*Caused by:* The toxin produced by the bacterium *Clostridium botulinum.* This is among the most poisonous toxins known to man. *Symptoms:* Paralysis and sometimes death.
Cholera (**KOL**-er-ah) is transmitted through contact with contaminated food or water.	*Caused by:* The bacterium *Vibrio cholerae.* *Symptoms:* Starts with diarrhea and can progress to profuse diarrhea, vomiting, and rapid dehydration that can be fatal if not treated.
E. coli is transmitted through contaminated foods that have not been properly cooked.	*Caused by:* The bacterium *Escherichia coli.* *Symptoms:* Bloody diarrhea and abdominal cramping that can be severe, or fatal, in the very young and the elderly.
Salmonellosis (**sal**-moh-nel-**LOH**-sis), also referred to as *salmonella*, is transmitted by food that is contaminated by feces.	*Caused by:* The bacterium *Salmonella.* *Symptoms:* Severe diarrhea, vomiting, abdominal cramps, and high fever.
Typhoid fever, also known as *enteric fever*, is caused by eating food that has been handled by a typhoid-carrier. A *carrier* is someone who is infected with the bacteria but is not sick.	*Caused by:* The bacteria *Salmonella typhi.* *Symptoms:* Headache, delirium, cough, watery diarrhea, rash, and a high fever.

The Liver

Liver disorders are a major concern because the functioning of the liver is essential to the digestive process.

- **Hepatitis** (**hep**-ah-**TYE**-tis) is an inflammation of the liver (**hepat** means liver, and **-itis** means inflammation). The five viral varieties of hepatitis are shown in Table 8.2.
- **Hepatomegaly** (**hep**-ah-toh-**MEG**-ah-lee) is the abnormal enlargement of the liver (**hepat/o** means liver, and **-megaly** means enlargement).
- **Jaundice** (**JAWN**-dis) is a yellow discoloration of the skin, mucous membranes, and the eyes. This condition is caused by greater-than-normal amounts of bilirubin in the blood.

Cirrhosis

Cirrhosis (sih-**ROH**-sis) is a progressive degenerative disease of the liver that is often caused by excessive alcohol use or by viral hepatitis B or C (**cirrh** means yellow or orange, and **-osis** means abnormal condition or disease). *Degenerative* means progressive deterioration resulting in the loss of tissue or organ function.

The progress of cirrhosis is marked by the formation of areas of scarred liver tissue that are filled with fat. The liver damage causes abnormal conditions throughout the other body systems (Figure 8.15).

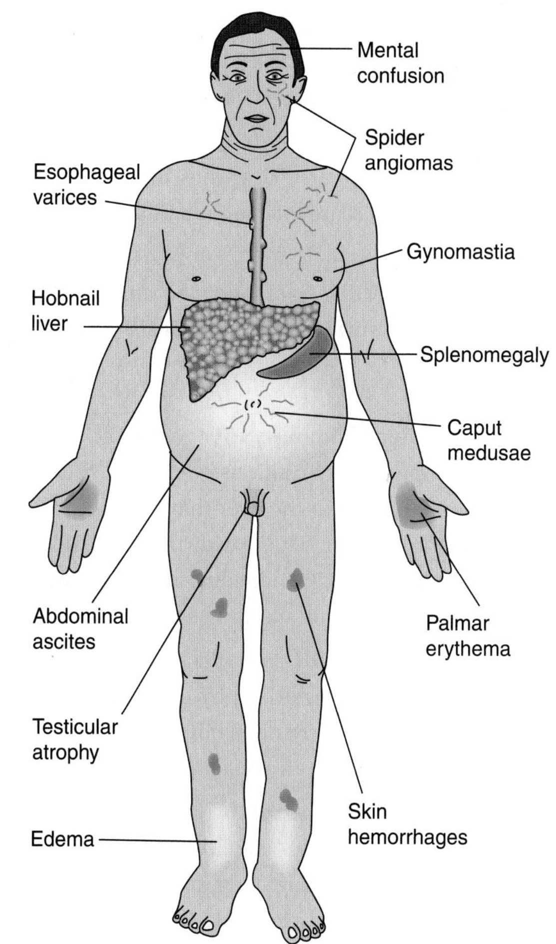

FIGURE 8.15 Clinical conditions associated with cirrhosis of the liver.

TABLE 8.2

HEPATITIS FROM A TO E

HAV	**Hepatitis A** which is caused by the HAV virus, is transmitted by contaminated food and water, and prevented by the hepatitis A vaccine.
HBV	**Hepatitis B virus** is a bloodborne disease that is transmitted through contact with blood and other body fluids that are contaminated with this virus. A vaccine is available to provide immunity against HBV.
HCV	**Hepatitis C virus** is a bloodborne disease that is spread through contact with blood and other body fluids that are contaminated with this virus. HVC is a described as a silent epidemic because it can be present in the body for years, and destroy the liver, before any symptoms appear. There is no vaccine available to prevent this form of hepatitis.
HDV	**Hepatitis D virus** is bloodborne disease that only occurs as a co-infection with B infection. Although there is no specific vaccine for HDV, hepatitis B vaccine should be given to prevent a HBV/HDV co-infection.
HEV	**Hepatitis E virus**, which is transmitted through contaminated food and water, is not common in the United States.

- **Ascites** (ah-**SIGH**-teez) is an abnormal accumulation of serous fluid in the peritoneal cavity. As used here, the term *serous* means a substance having a watery consistency.
- The term *caput medusae* describes the distended and engorged veins that are visible radiating from the umbilicus.
- The term *hobnail liver* describes the lumpy appearance of the liver surface due to cirrhosis.

Nonalcoholic Fatty Liver Disease

The term **nonalcoholic fatty liver disease** (NAFLD) describes a range of conditions characterized by an accumulation of fat within the liver that affect people who drink little or no alcohol. Those with this condition most commonly are middle-aged individuals who are obese and may also have diabetes and elevated cholesterol.

Steatosis (**stee**-ah-**TOH**-sis), which is the mildest type of this condition, is characterized by accumulations of fat within the liver that usually does not cause liver damage (**steat/o** means fat, and **-osis** means abnormal condition).

Nonalcoholic steatohepatitis (NASH), which is a more serious form of this condition, consists of fatty accumulations plus liver-damaging inflammation (**steat/o** means fat, **hepat** means liver, and **-itis** mean inflammation). In some cases, this will progress to cirrhosis, irreversible liver scarring, or liver cancer.

The Gallbladder

- **Cholangitis (koh-**lan-**JIGH**-tis) is an acute infection of the bile duct characterized by pain in the upper-right quadrant of the abdomen, fever, and jaundice (**choleang** means bile duct, and **-itis** means inflammation).
- **Cholecystalgia** (**koh**-lee-sis-**TAL**-jee-ah) is pain in the gallbladder (**cholecyst** means gallbladder, and **-algia** means pain).
- **Cholecystitis** (**koh**-lee-sis-**TYE**-tis) is inflammation of the gallbladder, usually associated with gallstones blocking the flow of bile (**cholecyst** means gallbladder, and **-itis** means inflammation).
- A **gallstone**, also known as *biliary calculus* or a *cholelith*, is a hard deposit formed in the gallbladder and bile ducts due to the concretion of bile components (plural, *calculi*). The formation of stones is discussed further in Chapter 9.
- **Cholelithiasis** (**koh**-lee-lih-**THIGH**-ah-sis) is the presence of gallstones in the gallbladder or bile ducts (**chole** means bile or gall, and **-lithiasis** means presence of stones).

The Pancreas

Disorders of the pancreas are discussed in Chapter 13.

DIAGNOSTIC PROCEDURES OF THE DIGESTIVE SYSTEM

- **Abdominal computed tomography** (CT) is a radiographic procedure that produces a detailed cross-section of the tissue structure within the abdomen, showing, for example, the presence of a tumor or obstruction. CT scans are discussed in Chapter 15.
- An **abdominal ultrasound** is a noninvasive test used to visualize internal organs by using very high frequency sound waves.
- An **anoscopy** (ah-**NOS**-koh-pee) is the visual examination of the anal canal and lower rectum (**an/o** means anus, and **-scopy** means visual examination). An *anoscope*, which is a short speculum, is used for this procedure. A *speculum* is an instrument used to enlarge the opening of any body cavity to facilitate inspection of its interior.
- A **capsule endoscopy** is a tiny video camera in a capsule that the patient swallows. For approximately 8 hours as it passes through the small intestine, this camera transmits images of the walls of the small intestine. The images are detected by sensor devices attached to the patient's abdomen and transmitted to a data recorder worn on the patient's belt.
- **Cholangiography** (koh-**LAN**-jee-**og**-rah-fee) is a radiographic examination of the bile ducts with the use of a contrast medium (**cholangi/o** means bile duct, and **-graphy** means the process of recording). This test is used to identify obstructions in the liver or bile ducts that slow or block the flow of bile from the liver. The resulting record is a *cholangiogram*.
- An **esophagogastroduodenoscopy** (eh-**sof**-ah-goh-**gas**-troh-**dew**-oh-deh-**NOS**-koh-pee) is an endoscopic procedure that allows direct visualization of the upper GI tract which includes the esophagus, stomach, and upper duodenum (**esophag/o** means esophagus, **gastr/o** means stomach, **duoden/o** means duodenum, and **-scopy** means visual examination).
- An **upper GI series** and a **lower GI series** are radiographic studies to examine the digestive system.

A contrast medium is required to make these structures visible. A *barium swallow* is used for the upper GI series, and a *barium enema* is used for the lower GI series.

- **Hemoccult test** (**HEE**-moh-kult), also known as the *fecal occult blood test*, is a laboratory test for hidden blood in the stools (**hem** means blood, and **-occult** means hidden). A test kit is used to obtain the specimens at home, and these are then evaluated in a laboratory or physician's office.
- **Stool samples** are specimens of feces that are examined for content and characteristics. For example, fatty stools might indicate the presence of pancreatic problems. Cultures of the stool sample can be examined in the laboratory for the presence of bacteria or *O & P*. This abbreviation stands for ova (parasite eggs) and parasites.

Endoscopic Procedures

An **endoscope** is an instrument used for visual examination of internal structures (**endo-** means within, and **-scope** means an instrument for visual examination). The following endoscopic examinations are used as preventive measure for the early detection of polyps that may be cancerous. *Polyps* are mushroom-like growths from the surface of mucous membrane. Not all polyps are malignant.

- **Colonoscopy** (**koh**-lun-**OSS**-koh-pee) is the direct visual examination of the inner surface of the entire colon from the rectum to the cecum (**colon/o** means colon, and **-scopy** means visual examination). A *virtual colonoscopy* uses x-rays and computers to produce two- and three-dimensional images of the colon.
- **Sigmoidoscopy** (**sig**-moi-**DOS**-koh-pee) is the endoscopic examination of the interior of the rectum, sigmoid colon, and possibly a portion of the descending colon (**sigmoid/o** means sigmoid colon, and **-scopy** is the visual examination).
- An **enema** is the placement of a solution into the rectum and colon to empty the lower intestine through bowel activity. An enema is part of the preparation for an endoscopic examination; however, enemas are also used to treat severe constipation.

TREATMENT PROCEDURES OF THE DIGESTIVE SYSTEM

Medications

- **Antacids**, which neutralize the acids in the stomach, are taken to relieve the discomfort of conditions such as pyrosis or to help peptic ulcers heal.
- **Acid reducers**, which decrease the amount of acid produced by the stomach, are used to treat the symptoms of conditions such as gastroesophageal reflux disease.
- An **antiemetic** (**an**-tih-ee-**MET**-ick) is a medication that is administered to prevent or relieve nausea and vomiting (**anti-** means against, **emet** means vomit, and **-ic** means pertaining to).
- **Laxatives** are medications, or foods, given to stimulate bowel movements. *Bulk-forming laxatives*, such as bran, treat constipation by helping fecal matter retain water and remain soft as it moves through the intestines.
- **Oral rehydration therapy** (ORT) is a treatment in which a solution of electrolytes is administered in a liquid preparation to counteract the dehydration that can accompany severe diarrhea, especially in young children.

The Oral Cavity and Esophagus

- A **dental prophylaxis** (**proh**-fih-**LACK**-sis) is the professional cleaning of the teeth to remove plaque and calculus. The term *prophylaxis* also refers to a treatment intended to prevent a disease or stop it from spreading. Examples include vaccination to provide immunity against a specific disease.
- A **gingivectomy** (**jin**-jih-**VECK**-toh-mee) is the surgical removal of diseased gingival tissue (**gingiv** means gingival tissue, and **-ectomy** means surgical removal).
- **Maxillofacial surgery** (mack-**sill**-oh-**FAY**-shul) is specialized surgery of the face and jaws to correct deformities, treat diseases, and repair injuries.
- **Palatoplasty** (**PAL**-ah-toh-**plas**-tee) is surgical repair of a cleft lip and/or palate (**palat/o** means palate, and **-plasty** means surgical repair) (see Figure 8.9).
- **Stomatoplasty** (**STOH**-mah-toh-**plas**-tee) is the surgical repair of the mouth (**stomat/o** means mouth or oral cavity, and **-plasty** means surgical repair).

The Stomach

- A **gastrectomy** (gas-**TRECK**-toh-mee) is the surgical removal of all or a part of the stomach (**gastr** means stomach, and **-ectomy** means surgical removal).
- **Nasogastric intubation** (**nay**-zoh-**GAS**-trick **in**-too-**BAY**-shun) is the placement of a feeding tube through the nose and into the stomach (**nas/o** means nose,

gastr means stomach, and -ic means pertaining to). This tube, which is placed temporarily, provides nutrition for patients who cannot take sufficient nutrients by mouth (see Figure 8.16).

- A **gastrostomy tube** (gas-**TROS**-toh-mee) is a surgically placed feeding tube from the exterior of the body into the stomach (gastr means stomach, and -ostomy means surgically creating an opening). This tube, which is placed permanently, provides nutrition for patients who cannot swallow or take sufficient nutrients by mouth (see Figure 8.16).
- **Total parenteral nutrition** (pah-**REN**-ter-al) is administered to patients who cannot, or should not, get their nutrition through eating. All of the patient's nutritional requirements are met through a nutritional liquid that is administered intravenously for 10–12 hours, once a day or five times a week. *Parenteral* means not in, or through, the digestive system.

Bariatric Surgery

Bariatric surgery is performed to treat morbid obesity by restricting the amount of food that can enter the stomach and be digested. These procedures limit food intake and force dietary changes that enable weight reduction.

- *Gastric bypass surgery* surgically makes the stomach smaller and causes food to bypass the first part of the small intestine. This procedure is not reversible.
- A *Gastric lap-band* procedure involves placing a band around the exterior of the stomach to restrict the amount of food that can enter the stomach. This procedure has the advantage of being reversible through the removal of the band.

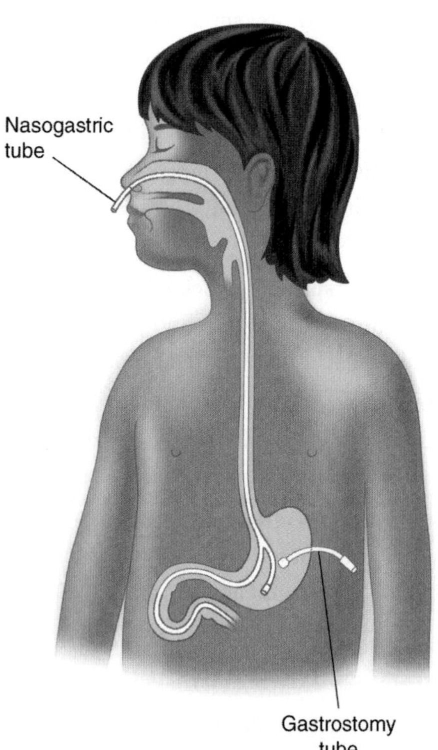

FIGURE 8.16 Nasogastric and gastrostomy tubes can be used to supply nutrition to a child who cannot eat by mouth.

The Intestines

- A **colectomy** (koh-**LECK**-toh-mee) is the surgical removal of all, or part of, the colon (col means colon, and -ectomy means surgical removal).
- A **diverticulectomy** (**dye**-ver-**tick**-you-**LECK**-toh-mee) is the surgical removal of a diverticulum (diverticul means diverticulum, and -ectomy means surgical removal).
- A **gastroduodenostomy** (**gas**-troh-**dew**-oh-deh-**NOS**-toh-mee) is the establishment of an anastomosis between the upper portion of the stomach, and the duodenum (gastr/o means stomach, duoden means first part of the small intestine, and -ostomy means surgically creating an opening). This procedure is performed to treat stomach cancer or to remove a malfunctioning pyloric valve (see Figure 8.17). An **anastomosis** (ah-**nas**-toh-**MOH**-sis) is a surgical connection between two hollow or tubular structures (plural, *anastomoses*).
- An **ileectomy** (**ill**-ee-**ECK**-toh-mee) is the surgical removal of the ileum (ile means the ileum, and -ectomy means surgical removal. Note: This term is spelled with a double *e*.)

Ostomies

An **ostomy** (**OSS**-toh-mee) is a surgical procedure to create an artificial opening between an organ and the body surface. This opening is called a *stoma*. Ostomy can be used alone as a noun to describe a procedure or as a suffix with the word part that describes the organ involved.

- An **ileostomy** (**ill**-ee-**OS**-toh-mee) is the surgical creation of an artificial excretory opening between the ileum, at the end of the small intestine, and the outside of the abdominal wall (ile means small intestine, and -ostomy means surgically creating an opening).

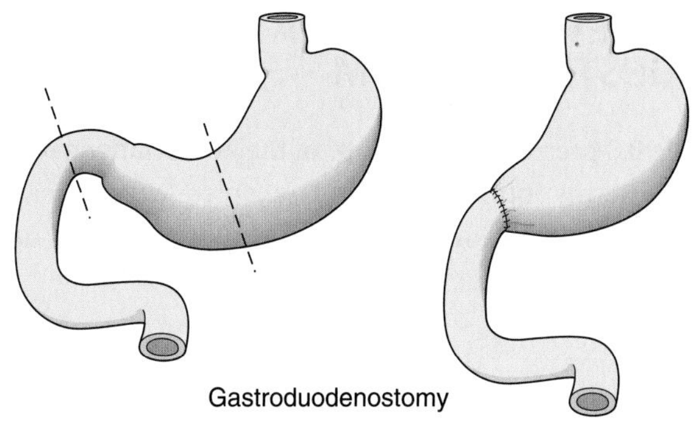

FIGURE 8.17 In a gastroduodenostomy, an anastomosis is formed where the stomach and duodenum are surgically joined.

- A **colostomy** (koh-**LAHS**-toh-mee) is the surgical creation of an artificial excretory opening between the colon and the body surface (col means colon, and -ostomy means surgically creating an opening). The segment of the intestine below the ostomy is usually removed, and the fecal matter flows through the stoma into a disposable bag. A colostomy can be temporary, to divert feces from an area that needs to heal (Figure 8.18).

The Rectum and Anus

- A **hemorrhoidectomy** (**hem**-oh-roid-**ECK**-toh-mee) is the surgical removal of hemorrhoids (hemorrhoid means piles, and -ectomy means surgical removal). *Rubber band ligation* is often used instead of surgery. Rubber bands cut off the circulation at the base of the hemorrhoid, causing it to eventually fall off. *Ligation* means the tying off of blood vessels or ducts.
- A **proctectomy** (prock-**TECK**-toh-mee) is the surgical removal of the rectum (proct means rectum, and -ectomy means surgical removal).
- **Proctopexy** (**PROCK**-toh-**peck**-see) is the surgical fixation of a prolapsed rectum to an adjacent tissue or organ (proct/o means rectum, and -pexy means surgical fixation). *Prolapse* means the falling or dropping down of an organ or internal part. This can be performed as a laparoscopic procedure in which a laparoscope and instruments are inserted into the abdomen through small incisions. A *laparoscope* is a specialized endoscope used for the examination and treatment of abdominal conditions.

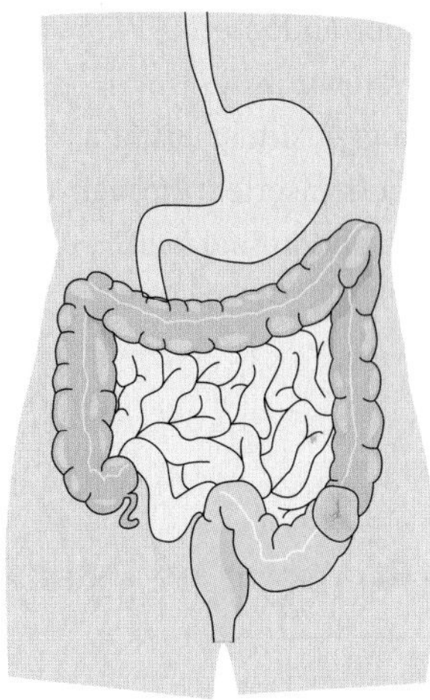

FIGURE 8.18 Colostomy sites are named for part of the bowel removed. Shown here is a sigmoid colostomy. The stoma is located at the end of the remaining intestine, which is shown in brown. The portion that has been removed is shown in blue.

- **Proctoplasty** (**PROCK**-toh-**plas**-tee) is the surgical repair of the rectum (proct/o means rectum, and -plasty means surgical repair).

The Liver

A **hepatectomy** (**hep**-ah-**TECK**-toh-mee) is the surgical removal of all or part of the liver (hepat means liver, and -ectomy means surgical removal).

Hepatorrhaphy (**hep**-ah-**TOR**-ah-fee) means surgical suturing of the liver (hepat/o means liver, and -rrhaphy means surgical suturing).

A **liver transplant** is an option for a patient whose liver has failed for a reason other than liver cancer. Because liver tissue regenerates, a *partial liver transplant*, in which only part of the organ is donated, can be adequate. A partial liver can be donated by a living donor whose blood and tissue types match.

The Gallbladder

- A **choledocholithotomy** (koh-**led**-oh-koh-lih-**THOT**-oh-mee) is an incision into the common bile duct for the removal of gallstones (choledoch/o means the common bile duct, lith means stone, and -otomy means surgical incision).
- A **cholecystectomy** (**koh**-lee-sis-**TECK**-toh-mee) is the surgical removal of the gallbladder. An *open cholecystectomy* is performed through an incision in the right

side of the upper abdomen. A *laparoscopic cholecystectomy*, also known as a *lap choley*, is the surgical removal of the gallbladder using a laparoscope and other instruments inserted through three or four small incisions in the abdominal wall.

ABBREVIATIONS RELATED TO THE DIGESTIVE SYSTEM

Table 8.3 presents an overview of the abbreviations related to the terms introduced in this chapter. Note: To avoid errors or confusion, always be cautious when using abbreviations.

TABLE 8.3

ABBREVIATIONS RELATED TO THE DIGESTIVE SYSTEM

bilirubin = BIL, Bil, bili	**BIL, Bil, bili** = bilirubin
cholecystectomy = CCE, chole	**CCE, chole** = cholecystectomy
cirrhosis = CIR, CIRR	**CIR, CIRR** = cirrhosis
colonoscopy = COL	**COL** = colonoscopy
colorectal carcinoma = CRC	**CRC** = colorectal carcinoma
esophagogastroduodenoscopy = EGD	**EGD** = esophagogastroduodenoscopy
esophageal varices = EV	**EV** = esophageal varices
gastroenteritis = GE	**GE** = gastroenteritis
ileocecal sphincter = ICS	**ICS** = ileocecal sphincter
inguinal hernia = IH	**IH** = inguinal hernia
intestinal obstruction = IO	**IO** = intestinal obstruction
jaundice = j, jaund	**j, jaund** = jaundice
morbid obesity = MO	**MO** = morbid obesity
peptic ulcers = PU	**PU** = peptic ulcers
temporomandibular disorders = TMD	**TMD** = temporomandibular disorders
total parenteral nutrition = TPN	**TPN** = total parenteral nutrition
ulcerative colitis = UC	**UC** = ulcerative colitis

CAREER OPPORTUNITIES

In addition to the medical specialties already discussed, some of the health occupations involving the treatment of the digestive system include:

- **Dental hygienist:** works under the supervision of a dentist, is licensed to remove stains and deposits from the teeth, exposes and develops x-rays, and assists the patient in learning about and maintaining good dental health
- **Dental assistant:** works under the supervision of a dentist, preparing patients for examinations, passing instruments during procedures, exposing and developing x-rays, sterilizing instruments, and/or performing receptionist and practice management duties
- **Dental laboratory technician:** following a written prescription from a dentist, fabricates and repairs dental appliances such as crowns, bridges, and orthodontic appliances
- **Registered Dietitian (RD):** licensed to assess patients' dietary needs, manage food service systems, and supervise and train personnel. Some specialties include:

    Pediatric dietitian

    Total parenteral nutrition (TPN) dietitian

    Renal (kidney) dietitian

    Diabetic patient care dietitian

    Weight management dietitian

- **Dietetic technician, registered (DTR):** works under the supervision of a dietitian to plan menus, prepare food, and provide basic dietary instruction
- **Dietetic assistant** or **food service worker:** assists in menu selection, food preparation and service, and cleanup
- **Sanitarian:** performs environmental health inspections, and encourages compliance with public standards for food safety, water purity, waste disposal, and air quality

HEALTH OCCUPATION PROFILE
CERTIFIED DENTAL ASSISTANT

Debbie Robinson is a certified dental assistant (CDA). *"The first time I thought about a career in dentistry was when I was 12 years old. I had such a great experience as a child going to the dentist. Everyone in the office was kind and helpful and made my visits a lot of fun. I searched out information on different professions in dentistry and found that becoming a dental assistant was a great track for me. I received my classroom and clinical training in a 1-year program in which I earned a certificate of completion. I took the National Board Exam and passed, so now my title is Certified Dental Assistant. Because of my great experiences as a child, I pursued a job in a pediatric dental office where I assist in treating children and individuals with special needs. Being a dental assistant provides me with the real satisfaction that I had hoped to find in my job."*

Study Break

An *eponym* is a term derived from someone's name. Many people believe that a common slang word associated with *defecation,* or the elimination of solid waste products, comes from the name of the inventor of the toilet, Thomas Crapper.

This is only partially true. There was indeed a Thomas Crapper, an English inventor and plumber of the nineteenth century who set about to improve the water closet (WC) already in common use at the time. Ironically, although he did hold nine patents of his own, he bought the patent for a device allowing a toilet to flush more effectively from its actual inventor, Albert Giblin. But the name of Crapper's company, T. Crapper—Chelsea, was emblazoned on new, improved toilets throughout England.

When American soldiers passed through England during World War I, they picked up the habit of using "crapper" as a slang term for the WC. Thomas Crapper thus achieved a dubious place in our language through an eponym that is frowned upon, but still in use, today.

Review Time

Write the answers to the following questions on a separate piece of paper or in your notebook. In addition, be prepared to take part in the classroom discussion.

1. ***Written Assignment:*** Using your own words, describe the differences between **anorexia nervosa** and **bulimia nervosa**.

   Discussion Assignment: Describe why both of these eating disorders are harmful to the patient's physical health.

2. ***Written Assignment:*** Using terms a patient would understand, describe how **hepatitis A** and **hepatitis B** are transmitted.

   Discussion Assignment: Health care workers are required to be immunized against hepatitis B. State why you think this immunization is so important.

3. ***Written Assignment:*** Using terms a physician would understand, describe the differences between an **ileostomy** and a **colostomy**.

   Discussion Assignment: Mr. Hernandez has a colostomy. Describe how fecal matter is removed from his body.

4. ***Written Assignment:*** Using terms the family would understand, describe the differences between a **cleft lip** and a **cleft palate**.

   Discussion Assignment: Think about how parents feel when their child is born with this type of defect. Describe their possible emotions, and state how a health care worker could help the family.

5. ***Written Assignment:*** Describe the differences between **gastroesophageal reflux disease** (GERD) and **esophageal varices**.

   Discussion Assignment: Do you think it is safe to ignore these conditions, or to self-medicate with heavily advertised over-the-counter products? (Be prepared to explain your view on this topic.)

continues

Optional Internet Activity

The goal of this activity is to help you learn more about medical terminology as it applies to the "real world." Select **one** *of these two options and follow the instructions.*

1. To learn more about foodborne diseases, search for the **Bad Bug Book** available on the U.S. Food and Drug Administration web site. Write a brief (one- or two-paragraph) report on something new you learned here and include the address of the web site where you found this information.
2. To learn more about the many types of **hepatitis**, go to the web site of the World Health Organization (WHO). Write a brief (one- or two-paragraph) report on something new you learned about any one type of hepatitis.

THE HUMAN TOUCH: CRITICAL THINKING ACTIVITY

The following story and questions are designed to stimulate critical thinking through class discussion or as a brief essay response. There are no right or wrong answers to these questions.

"Ugh, I hate waiting in that pizza line everyday! But it is totally worth it," ***Amber plopped down in the seat next to her friend Erin and took a big bite of her gooey pepperoni pizza, then a slurp from her soda.*** **"What do you have today? Oh gross, another whole-wheat turkey wrap. I don't know why you do that to yourself."** ***Erin looked down at the lunch that she had packed that morning: a turkey wrap, carrot sticks, four pretzels, and a non-fat strawberry yoghurt. She didn't understand how Amber could eat cafeteria pizza everyday and still look the way that she did, with her tiny waist and clear skin. The few times that Erin had given in and decided to buy pizza, she had felt bloated after lunch and her face had broken out.***

"I don't know how why you do that to yourself," ***Erin said as she pointed to Amber's pizza with a carrot stick.*** **"Don't you know it's not healthy to eat greasy food for lunch every day? You must have the world's fastest metabolism, though, because you still look so thin."** ***Erin tried to hide the hint of jealousy that she could detect in her own voice. If it was Amber's metabolism that was keeping her so thin, then Erin felt justified in being jealous. But she secretly suspected that Amber was keeping off the pounds in another way.***

"I'm just going to stop in the girls' lavatory on my way to class. See you there!" ***Amber bounced off before Erin had time to respond. She wanted to confront Amber about her suspicion, but wasn't sure how to bring it up without hurting her feelings. And what if she was wrong?***

continues

Suggested Discussion Topics

1. Discuss whether or not the school cafeteria should be serving foods such as pepperoni pizza and soda. Discuss the steps that the cafeteria staff might take to encourage students to select healthier choices for these meals.
2. What might Amber be doing to keep her weight down despite a diet heavy on pizza and soda? Include in your discussion the clue that is in the story. If you were in Erin's position, would you confront Amber? How could you do this in a way that would be helpful to Amber?
3. Discuss the potential damage Amber is doing to her body if she is vomiting to get rid of excess food.
4. What might happen to Amber if she stops the activities associated with bulimia but continues to consume excess calories?

STUDENT WORKBOOK AND StudyWARE™ CD-ROM

1. Go to your **Student Workbook** and complete the Learning Exercises for this chapter.

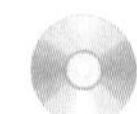

2. Go to the **StudyWARE™ CD-ROM** and have fun with the exercises and games for this chapter.

CHAPTER 9

THE URINARY SYSTEM

OVERVIEW OF STRUCTURES, COMBINING FORMS, AND FUNCTIONS OF THE URINARY SYSTEM

MAJOR STRUCTURES	RELATED COMBINING FORMS	PRIMARY FUNCTIONS
Kidneys	nephr/o, ren/o	Filter the blood to remove waste products, maintain electrolyte concentrations, and remove excess water to maintain the fluid volume within the body.
Renal Pelvis	pyel/o	Collects urine produced by the kidneys.
Urine	ur/o,urin/o	Liquid waste products to be excreted.
Ureters	ureter/o	Transport urine from the kidneys to the bladder.
Urinary Bladder	cyst/o	Stores urine until it is excreted.
Urethra	urethr/o	Transports urine from the bladder through the urethral meatus, where it is excreted.
Prostate	prostat/o	A gland of the male reproductive system that surrounds the male urethra. Disorders of this gland can disrupt the flow of urine.

VOCABULARY RELATED TO THE URINARY SYSTEM

This list contains essential word parts and medical terms for this chapter. These terms are pronounced on the student StudyWARE™ CD-ROM and Audio CDs that are available for use with this text. These and the other important **primary terms** are shown in boldface throughout the chapter. *Secondary terms*, which appear in *orange* italics, clarify the meaning of primary terms.

Word Parts

- ☐ -cele
- ☐ cyst/o
- ☐ dia-
- ☐ -ectasis
- ☐ glomerul/o
- ☐ lith/o
- ☐ -lysis
- ☐ nephr/o
- ☐ -pexy
- ☐ pyel/o
- ☐ -tripsy
- ☐ ur/o
- ☐ ureter/o
- ☐ urethr/o
- ☐ -uria

Medical Terms

- ☐ **ablation** (ab-**LAY**-shun)
- ☐ **anuria** (ah-**NEW**-ree-ah)
- ☐ **benign prostatic hypertrophy** (pros-**TAT**-ick high-**PER**-troh-fee)
- ☐ **catheterization** (**kath**-eh-ter-eye-**ZAY**-shun)
- ☐ **cystitis** (sis-**TYE**-tis)
- ☐ **cystocele** (**SIS**-toh-seel)
- ☐ **cystolith** (**SIS**-toh-lith)
- ☐ **cystopexy** (**sis**-toh-**peck**-see)
- ☐ **cystoscopy** (sis-**TOS**-koh-pee)
- ☐ **dialysis** (dye-**AL**-ih-sis)
- ☐ **diuresis** (**dye**-you-**REE**-sis)
- ☐ **enuresis** (**en**-you-**REE**-sis)
- ☐ **epispadias** (**ep**-ih-**SPAY**-dee-as)
- ☐ **extracorporeal shockwave lithotripsy** (**LITH**-oh-**trip**-see)
- ☐ **glomerulonephritis** (gloh-**mer**-you-loh-neh-**FRY**-tis)
- ☐ **hemodialysis** (**hee**-moh-dye-**AL**-ih-sis)
- ☐ **hydronephrosis** (**high**-droh-neh-**FROH**-sis)
- ☐ **hydroureter** (**high**-droh-you-**REE**-ter)
- ☐ **hyperproteinuria** (**high**-per-**proh**-tee-in-**YOU**-ree-ah)
- ☐ **hypoproteinemia** (**high**-poh-**proh**-tee-in-**EE**-mee-ah)
- ☐ **hypospadias** (**high**-poh-**SPAY**-dee-as)
- ☐ **incontinence** (in-**KON**-tih-nents)
- ☐ **interstitial cystitis** (**in**-ter-**STISH**-al sis-**TYE**-tis)
- ☐ **intravenous pyelogram** (**in**-trah-**VEE**-nus **PYE**-eh-loh-**gram**)
- ☐ **lithotomy** (lih-**THOT**-oh-mee)
- ☐ **nephrectasis** (neh-**FRECK**-tah-sis)
- ☐ **nephrolith** (**NEF**-roh-lith)
- ☐ **nephrolithiasis** (**nef**-roh-lih-**THIGH**-ah-sis)
- ☐ **nephrolysis** (neh-**FROL**-ih-sis)
- ☐ **nephropathy** (neh-**FROP**-ah-thee)
- ☐ **nephroptosis** (**nef**-rop-**TOH**-sis)
- ☐ **nephropyosis** (**nef**-roh-pye-**OH**-sis)
- ☐ **nephrostomy** (neh-**FROS**-toh-me)
- ☐ **nephrotic syndrome** (neh-**FROT**-ick)
- ☐ **neurogenic bladder** (new-roh-**JEN**-ick)
- ☐ **nocturia** (nock-**TOO**-ree-ah)
- ☐ **nocturnal enuresis** (**en**-you-**REE**-sis)
- ☐ **oliguria** (**ol**-ih-**GOO**-ree-ah)
- ☐ **percutaneous nephrolithotomy** (**per**-kyou-**TAY**-nee-us **nef**-roh-lih-**THOT**-oh-mee)
- ☐ **peritoneal dialysis** (**pehr**-ih-toh-**NEE**-al dye-**AL**-ih-sis)
- ☐ **polycystic kidney disease** (**pol**-ee-**SIS**-tick)
- ☐ **polyuria** (**pol**-ee-**YOU**-ree-ah)
- ☐ **prostate-specific antigen**
- ☐ **prostatism** (**PROS**-tah-tizm)
- ☐ **pyeloplasty** (**PYE**-eh-loh-**plas**-tee)
- ☐ **pyelotomy** (**pye**-eh-**LOT**-oh-mee)
- ☐ **suprapubic catheterization** (**soo**-prah-**PYOU**-bick **kath**-eh-ter-eye-**ZAY**-shun)
- ☐ **uremia** (you-**REE**-mee-ah)
- ☐ **ureterectasis** (you-**ree**-ter-**ECK**-tah-sis)
- ☐ **ureterolith** (you-**REE**-ter-oh-**lith**)
- ☐ **ureterorrhagia** (you-**ree**-ter-oh-**RAY**-jee-ah)
- ☐ **ureterorrhaphy** (**you**-ree-ter-**OR**-ah-fee)
- ☐ **urethritis** (**you**-reh-**THRIGH**-tis)
- ☐ **urethropexy** (you-**REE**-throh-**peck**-see)
- ☐ **urethrorrhagia** (you-**ree**-throh-**RAY**-jee-ah)
- ☐ **urethrostenosis** (you-**ree**-throh-steh-**NOH**-sis)
- ☐ **urethrostomy** (**you**-reh-**THROS**-toh-mee)
- ☐ **vesicovaginal fistula** (**ves**-ih-koh-**VAJ**-ih-nahl **FIS**-tyou-lah)
- ☐ **voiding cystourethrography** (**sis**-toh-you-ree-**THROG**-rah-fee)
- ☐ **Wilms tumor**

OBJECTIVES

On completion of this chapter, you should be able to:

1. Describe the major functions of the urinary system.
2. Name and describe the structures of the urinary system.
3. Recognize, define, spell, and pronounce terms related to the pathology and the diagnostic and treatment procedures of the urinary system.

FUNCTIONS OF THE URINARY SYSTEM

The urinary system performs many functions that are important in maintaining homeostasis. *Homeostasis* is the process through which the body maintains a constant internal environment (**home/o** means constant, and **-stasis** means control). These functions include:

- Maintaining the proper balance of water, salts, and acids in the body by filtering the blood as it flows through the kidneys.
- Constantly filtering the blood to remove urea and other waste materials from the bloodstream. **Urea** (you-**REE**-ah) is the major waste product of protein metabolism.
- Converting these waste products and excess fluids into **urine** in the kidneys and excreting them from the body via the urinary bladder.

STRUCTURES OF THE URINARY SYSTEM

The urinary system, also referred to as the **urinary tract**, consists of two kidneys, two ureters, one bladder, and a urethra (Figure 9.1). The adrenal glands, which are part of the endocrine system, are located on the top of the kidneys.

The Kidneys

The **kidneys** constantly filter the blood to remove waste products and excess water. These are excreted as urine, which is 95% water and 5% other wastes.

- The term **renal** (**REE**-nal) means pertaining to the kidneys (**ren** means kidney or kidneys, and **-al** means pertaining to).
- The two kidneys are located retroperitoneally with one on each side of the vertebral column below the diaphragm. *Retroperitoneal* means pertaining to being located behind the peritoneum. The *peritoneum* is the membrane that lines the abdominal cavity.
- The **renal cortex** (**REE**-nal **KOR**-tecks) is the outer region of the kidney. It contains over one million microscopic units called nephrons. The *cortex* is the outer portion of an organ.
- The **medulla** (meh-**DULL**-ah) is the inner region of the kidney; it contains most of the urine-collecting tubules. A *tubule* is a small tube.

Nephrons

A **nephron** (**NEF**-ron) is a functional unit of the kidney. These units form urine by the processes of filtration, reabsorption, and secretion (Figure 9.2). *Reabsorption* is the return to the blood of some of the substances that were removed during filtration.

- Each nephron contains a **glomerulus** (gloh-**MER**-you-lus), which is a cluster of capillaries surrounded by a cup-shaped membrane called the Bowman's capsule (plural, *glomeruli*).
- Blood enters the kidney through the renal artery and flows into the nephrons. After being filtered in the capillaries of the glomerulus, the blood leaves the kidney through the renal vein.
- Waste products that were filtered out of the blood remain behind in the kidney where they pass through a series of urine-collecting tubules. When this process has been completed, the urine is transported to the renal pelvis where it is collected in preparation for entry into the ureters.
- **Urochrome** (**YOU**-roh-krome) is the pigment that gives urine its normal yellow-amber or straw color (**ur/o** means urine, and **-chrome** means color). The color of urine can be influenced by normal factors such as the amount of liquid consumed, and can also be changed by diseases and medications.

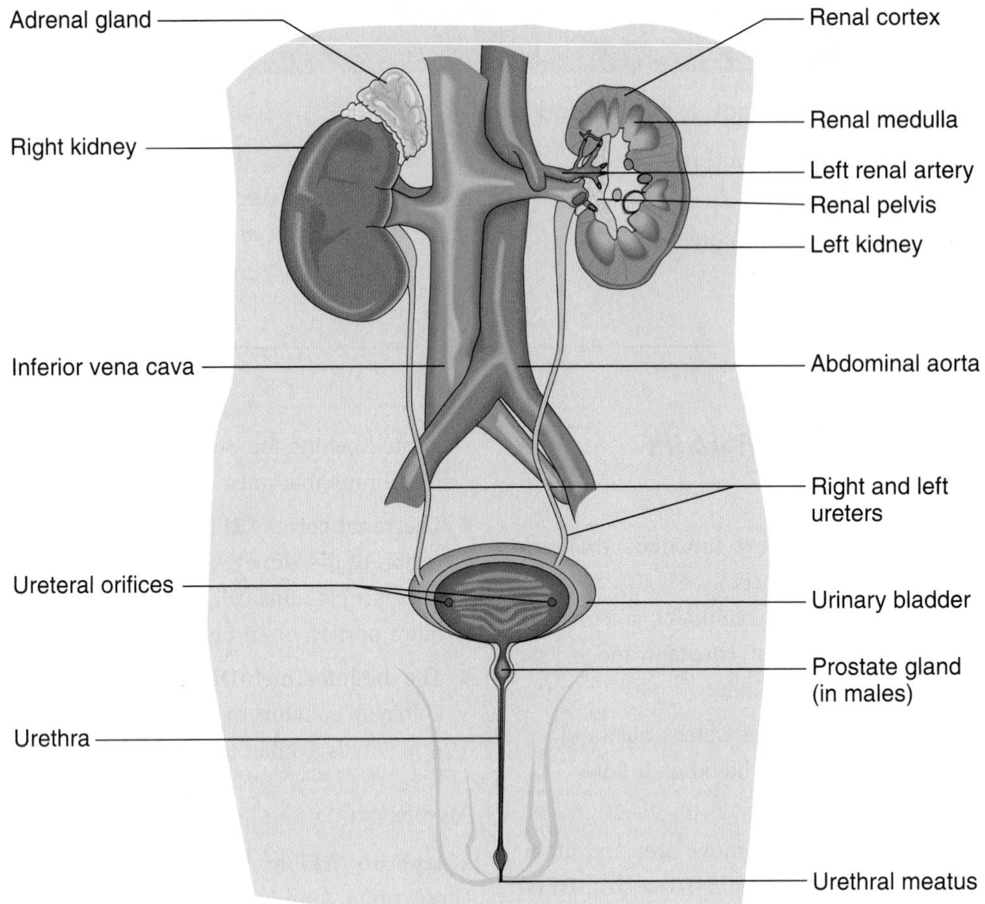

FIGURE 9.1 The primary structures of the urinary system as shown here in a male are the kidneys, ureters, urinary bladder, and urethra. The adrenal gland, positioned on top of each kidney, is a structure of the endocrine system. The prostrate gland, which is part of the male reproductive system, surrounds the urethra.

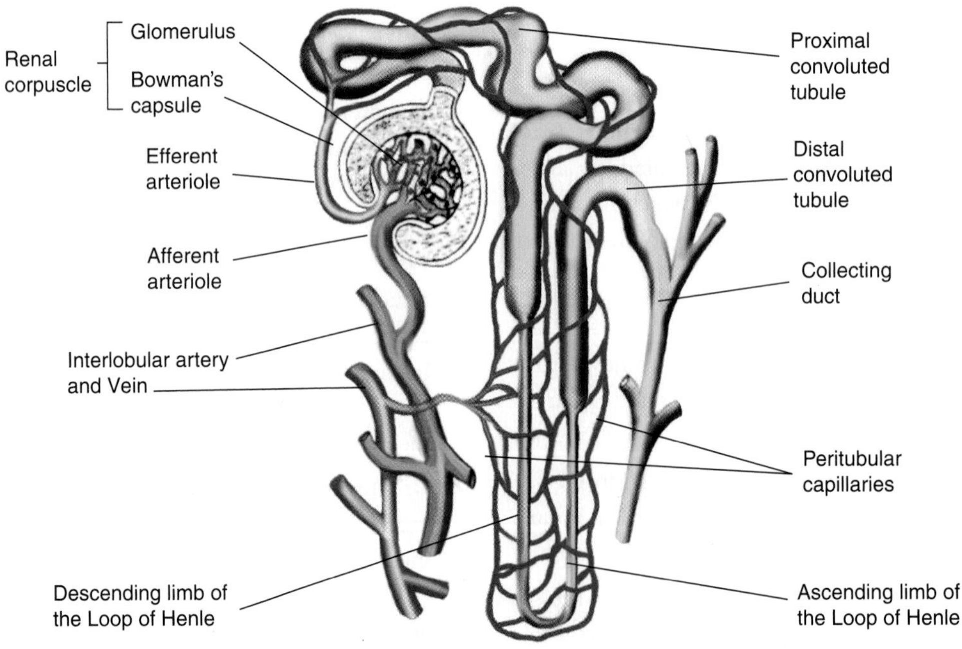

FIGURE 9.2 A nephron unit and its associated structures.

The Renal Pelvis

The **renal pelvis** is the funnel-shaped area within each kidney that is surrounded by renal cortex and medulla. This is where the newly formed urine collects before it flows into the ureters.

The Ureters

The **ureters** (you-**REE**-ters) are two narrow tubes, each about 10–12 inches long, which transport urine from the kidney to the bladder. *Peristalsis*, which is a series of wave-like contractions, moves urine down each ureter to the bladder. Urine drains from the ureters into the bladder through the *ureteral orifices* in the wall of the urinary bladder (see Figure 9.1).

The Urinary Bladder

The **urinary bladder** is a hollow muscular organ that is a reservoir for urine before it is excreted from the body (Figure 9.3).

- The bladder is located in the anterior portion of the pelvic cavity behind the pubic symphysis. The bladder stores about one pint of urine.
- Like the stomach, the bladder is lined with rugae, which are folds that allow it to expand and contract.

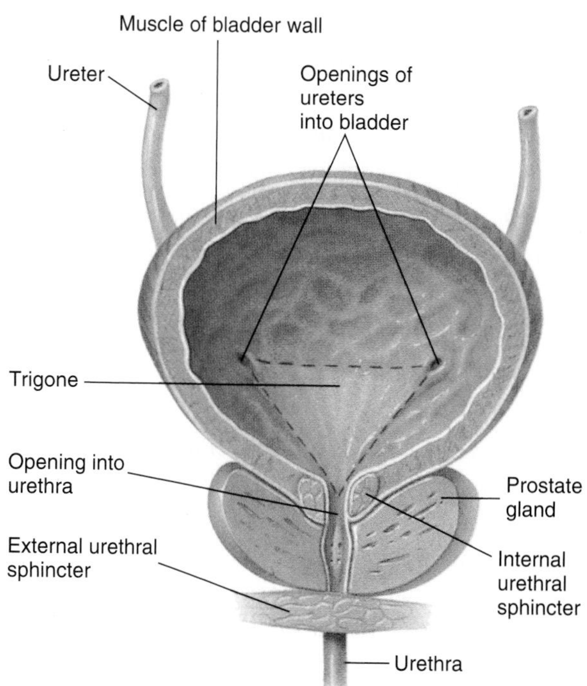

FIGURE 9.3 The structures of the urinary bladder in the male.

- The **trigone** (**TRY**-gon) is the smooth triangular area on the inner surface of the bladder located between the openings of the ureters and urethra (see Figure 9.3).

The Urethra

The **urethra** (you-**REE**-thrah) is the tube extending from the bladder to the outside of the body. Caution: The spellings of *ureter* and *urethra* are very similar!

- Two *urinary sphincters*, one located at either end of the urethra, control the flow of urine from the bladder into the urethra and out of the urethra through the urethral meatus. A *sphincter* is a ring-like muscle that closes a passageway (see Figure 9.3).
- The **urethral meatus** (you-**REE**-thrahl mee-**AY**-tus), also known as the *urinary meatus*, is the external opening of the urethra. *Meatus* means the external opening of a canal.
- The **female urethra** is approximately 1.5 inches long, and the urethral meatus is located between the clitoris and the opening of the vagina (see Chapter 14). In the female, the urethra conveys only urine.
- The **male urethra** is approximately 8 inches long, and the urethral meatus is located at the tip of the penis (see Figure 9.1). This urethra transports both urine and semen.
- The **prostate gland** (**PROS**-tayt), which is part of the male reproductive system, surrounds the urethra (see Figure 9.3). Most disorders of the prostate affect the male's ability to urinate.

THE EXCRETION OF URINE

Urination, also known as *voiding* or *micturition*, is the normal process of excreting urine.

- As the bladder fills up with urine, pressure is placed on the base of the urethra, resulting in the urge to **urinate** or *micturate*.
- Urination requires the coordinated contraction of the bladder muscles and relaxation of the sphincters. This action forces the urine through the urethra and out through the urinary meatus.

MEDICAL SPECIALTIES RELATED TO THE URINARY SYSTEM

- A **nephrologist** (neh-**FROL**-oh-jist) is a physician who specializes in diagnosing and treating diseases and disorders of the kidneys (**nephr** means kidney, and **-ologist** means specialist).

- A **urologist** (you-**ROL**-oh-jist) is a physician who specializes in diagnosing and treating diseases and disorders of the urinary system of females and the genitourinary system of males (**ur** means urine, and **-ologist** means specialist). The term *genitourinary* refers to both the genital and urinary organs.

PATHOLOGY OF THE URINARY SYSTEM

Renal Failure

Renal failure, also known as *kidney failure*, is the inability of one or both of the kidneys to perform their functions. The body cannot replace damaged nephrons, and when too many nephrons have been destroyed, the result is kidney failure.

- **Uremia** (you-**REE**-mee-ah), also known as *uremic poisoning*, is a toxic condition resulting from renal failure in which kidney function is compromised and urea is retained in the blood (**ur** means urine, and **-emia** means blood condition).
- **Acute renal failure** (ARF) has sudden onset and is characterized by uremia. It can be fatal if not reversed promptly. This condition can be caused by many factors, including a sudden drop in blood volume or blood pressure due to injury or surgery.
- **Chronic renal failure** is the progressive loss of renal function, sometimes leading to uremia, which is caused by a variety of conditions such as kidney disease, diabetes mellitus, or hypertension.
- **End-stage renal disease** (ESRD) refers to the late stages of chronic renal failure in which there is irreversible loss of the function of both kidneys. Without dialysis or a kidney transplant, this condition is fatal.
- **Hemolytic uremic syndrome** (**hee**-moh-**LIT**-ick you-**REE**-mick) is a condition in which *hemolytic anemia* and *thrombocytopenia* cause acute renal failure and possibly death. This syndrome can be the result of an *Escherichia coli* (*E. coli*) infection in young children and the elderly. (These blood disorders are discussed in Chapter 5, and *Escherichia coli* is discussed in Chapter 8.)

Nephrotic Syndrome

Nephrotic syndrome (neh-**FROT**-ick) is a condition in which very high levels of protein are lost in the urine and abnormally low levels of protein are present in the blood (**nephr/o** means kidney, and **-tic** means pertaining to). This is the result of damage to the kidney's glomeruli.

Nephrosis (neh-**FROH**-sis) is any degenerative kidney disease causing nephrotic syndrome *without* inflammation (**nephr** means kidney, and **-osis** means abnormal condition or disease). The following are characteristics of diseases that are caused by the malfunctioning of the kidneys.

- **Anuria** (ah-**NEW**-ree-ah) is the absence of urine formation by the kidneys (**an-** means without, and **-uria** means urine).
- **Edema** (eh-**DEE**-mah) is excessive fluid in the body tissues.
- **Hyperproteinuria** (**high**-per-**proh**-tee-in-**YOU**-ree-ah) is the presence of abnormally high concentrations of protein in the *urine* (**hyper-** means excessive, **protein** means protein, and **-uria** means urine). This condition is often associated with *hypoproteinemia*.
- **Hypoproteinemia** (**high**-poh-**proh**-tee-in-**EE**-mee-ah) is the presence of abnormally low concentrations of protein in the *blood* (**hypo-** means deficient or decreased, **protein** means protein, and **-emia** means blood condition). This condition is often associated with *hyperproteinuria*.
- Hypertension and high cholesterol, which are discussed in Chapter 5, are also part of the nephrotic syndrome.

Nephropathy

The term **nephropathy** (neh-**FROP**-ah-thee) means any disease of the kidney (**nephr** means kidney, and **-pathy** means disease). This definition includes both degenerative and inflammatory conditions.

- *Diabetic nephropathy* is a kidney disease characterized by hyperproteinuria, which is the result of thickening and hardening of the glomeruli caused by long-term diabetes mellitus.

The Kidneys

- **Hydronephrosis** (**high**-droh-neh-**FROH**-sis) is the dilation (swelling) of one or both kidneys (**hydr/o** means water, **nephr** means kidney, and **-osis** means abnormal condition or disease). This condition can be caused by problems associated with the backing up of urine due to an obstruction such as a stricture in the ureter or blockage in the opening from the bladder to the urethra, or in the urethra itself (Figure 9.4). A *stricture* is an abnormal band of tissue that narrows or completely blocks a body passage.

- **Nephrectasis** (neh-**FRECK**-tah-sis) is the distention of the pelvis of the kidney (**nephr** means kidney, and **-ectasis** means enlargement or stretching). *Distention* means enlarged or stretched.

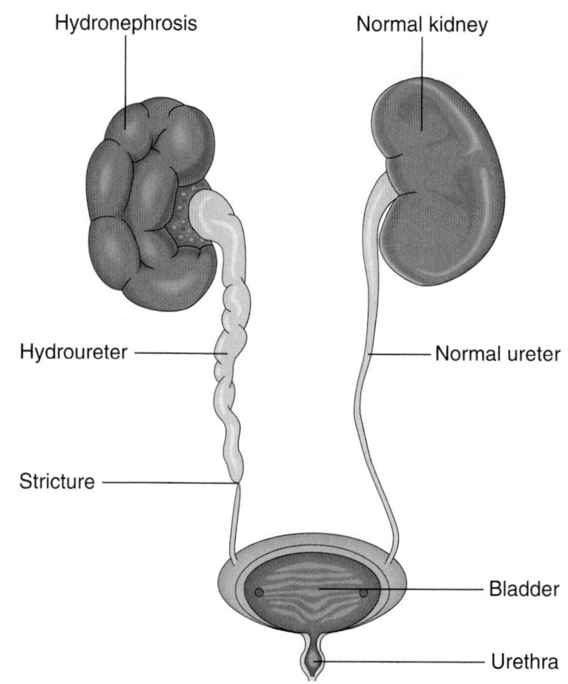

FIGURE 9.4 A stricture of the ureter can cause both hydronephrosis and hydroureter.

- **Nephritis** (neh-**FRY**-tis) is an inflammation of the kidney or kidneys (**nephr** means kidney, and **-itis** means inflammation). The two most common causes of nephritis are infection or an autoimmune disease.
- **Glomerulonephritis** (gloh-**mer**-you-loh-neh-**FRY**-tis), also known as *Bright's disease*, is a type of kidney disease caused by inflammation of the glomeruli that causes red blood cells and proteins to leak into the urine (**glomerul/o** means glomeruli, **nephr** means kidney, and **-itis** means inflammation).
- **Nephroptosis** (**nef**-rop-**TOH**-sis), also known as a *floating kidney*, is the prolapse of a kidney (**nephr/o** means kidney, and **-ptosis** means droop or prolapse). *Prolapse* means slipping or falling out of place.
- **Nephropyosis** (**nef**-roh-pye-**OH**-sis), also known as *pyonephrosis*, is suppuration of the kidney (**nephr/o** means kidney, **py** means pus, and **-osis** means abnormal condition or disease). *Suppuration* means the formation or discharge of pus.
- **Polycystic kidney disease** (**pol**-ee-**SIS**-tick) is a genetic disorder characterized by the growth of numerous fluid-filled cysts in the kidneys (**poly-** means many, **cyst** means cyst, and **-ic** means pertaining to). These cysts, which slowly replace much of the mass of the kidney, reduce the kidney function, and this eventually leads to kidney failure (Figure 9.5).

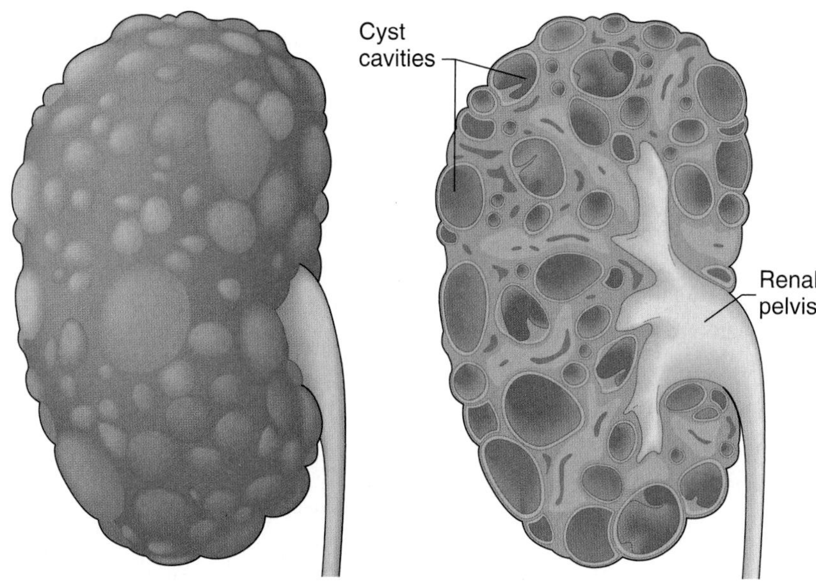

FIGURE 9.5 Polycystic kidney disease: On the left is the exterior of a kidney with polycystic disease. On the right is a cross-section through a kidney with polycystic disease.

- **Renal colic** (**REE**-nal **KOLL**-ick) is an acute pain in the kidney area that is caused by blockage during the passage of a kidney stone. *Colic* means spasmodic pains in the abdomen.
- A **Wilms tumor** is a malignant tumor of the kidney that occurs in young children. There is a high cure rate for this condition when this condition is treated promptly.

Stones

A **stone**, also known as *calculus*, is an abnormal mineral deposit that has formed within the body (plural, *calculi*). These stones vary in size from small sand-like granules to the size of marbles and are named for the organ or tissue where they are located. In the urinary system, stones are formed when waste products in the urine crystallize.

The term **nephrolithiasis** (**nef**-roh-lih-**THIGH**-ah-sis) describes the presence of stones in the kidney (**nephr/o** means kidney, and **-lithiasis** means the presence of stones). As these stones travel with the urine, they are named for the location where they become lodged (Figure 9.6).

- A **nephrolith** (**NEF**-roh-lith), also known as *renal calculus* or a *kidney stone*, is found in the kidney (**nephr/o** means kidney, and **-lith** means stone).
- A **ureterolith** (you-**REE**-ter-oh-**lith**) is a stone located anywhere along the ureter (**ureter/o** means ureter, and **-lith** means stone).
- A **cystolith** (**SIS**-toh-lith) is a stone located within the urinary bladder (**cyst/o** means bladder, and **-lith** means stone).

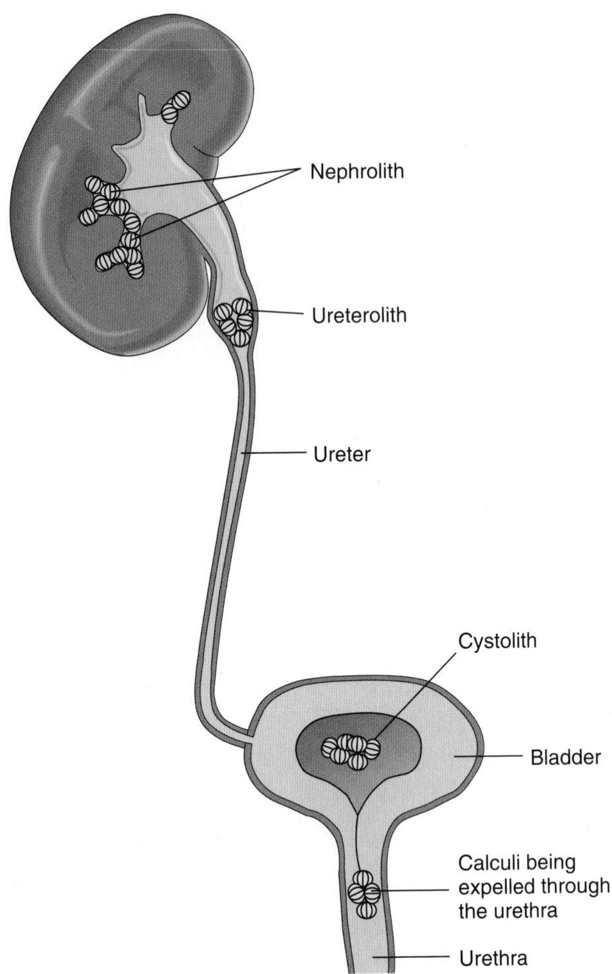

FIGURE 9.6 Potential locations of renal calculi (stones) as they move through the urinary system.

The Ureters

- **Hydroureter** (**high**-droh-you-**REE**-ter) is the distention of the ureter with urine that cannot flow because the ureter is blocked (**hydr/o** means water, and **-ureter** means ureter) (see Figure 9.4).
- **Ureterectasis** (you-**ree**-ter-**ECK**-tah-sis) is the distention of a ureter (**ureter** means ureter, and **-ectasis** means enlargement).
- **Ureterorrhagia** (you-**ree**-ter-oh-**RAY**-jee-ah) is the discharge of blood from the ureter (**ureter/o** means ureter, and **-rrhagia** means bleeding).

Urinary Tract Infections

A **urinary tract infection** (UTI) usually begins in the bladder; however, these infections can affect all, or parts, of the urinary system (Figure 9.7A). These infections occur more frequently in women because of the urethra is short and located near the openings to the vagina and rectum.

- **Urethritis** (**you**-reh-**THRIGH**-tis) is an inflammation of the urethra (**urethr** means urethra, and **-itis** means inflammation) (see Figure 9.7B).
- **Cystitis** (sis-**TYE**-tis) is an inflammation of the bladder (**cyst** mean bladder, and **-itis** means inflammation) (see Figure 9.7C).
- **Pyelitis** (**pye**-eh-**LYE**-tis) is an inflammation of the renal pelvis (**pyel** means renal pelvis, and **-itis** means inflammation) (see Figure 9.7D).
- **Pyelonephritis** (**pye**-eh-loh-neh-**FRY**-tis) is an inflammation of both the renal pelvis and of the kidney (**pyel/o** means renal pelvis, **nephr** means kidney, and **-itis** means inflammation). This is usually caused by a bacterial infection that has spread upward from the bladder (see Figure 9.7E).

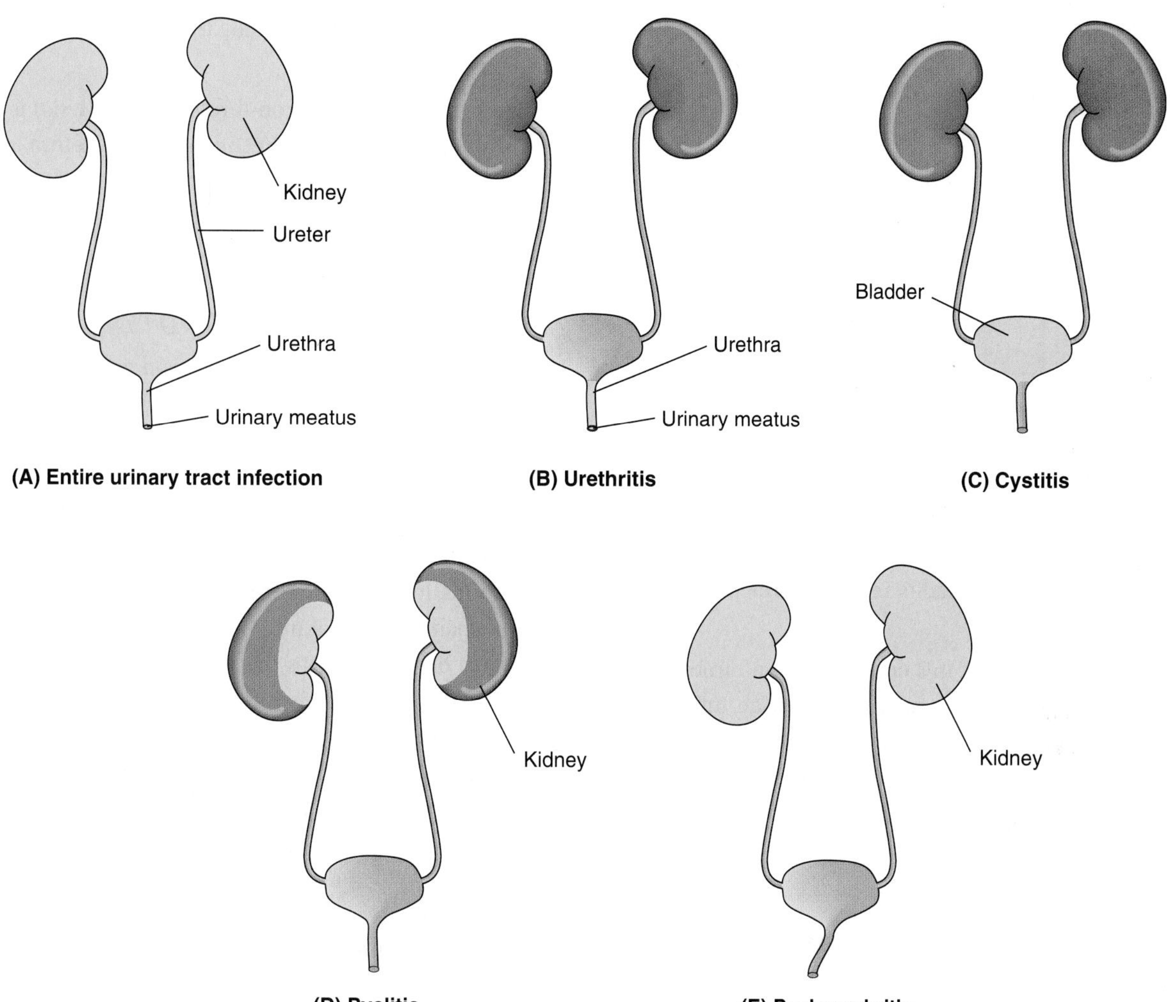

FIGURE 9.7 Infections of the urinary tract: (A) Entire urinary tract infection; (B) Urethritis; (C) Cystitis; (D) Pyelitis; and (E) Pyelonephritis.

The Urinary Bladder

- **Cystalgia** (sis-**TAL**-jee-ah) and *cystodynia* both mean pain in the urinary bladder (**cyst** means bladder, and **-algia** means pain).
- A **cystocele** (**SIS**-toh-seel), also known as a *fallen bladder*, is a hernia of the bladder through the vaginal wall (**cyst/o** means bladder, and **-cele** means hernia).
- **Interstitial cystitis** (**in**-ter-**STISH**-al sis-**TYE**-tis) is a chronic inflammation within the walls of the bladder. The symptoms of this condition are similar to those of cystitis; however, they do not respond to traditional treatment. *Interstitial* means relating to spaces within a tissue or organ.
- **Trigonitis** (**tryg**-oh-**NYE**-tis) is an inflammation of the urinary bladder that is localized in the region of the trigone (**trigon** means trigone, and **-itis** means inflammation).
- A **vesicovaginal fistula** (**ves**-ih-koh-**VAJ**-ih-nahl **FIS**-tyou-lah) is an abnormal opening between the bladder and vagina that allows the constant flow of urine from the bladder into the vagina (**vesic/o** means bladder, **vagin** means vagina, and **-al** means pertaining to). A *fistula* is an abnormal passage between two internal organs (Figure 9.8).

Neurogenic Bladder

Neurogenic bladder (new-roh-**JEN**-ick) is a urinary problem caused by interference with the normal nerve pathways associated with urination (**neur/o** means nervous system, and **-genic** means created by).

- Depending on the type of neurological disorder causing the problem, the bladder may empty spontaneously, resulting in incontinence. As used here, *incontinence* means the inability to control the voiding of urine. In contrast, the problem can prevent the bladder from

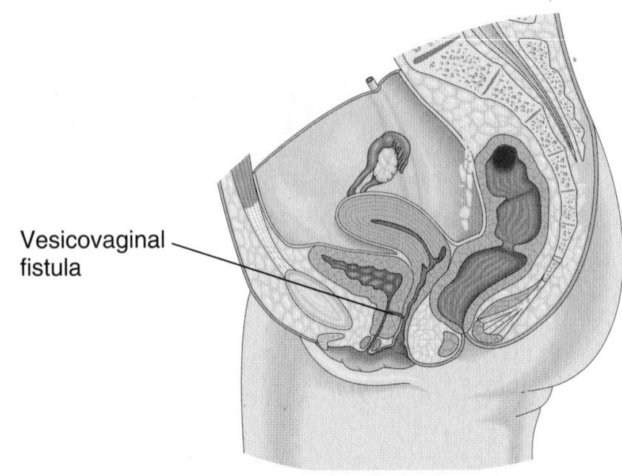

FIGURE 9.8 A vesicovaginal fistula allows urine to flow into the vagina.

emptying at all. This results in urinary retention with overflow leakage.

- Some of the causes of this condition are a tumor of the nervous system, trauma, neuropathy, or an inflammatory condition such as multiple sclerosis. *Neuropathy* is a peripheral nervous system disorder affecting nerves anywhere except the brain or the spinal cord.

The Urethra

- **Urethrorrhagia** (you-**ree**-throh-**RAY**-jee-ah) is bleeding from the urethra (**urethr/o** means urethra, and **-rrhagia** means bleeding).
- **Urethrorrhea** (you-**ree**-throh-**REE**-ah) is an abnormal discharge from the urethra (**urethr/o** means urethra, and **-rrhea** means flow or discharge). This condition is associated with some sexually transmitted diseases (see Chapter 14).
- **Urethrostenosis** (you-**ree**-throh-steh-**NOH**-sis) is narrowing of the urethra (**urethr/o** means urethra, and **-stenosis** means tightening or narrowing). This condition occurs almost exclusively in men and is often associated with prostate enlargement.

Abnormal Urethral Openings

- **Epispadias** (**ep**-ih-**SPAY**-dee-as) is a congenital abnormality of the urethral opening. In the male with epispadias, the urethral opening is located on the upper surface of the penis. In the female with epispadias, the urethral opening is in the region of the clitoris.
- **Hypospadias** (**high**-poh-**SPAY**-dee-as) is a congenital abnormality of the urethral opening. In the male with hypospadias, the urethral opening is on the under surface of the penis. In the female with hypospadias, the urethral opening is into the vagina.
- **Paraspadias** (**par**-ah-**SPAY**-dee-as) is a congenital abnormality in males in which the urethral opening is on the side of the penis.

The Prostate Gland

- **Benign prostatic hypertrophy** (pros-**TAT**-ick high-**PER**-troh-fee), also known as an *benign prostatic hyperplasia*, *enlarged prostate*, or *prostatomegaly*, is an abnormal enlargement of the prostate gland that occurs most often in men over age 50 (see Figure 9.9). This condition can make urination difficult.

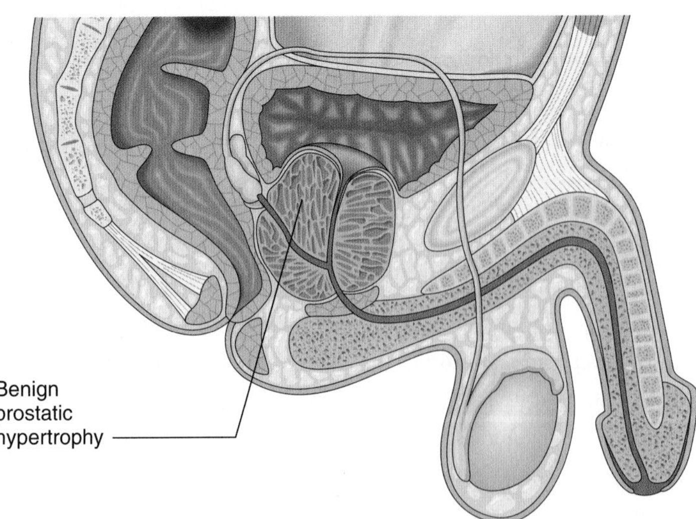

FIGURE 9.9 In benign prostatic hypertrophy, the enlarged prostate presses against the bladder and slows the flow of urine through the urethra.

Hypertrophy is the general increase in bulk of a body part or organ that is not due to tumor formation.

- **Prostatism** (**PROS**-tah-tizm) is the condition of having symptoms resulting from compression or obstruction of the urethra due to benign prostatic hypertrophy (**prostat** means prostate gland, and **-ism** means condition of). This can produce difficulties with urination and with urinary retention.
- **Prostate cancer** is one of the most common cancers among men. The disease can grow slowly with no symptoms, or it can grow aggressively and spread throughout the body.
- **Prostatitis** (**pros**-tah-**TYE**-tis) is an inflammation of the prostate gland (**prostat** means prostate gland, and **-itis** means inflammation).

Urination

- **Diuresis** (**dye**-you-**REE**-sis) is the increased output of urine (**diur** means increasing the output of urine, and **-esis** means an abnormal condition).
- **Dysuria** (dis-**YOU**-ree-ah) is difficult or painful urination (**dys-** means painful, and **-uria** means urination). This condition is frequently associated with urinary tract infections.
- **Enuresis** (**en**-you-**REE**-sis) is the involuntary discharge of urine (**en-** means into, and **-uresis** means urination).
- **Nocturnal enuresis** (nock-**TER**-nal **en**-you-**REE**-sis) is urinary incontinence during sleep. It is also known as *bed-wetting*. *Nocturnal* means pertaining to night.
- **Nocturia** (nock-**TOO**-ree-ah) is excessive urination during the night (**noct** means night, and **-uria** means urination).
- **Oliguria** (**ol**-ih-**GOO**-ree-ah) means scanty urination (**olig** means scanty, and **-uria** means urination). Oliguria is the opposite of *polyuria*.
- **Polyuria** (**pol**-ee-**YOU**-ree-ah) means excessive urination (**poly-** means many, and **-uria** means urination). Polyuria is the opposite of *oliguria*.
- **Urinary hesitancy** is difficulty in starting a urinary stream. This condition is most common in older men with enlarged prostate glands. In younger people, the inability to urinate when another person is present is known as *bashful bladder syndrome*.
- **Urinary retention** is the inability to empty the bladder. This condition is also more common in men, and is frequently associated with an enlarged prostate gland.

Incontinence

Incontinence (in-**KON**-tih-nents) means the inability to control the excretion of urine and feces.

- **Urinary incontinence** is the inability to control the voiding of urine.
- **Stress incontinence** is the inability to control the voiding of urine under physical stress such as running, sneezing, laughing, or coughing.
- **Overactive bladder** (OAB), also known as *urge incontinence*, occurs when the detrusor muscle in the wall of the bladder is too active (see Figure 9.3). Symptoms can include urinary frequency, urgency, and accidental urination due to a sudden and unstoppable need to urinate.

DIAGNOSTIC PROCEDURES OF THE URINARY SYSTEM

- **Urinalysis** (**you**-rih-**NAL**-ih-sis) is the examination of urine to determine the presence of abnormal elements (**urin** means urine, and **-analysis** means a study of the parts). These tests are discussed further in Chapter 15.
- A **bladder ultrasound** is the use of a handheld ultrasound transducer to measure the amount of urine remaining in the bladder after urination. A normal bladder holds between 300 and 400 ccs of urine. When more than this amount is still present after urination, the bladder is described as being distended (enlarged).
- **Catheterization** (**kath**-eh-ter-eye-**ZAY**-shun) is the insertion of a tube into the bladder in order to procure a sterile specimen for diagnostic purposes. It is also used to remove urine from the bladder when the patient is unable to urinate for other reasons. Another use is to place medication into the bladder.
- **Cystography** (sis-**TOG**-rah-fee) is a radiographic examination of the bladder after instillation of a contrast medium via a urethral catheter (**cyst/o** means bladder, and **-graphy** means the process of creating a picture or record). The resulting film is a *cystogram*.
- **Cystoscopy** (sis-**TOS**-koh-pee) is the visual examination of the urinary bladder using a cystoscope (**cyst/o** means bladder, and **-scopy** means visual examination) (Figure 9.10). A specialized *cystoscope* is also for treatment procedures such as the removal of tumors or the reduction of an enlarged prostate gland.
- An **intravenous pyelogram** (**in**-trah-**VEE**-nus **PYE**-eh-loh-**gram**), also known as *excretory urography*, is a radiographic study of the kidneys and ureters (**pyel/o**

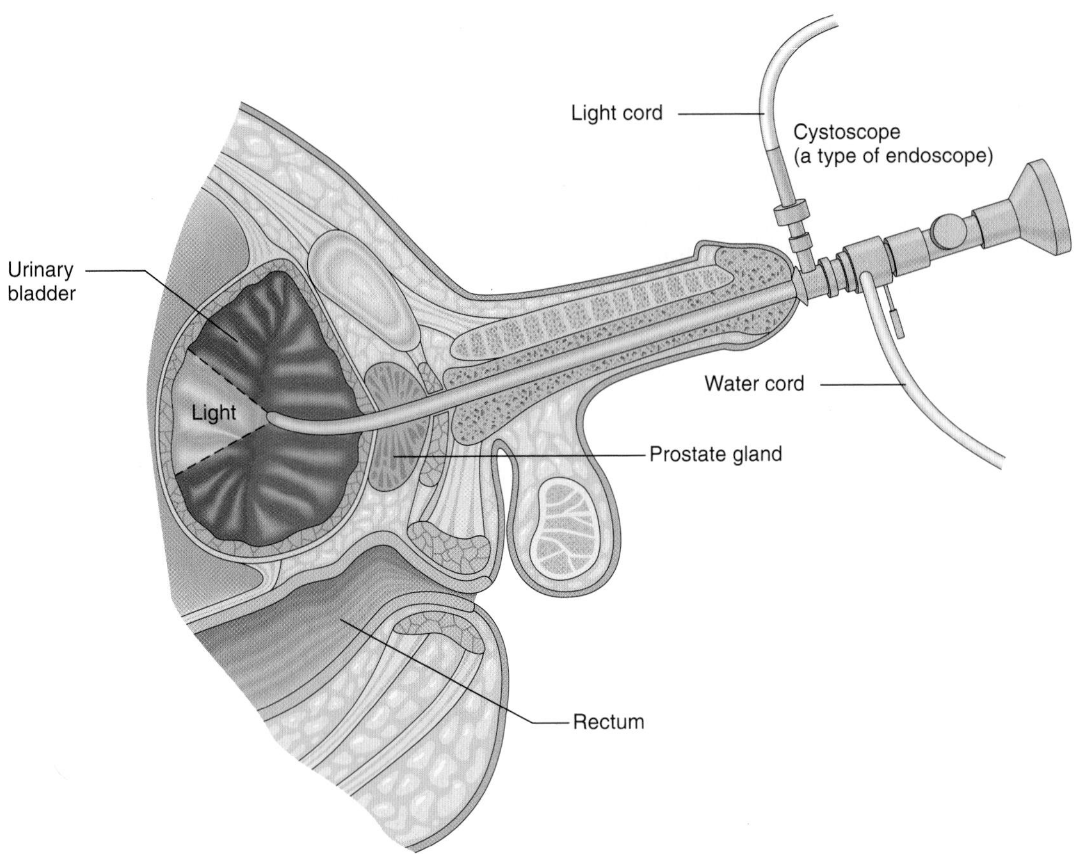

FIGURE 9.10 Use of a cystoscope to examine the interior of the bladder in a male.

means renal pelvis, and **-gram** means a picture or record). A contrast medium is administered intravenously to clearly define these structures in the resulting image. This examination is used to diagnose changes in the urinary tract resulting from kidney stones, infections, enlarged prostate, tumors, and internal injuries after an abdominal trauma (Figure 9.11).

- **Computed tomography**, also known as a *CAT scan*, is more commonly used as a primary tool for evaluation of the urinary system because it can be rapidly performed and provides additional imaging of the abdomen, which may reveal other potential sources for the patient's symptoms.
- A **KUB** (Kidneys, Ureters, Bladder) is a radiographic study of these structures without the use of a contrast medium. This study is also referred to as a *flat-plate of the abdomen*.
- **Retrograde urography** is a radiograph of the urinary system taken after dye has been placed in the urethra through a sterile catheter and caused to flow upward (backward) through the urinary tract.
- **Voiding cystourethrography** (**sis**-toh-you-ree-**THROG**-rah-fee) is a diagnostic procedure in which a

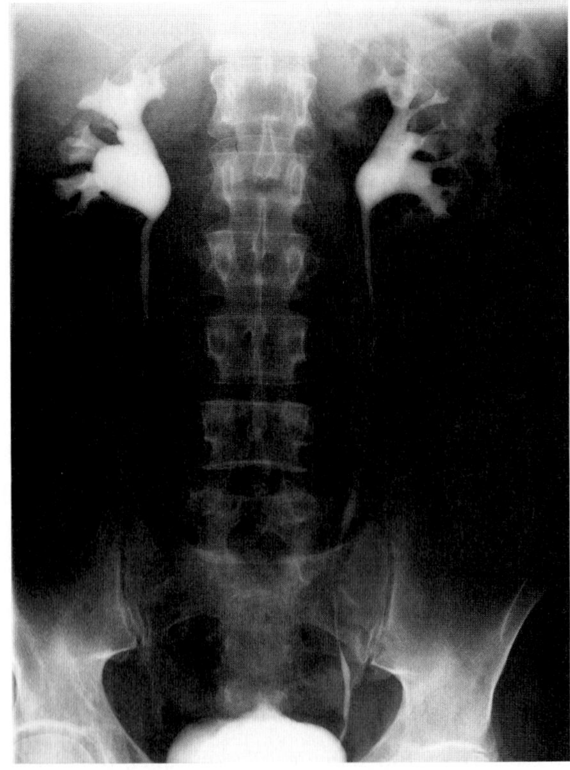

FIGURE 9.11 An intravenous pyelogram (IVP) showing the internal structures of the kidneys and ureters.

fluoroscope is used to examine the flow of urine from the bladder and through the urethra (**cyst/o** means bladder, **urethr/o** means urethra, and **-graphy** means the process of producing a picture or record). This procedure is often performed after cystography.

Diagnostic Procedures of the Prostate Gland

- A **digital rectal examination** is performed on men to screen for prostate enlargement, infection, and indications of prostate cancer. As used here, the term *digital* means performed with a gloved finger placed in the rectum to palpate the prostate gland. *Palpate* means the use of the hands to examine a body part.
- The **prostate-specific antigen** blood test is used to screen for prostate cancer. Commonly referred to as the *PSA test*, it measures the amount of prostate-specific antigen that is present in a blood specimen. The *prostate-specific antigen* is a protein produced by the cells of the prostate gland. The higher a man's PSA level, the more likely it is that cancer is present.

TREATMENT PROCEDURES OF THE URINARY SYSTEM

Medications

- **Diuretics** (**dye**-you-**RET**-icks) are medications administered to increase urine secretion in order to rid the body of excess water and salt.

Dialysis

Dialysis (dye-**AL**-ih-sis) is a procedure to remove waste products from the blood of a patient whose kidneys no longer function (**dia-** means complete or through, and **-lysis** means separation). The two types of dialysis in common use are hemodialysis and peritoneal dialysis.

Hemodialysis

Hemodialysis (**hee**-moh-dye-**AL**-ih-sis) is the process by which waste products are filtered directly from the patient's blood (**hem/o** means blood, **dia** means complete or through, and **-lysis** means separation). Treatment is performed on a hemodialysis unit which is commonly referred to as an *artificial kidney* (Figure 9.12).

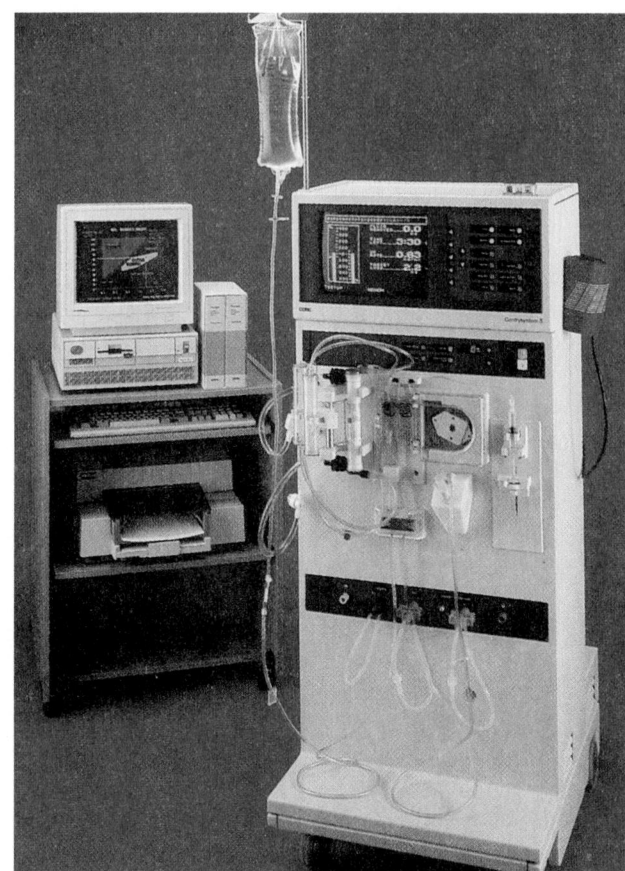

FIGURE 9.12 In a hemodialysis unit, waste is filtered from the patient's blood. Then the filtered blood is returned to the patient's body.

- A shunt implanted in the patient's arm is connected to the hemodialysis unit and arterial blood flows through the filters of the unit. A *shunt* is an artificial passage that allows the blood to flow between the body and the hemodialysis unit.
- The filters contain *dialysate*, which is a solution made up of water and electrolytes. This solution cleanses the blood by removing waste products and excess fluids. *Electrolytes* are the salts that conduct electricity and are found in the body fluid, tissue, and blood.
- The cleansed blood is returned to the body through a vein.
- These treatments each take several hours and must be repeated about three times a week.

Peritoneal Dialysis

In **peritoneal dialysis** (**pehr**-ih-toh-**NEE**-al dye-**AL**-ih-sis) the lining of the peritoneal cavity acts as the filter to remove waste from the blood. The dialysate solution flows into the peritoneal cavity and the fluid is exchanged through a catheter implanted in the abdominal wall. This type of dialysis is used for renal failure and certain types of poisoning (Figure 9.13).

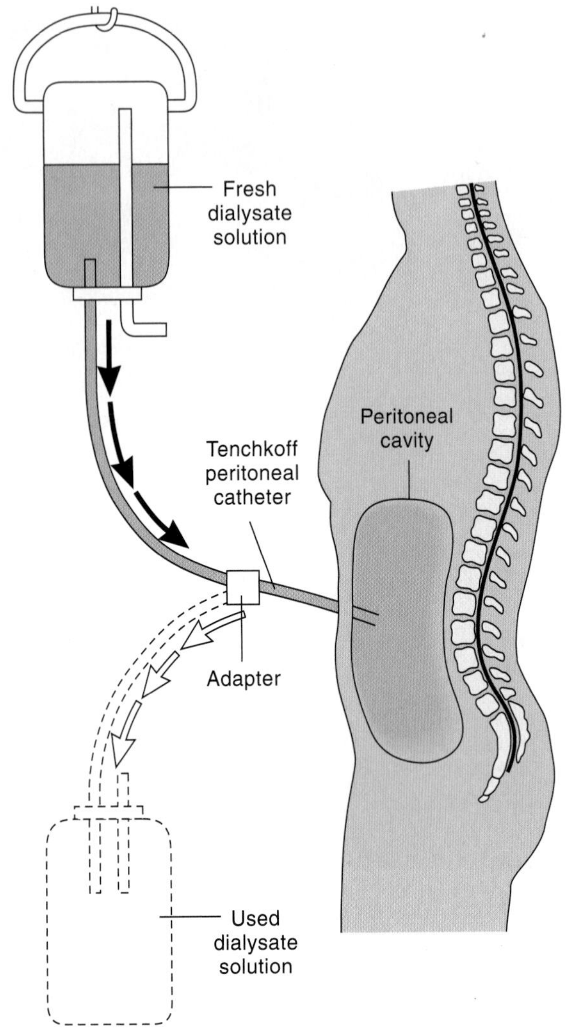

FIGURE 9.13 Peritoneal dialysis removes waste through a fluid exchange in the peritoneal cavity.

- *Continuous ambulatory peritoneal dialysis* provides ongoing dialysis as the patient goes about his or her daily activities. In this procedure, a dialysate solution is instilled from a plastic container worn under the patient's clothing. About every 4 hours, the used solution is drained back into this bag and the bag is discarded. A new bag is then attached, the solution is instilled, and the process continues.
- *Continuous cycling peritoneal dialysis* uses a machine to cycle the dialysate fluid during the night while the patient sleeps.

The Kidneys

- **Nephrolysis** (neh-**FROL**-ih-sis) is the freeing of a kidney from adhesions (**nephr/o** means kidney, and **-lysis** means setting free). An *adhesion* is a band of fibers that holds structures together abnormally.
- Note: The suffix **-lysis** means setting free; however, it also means destruction. Therefore, the term *nephrolysis* can also describe a pathologic condition in which there is the destruction of renal cells.
- A **nephropexy** (**NEF**-roh-**peck**-see), also known as *nephrorrhaphy*, is the surgical fixation of a floating kidney (**nephr/o** means kidney, and **-pexy** means surgical fixation).
- A **nephrostomy** (neh-**FROS**-toh-mee) is the establishment of an opening from the pelvis of the kidney to the exterior of the body (**nephr** means kidney and **-ostomy** means creating an opening). In a kidney affected by hydronephrosis, this allows bypassing of the ureter because the urine from the kidney is drained directly through the back.
- **Pyeloplasty** (**PYE**-eh-loh-**plas**-tee) is the surgical repair of the renal pelvis (**pyel/o** means the renal pelvis, and **-plasty** means surgical repair).
- A **pyelotomy** (**pye**-eh-**LOT**-oh-mee) is a surgical incision into the renal pelvis (**pyel** means the renal pelvis, and **-otomy** means surgical incision). This procedure is performed to correct an obstruction of the junction between the renal pelvis and the ureter.
- **Renal transplantation**, commonly known as a *kidney transplant*, is the grafting of a donor kidney into the body to replace the recipient's failed kidneys. A single transplanted kidney, from either a living or nonliving donor, is capable of adequately performing all kidney functions (Figure 9.14).

Removal of Kidney Stones

- **Extracorporeal shockwave lithotripsy** (ESWL) is the destruction of stones with the use of high-energy ultrasonic waves traveling through water or gel (Figure 9.15). The fragments of these stones are then excreted in the urine. *Extracorporeal* means situated or occurring outside the body. **Lithotripsy** (**LITH**-oh-**trip**-see) means to crush a stone (**lith/o** means stone, and **-tripsy** means to crush).
- A **nephrolithotomy** (**nef**-roh-lih-**THOT**-oh-mee) is the surgical removal of a nephrolith (kidney stone) through an incision in the kidney (**nephr/o** means kidney, **lith** means stone, and **-otomy** means surgical incision).
- A **percutaneous nephrolithotomy** (**per**-kyou-**TAY**-nee-us **nef**-roh-lih-**THOT**-oh-mee) is performed by making

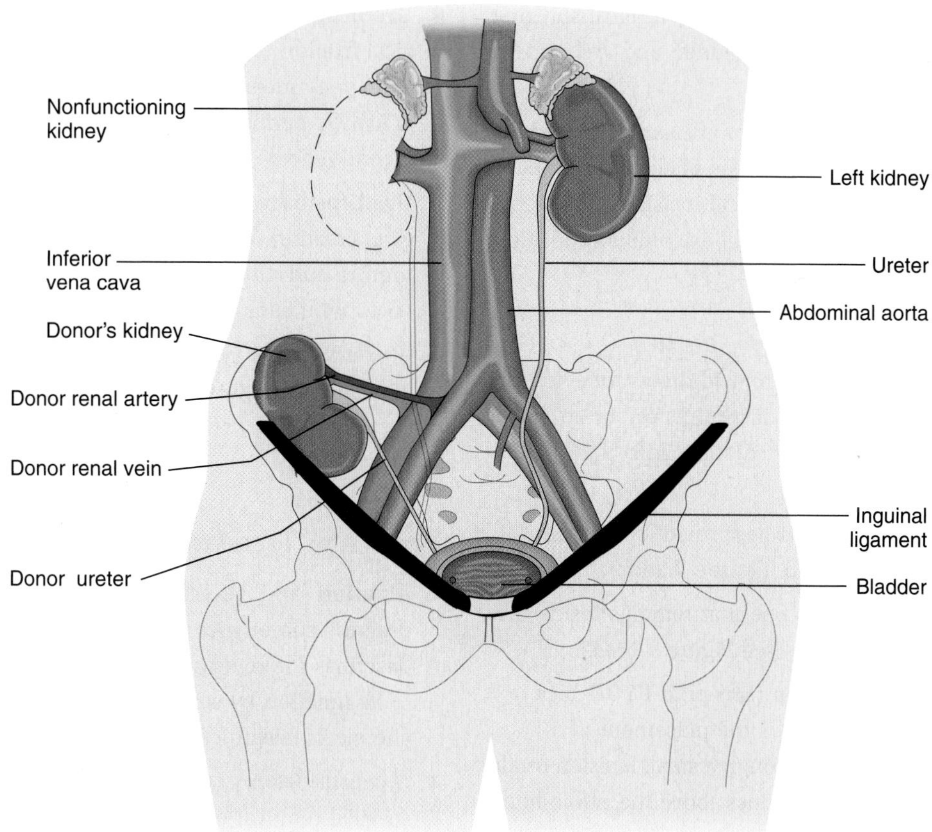

FIGURE 9.14 In a kidney transplant, the nonfunctioning kidney is not removed. Instead, the donor kidney and its associated structures are sutured into place at a lower point in the abdomen.

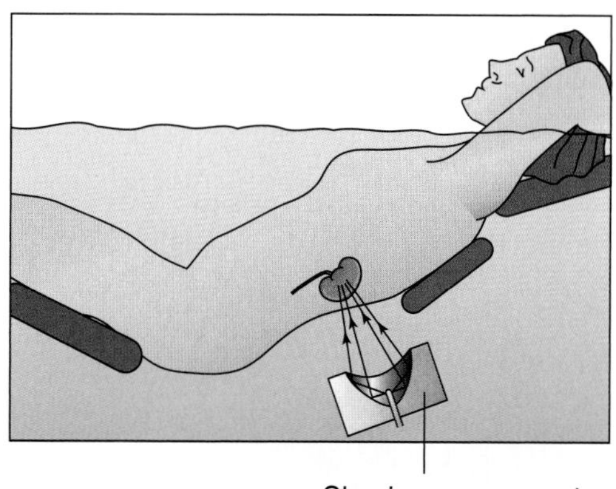

FIGURE 9.15 Lithotripsy utilizes shock waves traveling through water or a gel to destroy kidney stones.

a small incision in the back and inserting a nephroscope to crush and remove a kidney stone. *Percutaneous* means performed through the skin. A *nephroscope* is a specialized endoscope used in the treatment of the kidneys.

The Ureters

- A **ureterectomy** (**you**-ree-ter-**ECK**-toh-mee) is the surgical removal of a ureter (**ureter** means ureter, and **-ectomy** means surgical removal).
- **Ureteroplasty** (you-**REE**-ter-oh-**plas**-tee) is the surgical repair of a ureter (**ureter/o** means ureter, and **-plasty** means surgical repair).
- **Ureterorrhaphy** (**you**-ree-ter-**OR**-ah-fee) is the surgical suturing of a ureter (**ureter/o** means ureter, and **-rrhaphy** means surgical suturing).

The Urinary Bladder

- A **cystectomy** (sis-**TECK**-toh-mee) is the surgical removal of all or part of the urinary bladder (**cyst** means bladder, and **-ectomy** means surgical removal).
- **Cystopexy** (**sis**-toh-**peck**-see) is the surgical fixation of the bladder to the abdominal wall (**cyst/o** means bladder, and **-pexy** means surgical fixation).

- **Cystorrhaphy** (sis-**TOR**-ah-fee) is the surgical suturing of the bladder (**cyst/o** means bladder, and **-rrhaphy** means surgical suturing).
- A **lithotomy** (lih-**THOT**-oh-mee) is a surgical incision for the removal of a stone from the bladder (**lith** means stone, and **-otomy** means surgical incision). This term also is used to describe a physical examination position (see Chapter 15).

Catheterization

Catheterization is performed to withdraw urine for diagnostic purposes, to control incontinence, or to place fluid, such as a chemotherapy solution, into the bladder (Figure 9.16).

- **Urethral catheterization** is performed by inserting a tube along the urethra and into the bladder.
- An **indwelling catheter** is one that remains inside the body for a prolonged time (see Figure 9.16A).
- **Suprapubic catheterization** (**soo**-prah-**PYOU**-bick **kath**-eh-ter-eye-**ZAY**-shun) is the placement of a catheter into the bladder through a small incision made through the abdominal wall just above the pubic bone (see Figure 9.16B).

The Urethra

- A **meatotomy** (**mee**-ah-**TOT**-oh-mee) is a surgical incision made in the urinary meatus to enlarge the opening (**meat** means meatus, and **-otomy** means surgical incision).
- **Urethropexy** (you-**REE**-throh-**peck**-see) is the surgical fixation of the urethra (**urethr/o** means urethra, and **-pexy** means surgical fixation). This procedure is usually performed to correct urinary stress incontinence.
- **Urethrostomy** (**you**-reh-**THROS**-toh-mee) is the surgical creation of a permanent opening between the urethra and the skin (**urethr** means urethra, and **-ostomy** means creating an opening).
- A **urethrotomy** (**you**-reh-**THROT**-oh-mee) is a surgical incision into the urethra for relief of a stricture (**urethr** means urethra, and **-otomy** means surgical incision).

Prostate Treatment

- **Ablation** (ab-**LAY**-shun), which is the term used to describe some types of treatment of prostate cancer, describes the removal of a body part or the destruction of its function by surgery, hormones, drugs, heat, chemicals, electrocautery, or other methods.
- A **prostatectomy** (**pros**-tah-**TECK**-toh-mee) is the surgical removal of all or part of the prostate gland (**prostat** means prostate, and **-ectomy** means surgical removal). This procedure is performed to treat prostate cancer or to reduce an enlarged prostate gland.
- A *radical prostatectomy*, which is performed through the abdomen, is the surgical removal of the entire prostate gland, the seminal vesicles, and some surrounding tissues.

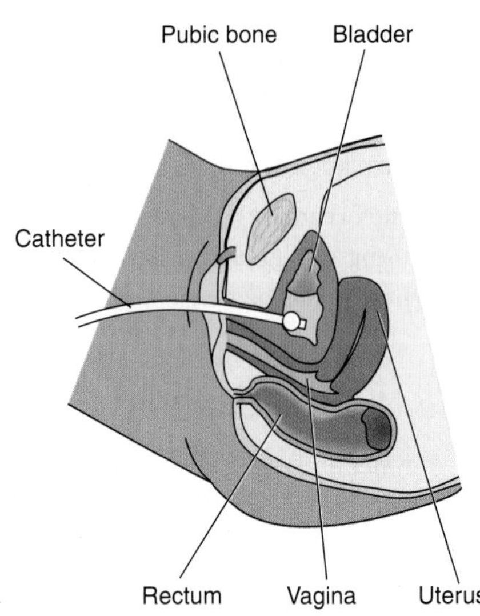

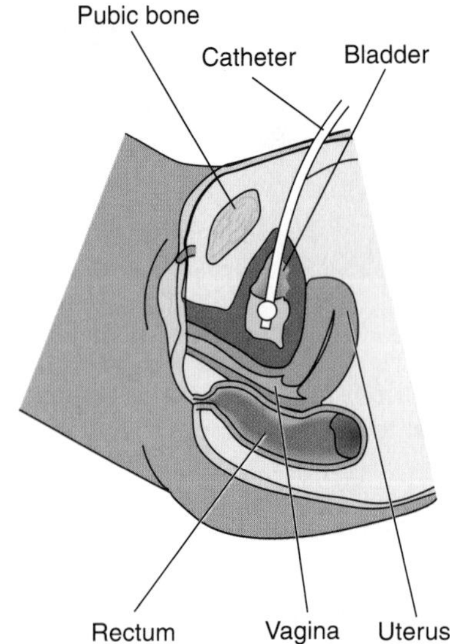

FIGURE 9.16 Types of urinary catheterization. (A) An indwelling catheter. (B) A suprapubic catheter.

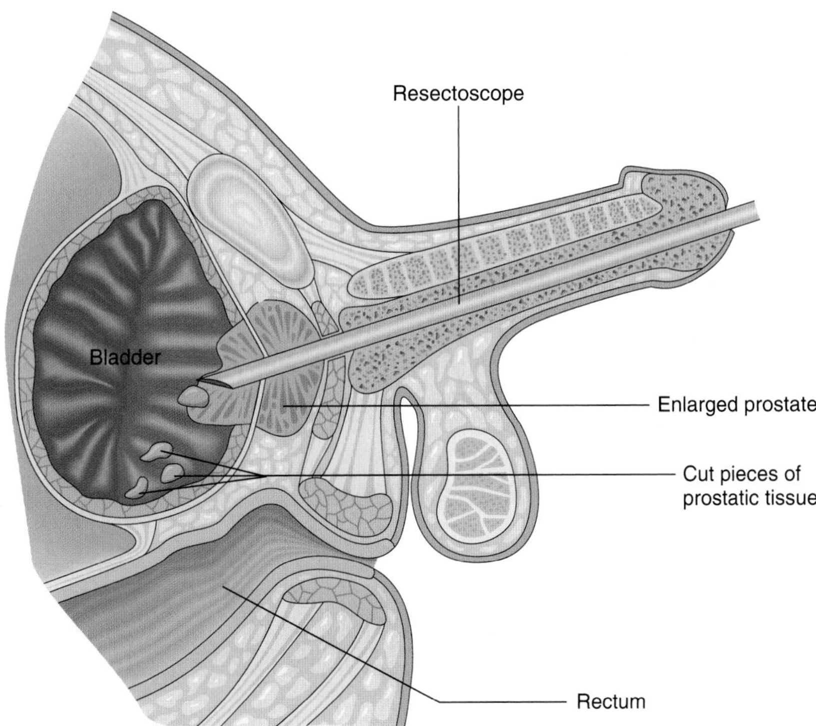

FIGURE 9.17 A transurethral prostatectomy (TURP) being performed to relieve benign prostatic hypertrophy.

- A **transurethral prostatectomy**, also known as a *TURP*, is the removal of an overgrowth of tissue from the prostate gland through a resectoscope (Figure 9.17). A *resectoscope* is a specialized endoscopic instrument that resembles a cystoscope.
- *Radiation therapy* and *hormone therapy* are additional treatments used to control prostate cancer.

Urinary Incontinence Treatment

- **Kegel exercises**, which were named for Dr. Arnold Kegel, are a series of pelvic muscle exercises used to strengthen the muscles of the pelvic floor to control urinary stress incontinence in women.
- **Bladder retraining** is a program of urinating on a schedule with increasingly longer time intervals between scheduled urination. The goal is to reestablish voluntary bladder control and to break the cycle of frequency, urgency, and urge incontinence.

ABBREVIATIONS RELATED TO THE URINARY SYSTEM

Table 9.1 presents an overview of the abbreviations related to the terms introduced in this chapter. Note: To avoid errors or confusion, always be cautious when using abbreviations.

TABLE 9.1

ABBREVIATIONS RELATED TO THE URINARY SYSTEM

benign prostatic hypertrophy = BPH	**BPH** = benign prostatic hypertrophy
catheterization = cath	**cath** = catheterization
chronic renal failure = CRF	**CRF** = chronic renal failure
cystoscopy = cysto	**cysto** = cystoscopy
intravenous pyelogram = IVP	**IVP** = intravenous pyelogram
polycystic kidney disease = PKD	**PKD** = polycystic kidney disease

Career Opportunities

In addition to the medical specialties already discussed, some of the health occupations involving the treatment of the urinary system include:

- **Dialysis technician:** operates the hemodialysis equipment, also provides emotional support and nutritional counseling for dialysis patients
- **Urology** (or **renal) licensed practical nurse** or **certified nursing assistant:** provides care and information to patients with disorders of the kidneys, urinary tract, and male reproductive organs, including infections, kidney and bladder stones, and cancers

Health Occupation Profile

Urologist

Dr. Arthur Sonneland, M.D., is a urologist specializing in diseases of the urogenital system. *"About half of my work time is spent performing surgery on the prostate, bladder, or kidneys. I also do surgical repairs to help control female incontinence. The other half of my practice is consulting with patients in the office.*

"My father was also a urologist, so it was probably natural for me to follow in his footsteps. Urology may not be the most popular field for medical students looking for a possible career. But I've found it to be a fascinating surgical specialty, with a wide variety of diseases to treat and yet a sane lifestyle (most of the time), with very little nighttime emergency duty."

Study Break

Most human infants are "potty trained" at around age 2 or 3 years. Until that time, babies are clothed in diapers to absorb their urinary output and other excretions. The average baby will go through 5,000–6,000 diaper changes! The majority of parents today use disposable diapers, so we tend to forget that these are a somewhat recent invention.

Over the course of time, many different methods of diapering a baby have been used:

- **Native Americans packed the soft insides of milkweed around their babies' bottoms before strapping the child onto a papoose board.**
- **Eskimos gathered moss during the summer and placed it inside the animal skins in which the mothers carried their babies.**
- **Cotton diapers, still in use today, are what our term *diaper* (meaning a diamond-patterned fabric) comes from. The invention of the safety pin in the 19th century helped make cotton diapers practical.**

REVIEW TIME

Write the answers to the following questions on a separate piece of paper or in your notebook. In addition, be prepared to take part in the classroom discussion.

1. ***Written Assignment:*** Using terms a physician would understand, describe the difference between **hemodialysis** and **peritoneal dialysis**.

   Discussion Assignment: How would being on hemodialysis, as compared with peritoneal dialysis, affect the patient's quality of life?

2. ***Written Assignment:*** Using terms a patient would understand, describe the difference between a **nephrolithotomy** and **extracorporeal shockwave lithotripsy** (ESWL) for the removal of a kidney stone.

   Discussion Assignment: What is the medical term for a stone lodged in a ureter? Joe Morrison has a stone lodged in the left ureter. If this stone is not removed, what other condition is likely to develop?

3. ***Written Assignment:*** Describe the difference between **epispadias** and **hypospadias** in the male.

   Discussion Assignment: How do these two conditions affect the female?

4. ***Written Assignment:*** Describe the differences between **acute renal failure** and **chronic renal failure**.

   Discussion Assignment: What are some of the causes of acute renal failure?

5. ***Written Assignment:*** Describe the difference between a **cystocele** and a **vesicovaginal fissure**.

   Discussion Assignment: What are some of the possible complications that might result from either of these conditions if it has not been repaired?

Optional Internet Activity

The goal of this activity is to help you learn more about medical terminology as it applies to the "real world." Select **one** *of these two options and follow the instructions.*

1. Search for information about a **kidney transplant**. Write a brief (one- or two-paragraph) report on something new you learned here and include the address of the web site where you found this information.
2. To learn more about **bladder diseases**, go to MedLinePlus, which is a service of the National Institutes of Health. Write a brief (one- or two-paragraph) report on something new you learned here.

THE HUMAN TOUCH: CRITICAL THINKING ACTIVITY

The following story and questions are designed to stimulate critical thinking through class discussion or as a brief essay response. There are no right or wrong answers to these questions.

"Mom, they want me to play for the National Women's Hockey League!" ***Josie yelled as she ran into the living room. She had just finished practice, and the scouts had told her afterwards how impressed they were with her moves. Finally, her lifelong dream of winning an Olympic gold medal for Canada might actually come true! She'd had to make some sacrifices, like living at home after***

continues

high school, but it looked like that would all pay off. As soon as she saw the looks on the faces of her parents, her smile disappeared.

"Honey, we just got back from the doctor. It turns out that your brother's recurrent bouts of pyelonephritis have led to irreversible renal damage. The nephrologist is recommending that Xavier have a kidney transplant," ***her mom explained with a pained look.*** **"We know that he has a better chance if he has a related donor, but he could always go on hemodialysis and wait for a cadaver donor ..."**

Josie saw her dreams of a hockey career fade away. After Xavier's third bout with nephrotic syndrome, her whole family had been tested for compatibility in case he needed a transplant. Josie was the only one eligible, with a negative cross-match. The doctors had explained to her then what it would mean if she decided to donate one of her kidneys, but Josie had brushed it off, assuming that her brother would get better. Now the voices of the doctors came back to her **"No contact sports after a nephrectomy,"** ***she heard them say.*** **"There's too big a risk of rupturing the remaining kidney."**

Josie was faced with the toughest decision of all: she loved Xavier, but hockey was her life.

Suggested Discussion Topics

1. Discuss the long-term repercussions of being a living organ donor.
2. Imagine that you are Josie's mom or dad and one of your children has the opportunity to save the life of another one of your children. Would you encourage him or her to donate an organ?
3. If Josie decides to donate her kidney and then later chooses to continue playing hockey, what advice should her parents give her?
4. What options might be open to Josie's brother other than having his sister donate a kidney?

STUDENT WORKBOOK AND StudyWARE™ CD-ROM

1. Go to your **Student Workbook** and complete the Learning Exercises for this chapter.

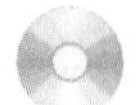

2. Go to the **StudyWARE™ CD-ROM** and have fun with the exercises and games for this chapter.

CHAPTER 10

THE NERVOUS SYSTEM

OVERVIEW OF STRUCTURES, COMBINING FORMS, AND FUNCTIONS OF THE NERVOUS SYSTEM

MAJOR STRUCTURES	RELATED COMBINING FORMS	PRIMARY FUNCTIONS
Brain	cerebr/o, encephal/o	Coordinates all body activities by receiving and transmitting messages throughout the body.
Spinal Cord	myel/o	Transmits nerve impulses between the brain, arms and legs, and lower part of the body.
Nerves	neur/i, neur/o	Receive and transmit messages to and from all parts of the body.
Sensory Organs and Receptors		Receive external stimulation and transmit these stimuli to the sensory neurons.
Eyes (sight)		See Chapter 11.
Ears (hearing)		See Chapter 11.
Nose (smell)		See Chapter 7.
Skin (touch)		See Chapter 12.
Tongue (taste)		See Chapter 8.

VOCABULARY RELATED TO THE NERVOUS SYSTEM

This list contains essential word parts and medical terms for this chapter. These terms are pronounced on the student StudyWARE™ CD-ROM and Audio CDs that are available for use with this text. These and the other important **primary terms** are shown in boldface throughout the chapter. *Secondary terms*, which appear in *orange* italics, clarify the meaning of primary terms.

Word Parts

- ☐ **caus/o**
- ☐ **concuss/o**
- ☐ **contus/o**
- ☐ **encephal/o**
- ☐ **-esthesia**
- ☐ **esthet/o**
- ☐ **-graphy**
- ☐ **klept/o**
- ☐ **-mania**
- ☐ **mening/o**
- ☐ **myel/o**
- ☐ **neur/i, neur/o**
- ☐ **-phobia**
- ☐ **psych/o**
- ☐ **-tropic**

Medical Terms

- ☐ **acrophobia** (**ack**-roh-**FOH**-bee-ah)
- ☐ **Alzheimer's disease** (**ALTZ**-high-merz)
- ☐ **amyotrophic lateral sclerosis** (ah-**my**-oh-**TROH**-fick)
- ☐ **anesthetic** (**an**-es-**THET**-ick)
- ☐ **anesthetist** (ah-**NES**-theh-tist)
- ☐ **anxiety disorders**
- ☐ **autism** (**AW**-tizm)
- ☐ **Bell's palsy**
- ☐ **carotid ultrasonography** (**ul**-trah-son-**OG**-rah-fee)
- ☐ **causalgia** (kaw-**ZAL**-jee-ah)
- ☐ **cerebral contusion** (**SER**-eh-bral kon-**TOO**-zhun)
- ☐ **cerebral palsy** (**SER**-eh-bral **PAWL**-zee)
- ☐ **cerebrovascular accident** (**ser**-eh-broh-**VAS**-kyou-lar)
- ☐ **cervical radiculopathy** (rah-**dick**-you-**LOP**-ah-thee)
- ☐ **claustrophobia** (**klaws**-troh-**FOH**-bee-ah)
- ☐ **cognition** (kog-**NISH**-un)
- ☐ **coma** (**KOH**-mah)
- ☐ **concussion** (kon-**KUSH**-un)
- ☐ **cranial hematoma** (**hee**-mah-**TOH**-mah)
- ☐ **delirium** (dee-**LIR**-ee-um)
- ☐ **delirium tremens** (dee-**LIR**-ee-um **TREE**-mens)
- ☐ **delusion** (dee-**LOO**-zhun)
- ☐ **dementia** (dee-**MEN**-shee-ah)
- ☐ **dura mater** (**DOO**-rah **MAH**-ter)
- ☐ **dyslexia** (dis-**LECK**-see-ah)
- ☐ **echoencephalography** (**eck**-oh-en-**sef**-ah-**LOG**-rah-fee)
- ☐ **electroencephalography** (ee-**leck**-troh-en-**sef**-ah-**LOG**-rah-fee)
- ☐ **encephalitis** (**en**-sef-ah-**LYE**-tis)
- ☐ **epidural anesthesia** (**ep**-ih-**DOO**-ral **an**-es-**THEE**-zee-ah)
- ☐ **epilepsy** (**EP**-ih-**lep**-see)
- ☐ **factitious disorder** (fack-**TISH**-us)
- ☐ **Guillain-Barré syndrome** (gee-**YAHN**-bah-**RAY** **SIN**-drohm)
- ☐ **hallucination** (hah-**loo**-sih-**NAY**-shun)
- ☐ **hemorrhagic stroke** (**hem**-oh-**RAJ**-ick)
- ☐ **hydrocephalus** (high-droh-**SEF**-ah-lus)
- ☐ **hyperesthesia** (**high**-per-es-**THEE**-zee-ah)
- ☐ **hypochondriasis** (**high**-poh-kon-**DRY**-ah-sis)
- ☐ **ischemic stroke** (iss-**KEE**-mick)
- ☐ **lethargy** (**LETH**-ar-jee)
- ☐ **meningitis** (**men**-in-**JIGH**-tis)
- ☐ **meningocele** (meh-**NING**-goh-**seel**)
- ☐ **migraine headache** (**MY**-grayn)
- ☐ **multiple sclerosis** (skleh-**ROH**-sis)
- ☐ **myelitis** (**my**-eh-**LYE**-tis)
- ☐ **myelography** (**my**-eh-**LOG**-rah-fee)
- ☐ **narcolepsy** (**NAR**-koh-**lep**-see)
- ☐ **neurotransmitters** (**new**-roh-trans-**MIT**-erz)
- ☐ **obsessive-compulsive disorder**
- ☐ **panic attack**
- ☐ **paresthesia** (**pair**-es-**THEE**-zee-ah)
- ☐ **Parkinson's disease**
- ☐ **peripheral neuropathy** (new-**ROP**-ah-thee)
- ☐ **posttraumatic stress disorder**
- ☐ **Reye's syndrome**
- ☐ **schizophrenia** (**skit**-soh-**FREE**-nee-ah)
- ☐ **sciatica** (sigh-**AT**-ih-kah)
- ☐ **shaken baby syndrome**
- ☐ **syncope** (**SIN**-koh-pee)
- ☐ **trichotillomania** (**trick**-oh-**till**-oh-**MAY**-nee-ah)
- ☐ **trigeminal neuralgia** (try-**JEM**-ih-nal new-**RAL**-jee-ah)

OBJECTIVES

On completion of this chapter, you should be able to:

1. Describe the functions and structures of the nervous system.
2. Identify the major divisions of the nervous system and describe the structures of each by location and function.
3. Identify the medical specialists who treat disorders of the nervous system.
4. Recognize, define, spell, and pronounce terms related to the pathology and the diagnostic and treatment procedures of the nervous system.
5. Recognize, define, spell, and pronounce terms related to the pathology and the diagnostic and treatment procedures of mental health disorders.

FUNCTIONS OF THE NERVOUS SYSTEM

The nervous system, with the brain as its center, coordinates and controls all bodily activities. When the brain ceases functioning, the body dies.

STRUCTURES OF THE NERVOUS SYSTEM

The major structures of the nervous system are the nerves, brain, spinal cord, and sensory organs. The sensory organs, which are the eyes, ears, nose, skin, and tongue, are discussed in other chapters.

Divisions of the Nervous System

For descriptive purposes, the nervous system is divided into two primary parts: the central and peripheral nervous systems (see Figure 10.1).

- The **central nervous system** (CNS) includes the brain and spinal cord. The functions of the central nervous system are to receive and process information, and to regulate all bodily activity.
- The **peripheral nervous system** (PNS) includes the 12 pairs of cranial nerves extending from the brain and the 31 pairs of peripheral spinal nerves extending outward from the spinal cord. The function of the peripheral nervous system is to transmit nerve signals to, and from, the central nervous system.

The Nerves

A **nerve** is one or more bundles of neurons that connect the brain and the spinal cord with other parts of the body. A **tract** is a bundle or group of nerve fibers located within the brain or spinal cord.

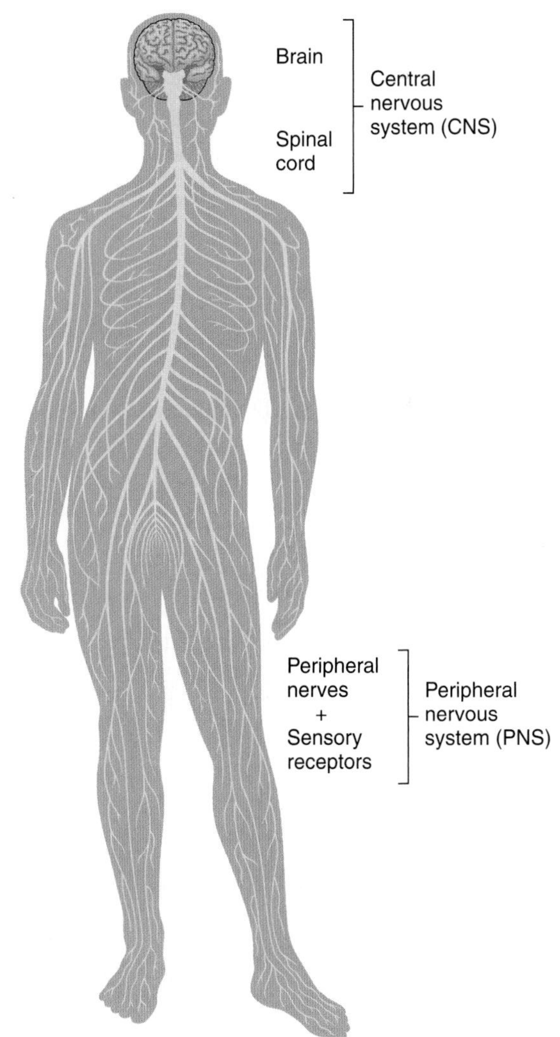

FIGURE 10.1 The structural organization of the central and peripheral nervous systems.

- **Ascending nerve tracts** carry nerve impulses *toward* the brain.
- **Descending nerve tracts** carry nerve impulses *away from* the brain.
- A **ganglion** (**GANG**-glee-on) is a nerve center made up of a cluster of nerve cell bodies outside the central nervous system (plural, *ganglia* or *ganglions*). Note: The term ganglion also describes a benign, tumor-like cyst.
- The term **innervation** (**in**-err-**VAY**-shun) means the supply of nerves to a specific body part.
- A **plexus** (**PLECK**-sus) is a network of intersecting spinal nerves (plural, *plexuses*) (see Figure 10.9). This term also describes a network of intersecting blood or lymphatic vessels.
- **Receptors** are sites in the sensory organs (eyes, ears, skin, nose, and taste buds) that receive external stimulation. The receptors send the stimulus through the sensory neurons to the brain for interpretation.
- A **stimulus** is anything that excites (activates) a nerve and causes an impulse (plural, *stimuli*). An *impulse* is a wave of excitation transmitted through nerve fibers and neurons.

The Reflexes

A **reflex** (**REE**-flecks) is an automatic, involuntary response to some change, either inside or outside the body. Examples of reflex actions include:

- Changes in the heart rate, breathing rate, and blood pressure.
- Coughing and sneezing.
- Responses to painful stimuli.

Deep tendon reflexes are discussed in Chapter 4.

The Neurons

Neurons (**NEW**-ronz) are the basic cells of the nervous system that allow different parts of the body to communicate with each other.

- The body has billions of neurons carrying nerve impulses throughout the body via an electrochemical process. This process creates patterns of neuron electrical activity known as *brain waves*. Different types of brain waves are produced during periods of intense activity, rest, and sleep.
- The three types of neurons are described according to their function. The system of naming the neurons is summarized in Table 10.1. The *memory aid* **A-C-E** will help you remember their names, and **S-A-M** will help you remember their functions.

Neuron Parts

Each neuron consists of a cell body, several dendrites, a single axon, and terminal end fibers (Figure 10.2).

- The **dendrites** (**DEN**-drytes) are the root-like processes that receive impulses and conduct them to the cell body. A *process* is a structure that extends out from the cell body.
- The **axon** (**ACK**-son) is a process that extends away from the cell body and conducts impulses away from the nerve cell. An axon can be more than three feet long. Many, but not all, axons are protected by a myelin sheath, which is a white fatty tissue covering.

TABLE 10.1
TYPES OF NEURONS AND THEIR FUNCTIONS

Types of Neurons	Neuron Functions
"ACE"	**"SAM"**
Afferent neurons (**AF**-er-ent) *Afferent* means toward.	Also known as *sensory neurons*, these neurons emerge from sensory organs and the skin to carry the impulses from the sensory organs *toward* the brain and spinal cord.
Connecting neurons	Also known as *associative neurons*, these neurons link sensory and motor neurons.
Efferent neurons (**EF**-er-ent) *Efferent* means away from.	Also known as *motor neurons*, these neurons carry impulses *away from* the brain and spinal cord and toward the muscles and glands.

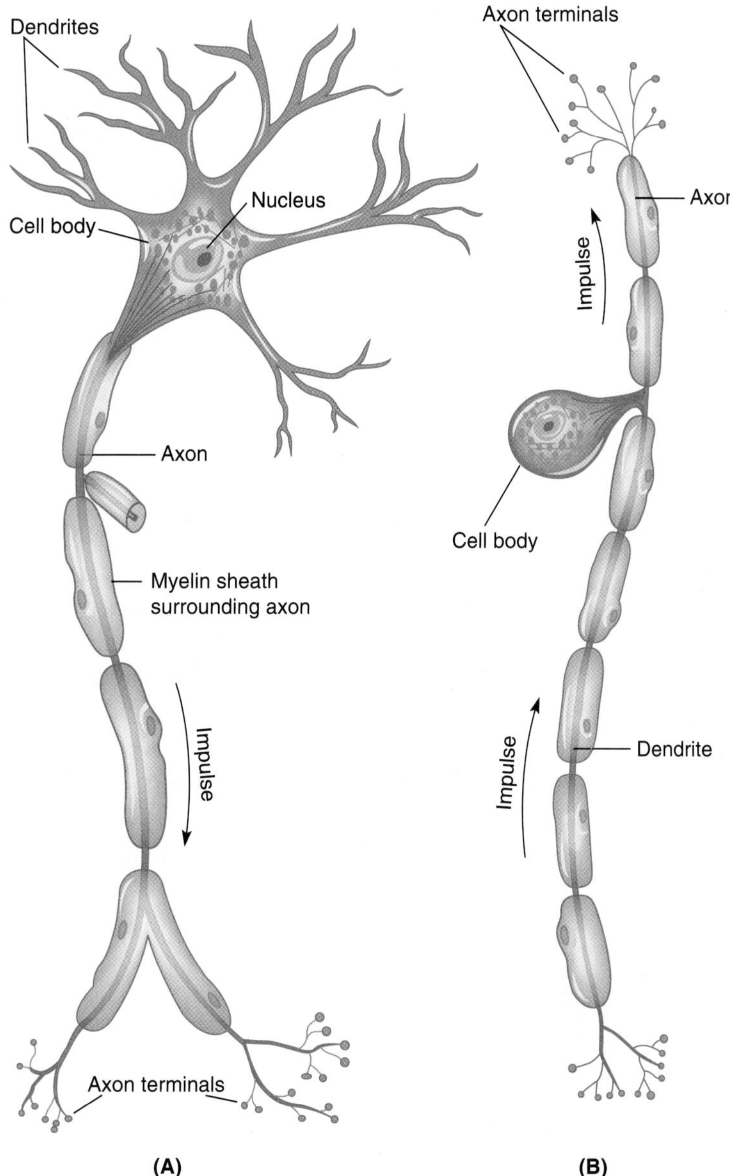

FIGURE 10.2 The structure of two type of neurons. (A) Motor neurons. (B) Sensory neurons.

- **Terminal end fibers** are the branching fibers at the end of the axon that lead the nervous impulse from the axon to the synapse.
- A **synapse** (**SIN**-apps) is the space between two neurons or between a neuron and a receptor organ. A single neuron can have a few, or several hundred, synapses.

Neurotransmitters

Neurotransmitters (**new**-roh-trans-**MIT**-erz) are chemical substances that make it possible for messages to cross from the synapse of a neuron to the target receptor. There are between 200 and 300 known neurotransmitters, and each has a specialized function. Examples of neurotransmitters and their roles are shown below.

- *Acetylcholine* is released at some synapses in the spinal cord and at neuromuscular junctions; it influences muscle action.
- *Dopamine* is released within the brain. It is believed to be involved in mood and thought disorders and in abnormal movement disorders such as Parkinson's disease.
- *Endorphins* are naturally occurring substances that are produced by the brain to help relieve pain.
- *Norepinephrine*, which is released at synaptic nerve endings, responds to hypotension and physical stress.

- *Serotonin*, which is released in the brain, has roles in sleep, hunger, and pleasure recognition. It is also sometimes linked to mood disorders.

Glial Cells

Glial cells provide support and protection for neurons, and their four main functions are: (1) to surround neurons and hold them in place, (2) to supply nutrients and oxygen to neurons, (3) to insulate one neuron from another, and (4) to destroy and remove dead neurons.

The Myelin Sheath

A **myelin sheath** (**MY**-eh-lin) is the protective covering made up of glial cells. This white sheath forms the white matter of the brain, and covers some parts of the spinal cord and the axon of most peripheral nerves (see Figure 10.2).

- The portion of the nerve fibers that are myelinated are known as *white matter*. The term *myelinated* means having a myelin sheath. It is the color of this covering that makes these fibers white.
- The portion of the nerve fibers that are unmyelinated are known as *gray matter*. The term *unmyelinated* means lacking a myelin sheath. It is the lack of the myelin sheath that creates the gray color of the brain and spinal cord.

THE CENTRAL NERVOUS SYSTEM

The **central nervous system** is made up of the brain and spinal cord. These structures are protected externally by the bones of the cranium and the vertebrae of the spinal column, which are discussed in Chapter 3. Within these bony structures, the brain and spinal cord are further protected by the meninges and the cerebrospinal fluid (Figure 10.3).

The Meninges

The **meninges** (meh-**NIN**-jeez) are the system of membranes that enclose the brain and spinal cord of the central nervous (singular *meninx*). The meninges consist of three layers of connective tissue. These are the dura mater, arachnoid membrane, and the pia mater (see Figure 10.3).

The Dura Mater

The **dura mater** (**DOO**-rah **MAH**-ter) is the thick, tough, outermost membrane of the meninges. *Dura* means hard, and *mater* means mother.

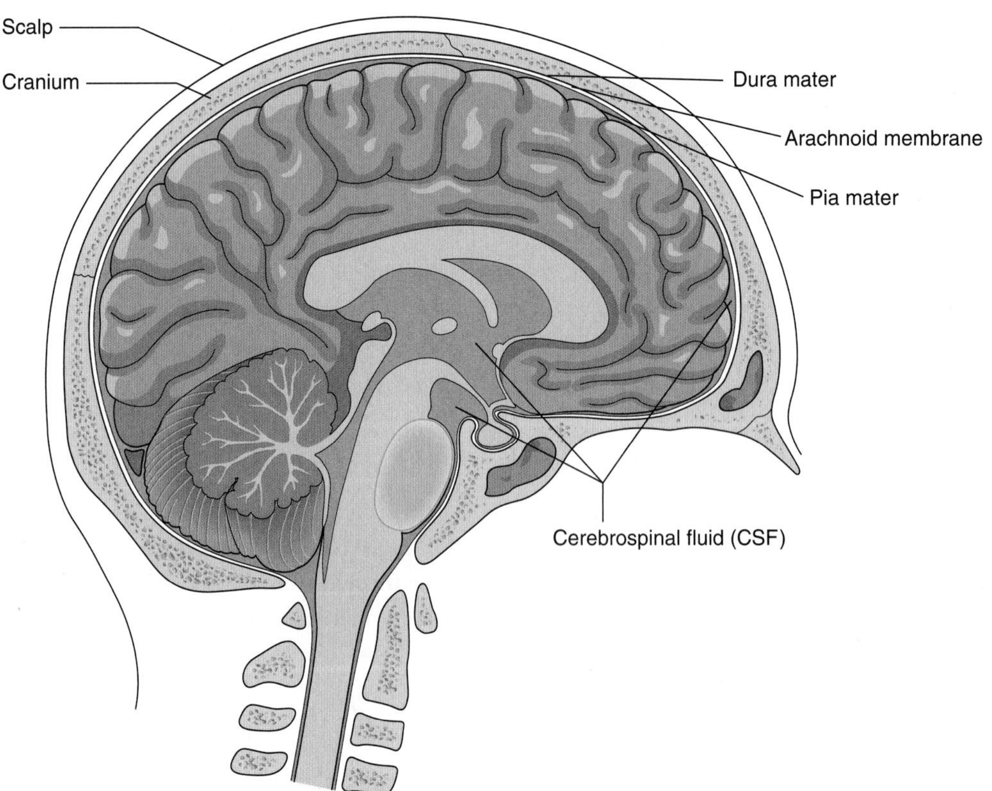

FIGURE 10.3 A cross-section of the brain showing the protective coverings. The cerebrospinal fluid is shown in pink.

- The inner surface of cranium (skull) is lined with dura mater.
- The inner surface of the vertebral column is known as the *epidural space*. This space, which is located between the walls of the vertebral column and the dura mater of the meninges, contains fat and supportive connective tissues to cushion the dura mater.
- In both the skull and vertebral column, the *subdural space* is located between the dura mater and the arachnoid membrane.

The Arachnoid Membrane

The **arachnoid membrane** (ah-**RACK**-noid), which resembles a spider web, is the second layer of the meninges and is located between the dura mater and the pia mater. *Arachnoid* means having to do with spiders.

- The arachnoid membrane is loosely attached to the other meninges to allow space for fluid to flow between the layers.
- The *subarachnoid space*, which is located below the arachnoid membrane and above the pia mater, contains cerebrospinal fluid.

The Pia Mater

The **pia mater** (**PEE**-ah **MAH**-ter), which is the third layer of the meninges, is located nearest to the brain and spinal cord. It consists of delicate connective tissue that contains a rich supply of blood vessels. *Pia* means tender or delicate, and *mater* means mother.

Cerebrospinal Fluid

Cerebrospinal fluid (**ser**-eh-broh-**SPY**-nal), also known as *spinal fluid*, is produced by special capillaries within the four ventricles located in the middle region of the cerebrum (see Figures 10.3 and 10.4). Cerebrospinal fluid is a clear, colorless, and watery fluid that flows throughout the brain and around the spinal cord. The functions of this fluid are to:

- Cool and cushion these organs from shock or injury.
- Nourish the brain and spinal cord by transporting nutrients and chemical messengers to these tissues.

The Parts of the Brain

The brain parts are shown in Figures 10.4 through 10.7. The body functions that are controlled by these brain parts

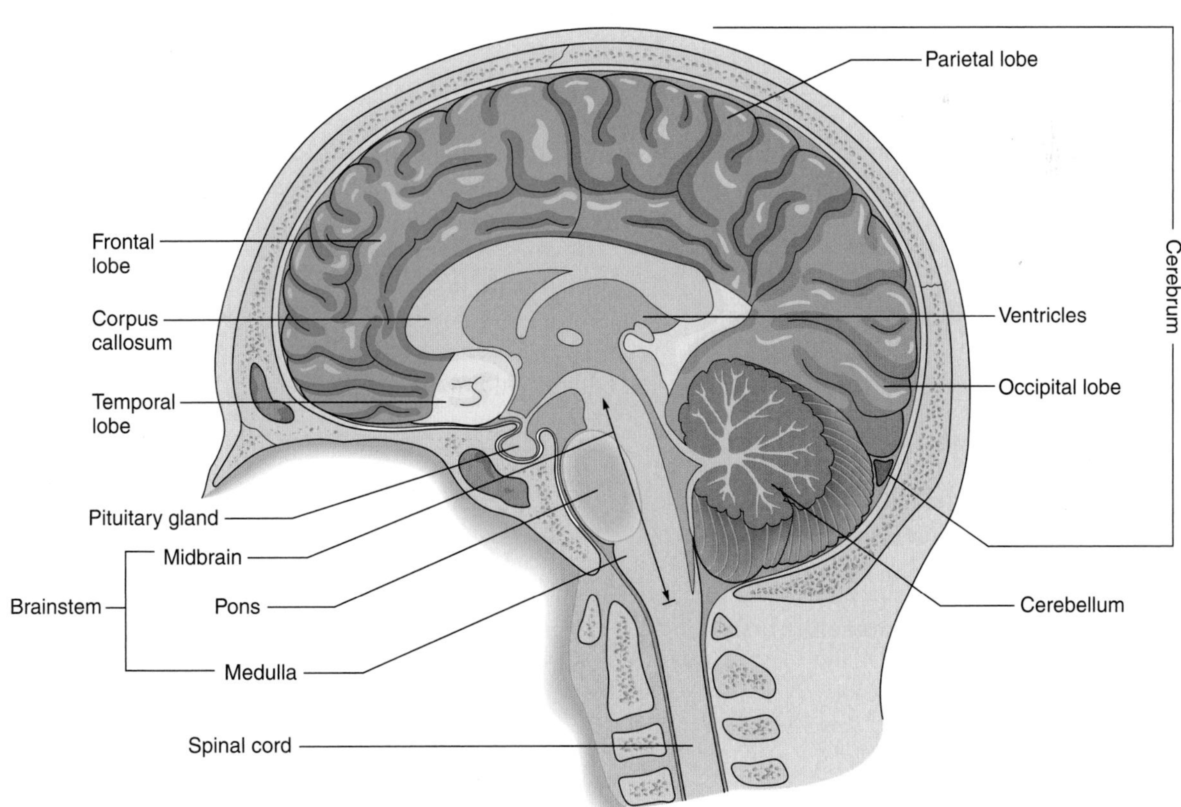

FIGURE 10.4 A cross-section showing the major parts of the brain.

are summarized in Table 10.2. Notice that the functions most essential to the support of life are located within the most protected portions of the brain.

The Cerebrum

The **cerebrum** (seh-**REE**-brum) is the largest and uppermost portion of the brain. It is responsible for all thought, judgment, memory, and emotion, as well as for controlling and integrating motor and sensory functions. Note that *cerebrum* and *cerebellum* are similar words, but refer to very different parts of the brain. Memory aid: The cere*bel*lum is *bel*ow the cerebrum.

- The term **cerebral** (**SER**-eh-bral) means pertaining to the cerebrum or to the brain (**cerebr** means brain, and **-al** means pertaining to).
- The *cerebral cortex*, which is made up of gray matter, is the outer layer of the cerebrum and is arranged in deep folds known as fissures. As used here, a *fissure* is a normally occurring deep groove. Skin fissures, which are crack-like sores, are discussed in Chapter 12.

The Cerebral Hemispheres

The cerebrum is divided to create two **cerebral hemispheres** that are connected at the lower midpoint by the *corpus callosum* (Figure 10.5).

- The *left cerebral hemisphere* controls the majority of functions on the right side of the body. An injury to the left hemisphere produces sensory and motor deficits on the right side of the body.
- The *right cerebral hemisphere* controls most of functions on the left side of the body. An injury to the right hemisphere produces sensory and motor deficits on the left side of the body.
- The crossing of nerve fibers that makes this arrangement possible occurs in the brain stem (see Figure 10.4).

The Cerebral Lobes

Each cerebral hemisphere is subdivided to create pairs of **cerebral lobes**. Each lobe is named for the bone of the cranium that covers it (Figure 10.6).

- The *frontal lobe* controls skilled motor functions, memory, and behavior.

TABLE 10.2

BRAIN PARTS AND THEIR FUNCTIONS

Brain Part	Functions
The **cerebrum**, which is the largest and uppermost part of the brain, consists of four lobes.	Controls the highest level of thought, including judgment, memory, association, and critical thinking. It also processes sensations and controls all voluntary muscle activity.
The **thalamus** is located below the cerebrum.	Relays sensory stimuli from the spinal cord and midbrain to the cerebral cortex. The thalamus suppresses some stimuli and magnifies others.
The **hypothalamus** is located below the thalamus	Controls vital bodily functions (Table 10.3).
The **cerebellum** is located in the lower back of the cranium below the cerebrum.	Coordinates muscular activity and balance for smooth and steady movements.
The **brainstem** is located in the base of the brain and forms the connection between the brain and spinal cord. It consists of the: ▪ midbrain ▪ pons ▪ medulla	Controls the functions necessary for survival (breathing, digestion, heart rate, and blood pressure), and for arousal (being awake and alert).

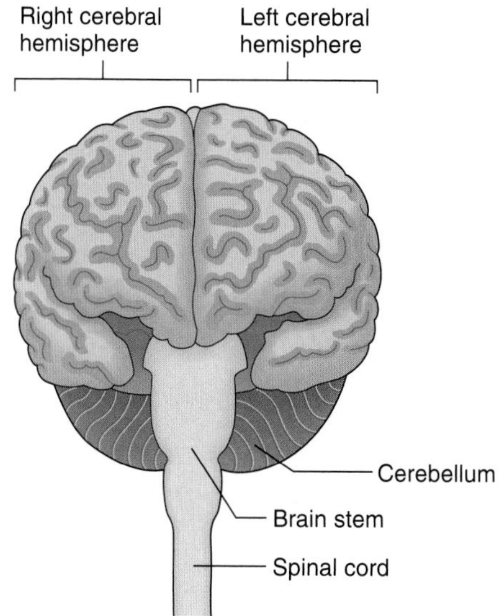

FIGURE 10.5 An anterior view showing how the brain is divided into right and left hemispheres.

- The *parietal lobe* receives and interprets nerve impulses from sensory receptors in the tongue, skin, and muscles.
- The *occipital lobe* controls eyesight.
- The *temporal lobe* controls the senses of hearing and smell, and the ability to create, store, and access new information.

The Thalamus

The **thalamus** (**THAL**-ah-mus), which is located below the cerebrum, produces sensations by relaying impulses to and from the cerebrum and the sense organs of the body (Figure 10.7).

The Hypothalamus

The **hypothalamus** (**high**-poh-**THAL**-ah-mus) is located below the thalamus (see Figure 10.7). The seven major regulatory functions of the hypothalamus are summarized in Table 10.3.

The Cerebellum

The **cerebellum** (**ser**-eh-**BELL**-um) is the second-largest part of the brain. It is located at the back of the head below the posterior portion of the cerebrum (see Figures 10.4–10.7).

- The cerebellum receives incoming messages regarding movement within joints, muscle tone, and positions of the body. From here, messages are relayed to the different parts of the brain that control the motions of skeletal muscles.
- The general functions of the cerebellum are to produce smooth, coordinated movements, to maintain equilibrium, and to sustain normal postures.

The Brainstem

The **brainstem** is the stalk-like portion of the brain that connects the cerebral hemispheres with the spinal cord. It is made up of three parts: the midbrain, pons, and medulla (see Figures 10.3 and 10.7).

- The **midbrain** and **pons (PONZ)** provide conduction pathways to and from the higher and lower centers in the brain. They also control reflexes for movements of the eyes and head in response to visual and auditory stimuli. (*Pons* is the Latin word for bridge.)
- The **medulla** (meh-**DULL**-ah), which is located at the lowest part of the brainstem, is connected to the spinal

TABLE 10.3

REGULATORY FUNCTIONS OF THE HYPOTHALAMUS

1.	Regulates and integrates the autonomic nervous system, including controlling heart rate, blood pressure, respiratory rate, and digestive tract activity.
2.	Regulates emotional responses, including fear and pleasure.
3.	Regulates body temperature.
4.	Regulates food intake by controlling hunger sensations.
5.	Regulates water balance by controlling thirst sensations.
6.	Regulates sleep-wakefulness cycles.
7.	Regulates the pituitary gland and endocrine system activity (see Chapter 13).

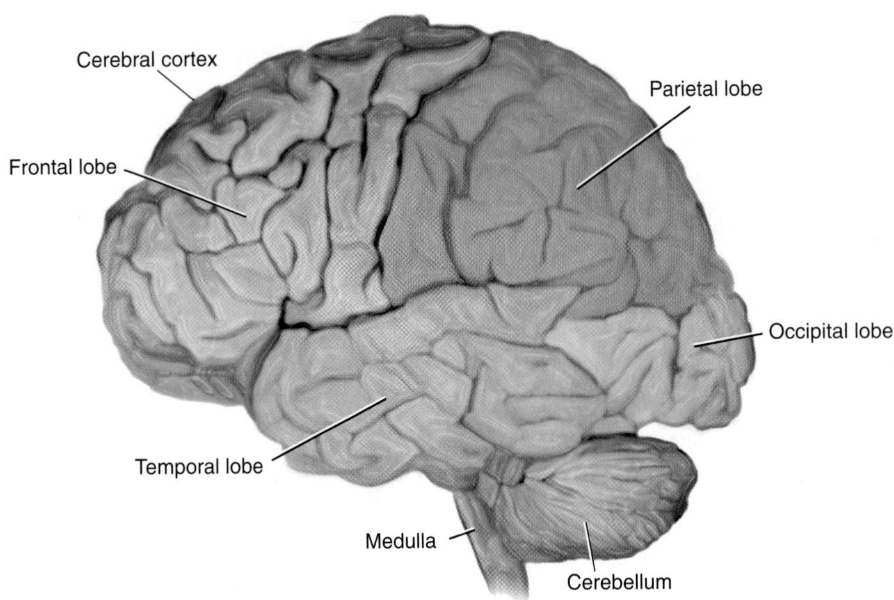

FIGURE 10.6 A left lateral view of the exterior of the brain showing the four cerebral lobes plus the medulla and the cerebellum.

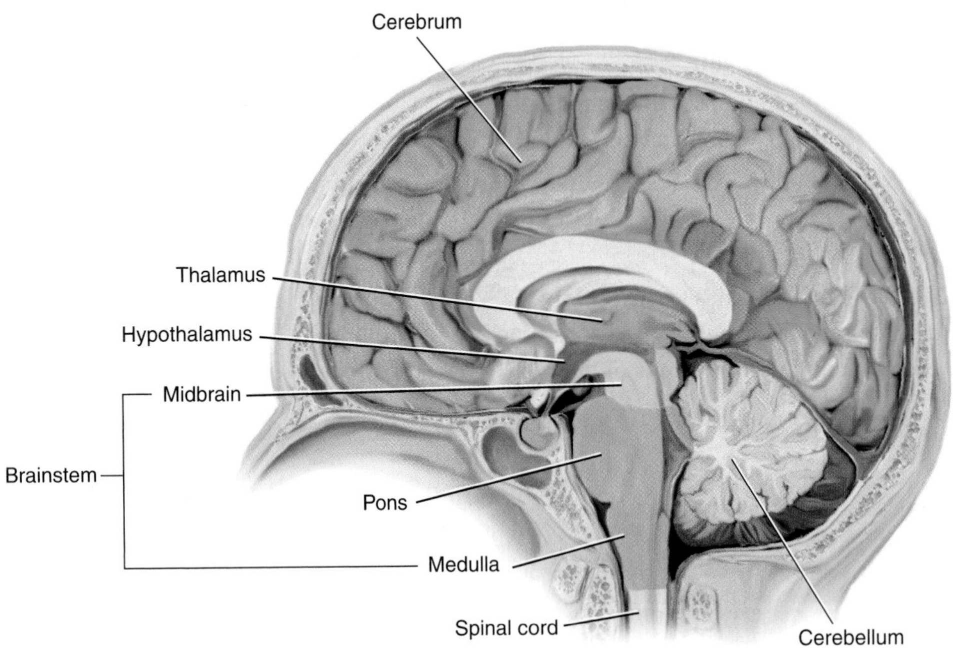

FIGURE 10.7 A schematic representation of the inner structures of the brain.

cord. It controls basic survival functions, including the muscles that make possible respiration, heart rate, and blood pressure, as well as reflexes for coughing, sneezing, swallowing, and vomiting.

The Spinal Cord

The **spinal cord** is a long, fragile tube-like structure that begins at the end of the brain stem and continues down almost to the bottom of the spinal column (see Figure 10.1).

- The spinal cord contains all the nerves that affect the limbs and lower part of the body, and serves as the pathway for impulses traveling to and from the brain.
- The spinal cord is surrounded and protected by cerebrospinal fluid and the meninges.

THE PERIPHERAL NERVOUS SYSTEM

The **peripheral nervous system** consists of the 12 pairs of cranial nerves that extend from the brain, plus 31 pairs of spinal nerves that extending from the spinal cord. *Peripheral* means pertaining to body parts that are away from the center of the body.

Three types of specialized peripheral nerves transmit signals to and from the central nervous system. These are autonomic, sensory, and somatic nerve fibers.

- *Autonomic nerve fibers* carry instructions to the organs and glands and from the autonomic nervous system.
- *Sensory nerve fibers* receive external stimuli, such as how something feels, and transmit this information to the brain where it is interpreted. *Somatic nerve fibers*, which are also known as *motor nerve fibers*, convey information that controls the body's voluntary muscular movements.

The Cranial Nerves

The 12 pairs of **cranial nerves** originate from the undersurface of the brain. The two nerves of a pair are identical in function and structure, and each nerve of a pair serves half of the body.

These cranial nerves are identified by Roman numerals and are named for the area or function they serve (Figure 10.8).

The Peripheral Spinal Nerves

The 31 pairs of **peripheral spinal nerves** are grouped together, and named, based on the region of the body they innervate, as shown in Figure 10.9.

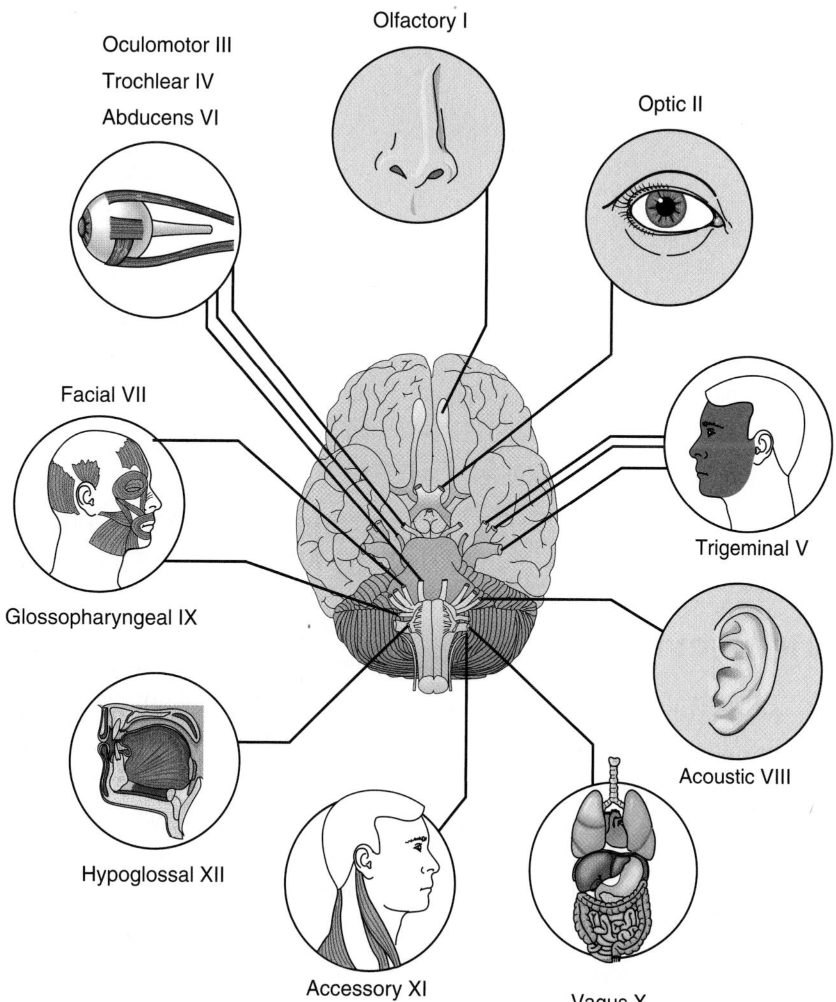

FIGURE 10.8 Cranial nerves are identified with Roman numerals and are named for the area, or function, they serve.

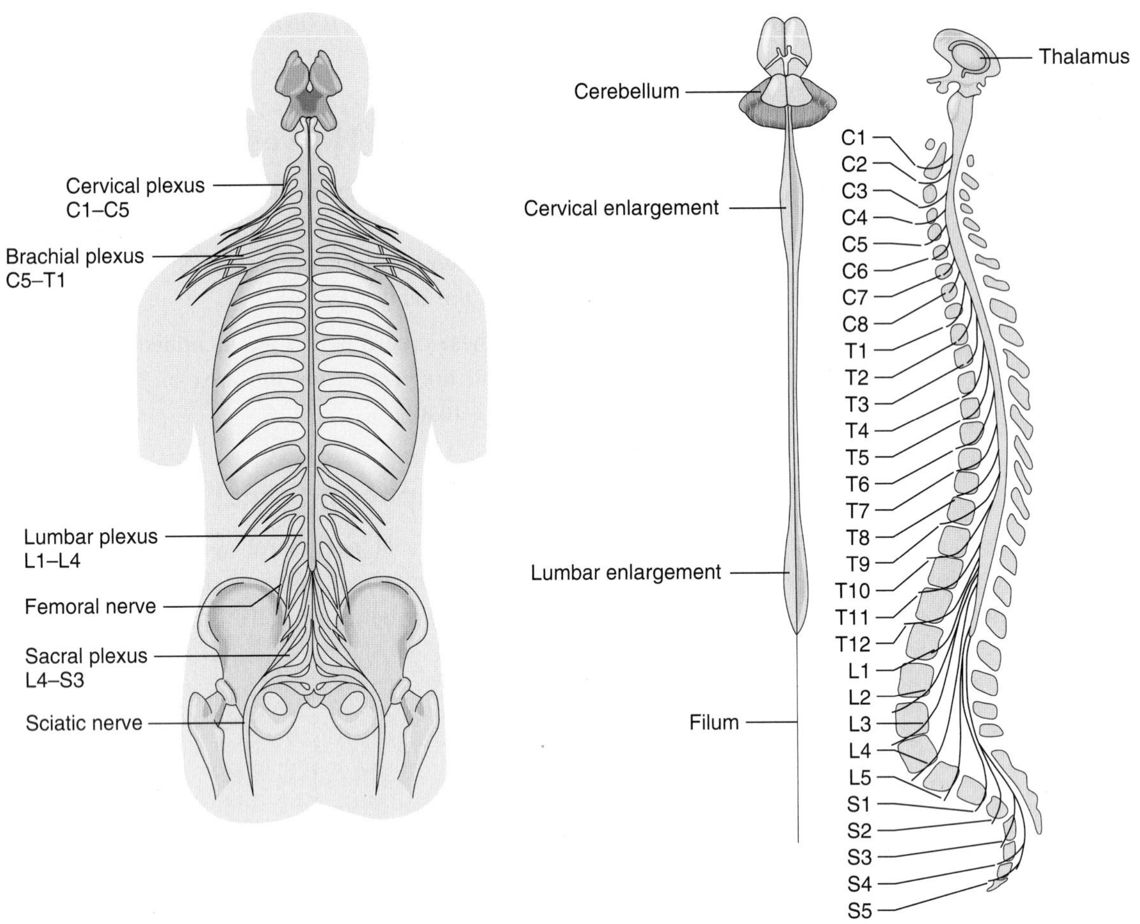

FIGURE 10.9 The spinal cord and nerves. Most spinal cord plexuses are named for the corresponding vertebrae.

- Within each region, the nerves are referred to by number. The cervical nerves are C1–C8, the thoracic nerves are T1–T12, the lumbar nerves are L1–L5, and the sacral nerves are S1–S5.
- Spinal nerves sometimes join with others to form a plexus to innervate a certain area. The lumbar plexus, as shown in Figure 10.9, is made up of the first four lumbar nerves (L1–L4) and serves the lower back.

THE AUTONOMIC NERVOUS SYSTEM

The **autonomic nervous system**, which is organized into two divisions, controls the involuntary actions of the body such as the functioning of internal organs (Figures 10.10 and 10.11). In order to maintain homeostasis within the body, each division balances the activity of the other division. *Homeostasis* is the process of maintaining the constant internal environment of the body.

- The **sympathetic nervous system** prepares the body for emergencies and stress by increasing the breathing rate, heart rate, and blood flow to muscles (Figure 10.10).
- The **parasympathetic nervous system** returns the body to normal after a response to stress (Figure 10.11). It also maintains normal body functions during ordinary circumstances that are not emotionally or physically stressful.

MEDICAL SPECIALTIES RELATED TO THE NERVOUS SYSTEM

- An **anesthesiologist** (**an**-es-**thee**-zee-**OL**-oh-jist) is a physician who specializes in administering anesthetic agents before and during surgery (**an-** means without, **esthesi** means feeling, and **-ologist** means specialist).
- An **anesthetist** (ah-**NES**-theh-tist) is a medical professional who specializes in administering anesthesia, but is not a physician, for example, a nurse anesthetist (**an-** means without, **esthet** means feeling, and **-ist** means specialist).
- A **neurologist** (new-**ROL**-oh-jist) is a physician who specializes in diagnosing and treating diseases and disorders of the nervous system (**neur** means nerve, and **-ologist** means specialist).

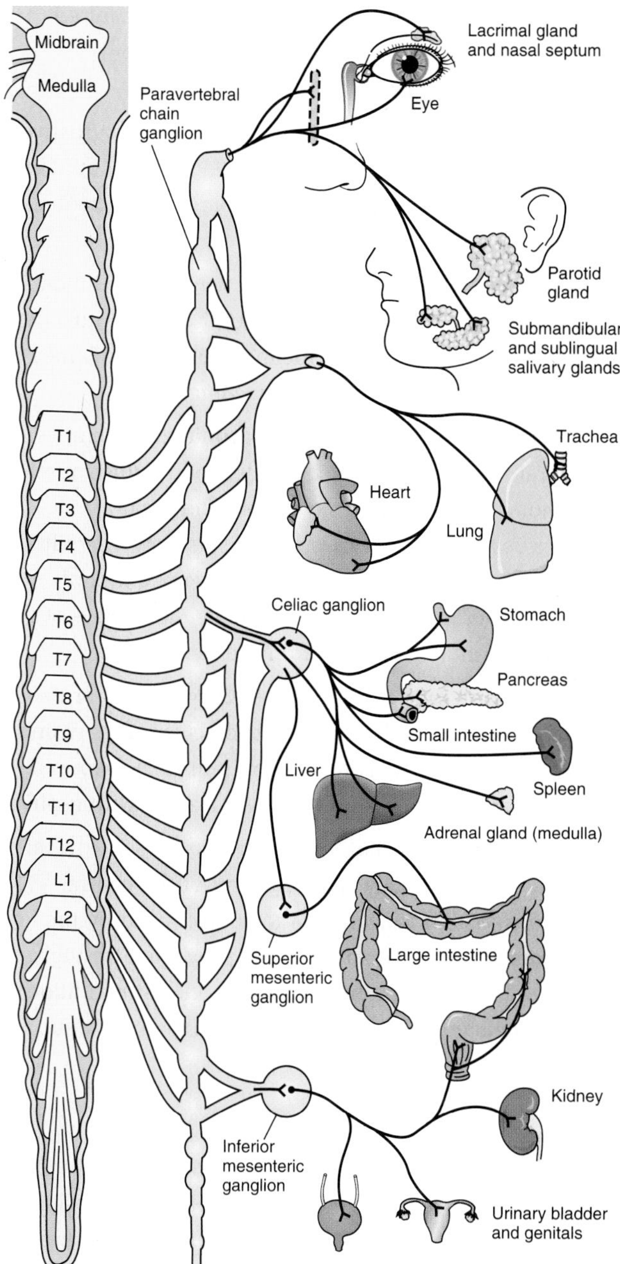

FIGURE 10.10 The nerve pathways of the sympathetic division of the autonomic nervous system.

- A **neurosurgeon** is a physician who specializes in surgery of the nervous system.
- A **psychiatrist** (sigh-**KYE**-ah-trist) is a physician who specializes in diagnosing and treating chemical dependencies, emotional problems, and mental illness (**psych** means mind, and **-iatrist** means specialist).
- A **psychologist** (sigh-**KOL**-oh-jist) holds an advanced degree, but is not a medical doctor (MD). This specialist evaluates and treats emotional problems and mental illness (**psych** means mind, and **-ologist** means specialist).

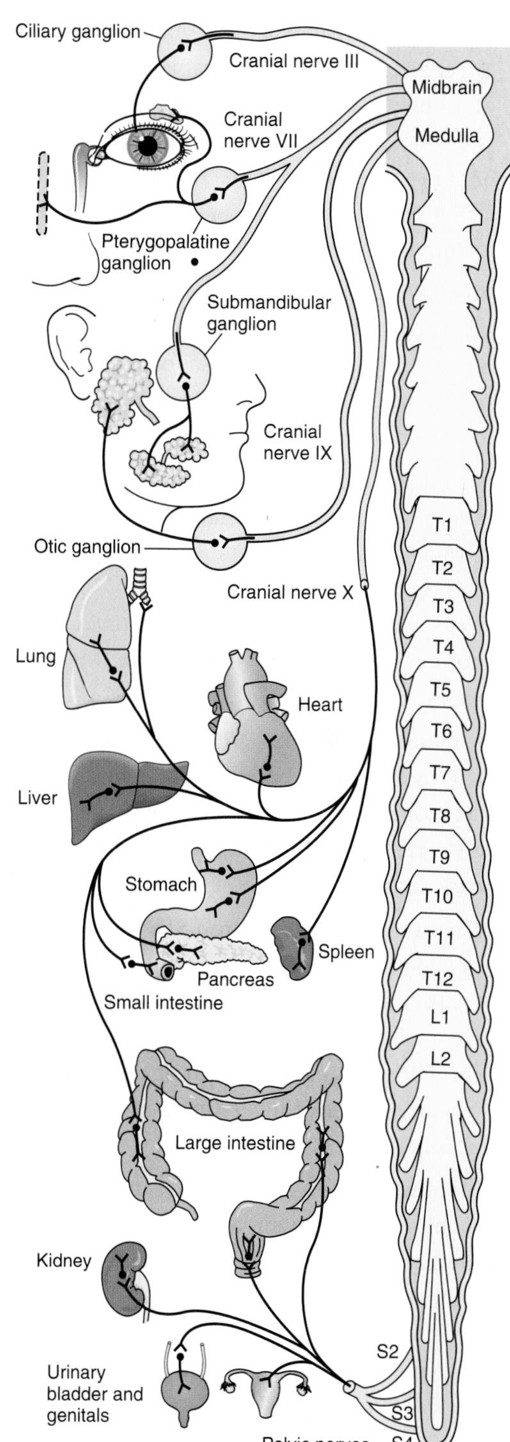

FIGURE 10.11 The nerve pathways of the parasympathetic division of the autonomic nervous system.

PATHOLOGY OF THE NERVOUS SYSTEM

The Head and Meninges

- **Cephalalgia** (**sef**-ah-**LAL**-jee-ah), also known as a *headache*, is pain in the head (**cephal** means head, and **-algia** means pain).

- A **migraine headache** (**MY**-grayn), which can be preceded by a warning aura, is characterized by throbbing pain on one side of the head. As used here, a *warning aura* is a sensation perceived by the patient that precedes a migraine. These headaches, which affect primarily women, are accompanied by nausea, vomiting, and sensitivity to light or sound.
- **Cluster headaches** are intensely painful headaches that affect one side of the head and may be associated with tearing of the eyes and nasal congestion. These headaches, which affect primarily men, are named for their repeated occurrence in groups or clusters.
- An **encephalocele** (en-**SEF**-ah-loh-**seel**), also known as a *craniocele*, is a congenital herniation of brain tissue through a gap in the skull (**encephal/o** means brain, and **-cele** means hernia). *Congenital* means present at birth, and *herniation* means protrusion of a structure from its normal position. Compare this with a *meningocele*.
- A **meningocele** (meh-**NING**-goh-**seel**) is the congenital herniation of the meninges through a defect in the skull or spinal column (**mening/o** means meninges, and **-cele** means hernia). Compare this with an *encephalocele*.
- **Hydrocephalus** (high-droh-**SEF**-ah-lus) is a condition in which excess cerebrospinal fluid accumulates in the ventricles of the brain (**hydr/o** means water, **cephal** means head, and **-us** is a singular noun ending). This condition can occur at birth or develop later on in life from obstructions related to meningitis, brain tumors, or other causes.
- **Meningitis** (**men**-in-**JIGH**-tis) is an inflammation of the meninges of the brain and spinal cord (**mening** means meninges, and **-itis** means inflammation). This condition, which can be fatal, is usually caused by a bacterial or viral infection and is characterized by fever, vomiting, intense headache, and a stiff neck. Compare with *encephalitis*.

Disorders of the Brain

- **Alzheimer's disease** (**ALTZ**-high-merz) is a group of disorders involving the parts of the brain that control thought, memory, and language. It is marked by progressive deterioration that affects both the memory and reasoning capabilities of an individual.
- The term **cognition** (kog-**NISH**-un) describes the mental activities associated with thinking, learning, and memory. *Mild cognitive impairment* is a memory disorder, usually associated with recently acquired information, that may be an early predictor of Alzheimer's disease.
- **Dementia** (dee-**MEN**-shee-ah) is a slowly progressive decline in mental abilities, including memory, thinking, and judgment, that is often accompanied by personality changes.
- **Encephalitis** (**en**-sef-ah-**LYE**-tis), which is an inflammation of the brain, can be caused by a viral infection such as rabies (**encelphal** means brain, and **-itis** means inflammation). Compare with *meningitis*.
- **Parkinson's disease** (PD) is a chronic, degenerative central nervous disorder characterized by fine muscle tremors, rigidity, and a slow or shuffling gait.*Gait* describes the manner of walking. This slow or shuffling gait is caused by the gradually progressive loss of control over movements due to inadequate levels of the neurotransmitter dopamine in the brain.
- **Reye's syndrome** (RS) is a potentially serious or deadly disorder in children that is characterized by vomiting and confusion. This syndrome usually follows a viral illness in which the child was treated with aspirin.
- **Tetanus** (**TET**-ah-nus), also known as *lockjaw*, is an acute and potentially fatal infection of the central nervous system caused by a toxin produced by the tetanus bacteria. Tetanus can be prevented through immunization. Without this protection, this condition is typically acquired through a deep puncture wound.

Brain Injuries

- **Amnesia** (am-**NEE**-zee-ah) is a memory disturbance characterized by a total or partial inability to recall past experiences. This condition can be caused by a brain injury, illness, or a psychological disturbance.
- A **concussion** (kon-**KUSH**-un) is a violent shaking up or jarring of the brain (**concuss** means shaken together, and **-ion** means condition or state of). A concussion may result in a temporary loss of awareness and function. Compare with a *cerebral contusion*.
- A **cerebral contusion** (**SER**-eh-bral kon-**TOO**-zhun) is the bruising of brain tissue as the result of a head injury that causes the brain to bounce against the rigid bone of the skull (**contus** means bruise, and **-ion** means condition). Compare with *concussion*.
- A **cranial hematoma** (**hee**-mah-**TOH**-mah) is a collection of blood trapped in the tissues of the brain (**hemat** means blood, and **-oma** means tumor). Named

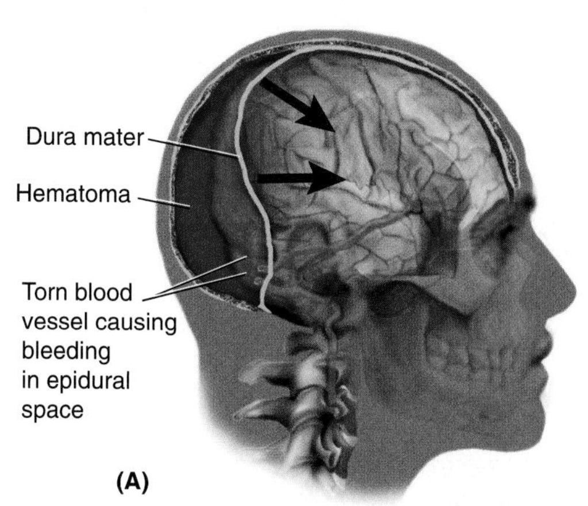

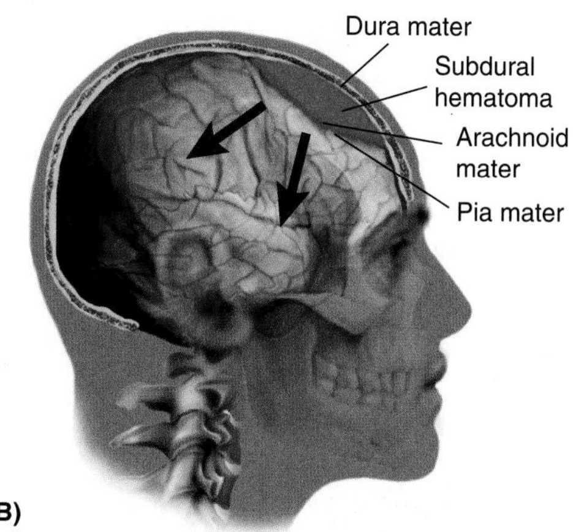

FIGURE 10.12 Cranial hematomas. (A) Epidural hematoma. (B) Subdural hematoma.

for their location, the types of cranial hematomas include an *epidural hematoma* located above the dura mater or a *subdural hematoma*, which is located below the dura mater (Figure 10.12).

Traumatic Brain Injury

A **traumatic brain injury** is a blow to the head or a penetrating head injury that damages the brain. Not all blows to the head result in damage to the brain. When an injury does occur, it can range from mild, with only a brief change in mental status, to severe, with longer lasting effects.

- The term *coup* describes an injury occurring within the skull near the point of impact, such as hitting the windshield in an auto accident. A *contrecoup*, also described as a *counter blow*, is an injury that occurs beneath the skull opposite to the area of impact (Figure 10.13).
- **Shaken baby syndrome** describes the results of a child being violently shaken by someone. This action can cause brain injury, blindness, fractures, seizures, paralysis, and death.

Levels of Consciousness

Levels of consciousness (LOC) are terms used to describe alterations of consciousness caused by injury, disease, or substances such as medication, drugs, or alcohol.

- Being **conscious** is the state of being awake, alert, aware, and responding appropriately.
- Being **unconscious** is a state of being unaware and unable to respond to any stimuli including pain.
- **Lethargy** (**LETH**-ar-jee) is a lowered level of consciousness marked by listlessness, drowsiness, and apathy. As used here, *apathy* means indifference and a reduced level of activity. The term *lethargic* refers to a person who is at this level of consciousness.
- A **stupor** (**STOO**-per) is an unresponsive state from which a person can be aroused only briefly and with vigorous, repeated attempts.
- **Syncope** (**SIN**-koh-pee), also known as *fainting*, is the brief loss of consciousness caused by the decreased flow of blood to the brain.
- A **coma** (**KOH**-mah) is a profound (deep) state of unconsciousness marked by the absence of spontaneous eye movements, no response to painful stimuli, and the lack of speech. The term *comatose* refers to a person who is in a coma.
- A **persistent vegetative state** is a type of coma in which the patient exhibits alternating sleep and wake cycles; however, due to severe damage to certain areas of the brain, the person is unconscious even when appearing to be awake.

Delirium

Delirium (dee-**LIR**-ee-um) is an acute condition of confusion, disorientation, disordered thinking and memory, agitation, and hallucinations.

This condition is usually caused by a treatable physical condition, such as a high fever. An individual suffering from this condition is described as being *delirious*.

Brain Tumors

A **brain tumor** is an abnormal growth located inside the skull (Figure 10.14).

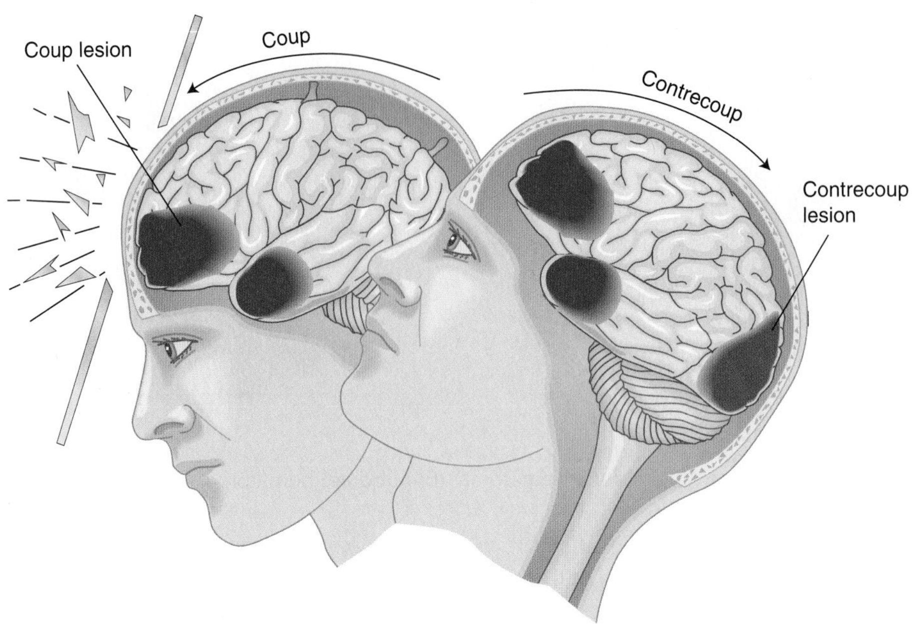

FIGURE 10.13 Coup and contrecoup brain injuries.

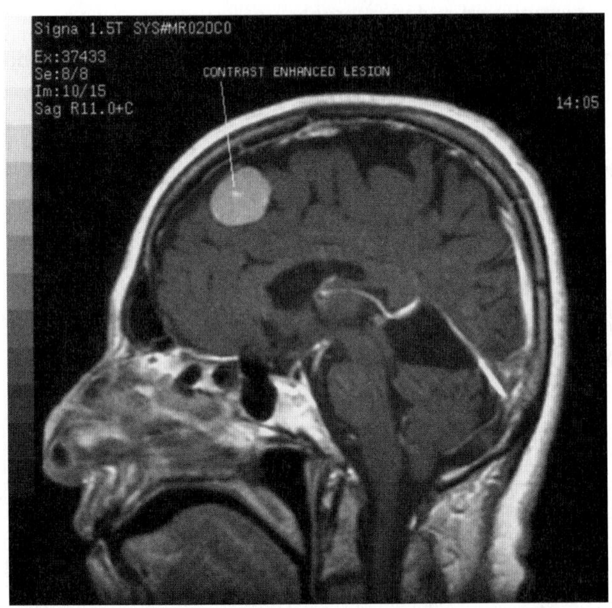

FIGURE 10.14 A brain tumor visualized by magnetic resonance imaging (MRI).

- An invasive *malignant brain tumor* destroys brain tissue. When this cancer originates in the brain, it is considered to be the primary site. If this cancer metastasizes (spreads) to the brain from another body system, it is considered to be a secondary site.
- A *benign brain tumor* does not invade the brain tissue; however, because this growth is surrounded by rigid bone, as the tumor enlarges, it can damage the brain tissue by placing pressure against the tissues and by increasing the intracranial pressure.
- **Intracranial pressure** is the amount of pressure inside the skull (**intra-** means within, **crani** means cranium, and **-al** means pertaining to). Elevated intracranial pressure can be due to a tumor, an injury, or improper drainage of cerebrospinal fluid.

Strokes

A stroke, or CVA, is properly known as a **cerebrovascular accident** (**ser**-eh-broh-**VAS**-kyou-lar). This condition is damage to the brain that occurs when the blood flow to the brain is disrupted because a blood vessel is either blocked or has ruptured. The location of the disruption determines the symptoms that will be present. Damage to the right side of the brain produces symptoms on the left side of the body. Damage to the left side of the brain produces symptoms on the right side of the body (Figure 10.15).

Ischemic Stroke

An **ischemic stroke** (iss-**KEE**-mick), which is the most common type of stroke in older people, occurs when the flow of blood to the brain is blocked. This type of stroke may be caused by narrowing of the carotid artery or by a cerebral thrombosis. A *cerebral thrombosis* occurs when a blood clot blocks an artery that supplies blood to the

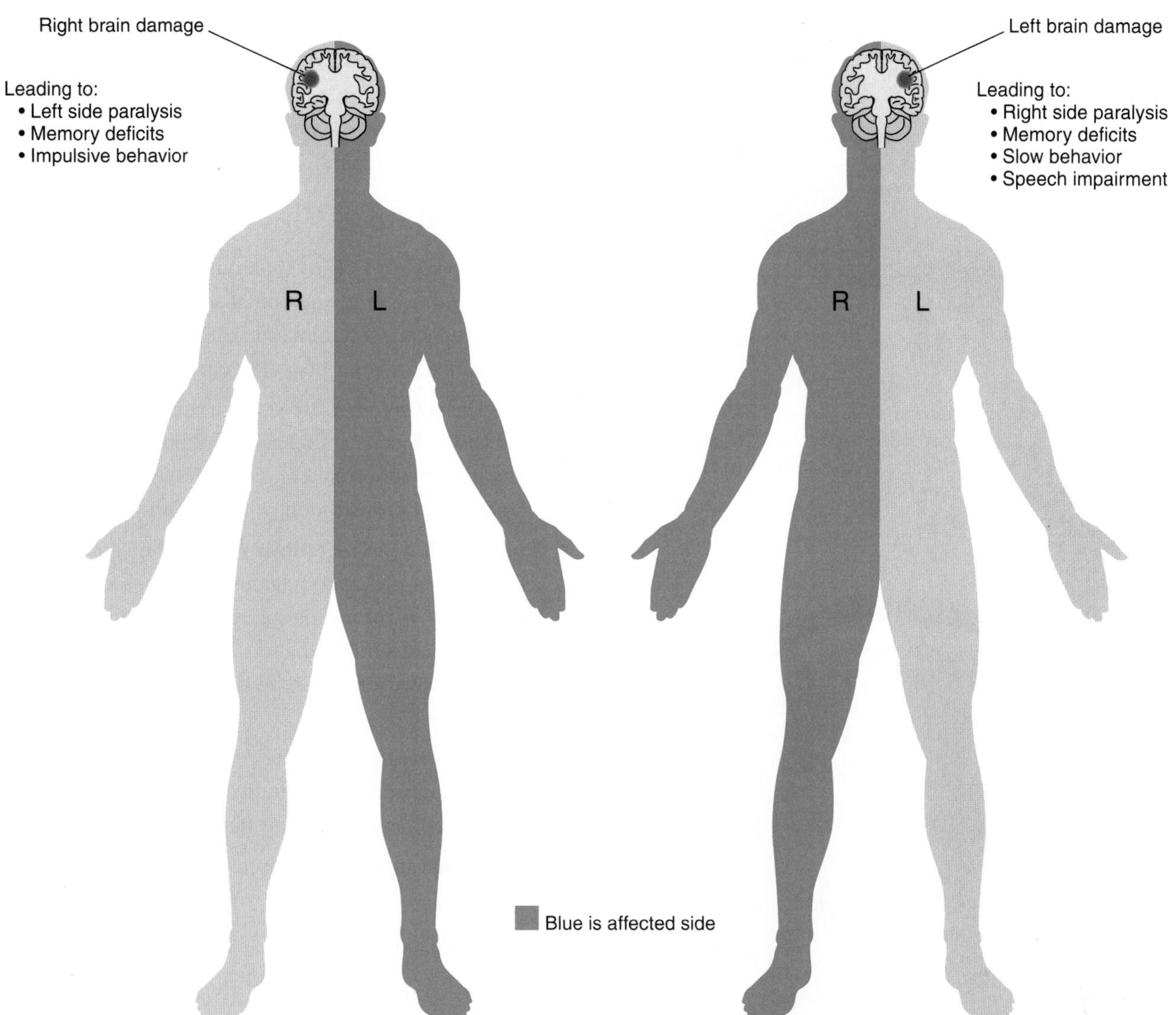

FIGURE 10.15 The location of the damage caused by a cerebrovascular accident depends upon which side of the brain is affected.

cerebrum. This blockage damages the controls of movement, senses, and speech.

- A **transient ischemic attack** (TIA), pronounced as *T-I-A*, is the temporary interruption in the blood supply to the brain. *Transient* means passing quickly, and *ischemic* means pertaining to the disruption of the blood supply. Symptoms of a TIA include numbness, blurred vision, dizziness, or loss of balance. A TIA passes in less than an hour; however, this incident is often a warning sign that the individual is at risk for a more serious and debilitating stroke.
- **Aphasia** (ah-**FAY**-zee-ah), which is often caused by brain damage associated with a stroke, is the loss of the ability to speak, write, and/or comprehend the written or spoken word (**a-** means without, and **-phasia** means speech).

Hemorrhagic Stroke

A **hemorrhagic stroke** (**hem**-oh-**RAJ**-ick), also known as a *bleed*, occurs when a blood vessel in the brain leaks. A bleed also occurs when an aneurysm within the brain ruptures. An *aneurysm* is a localized, weak, balloon-like enlargement of an artery wall. This type of stroke is less common than ischemic strokes and is often fatal. A hemorrhagic stroke affects the area of the brain damaged by the leaking blood (Figures 10.16 and 10.17).

Sleep Disorders

- **Insomnia** is the prolonged or abnormal inability to sleep. This condition is usually a symptom of another problem such as depression, pain, or excessive caffeine

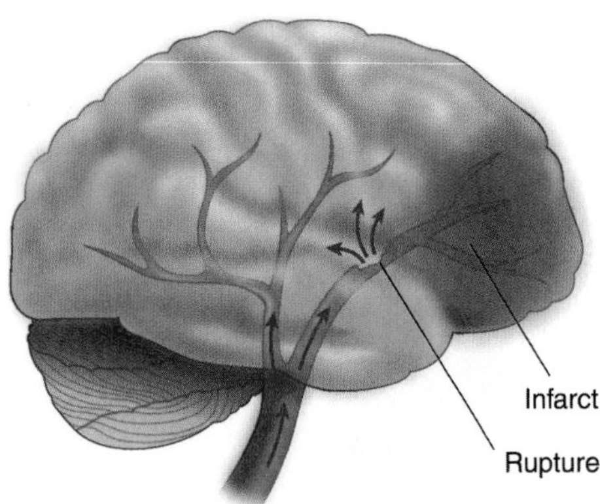

FIGURE 10.16 In a hemorrhagic stroke, the rupture of a blood vessel causes decreased blood flow to an area of the brain tissue. An *infarct* is a localized area of dead tissue caused by a lack of blood.

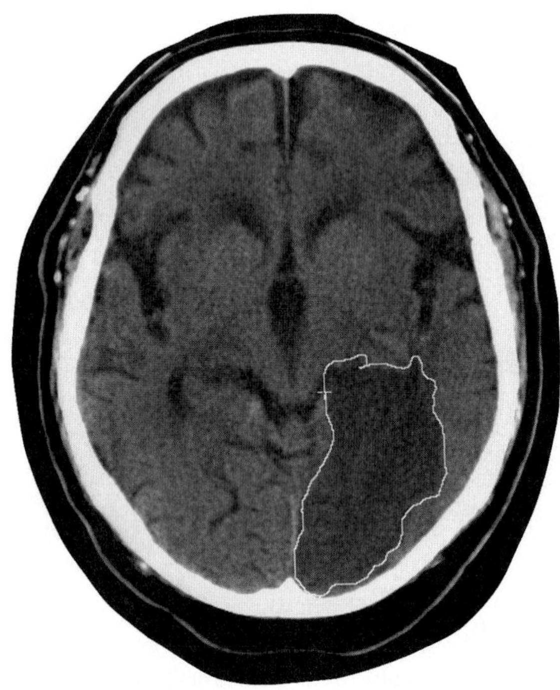

FIGURE 10.17 Magnetic resonance image of a brain with the area of a bleed visible in the lower right.

(**in**- means without, **somn** means sleep, and **-ia** means abnormal condition).

- **Narcolepsy** (**NAR**-koh-**lep**-see) is a sleep disorder consisting of sudden and uncontrollable brief episodes of falling asleep during the day (**narc/o** means stupor, and **-lepsy** means seizure).
- **Sleep deprivation** is a sufficient lack of restorative sleep over cumulative period so as to cause physical or psychiatric symptoms and affect routine performance or tasks.
- **Somnambulism** (som-**NAM**-byou-lizm), also known as *sleepwalking* or *noctambulism*, is the condition of walking or performing some other activity without awakening (**somn** means sleep, **ambul** means to walk, and **-ism** means condition of).

The Spinal Cord

- **Myelitis** (**my**-eh-**LYE**-tis) is an inflammation of the spinal cord (**myel** means spinal cord and bone marrow, and **-itis** means inflammation). The term *myelitis* also means inflammation of bone marrow.
- A **myelosis** (**my**-eh-**LOH**-sis) is a tumor of the spinal cord (**myel** means spinal cord and bone marrow, and **-osis** means abnormal condition). *Myelosis* also means an abnormal proliferation of bone marrow tissue.
- **Poliomyelitis** (**poh**-lee-oh-**my**-eh-**LYE**-tis), also known as *polio*, is a highly contagious viral disease (**poli/o** means gray, **myel** means spinal cord and bone marrow, and **-itis** means inflammation). There is no known cure for polio; however, it can be prevented through vaccination.
- *Post-polio syndrome* is the recurrence later in life of some polio symptoms in individuals who have had childhood poliomyelitis and have recovered from it.
- **Spinal cord injuries** are discussed in Chapter 4 under Paralysis.

Pinched Nerves

Radiculitis (rah-**dick**-you-**LYE**-tis), also known as a *pinched nerve*, is an inflammation of the root of a spinal nerve that causes pain and numbness radiating down the affected limb (**radicul** means root or nerve root, and **-itis** means inflammation). This term usually applies to that portion of the root that lies between the spinal cord and the intervertebral canal of the spinal column. Figure 3.20 shows one cause of this condition.

- **Cervical radiculopathy** (rah-**dick**-you-**LOP**-ah-thee) is nerve pain caused by pressure on the spinal nerve roots in the neck region (**radicul/o** means nerve root, and **-pathy** means disease).
- **Lumbar radiculopathy** is nerve pain in the lower back caused by muscle spasms or by nerve root irritation from the compression of vertebral disks such as a herniated disk.

Multiple Sclerosis

Multiple sclerosis (skleh-**ROH**-sis) is a progressive autoimmune disorder characterized by inflammation that causes demyelination of the myelin sheath. This scars the brain, spinal cord, and optic nerves and disrupts the transmission of nerve impulses. This damage leaves the patient with varying degrees of pain plus physical and cognitive problems.

- *Demyelination* is the loss of patches of the protective myelin sheath.
- The disease is characterized by periods of *exacerbations*, which are episodes of worsening symptoms that are also referred to as *flares*. Between these episodes, the patient may be in remission. *Remission* is a time during which the symptoms ease, but the disease has not been cured.

Nerves

- **Amyotrophic lateral sclerosis** (ah-**my**-oh-**TROH**-fick), also known as *Lou Gehrig's disease*, is a rapidly progressive neurological disease that attacks the nerve cells responsible for controlling voluntary muscles. Patients affected with this condition become progressively weaker until they are completely paralyzed and die.
- **Bell's palsy** is the temporary paralysis of the seventh cranial nerve that causes paralysis only of the affected side of the face. In addition, paralysis symptoms can include the inability to close the eye, pain, tearing, drooling, hypersensitivity to sound in the affected ear, and impairment of taste.
- **Guillain-Barré syndrome** (gee-**YAHN**-bah-**RAY**), also known as *infectious polyneuritis*, is an inflammation of the myelin sheath of peripheral nerves, characterized by rapidly worsening muscle weakness that can lead to temporary paralysis. This condition is an autoimmune reaction that can occur after certain viral infections or an immunization.
- **Sciatica** (sigh-**AT**-ih-kah) is inflammation of the sciatic nerve that results in pain, burning, and tingling along the course of the affected sciatic nerve through the thigh, leg, and foot (see Figure 10.9).
- **Trigeminal neuralgia** (try-**JEM**-ih-nal new-**RAL**-jee-ah) is characterized by severe lightning-like pain due to an inflammation of the fifth cranial nerve. These sudden, intense, brief attacks of sharp pain affect the cheek, lips, and gums only on the side of the face innervated by the affected nerve.

Cerebral Palsy

Cerebral palsy (**SER**-eh-bral **PAWL**-zee) is a condition characterized by poor muscle control, spasticity, speech defects, and other neurologic deficiencies due to damage that affects the cerebrum.*Spasticity* is a condition in which certain muscles are continuously contracted. *Palsy* means paralysis of a body part that is often accompanied by loss of feeling and uncontrolled body movements, such as shaking.

- Cerebral palsy occurs most frequently in premature or low-birthweight infants.
- Cerebral palsy is usually caused by an injury that occurs during pregnancy, birth, or soon after birth.

Epilepsy and Seizures

Epilepsy (**EP**-ih-**lep**-see) is a chronic neurological condition characterized by recurrent episodes of seizures of varying severity. Also known as a *seizure disorder*, epilepsy can usually be controlled with medication.

A **seizure** (**SEE**-zhur) is a sudden surge of electrical activity in the brain that affects how a person feels or acts for a short time. Some seizures can hardly be noticed, whereas others cause a brief loss of consciousness. Seizures are symptoms of different disorders that can affect the brain and also can be caused by extreme high fever, brain injury, or brain lesions.

Abnormal Sensations

- **Causalgia** (kaw-**ZAL**-jee-ah) is persistent, severe burning pain that usually follows an injury to a sensory nerve (**caus** means burning, and **-algia** means pain).
- **Complex regional pain syndrome**, also known as *reflex sympathetic dystrophy syndrome*, is pain that occurs after an injury to an arm or a leg, a heart attack, stroke, or other medical problem. This condition is a form of causalgia with burning pain that is much worse than would be expected due to the injury.
- **Hyperesthesia** (**high**-per-es-**THEE**-zee-ah) is a condition of abnormal and excessive sensitivity to touch, pain, or other sensory stimuli (**hyper-** means excessive, and **-esthesia** means sensation or feeling).
- **Paresthesia** (**pair**-es-**THEE**-zee-ah) refers to a burning or prickling sensation that is usually felt in the hands, arms, legs, or feet, but can also occur in other parts of the body (**par-** means abnormal, and **-esthesia** means sensation or feeling). These sensations may constitute the first symptoms of peripheral neuropathy or it may be a drug side effect.
- **Peripheral neuropathy** (new-**ROP**-ah-thee), also known as *peripheral neuritis*, is a disorder of the nerves that carry information to and from the brain and

spinal cord. This produces pain, the loss of sensation, and the inability to control muscles, particularly in the arms or legs.

- **Restless legs syndrome** (RLS) is a neurological disorder characterized by uncomfortable feelings in the legs, producing a strong urge to move them. The sensation is usually most noticeable at night or when trying to rest.

DIAGNOSTIC PROCEDURES OF THE NERVOUS SYSTEM

- **Magnetic resonance imaging** (MRI) and **computed tomography** (CT) are important neuroimaging tools because they facilitate the examination of the soft tissue structures of the brain and spinal cord (see Figures 10.14 and 10.17). These diagnostic techniques are discussed further in Chapter 15.
- **Carotid ultrasonography** (**ul**-trah-son-**OG**-rah-fee) is an ultrasound study of the carotid artery (**ultra-** means beyond, **son/o** means sound, and **-graphy** means the process of producing a picture or record). This diagnostic test is performed to detect plaque buildup in the artery to predict or diagnose an ischemic stroke.
- **Echoencephalography** (**eck**-oh-en-**sef**-ah-**LOG**-rah-fee) is the use of ultrasound imaging to diagnose a shift in the midline structures of the brain (**ech/o** means sound, **encephal/o** means brain, and **-graphy** means the process of producing a picture or record).
- **Electroencephalography** (ee-**leck**-troh-en-**sef**-ah-**LOG**-rah-fee) is the process of recording the electrical activity of the brain through the use of electrodes attached to the scalp (**electr/o** means electric, **encephal/o** means brain, and **-graphy** means the process of producing a picture or record). The resulting record is an *electroencephalogram*. This electrical activity may also be displayed on a monitor as brain waves.
- **Myelography** (**my**-eh-**LOG**-rah-fee) is a radiographic study of the spinal cord after the injection of a contrast medium through a lumbar puncture (**myel/o** means spinal cord, and **-graphy** means the process of producing a picture or record). The resulting record is a *myelogram*.
- A **lumbar puncture**, also known as a *spinal tap*, is the process of obtaining a sample of cerebrospinal fluid by inserting a needle into the subarachnoid space of the lumbar region to withdraw fluid. Changes in the composition of the cerebrospinal fluid can be an indication of injury, infection, or disease.

TREATMENT PROCEDURES OF THE NERVOUS SYSTEM

Sedative and Hypnotic Medications

- **Amobarbital** (**am**-oh-**BAR**-bih-tal) is a barbiturate used as a sedative and hypnotic.
- A **hypnotic** depresses the central nervous system and usually produces sleep.
- An **anticonvulsant** (**an**-tih-kon-**VUL**-sant) is administered to prevent seizures such as those associated with epilepsy.
- **Barbiturates** (bar-**BIT**-you-raytz) are a class of drugs whose major action is a calming or depressed effect on the central nervous system.
- **Phenobarbital** (**fee**-noh-**BAR**-bih-tal) is a barbiturate used as a sedative and as an anticonvulsant.
- A **sedative** depresses the central nervous system to produce calm and diminished responsiveness without producing sleep. *Sedation* is the effect produced by a sedative.

Anesthesia

Anesthesia (**an**-es-**THEE**-zee-ah) is the absence of normal sensation, especially sensitivity to pain, that is induced by the administration of an anesthetic (**an-** means without, and **-esthesia** means feeling).

- An **anesthetic** (**an**-es-**THET**-ick) is the medication used to induce anesthesia. The anesthetic may be topical, local, regional, or general (**an-** means without, **esthet** means feeling, and **-ic** means pertaining to).
- *Topical anesthesia* numbs only the tissue surface and is applied as a liquid, ointment, or spray.
- *Local anesthesia* causes the loss of sensation in a limited area by injecting an anesthetic solution near that area.
- *Regional anesthesia*, the temporary interruption of nerve conduction, is produced by injecting an anesthetic solution near the nerves to be blocked.
- **Epidural anesthesia** (**ep**-ih-**DOO**-ral **an**-es-**THEE**-zee-ah) is regional anesthesia produced by injecting a local anesthetic into the epidural space of the lumbar or sacral region of the spine. When administered during childbirth, it numbs the nerves from the uterus and birth passage without stopping labor (Figure 10.18).
- *Spinal anesthesia* is produced by injecting an anesthetic into the subarachnoid space that is located below

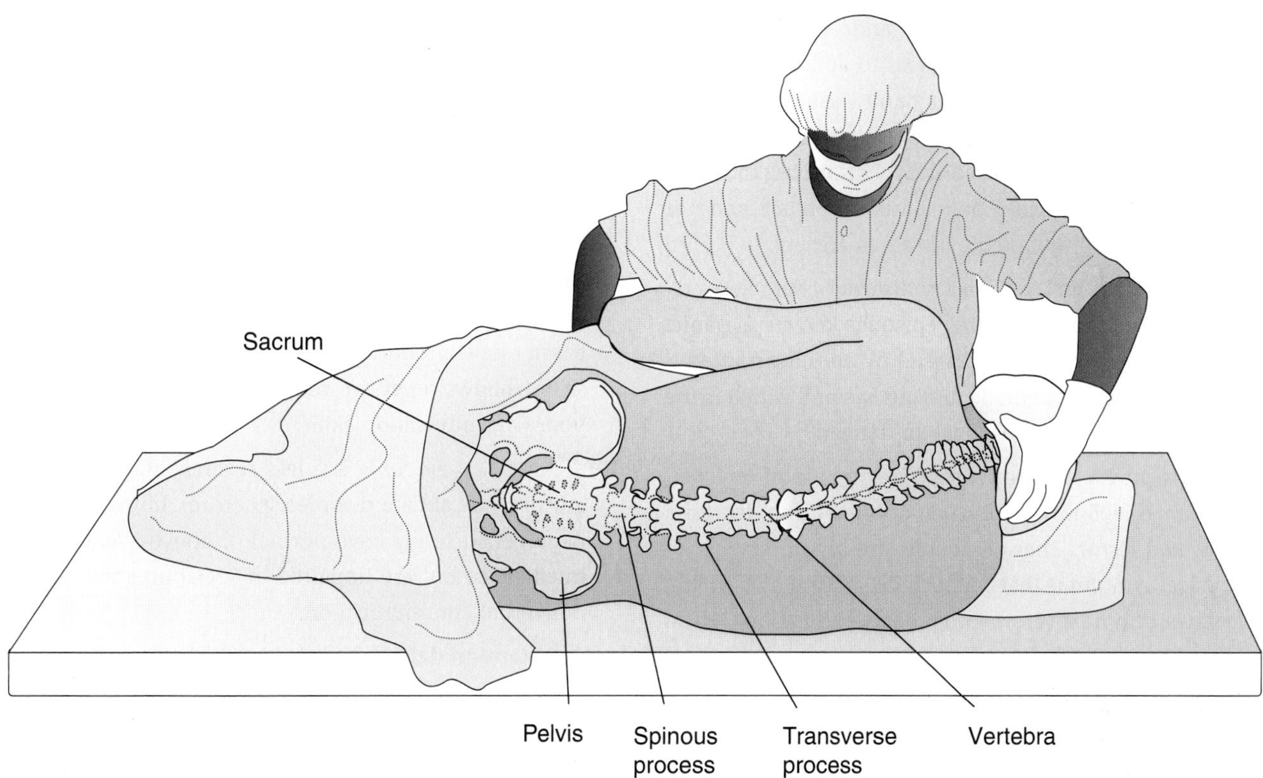

FIGURE 10.18 Epidural anesthesia administered during childbirth numbs the nerves from the uterus and birth passage without stopping labor.

the arachnoid membrane and above the pia mater that surrounds the spinal cord.

- *General anesthesia* involves the total loss of body sensation and consciousness induced by anesthetic agents administered primarily by inhalation or intravenous injection.

The Brain

- A **lobectomy** (loh-**BECK**-toh-mee) is surgical removal of a portion of the brain to treat brain cancer or seizure disorders that cannot be controlled with medication.
- A **thalamotomy** (**thal**-ah-**MOT**-oh-mee) is a surgical incision into the thalamus (**thalam** means thalamus, and **-otomy** means surgical incision). This procedure, which destroys brain cells, is primarily performed to quiet the tremors of Parkinson's disease.

Nerves

- **Neuroplasty** (**NEW**-roh-**plas**-tee) is the surgical repair of a nerve or nerves (**neur/o** means nerve, and **-plasty** means surgical repair).
- **Neurorrhaphy** (new-**ROR**-ah-fee) is surgically suturing together the ends of a severed nerve (**neur/o** means nerve, and **-rrhaphy** means surgical suturing).
- A **neurotomy** (new-**ROT**-oh-mee) is a surgical incision or the dissection of a nerve (**neur** means nerve, and **-otomy** means a surgical incision).

MENTAL HEALTH

Although described as being disorders of mental health, the causes of the following conditions also include congenital abnormalities, physical changes, substance abuse, medications, or any combination of these factors.

Anxiety Disorders

Anxiety disorders are mental conditions characterized by excessive, irrational dread of everyday situations, or fear that is out of proportion to the real danger in a situation. Without treatment, an anxiety disorder can become chronic.

- A **generalized anxiety disorder** is characterized by chronic anxiety plus exaggerated worry and tension even when there is little or nothing to provoke these feelings. Physical symptoms associated with this condition include muscle tension, sleep disturbance, and restlessness.
- **Obsessive-compulsive disorder** is an anxiety disorder characterized by recurrent, unwanted *obsessions*

(repetitive thoughts or impulses) and/or recurrent *compulsions* (unwanted impulses to act). Repetitive compulsive behaviors, such as hand washing, are often performed with the hope of preventing obsessive thoughts or making them go away. Performing these so-called "rituals" provides only temporary relief, and not performing them markedly increases anxiety.

- A **panic disorder** is an anxiety disorder characterized by unexpected and repeated episodes known as panic attacks. These attacks are caused by an unwarranted arousal of the sympathetic nervous system, which is the body's fight or flight response to danger.
- A **panic attack** is characterized by a group of intense emotional feelings that include apprehension, fearfulness, and terror. These emotions are accompanied by physical symptoms that can include shortness of breath, feelings of unreality, sweating, heart palpitations, chest pain, and choking sensations.
- **Posttraumatic stress disorder** (PTSD) may develop after an event involving actual or threatened death or injury to the individual or someone else, during which the person felt intense fear, helplessness, or horror. Military service, a natural disaster, or a hostage situation can cause this disorder, with symptoms including diminished responsiveness to stimuli, anxiety, sleep disorders, persistent reliving of the event, and difficulty concentrating.

Phobias

A **phobia** (**FOH**-bee-ah) is a persistent irrational fear of a specific thing or situation, strong enough to cause significant distress, to interfere with functioning, and to lead to the avoidance of the thing or situation that causes this reaction. There are countless types of phobias, and they are named by adding **-phobia** to the name of the object.

- **Acrophobia** (**ack**-roh-**FOH**-bee-ah) is an excessive fear of being in high places (**acr/o** means top, and **-phobia** means abnormal fear).
- **Agoraphobia** (**ag**-oh-rah-**FOH**-bee-ah) is an excessive fear of situations in which having a panic attack seems likely and/or dangerous or embarrassing. An example is a person who fears leaving the familiar setting of home and going out in public because social situations may provoke anxiety (**agor/a** means marketplace, and **-phobia** means abnormal fear).
- **Arachnophobia** (ah-**rach**-noh-**FOH**-bee-ah) is an excessive fear of spiders (**arachn/o** means spider, and **-phobia** means abnormal fear).
- **Claustrophobia** (**klaws**-troh-**FOH**-bee-ah) is an abnormal fear of being in narrow or enclosed spaces (**claustr/o** means barrier, and **-phobia** means abnormal fear).

Developmental Disorders

- **Autism** (**AW**-tizm), also known as *autistic disorders*, describes a group of conditions in which a young child cannot develop normal social relationships, compulsively follows repetitive routines, and frequently has poor communication skills.
- *Asperger's syndrome* is a less severely affected subgroup of the autism disorder spectrum. Individuals with Asperger's usually have normal or above-average intelligence but are impaired in social interactions and nonverbal communication.
- An **attention deficit disorder** (ADD) is characterized by a short attention span and impulsive behavior that is inappropriate for the child's developmental age. The term *attention deficit/hyperactivity disorder* (ADHD) is sometimes used if there is a consistently high level of activity. *Hyperactivity* is restlessness or a continuing excess of movement. These conditions may persist into adulthood.
- **Dyslexia** (dis-**LECK**-see-ah), also known as a *developmental reading disorder*, is a learning disability characterized by substandard reading achievement due to the inability of the brain to process symbols.
- **Learning disabilities** are disorders found in children of normal intelligence who have difficulties in learning specific skills such as processing language or grasping mathematical concepts.
- A diagnosis of **mental retardation** is based on three criteria: (1) significant below-average intellectual functioning; (2) significant deficits in adaptive functioning; and (3) onset during the developmental period of life, which is before age 18.

Dissociative Disorders

Dissociative disorders occur when normal thought is separated from consciousness.

- **Dissociative identity disorder**, formerly known as *multiple personality disorder*, is a mental illness characterized by the presence of two or more distinct personalities, each with its own characteristics, which appear to exist within the same individual.

Factitious Disorders

A **factitious disorder** (fack-**TISH**-us) is a condition in which an individual acts as if he or she has a physical or mental illness when he or she is not really sick. The term *factitious* means artificial, self-induced, or not naturally occurring. Visible symptoms are self-inflicted and the motivation is the patient's desire to receive attention and sympathy.

- A **factitious disorder by proxy** is a form of child abuse. Although seeming very concerned about the child's well-being, the mentally ill parent will falsify an illness in a child by making up, or inducing symptoms, and then seeking medical treatment, even surgery, for the child.

Impulse-Control Disorders

Impulse-control disorders are a group of psychiatric disorders characterized by the inability to resist an impulse despite potential negative consequences. In additional to the examples listed below, this disorder includes compulsive shopping and gambling.

- **Kleptomania** (**klep**-toh-**MAY**-nee-ah) is a disorder characterized by repeatedly stealing objects neither for personal use nor for their monetary value (**klept/o** means to steal, and **-mania** means madness).
- **Pyromania** (**pye**-roh-**MAY**-nee-ah) is a disorder characterized by repeated, deliberate fire setting (**pyr/o** means fire, and **-mania** means madness).
- **Trichotillomania** (**trick**-oh-**till**-oh-**MAY**-nee-ah) is a disorder characterized by the repeated pulling out of one's own hair (**trichotill/o** means related to hair, and **-mania** means madness).

Mood Disorders

- A **bipolar disorder** is a condition characterized by cycles of severe mood changes shifting from highs (manic behavior) and severe lows (depression) that affect a person's attitude, energy, and ability to function.
- **Manic behavior** includes an abnormally elevated mood state, including inappropriate elation, increased irritability, severe insomnia, poor judgment, and inappropriate social behavior.
- **Depression** is a common mood disorder characterized by lethargy and sadness, as well as the loss of interest or pleasure in normal activities. Severe depression may lead to feelings of worthlessness and thoughts of death or suicide.
- **Dysthymia** (dis-**THIGH**-mee-ah), also known as a *dysthymic disorder*, is a low-grade chronic depression with symptoms that are milder than those of severe depression but are present on a majority of days for 2 or more years (**dys-** means bad, **thym** means mind, and **-ia** means condition).
- **Seasonal affective disorder** (SAD) is a seasonal bout of depression associated with the decrease in hours of daylight during winter months.

Personality Disorders

A **personality disorder** is a chronic pattern of inner experience and behavior that causes serious problems with relationships and work. This pattern is pervasive and inflexible, has an onset in adolescence or early adulthood, is stable over time, and leads to distress or impairment.

- An *antisocial personality disorder* is a pattern of disregard for, and violation of, the rights of others. This pattern brings the individual into continuous conflict with society.
- A *borderline personality disorder* is characterized by impulsive actions, often with the potential for self-harm, as well as mood instability and chaotic relationships.
- A *narcissistic personality disorder* is a pattern of extreme preoccupation with the self and complete lack of empathy for others. *Empathy* is the ability to understand another person's mental and emotional state without becoming personally involved.

Psychotic Disorders

A **psychotic disorder** (sigh-**KOT**-ick) is characterized by the loss of contact with reality and deterioration of normal social functioning.

- **Catatonic behavior** (**kat**-ah-**TON**-ick) is marked by a lack of responsiveness, stupor, and a tendency to remain in a fixed posture.
- A **delusion** (dee-**LOO**-zhun) is a false personal belief that is maintained despite obvious proof or evidence to the contrary. The belief is not one ordinarily accepted by other members of the individual's culture or religious faith.
- A **hallucination** (hah-**loo**-sih-**NAY**-shun) is a sensory perception (sight, touch, sound, smell, or taste) experienced in the absence of an external stimulation.

- **Schizophrenia** (**skit**-soh-**FREE**-nee-ah) is a psychotic disorder usually characterized by withdrawal from reality, illogical patterns of thinking, delusions, and hallucinations, and accompanied in varying degrees by other emotional, behavioral, or intellectual disturbances.

Somatoform Disorders

A **somatoform disorder** (soh-**MAT**-oh-**form**) is characterized by physical complaints or concerns about one's body that are out of proportion to any physical findings or disease.

- A **conversion disorder** is characterized by serious temporary or ongoing changes in function, such as paralysis or blindness, that are triggered by psychological factors rather than by any physical cause.
- **Hypochondriasis** (**high**-poh-kon-**DRY**-ah-sis) is characterized by fearing that one has a serious illness despite appropriate medical evaluation and reassurance. A person exhibiting this syndrome is known as a *hypochondriac*.
- **Malingering** (mah-**LING**-ger-ing) is characterized by the intentional creation of false or grossly exaggerated physical or psychological symptoms. In contrast to a factitious disorder, this condition is motivated by incentives such as avoiding work.

Substance-Related Disorders

Substance abuse is the addictive use of tobacco, alcohol, medications, or illegal drugs. This abuse leads to significant impairment in functioning, danger to one's self or others, and recurrent legal and/or interpersonal problems (Figure 10.19).

- **Alcoholism** (**AL**-koh-hol-izm) is chronic alcohol dependence with specific signs and symptoms upon withdrawal. *Withdrawal* is a psychological or physical syndrome (or both) caused by the abrupt cessation (stopping) of the use of alcohol or a drug in an addicted individual.
- **Delirium tremens** (dee-**LIR**-ee-um **TREE**-mens) is a disorder involving sudden and severe mental changes or seizures caused by abruptly stopping the use of alcohol.

Medications to Treat Mental Disorders

- An **antidepressant** is administered to prevent or relieve depression. Some of these medications are also used to treat obsessive-compulsive and generalized anxiety disorders and to help relieve chronic pain.

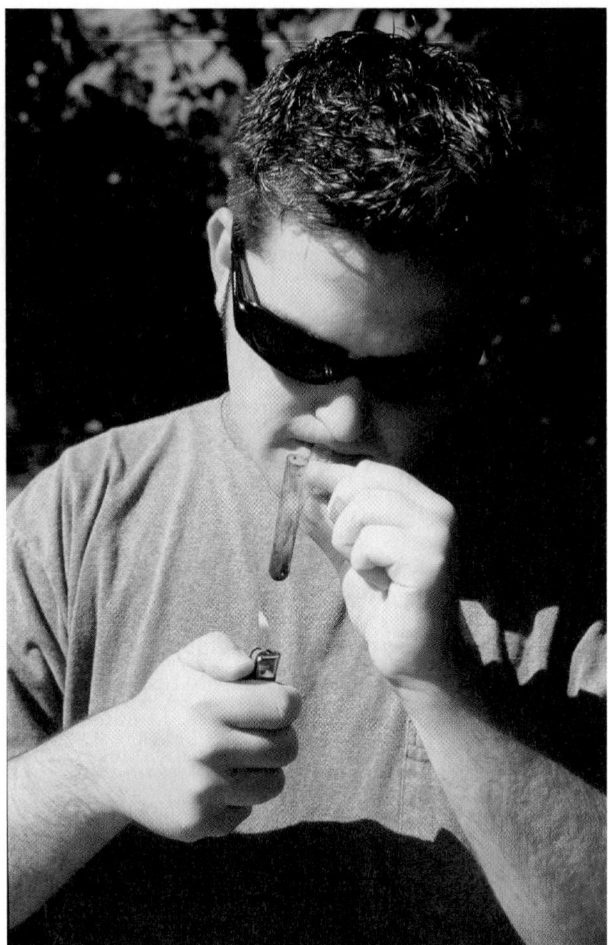

FIGURE 10.19 Substance abuse includes the use of illegal drugs.

- An **antipsychotic drug** (**an**-tih-sigh-**KOT**-ick) is administered to treat symptoms of severe disorders of thinking and mood that are associated with neurological and psychiatric illnesses such as schizophrenia, mania, and delusional disorders (**anti-** means against, **psych/o** means mind, and **-tropic** means having an affinity for).
- An **anxiolytic drug** (**ang**-zee-oh-**LIT**-ick), also known as an *antianxiety drug* or *tranquilizer*, is administered to temporarily relieve anxiety and to reduce tension (**anxi/o** means anxiety, and **-lytic** means to destroy).
- **Mood stabilizing drugs**, such as lithium, are used to treat mood instability and bipolar disorders.
- A **psychotropic drug** (**sigh**-koh-**TROP**-pick) acts primarily on the central nervous system, where it produces temporary changes affecting the mind, emotions, and behavior (**psych/o** means mind, and **-tropic** means having an affinity for). These drugs are used as

medications to control pain, and to treat narcolepsy and attention disorders.

- A **stimulant** works by increasing activity in certain areas of the brain to increase concentration and wakefulness. Drug therapies using stimulants have been effective in treating ADHD and narcolepsy. The overuse of stimulants, including caffeine, can cause sleeplessness and palpitations.

Psychological Therapies to Treat Mental Disorders

In addition to drug treatments, mental disorders are often treated with individual or group therapy by a qualified psychotherapist.

- **Psychoanalysis** (**sigh**-koh-ah-**NAL**-ih-sis) is based on the idea that mental disorders have underlying causes stemming from childhood and can only be overcome by gaining insight into one's feelings and patterns of behavior.
- **Behavioral therapy** focuses on changing behavior by identifying problem behaviors, replacing them with appropriate behaviors, and using rewards or other consequences to make the changes.
- **Cognitive therapy** focuses on changing cognitions or thoughts that are affecting a person's emotions and actions. These are identified and then are challenged through logic, gathering evidence, and/or testing in action. The goal is to change problematic beliefs.
- *Cognitive-behavioral therapy* combines the techniques of cognitive and behavioral therapy.
- **Hypnotherapy** is the use of hypnosis to produce a relaxed state of focused attention in which the patient may be more willing to believe and act on suggestions.

ABBREVIATIONS RELATED TO THE NERVOUS SYSTEM

Table 10.4 presents an overview of the abbreviations related to the terms introduced in this chapter. Note: To avoid errors or confusion, always be cautious when using abbreviations.

TABLE 10.4
ABBREVIATIONS RELATED TO THE NERVOUS SYSTEM

Alzheimer's disease = AD	**AD** = Alzheimer's disease
amyotrophic lateral sclerosis = ALS	**ALS** = amyotrophic lateral sclerosis
attention deficit hyperactivity disorder = ADHD	**ADHD** = attention deficit hyperactivity disorder
cerebral palsy = CP	**CP** = cerebral palsy
cerebrospinal fluid = CSF	**CSF** = cerebrospinal fluid
electroencephalography = ECG	**ECG** = electroencephalography
epidural anesthesia = EPAN	**EPAN** = epidural anesthesia
intracranial pressure = ICP	**ICP** = intracranial pressure
levels of consciousness = LOC	**LOC** = levels of consciousness
multiple sclerosis = MS	**MS** = multiple sclerosis
obsessive-compulsive disorder = OCD	**OCD** = obsessive-compulsive disorder

Career Opportunities

In addition to the medical specialties already discussed, some of the health occupations involving the treatment of the nervous system include:

- **Electroencephalographic (EEG) technologist:** operates an electroencephalograph (EEG machine) that records electrical activity of the brain for diagnosis and evaluation
- **Electroneurodiagnostic technologist:** in addition to performing resting EEGs, performs nerve conduction tests, measures sensory and physical responses to specific stimuli, and conducts sleep studies and ambulatory monitoring
- **Polysomnographic technologist:** administers sleep disorder evaluations
- **Social worker:** trained to help people make adjustments in their lives or to refer them to community resources for assistance; also called case managers, counselors, or sociologists. Some specialties include:

Child welfare and family counseling	Health care social work
Correctional (prison) counseling	Occupational social work
Geriatrics and hospice work	Psychiatric social work

- **Social services assistant:** aids social workers by maintaining records and performing other administrative tasks, often for a government agency
- **Psychiatric or mental health technician, assistant** and **aid:** work under the supervision of a psychiatrist or psychologist to help patients with care and rehabilitation. They may also observe and report behavior.
- **Art, music**, and **dance therapists:** use creative arts for nonverbal expression of feelings, and for communication and social integration. They may work with patients suffering from mental disorders, emotional trauma, or other social, psychological, or physical problems.
- **Recreational therapist:** uses creative arts and other activities, such sports and field trips, to improve the physical, emotional, and mental well-being of individuals with disabilities or illness

HEALTH OCCUPATION PROFILE

MENTAL HEALTH WORKER

Shawn Goldwyn, who holds a bachelor's degree in social work (BSW), is a mental health worker in a psychiatric hospital. *"In my job, I help people who are experiencing some form of mental crisis. Some of my patients have hallucinations or hear voices telling them to hurt themselves or others. Others have experienced severe trauma in their lives, have chemical imbalances that make them extremely aggressive or uninhibited, or are so profoundly depressed that suicide feels like the only option.*

"My job is to make sure they are in a safe and supportive environment. Sometimes, I help run groups to teach different coping skills and ways to manage anger, anxiety, or depression. Most of the time, I sit and listen to them talk.

"I have always been a good listener. In high school, friends would seek me out to tell me their problems. This job is perfect for someone with lots of patience and understanding. It also helps to be flexible. Some days are very chaotic, and I never know what will happen next; other days are quieter and more predictable. Every day is different, and I like that."

STUDY BREAK

We all know that hitting your funny bone is not really funny.

The sudden, sharp pain we associate with the "funny bone" comes from the *ulnar nerve.* Why does it hurt so much when it is hit? The ulnar nerve is a long one, running from the spinal cord to the fingertips. In most places along the way, it is protected by muscle or fat. But when it runs past the elbow joint, it is close to the skin. When you accidentally hit your elbow (which is easy to do, because it sticks out), you hit the ulnar nerve against the bone, causing a sharp pain or tingling sensation.

The ankle also has a nerve that runs close to the surface and can cause similar pain. But because the ankle doesn't move about as widely as the elbow, it is less likely to be bumped sharply.

And why do we call the bone that carries the ulnar nerve to the elbow a funny bone? Because it's scientific name, the *humerus,* sounds a lot like the word *humorous.*

Review Time

Write the answers to the following questions on a separate piece of paper or in your notebook. In addition, be prepared to take part in the classroom discussion.

1. ***Written Assignment:*** Using terms a physician would understand, describe the difference between an **encephalocele** and a **meningocele**.

   Discussion Assignment: Discuss how the word parts tell you what these terms mean.

2. ***Written Assignment:*** Describe the difference between a **concussion** and a **cerebral contusion**.

   Discussion Assignment: Describe how each type of injury could occur.

3. ***Written Assignment:*** Using terms a patient would understand, describe the difference between a **panic attack** and a **heart attack**.

   Discussion Assignment: How would each condition affect the treatment necessary?

4. ***Written Assignment:*** Research and report on the full name and dates of the person for whom **Alzheimer's disease** is named.

   Discussion Assignment: Mr. Greene has just been diagnosed with Alzheimer's disease. Since this is a progressive disease, what should his family be prepared to face in the months and years ahead?

5. ***Written Assignment:*** Describe the difference between an **ischemic stroke** and a **hemorrhagic stroke**.

   Discussion Assignment: Why is receiving treatment quickly so important for a stroke patient?

Optional Internet Activity

The goal of this activity is to help you learn more about medical terminology as it applies to the "real world." Select **one** *of these two options and follow the instructions.*

1. Search for information about **Alzheimer's disease**. Write a brief (one- or two-paragraph) report on something new you learned here and include the address of the web site where you found this information.
2. To learn more about **brain injuries**, look for the Brain Injuries Association, or similar organization, that specializes in education and support for those suffering from cerebral trauma. Explore the site and then write a brief (one- or two-paragraph) report on something new you learned here.

The Human Touch: Critical Thinking Activity

The following story and questions are designed to stimulate critical thinking through class discussion or as a brief essay response. There are no right or wrong answers to these questions.

The phone call came on Mrs. Burrow's cell phone while she was in a meeting. Since the phone was turned off, the high school secretary left a brief message explaining that her daughter Susanna had been absent all week and that any further unexcused absences would affect her grades.

continues

Mrs. Burrow was shocked to hear that her 16-year-old daughter had been skipping school, although she had noticed that Susanna had been quiet and oddly withdrawn lately. In fact, she'd been reluctant to talk at all and often got upset over perfectly normal comments.

Returning home from work at lunchtime, Mrs. Burrow opened the door of her daughter's room. She was surprised to find Susanna curled up in bed still sleeping. It was noon, and Susanna had slept through half of her classes already. Mrs. Burrow couldn't recall hearing about any problems at school and couldn't understand why Susanna was staying home to avoid it.

Sitting down on the bed, Mrs. Burrow patted her daughter's back gently through the covers. **"What's wrong, sweetie?"** *Susanna poked her head out from the covers and glared up at her mother.* **"I don't want to go to school! I can't do anything right and it's boring. No one likes me because I'm so dumb and fat. I hate all of my teachers and classes. Just go away and leave me alone."**

Mrs. Burrow was very surprised by her daughter's words. In fact, thinking back on it now, it seemed that Susanna hadn't been doing things or going places with her friends. Instead she stayed alone in her room and didn't join in family activities. She also seemed to sleep a lot. Was it possible that Susanna was struggling with depression?

With a sigh, Mrs. Burrow left her daughter to sleep for now and went to the kitchen telephone. Taking out her health insurance card, she called the advice nurse to ask what the first step would be to get help for Susanna. She hoped that with time, and professional treatment, she would get her loving, bubbly daughter back.

Suggested Discussion Topics

1. Discuss which of the health care workers mentioned in this chapter might be able to help Susanna overcome her depression.
2. Many people refuse to take medication for depression. Discuss why someone would avoid taking something that might help them feel better.
3. Imagine that Susanna is one of your friends. She hasn't been much fun to be around recently. She never wants to do anything, and you've heard her talk about wanting to die. You are worried. Discuss what, if anything, you could do to help her.
4. Discuss how you can learn about the resources that are available in your school or community to help someone who is depressed and/or suicidal.

STUDENT WORKBOOK AND StudyWARE™ CD-ROM

1. Go to your **Student Workbook** and complete the Learning Exercises for this chapter.

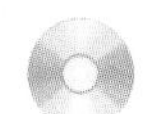

2. Go to the **StudyWARE™ CD-ROM** and have fun with the exercises and games for this chapter.

11

CHAPTER

Special Senses: The Eyes and Ears

Overview of Structures, Combining Forms, and Functions of the Eyes and Ears

Major Structures	Related Combining Forms	Primary Functions
Eyes	opt/i, opt/o, optic/o, ophthalm/o	Receptor organs for the sense of sight.
Iris	ir/i, ir/o, irid/o, irit/o	Controls the amount of light entering the eye.
Lens	phac/o, phak/o	Focuses rays of light on the retina.
Retina	retin/o	Converts light images into electrical impulses and transmits them to the brain.
Lacrimal Apparatus	dacryocyst/o,lacrim/o	Accessory structures of the eyes that produce, store, and remove tears.
Ears	acous/o, acoust/o, audi/o, audit/o,ot/o	Receptor organs for the sense of hearing; also help to maintain balance.
Outer Ear	pinn/i	Transmits sound waves to the middle ear.
Middle Ear	myring/o, tympan/o	Transmits sound waves to the inner ear.
Inner Ear	labyrinth/o	Receives sound vibrations and transmits them to the brain.

VOCABULARY RELATED TO THE SPECIAL SENSES

This list contains essential word parts and medical terms for this chapter. These terms are pronounced on the student StudyWARE™ CD-ROM and Audio CDs that are available for use with this text. These and the other important **primary terms** are shown in boldface throughout the chapter. *Secondary terms*, which appear in *orange* italics, clarify the meaning of primary terms.

Word Parts

- ☐ **blephar/o**
- ☐ **-cusis**
- ☐ **irid/o**
- ☐ **kerat/o**
- ☐ **myring/o**
- ☐ **ophthalm/o**
- ☐ **-opia**
- ☐ **opt/o**
- ☐ **ot/o**
- ☐ **phak/o**
- ☐ **presby/o**
- ☐ **retin/o**
- ☐ **scler/o**
- ☐ **trop/o**
- ☐ **tympan/o**

Medical Terms

- ☐ **adnexa** (ad-**NECK**-sah)
- ☐ **amblyopia** (**am**-blee-**OH**-pee-ah)
- ☐ **ametropia** (**am**-eh-**TROH**-pee-ah)
- ☐ **anisocoria** (**an**-ih-so-**KOH**-ree-ah)
- ☐ **astigmatism** (ah-**STIG**-mah-tizm)
- ☐ **barotrauma** (**bar**-oh-**TRAW**-mah)
- ☐ **blepharoptosis** (**blef**-ah-roh-**TOH**-sis)
- ☐ **cataract** (**KAT**-ah-rakt)
- ☐ **chalazion** (kah-**LAY**-zee-on)
- ☐ **cochlear implant** (**KOCK**-lee-ar)
- ☐ **conjunctivitis** (kon-**junk**-tih-**VYE**-tis)
- ☐ **dacryoadenitis** (**dack**-ree-oh-ad-eh-**NIGH**-tis)
- ☐ **diplopia** (dih-**PLOH**-pee-ah)
- ☐ **ectropion** (eck-**TROH**-pee-on)
- ☐ **emmetropia** (em-eh-**TROH**-pee-ah)
- ☐ **entropion** (en-**TROH**-pee-on)
- ☐ **esotropia** (**es**-oh-**TROH**-pee-ah)
- ☐ **eustachitis** (**you**-stay-**KYE**-tis)
- ☐ **exotropia** (**eck**-soh-**TROH**-pee-ah)
- ☐ **fluorescein angiography** (**flew**-oh-**RES**-ee-in **an**-jee-**OG**-rah-fee)
- ☐ **glaucoma** (glaw-**KOH**-mah)
- ☐ **hemianopia** (**hem**-ee-ah-**NOH**-pee-ah)
- ☐ **hordeolum** (hor-**DEE**-oh-lum)
- ☐ **hyperopia** (**high**-per-**OH**-pee-ah)
- ☐ **infectious myringitis** (**mir**-in-**JIGH**-tis)
- ☐ **iridectomy** (**ir**-ih-**DECK**-toh-mee)
- ☐ **iritis** (eye-**RYE**-tis)
- ☐ **keratitis** (**ker**-ah-**TYE**-tis)
- ☐ **labyrinthectomy** (**lab**-ih-rin-**THECK**-toh-mee)
- ☐ **laser trabeculoplasty** (trah-**BECK**-you-loh-**plas**-tee)
- ☐ **mastoidectomy** (**mas**-toy-**DECK**-toh-mee)
- ☐ **myopia** (my-**OH**-pee-ah)
- ☐ **myringotomy** (**mir**-in-**GOT**-oh-mee)
- ☐ **nyctalopia** (**nick**-tah-**LOH**-pee-ah)
- ☐ **nystagmus** (nis-**TAG**-mus)
- ☐ **ophthalmoscopy** (**ahf**-thal-**MOS**-koh-pee)
- ☐ **optometrist** (op-**TOM**-eh-trist)
- ☐ **otitis media** (oh-**TYE**-tis **MEE**-dee-ah)
- ☐ **otomycosis** (**oh**-toh-my-**KOH**-sis)
- ☐ **otopyorrhea** (**oh**-toh-**pye**-oh-**REE**-ah)
- ☐ **otorrhagia** (**oh**-toh-**RAY**-jee-ah)
- ☐ **otosclerosis** (**oh**-toh-skleh-**ROH**-sis)
- ☐ **papilledema** (**pap**-ill-eh-**DEE**-mah)
- ☐ **periorbital edema**
- ☐ **presbycusis** (**pres**-beh-**KOO**-sis)
- ☐ **presbyopia** (**pres**-bee-**OH**-pee-ah)
- ☐ **pterygium** (teh-**RIJ**-ee-um)
- ☐ **radial keratotomy** (**ker**-ah-**TOT**-oh-mee)
- ☐ **retinopexy** (**RET**-ih-noh-**peck**-see)
- ☐ **scleritis** (skleh-**RYE**-tis)
- ☐ **stapedectomy** (**stay**-peh-**DECK**-toh-mee)
- ☐ **strabismus** (strah-**BIZ**-mus)
- ☐ **tarsorrhaphy** (tahr-**SOR**-ah-fee)
- ☐ **tinnitus** (tih-**NIGH**-tus)
- ☐ **tonometry** (toh-**NOM**-eh-tree)
- ☐ **tympanometry** (**tim**-pah-**NOM**-eh-tree)
- ☐ **tympanostomy tubes** (**tim**-pan-**OSS**-toh-mee)
- ☐ **vertigo** (**VER**-tih-go)
- ☐ **vitrectomy (vih-TRECK-toh-mee)**
- ☐ **xerophthalmia** (**zeer**-ahf-**THAL**-mee-ah)

OBJECTIVES

On completion of this chapter, you should be able to:

1. Describe the functions and structures of the eyes and their accessory structures.
2. Recognize, define, spell, and pronounce terms related to the pathology and diagnostic and treatment procedures of the eyes and vision.
3. Describe the functions and structures of the ears.
4. Recognize, define, spell, and pronounce terms related to the pathology and diagnostic and treatment procedures of the ears and hearing.

FUNCTIONS OF THE EYES

The eyes are the receptor organs of sight and their functions are to receive images and transmit them to the brain. The abbreviations relating to the eyes, with the Latin words from which they originated, are shown in Table 11.1.

STRUCTURES OF THE EYES

The structures of the eye include the eyeball and the adnexa that are attached to or surround the eyeball (Figure 11.1).

Adnexa of the Eyes

The **adnexa of the eyes**, also known as *adnexa oculi*, are the structures outside the eyeball, and these include the orbit, eye muscles, eyelids, eyelashes, conjunctiva, and lacrimal apparatus. **Adnexa** (ad-**NECK**-sah) means appendages or accessory structures of an organ.

The Orbit

The **orbit**, also known as the *eye socket*, is the bony cavity of the skull that contains and protects the eyeball and its associated muscles, blood vessels, and nerves.

Muscles of the Eye

Six major **eye muscles**, which are arranged in three pairs, are attached to each eye. These are the superior and inferior oblique muscles, the superior and inferior rectus muscles, and the lateral and medial rectus muscles (Figure 11.2). These muscles make a wide range of very precise eye movements possible.

The muscles of both eyes work together in coordinated movements that enable normal **binocular vision** (**bin-** means two, **ocul** means eye, and **-ar** means pertaining to). The term *binocular* refers the use of both eyes working together.

TABLE 11.1

ABBREVIATIONS RELATING TO THE EYES

OD	Right eye (*Oculus Dexter*)
OS	Left eye (*Oculus Sinister*)
OU	Each eye or both eyes (*Oculus Uterque*)

The Eyelids, Eyebrows, and Eye Lashes

The **upper** and **lower eyelids** of each eye help protect the eyeball from foreign matter, excessive light, and injuries due to other causes (see Figure 11.1).

- The **canthus** (**KAN**-thus) is the angle where the upper and lower eyelids meet (**canth** means corner of the eye, and **-us** is a singular noun ending) (plural, *canthi*).
- The **inner canthus** is where the eyelids meet *nearest* the nose.
- The **epicanthus** (**ep**-ih-**KAN**-thus) is a vertical fold of skin on either side of the nose.
- The **outer canthus** is where the eyelids meet *farthest from* the nose.
- The **tarsus** (**TAHR**-suhs), also known as the *tarsal plate*, is the framework within the upper and lower eyelids that provides the necessary stiffness and shape (**tars** means edge of the eyelid, and **-us** is a singular noun ending) (plural, *tarsi*). Note: *Tarsus* also refers to the seven tarsal bones of the instep.
- The **eyebrows** and **eyelashes** prevent foreign matter from reaching the eyes. The eyelashes consist of small hairs known as **cilia** (**SIL**-ee-ah). Cilia are also found in the nose.
- The edges of the eyelids contain oil-producing sebaceous glands. These glands are discussed in Chapter 12.

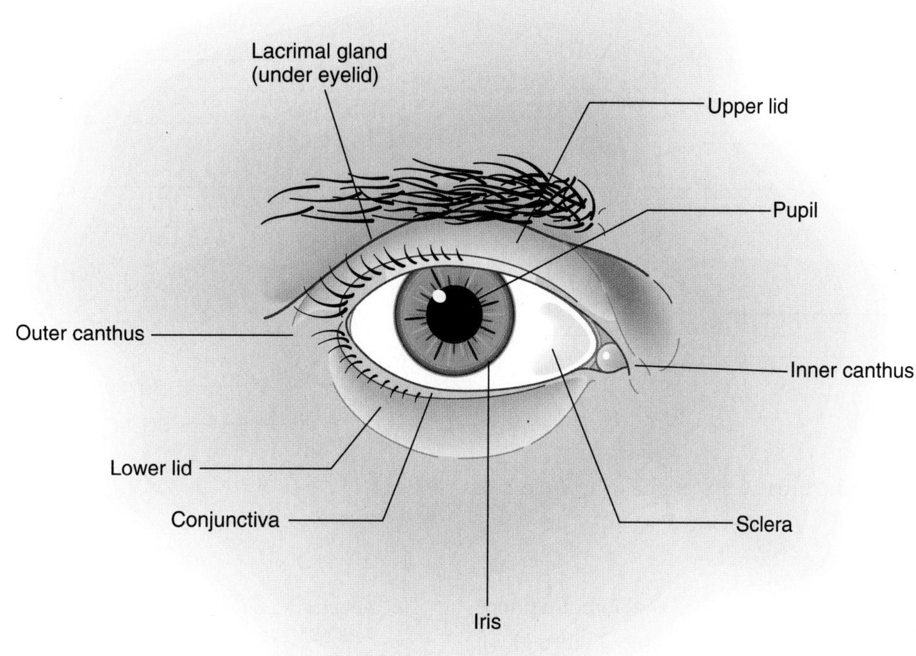

FIGURE 11.1 Major structures of the adnexa of the right eye.

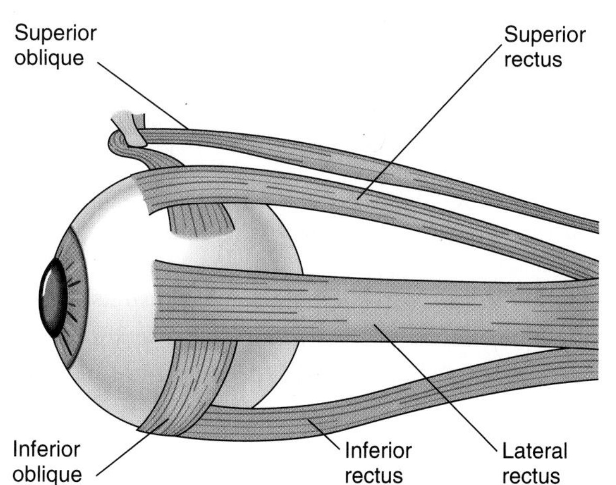

FIGURE 11.2 Six muscles, arranged as three pairs, make major eye movement possible. The medial rectus muscle is not visible here.

The Conjunctiva

The **conjunctiva** (**kon**-junk-**TYE**-vah) is the transparent mucous membrane that lines the underside of each eyelid and continues to form a protective covering over the exposed surface of the eyeball (plural, *conjunctivae*) (see Figure 11.1).

The Lacrimal Apparatus

The **lacrimal apparatus** (**LACK**-rih-mal), also known as the *tear apparatus*, consists of the structures that produce, store, and remove tears.

- The **lacrimal glands**, which secrete lacrimal fluid (tears), are located on the underside of the upper eyelid just above the outer corner of each eye (see Figure 11.1). *Lacrimation* is the secretion of tears.
- The function of **lacrimal fluid**, also known as *tears*, is to maintain moisture on the anterior surface of the eyeball. Blinking distributes the lacrimal fluid across the eye.
- The **lacrimal canal** (**LACK**-rih-mal) consists of a duct at the inner corner of each eye. These ducts collect tears and empty them into the lacrimal sacs. Crying is the overflowing of tears from the lacrimal canals.
- The **lacrimal sac**, also known the *tear sac*, is an enlargement of the upper portion of the lacrimal duct.
- The **lacrimal duct**, also known as the *nasolacrimal duct*, is the passageway that drains excess tears into the nose.

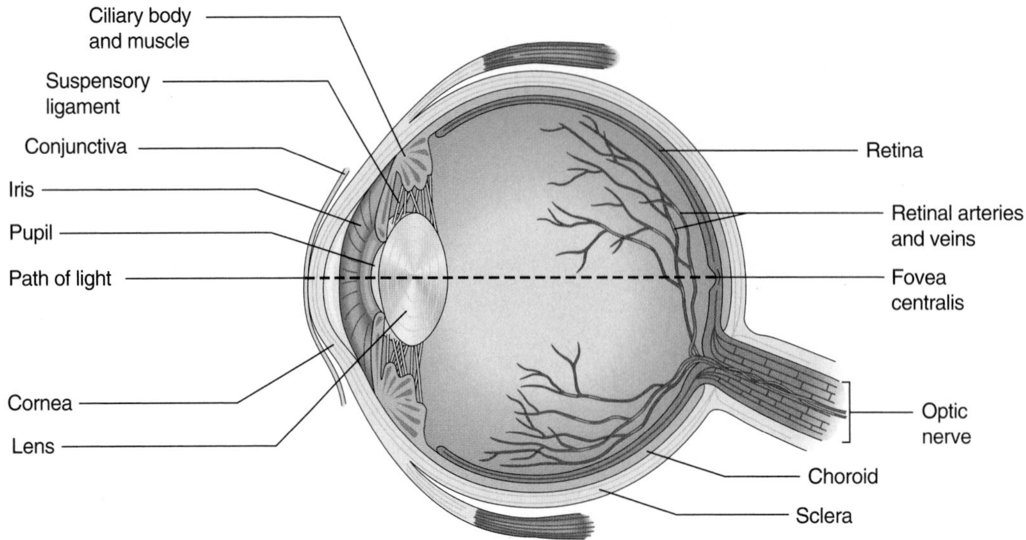

FIGURE 11.3 The structures of the eyeball shown in cross-section.

The Eyeball

The **eyeball**, also known as the *globe*, is a 1-inch sphere with only about one-sixth of its surface visible (Figure 11.3).

- The term **optic** means pertaining to the eye or sight (**opt** means sight, and **-ic** means pertaining to).
- **Ocular** (**OCK**-you-lar) means pertaining to the eye (**ocul** means eye, and **-ar** means pertaining to).
- **Extraocular** (**eck**-strah-**OCK**-you-lar) means outside the eyeball (**extra-** means on the outside, **ocul** means eye, and **-ar** means pertaining to).
- **Intraocular** (**in**-trah-**OCK**-you-lar) means within the eyeball (**intra-** means within, **ocul** means eye and **-ar** means pertaining to.)

Walls of the Eyeball

The walls of the eyeball are made up of three layers: the sclera, choroid, and retina (Figure 11.4).

- The **sclera** (**SKLEHR**-ah), also known as the *white of the eye*, maintains the shape of the eye and protects the delicate inner layers of tissue. This tough, fibrous tissue forms the outer layer of the eye, except for the part covered by the cornea. Note: The combining form **scler/o** means the white of the eye, and it also means hard.
- The **choroid** (**KOH**-roid), also known as the *choroid coat*, is the opaque middle layer of the eyeball that contains many blood vessels and provides the blood supply for the entire eye. *Opaque* means that light cannot pass through this substance.
- The **retina** (**RET**-ih-nah) is the sensitive innermost layer that lines the posterior segment of the eye. The retina receives nerve impulses and transmits them to the brain via the *optic nerve*. This is also known as the *second cranial nerve* and is discussed in Chapter 10 (see Figure 11.4).

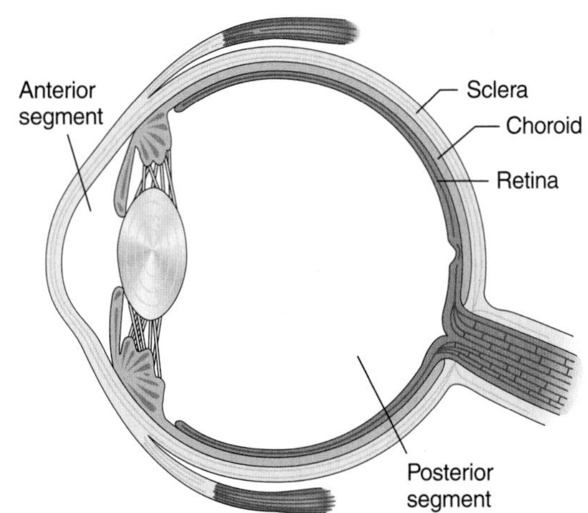

FIGURE 11.4 The walls of the eyeball are made up of the sclera, choroid, and retina.

Segments of the Eyeball

The interior of the eyeball is divided into the anterior and posterior segments (see Figures 11.4 and 11.5).

Anterior Segment of the Eye

The **anterior segment** makes up the front one-third of the eyeball. This segment is divided into anterior and posterior chambers (see Figures 11.5 and 11.6).

- The **anterior chamber** is located behind the cornea and in front of the iris. The **posterior chamber** is located behind the iris and in front of the ligaments

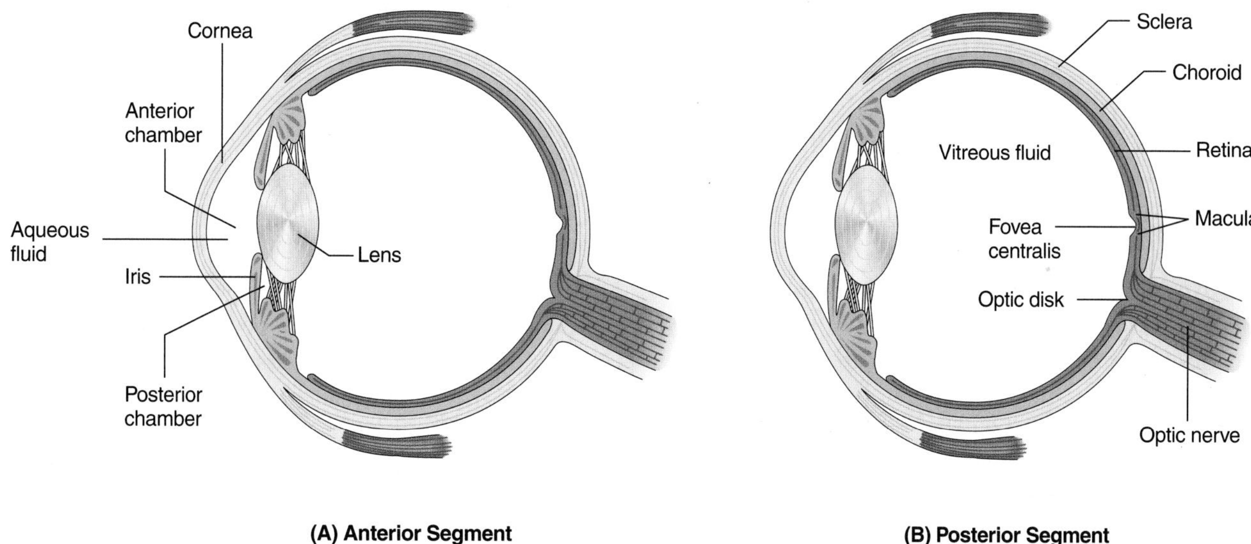

FIGURE 11.5 The segments of the eyeball. (A) The anterior segment is divided into anterior and posterior chambers. (B) The posterior segment.

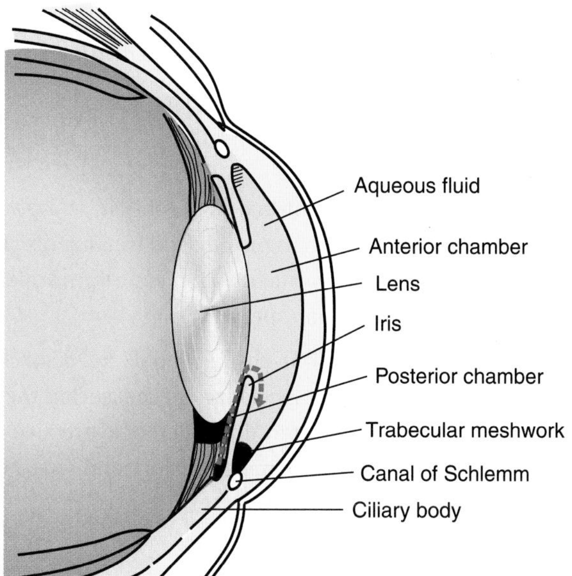

FIGURE 11.6 The flow of aqueous fluid in the anterior segment of the eye.

holding the lens in place. Note: Don't confuse the posterior chamber with the posterior segment.

- These chambers are filled with **aqueous fluid**, also known as *aqueous humor*. *Aqueous* means watery or containing water. As used here, a *humor* is any clear body liquid or semifluid substance.
- Aqueous fluid helps the eye maintain its shape and nourishes the intraocular structures. This fluid is constantly filtered and drained through the **trabecular meshwork** and the **canal of Schlemm** (Figure 11.6).
- **Intraocular pressure** (IOP) is a measurement of the fluid pressure inside the eye. The rate at which aqueous fluid enters and leaves the eye regulates this pressure.

Posterior Segment of the Eye

The **posterior segment**, which makes up the remaining two-thirds of the eyeball, is lined with the retina and filled with **vitreous gel** (**VIT**-ree-us). Also known as *vitreous humor*, this is a soft, clear, jelly-like mass that contains millions of fine fibers. These fibers, which are attached to the surface of the retina, help the eye maintain its shape (see Figures 11.3–11.5).

Structures of the Retina

- The **rods** and **cones** of the retina receive images that have passed through the lens of the eye. These images are converted into nerve impulses and transmitted to the brain via the optic nerve. *Rods* are the black and white receptors, and *cones* are the color receptors.
- The **macula** (**MACK**-you-lah), also known as the *macula lutea*, is a clearly defined yellow area in the center of the retina. This is the area of sharpest central vision.
- The **fovea centralis** (**FOH**-vee-ah sen-**TRAH**-lis) is a pit in the middle of the macula. Color vision is best in this area because it contains a high concentration of cones and no rods.
- The **optic disk**, also known as the *blind spot*, is a small region in the eye where the nerve endings of the retina

enter the optic nerve. This is called the blind spot because it does not contain any rods or cones to convert images into nerve impulses.

- The **optic nerve** transmits these nerve impulses from the retina to the brain.

The Uveal Tract

The **uveal tract** (**YOU**-vee-ahl) is the pigmented layer of the eye. It has a rich blood supply and consists of the choroid, ciliary body, and iris (see Figure 11.3).

The Ciliary Body

The **ciliary body** (**SIL**-ee-ehr-ee), which is located within the choroid, is a set of muscles and suspensory ligaments that adjust the thickness of the lens to refine the focus of light rays on the retina (see Figure 11.6).

- The ciliary body produces the aqueous fluid that fills the anterior segment of the eye.
- To focus on nearby objects, these muscles adjust the lens to make it *thicker*.
- To focus on distant objects, these muscles stretch the lens so it is *thinner*.

The Iris

The **iris** is the colorful muscular layer of the eye that surrounds the pupil (see Figure 11.3). The muscles within the iris control the amount of light that is allowed to enter the eye through the pupil.

- To *decrease* the amount of light, these circular muscles contract and make the pupil smaller.
- To *increase* the amount of light, the muscles dilate (relax) and make the pupil larger.

The Cornea, Pupil, and Lens

- The **cornea** (**KOR**-nee-ah) is the transparent outer surface of the eye covering the iris and pupil. It is the primary structure focusing light rays entering the eye (see Figure 11.3).
- The **pupil** is the black circular opening in the center of the iris that permits light to enter the eye.
- The **lens**, also known as the *crystalline lens*, is the clear, flexible, curved structure that focuses images on the retina. The lens is contained within a clear capsule located behind the iris and pupil.

Normal Action of the Eyes

- **Accommodation** (ah-**kom**-oh-**DAY**-shun) is the process whereby the eyes make adjustments for seeing objects at various distances. These adjustments include contraction (narrowing) and dilation (widening) of the pupil, movement of the eyes, and changes in the shape of the lens.
- **Convergence** (kon-**VER**-jens) is the simultaneous inward movement of the eyes toward each other. This occurs in an effort to maintain single binocular vision as an object comes nearer.
- **Emmetropia** (em-eh-**TROH**-pee-ah) is the normal relationship between the refractive power of the eye and the shape of the eye that enables light rays to focus correctly on the retina (**emmetr** means in proper measure, and **-opia** means vision condition).
- **Refraction**, also *refractive power*, is the ability of the lens to bend light rays so they focus on the retina. Normal refraction is shown in Figure 11.10A.
- **Visual acuity** (ah-**KYOU**-ih-tee) is the ability to distinguish object details and shape at a distance. *Acuity* means sharpness (see Figure 11.8A).

MEDICAL SPECIALTIES RELATED TO THE EYES

- An **ophthalmologist** (ahf-thal-**MOL**-oh-jist) is a physician who specializes in diagnosing and treating diseases and disorders of the eyes and vision (**ophthalm** means eye, and **-ologist** means specialist).
- An **optometrist** (op-**TOM**-eh-trist) holds a Doctor of Optometry degree and specializes in measuring the accuracy of vision to determine whether corrective lenses are needed (**opt/o** means vision, and **-metrist** means one who measures).

PATHOLOGY OF THE EYES AND VISION

The Eyelids

- **Blepharoptosis** (**blef**-ah-roh-**TOH**-sis), also known simply as *ptosis*, is drooping of the upper eyelid that is usually due to paralysis (**blephar/o** means eyelid, and **-ptosis** means drooping or sagging).
- A **chalazion** (kah-**LAY**-zee-on), also known as an *internal stye*, is a localized swelling inside the eyelid resulting from obstruction a sebaceous gland. Compare with a *hordeolum*.
- **Ectropion** (eck-**TROH**-pee-on) is the eversion of the edge of an eyelid (**ec-** mean out, **trop** means turn, and

-**ion** means condition). *Eversion* means turning outward. This usually affects the lower lid, thereby exposing the inner surface of the eyelid to irritation and preventing tears from draining properly (Figure 11.7A). Ectropion is the opposite of *entropion*.

- **Entropion** (en-**TROH**-pee-on) is the inversion of the edge of an eyelid (**en-** means in, **trop** means turn, and **-ion** means condition). *Inversion* means turning inward. This usually affects the lower eyelid and causing the eyelashes to rub against the cornea (Figure 11.7B). Entropion is the opposite of *ectropion*.
- A **hordeolum** (hor-**DEE**-oh-lum), also known as a *stye*, is a pus-filled lesion on the eyelid resulting from an infection in a sebaceous gland. Compare with a *chalazion*.
- **Periorbital edema** is swelling surrounding the eye or eyes (**peri-** means surrounding, **orbit** means eyeball, and **-al** means pertaining to). *Edema* means swelling of the tissues. This swelling can cause the eyes to be partially closed by the swollen eyelids. It can also give the face a bloated appearance. This swelling is associated with conditions including allergic reactions (Chapter 6), nephrotic syndrome (Chapter 9), and cellulitis (Chapter 12).

Additional Adnexa Pathology

- **Conjunctivitis** (kon-**junk**-tih-**VYE**-tis), also known as *pinkeye*, is an inflammation of the conjunctiva that is usually caused by an infection or allergy (**conjunctiv** means conjunctiva, and **-itis** means inflammation).
- **Dacryoadenitis** (**dack**-ree-oh-ad-eh-**NIGH**-tis) is an inflammation of the lacrimal gland that can be caused by a bacterial, viral, or fungal infection (**dacry/o** means tear, **aden** means gland, and **-itis** means inflammation). Signs and symptoms of this condition include sudden severe pain, redness, and pressure in the orbit of the eye.
- **Subconjunctival hemorrhage** is bleeding between the conjunctiva and the sclera. This common condition, which is usually caused by an injury, creates a red area over the white of the eye.
- **Xerophthalmia** (**zeer**-ahf-**THAL**-mee-ah), also known as *dry eye*, is drying of eye surfaces including the conjunctiva (**xer** means dry, **ophthalm** means eye, and **-ia** means abnormal condition). This condition is often associated with aging. In addition, it can be due to systemic diseases such as rheumatoid arthritis or to a lack of vitamin A.

Uveal Tract, Cornea, Iris, and Sclera

- **Iritis** (eye-**RYE**-tis), also known as *anterior uveitis*, is an inflammation of the uveal tract affecting primarily structures in the front of the eye (**ir** means iris, and **-itis** means inflammation). This condition can be acute or chronic.
- A **corneal abrasion** is an injury, such as a scratch or irritation, to the outer layers of the cornea. Compare with *corneal ulcer*.
- A **corneal ulcer** is a pitting of the cornea caused by an infection or injury. Although these ulcers heal with

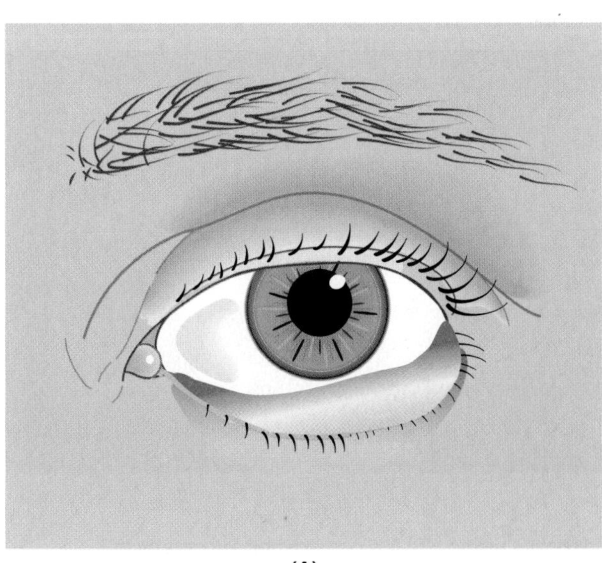

(A)

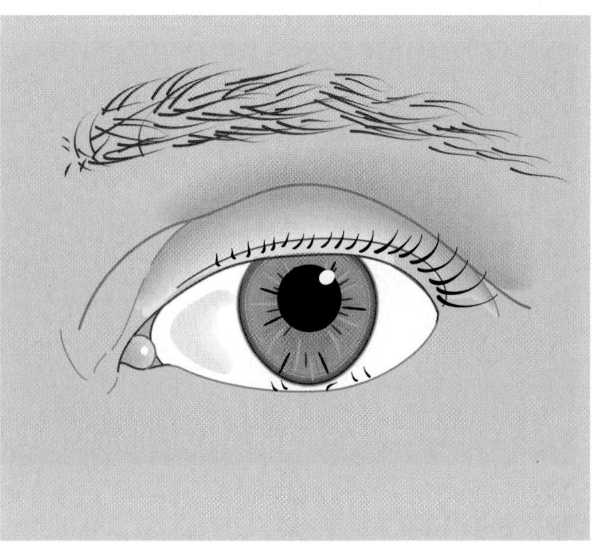

(B)

FIGURE 11.7 Disorders of the eyelid. (A) Ectropion. (B) Entropion.

treatment, they can leave a cloudy scar that impairs vision. Compare with *corneal abrasion*.

- **Keratitis** (**ker**-ah-**TYE**-tis) is an inflammation of the cornea (**kerat** means cornea, and **-itis** means inflammation). Note: **kerat/o** also means hard. This condition can be due to many causes including bacterial, viral, or fungal infections.
- A **pterygium** (teh-**RIJ**-ee-um) is a benign growth on the cornea that can become large enough to distort vision.
- **Scleritis** (skleh-**RYE**-tis) is an inflammation of the sclera (**scler** means white of eye, and **-itis** means inflammation). This condition is usually associated with infections, chemical injuries, or autoimmune diseases.
- **Synechia** (sigh-**NECK**-ee-ah) is an adhesion that binds the iris to an adjacent structure such as the lens or cornea (plural, *synechiae*). An *adhesion* holds structures together abnormally.

The Eye

- **Anisocoria** (**an**-ih-so-**KOH**-ree-ah) is a condition in which the pupils are unequal in size (**anis/o** means unequal, **cor** means pupil, and **-ia** means abnormal condition). This condition can be congenital or caused by a head injury, aneurysm, or pathology of the central nervous system.
- A **cataract** (**KAT**-ah-rakt) is the loss of transparency of the lens that causes a progressive loss of visual clarity. The formation of most cataracts is associated with aging; however, this condition can be congenital or due to an injury or disease (Figure 11.8B).
- **PERRLA** is an abbreviation meaning **P**upils are **E**qual, **R**ound, **R**esponsive to **L**ight and **A**ccommodation. This is a diagnostic observation, and any abnormality here could indicate a head injury or damage to the brain.

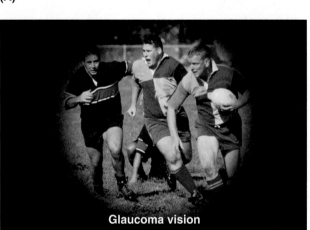

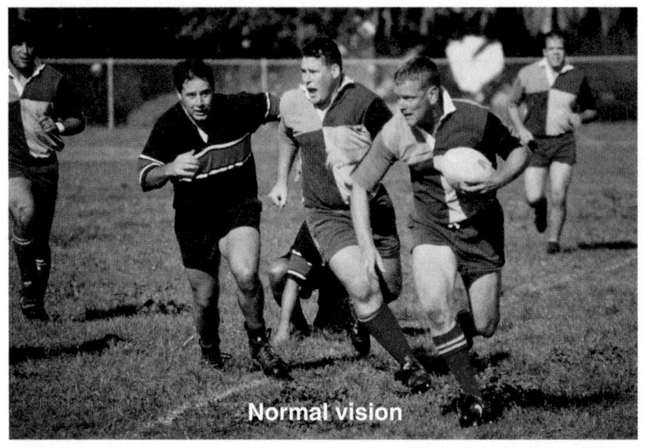

(A)

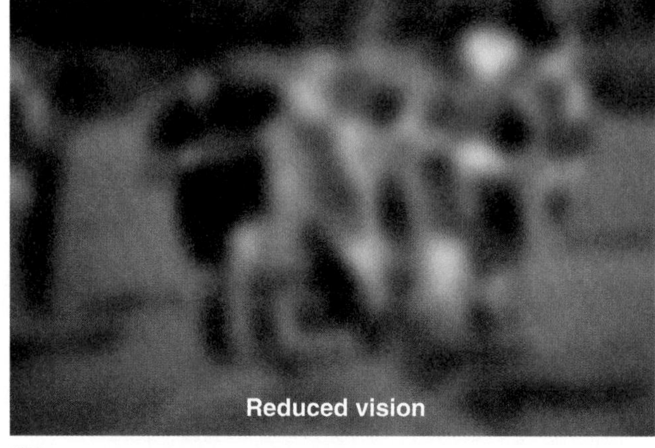

(B)

Glaucoma vision

(C)

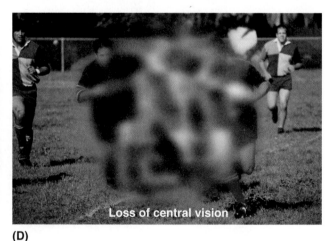

(D)

FIGURE 11.8 Normal vision and pathologic vision changes. (A) Normal vision. (B) Vision reduced by cataracts. (C) The loss of peripheral vision due to untreated glaucoma. (D) The loss of central vision due to macular degeneration.

- In a **retinal detachment**, also known as a *detached retina*, the retina is pulled away from its attachment to the choroid in the back of the eye (Figure 11.9).
- **Floaters**, also known as *vitreous floaters*, are particles of cellular debris that float in the vitreous fluid and cast shadows on the retina. Floaters occur normally with aging or in association with vitreous detachments, retinal tears, or intraocular inflammations.
- **Nystagmus** (nis-**TAG**-mus) is an involuntary, constant, rhythmic movement of the eyeball that can be congenital or caused by a neurological injury or drug use.
- **Papilledema** (**pap**-ill-eh-**DEE**-mah), also known as *choked disk*, is swelling and inflammation of the optic nerve at the point of entrance into the eye through the optic disk (**papill** means nipple-like, and **-edema** means swelling). This swelling is caused by increased intracranial pressure and can be due to a tumor pressing on the optic nerve.
- A **retinal tear** occurs when a hole develops in the retina as it is pulled away from its normal position. See *vitreous detachment.*
- **Retinitis pigmentosa** (**ret**-ih-**NIGH**-tis pig-men-**TOH**-sah) is a progressive degeneration of the retina that affects night and peripheral vision. It can be detected by the presence of dark pigmented spots in the retina.
- **Vitreous detachment** occurs as aging causes the vitreous gel to slowly shrink. With this shrinkage, the fine fibers within the gel pull on the retinal surface. Usually the fibers break, allowing the vitreous to separate and shrink from the retina. In most cases, this condition is not sight-threatening and does not require treatment; however, if the fibers pull hard enough on the retina, they can cause a retinal tear.

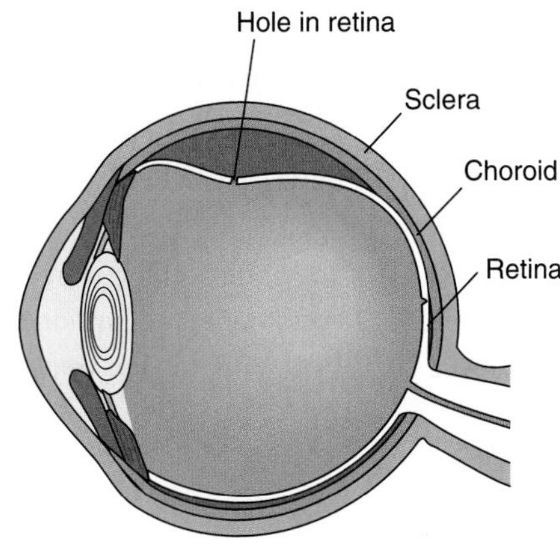

FIGURE 11.9 A retinal detachment.

Glaucoma

Glaucoma (glaw-**KOH**-mah) is a group of diseases characterized by increased intraocular pressure that cause damage to the retinal nerve fibers and the optic nerve (see Figure 11.8C). This increase in pressure is caused by a blockage in the flow of fluid out of the eye. If left untreated, this pressure can cause the loss of peripheral vision and eventually blindness.

- **Open-angle glaucoma**, also known as *chronic glaucoma*, is the most common form of this condition. Here the trabecular meshwork gradually becomes blocked, and this causes a buildup of pressure. Symptoms of this condition are not noticed by the patient until the optic nerve has been damaged; however, it can be detected earlier through regular eye examinations including tonometry and visual field testing. See Diagnostic Procedures of the Eyes.
- In **closed-angle glaucoma**, also known as *acute glaucoma*, the opening between the cornea and iris narrows so that fluid cannot reach the trabecular meshwork. This narrowing can cause a sudden increase in the intraocular pressure that produces severe pain, nausea, redness of the eye, and blurred vision. Without immediate treatment, blindness can occur in as little as 2 days.

Macular Degeneration

Macular degeneration (**MACK**-you-lar) is a gradually progressive condition in which the macula at the center of the retina is damaged, resulting in the loss of central vision, but not in total blindness (**macul** means spot, and **-ar** mean pertaining to). See Figure 11.8D.

- *Age-related macular degeneration* occurs most frequently in older people and is the leading cause of legal blindness in those over age 60.
- *Dry type macular degeneration*, which accounts for 90% of cases, is caused by the deterioration of the cells of the macula.
- *Wet type macular degeneration* is caused by the formation of new blood vessels that produce small hemorrhages, damaging the macula.

Functional Defects

- **Diplopia** (dih-**PLOH**-pee-ah), also known as *double vision*, is the perception of two images of a single object (**dipl** means double, and **-opia** means vision condition). It is sometimes a symptom of a serious underlying disorder such as multiple sclerosis or a brain tumor.

- **Hemianopia** (**hem**-ee-ah-**NOH**-pee-ah) is blindness in one-half of the visual field (**hemi-** mean half, **an-** means without, and **-opia** means vision).
- **Monochromatism** (**mon**-oh-**KROH**-mah-tizm), also known as *color blindness*, is the inability to distinguish colors(**mon/o** means one, **chromat** means color, and **-ism** means condition).
- **Nyctalopia** (**nick**-tah-**LOH**-pee-ah), also known as *night blindness*, is a condition in which an individual with normal daytime vision has difficulty seeing at night (**nyctal** means night, and **-opia** means vision condition).
- **Presbyopia** (**pres**-bee-**OH**-pee-ah) is the condition of common changes in the eyes that occur with aging (**presby** means old age, and **-opia** means vision condition). With age, near vision declines noticeably as the lens becomes less flexible and the muscles of the ciliary body become weaker. The result is that the eyes are no longer able to focus the image properly on the retina.

Strabismus

Strabismus (strah-**BIZ**-mus) is a disorder in which the eyes point in different directions or are not aligned correctly because the eye muscles are unable to focus together.

- **Esotropia** (**es**-oh-**TROH**-pee-ah), also known as *cross-eyes*, is strabismus characterized by an inward deviation of one or both eyes (**eso-** means inward, **trop** means turn, and **-ia** means abnormal condition). Esotropia is the opposite of *exotropia.*
- **Exotropia** (**eck**-soh-**TROH**-pee-ah), also known as *walleye*, is strabismus characterized by the outward deviation of one eye relative to the other (**exo-** means outward, **trop** means turn, and **-ia** means abnormal condition). Exotropia is the opposite of *esotropia.*

Refractive Disorders

A **refractive disorder** is a focusing problem that occurs when the lens and cornea do not bend light so that it focuses properly on the retina (Figure 11.10).

- **Ametropia** (**am**-eh-**TROH**-pee-ah) is any error of refraction in which images do not focus properly on the retina (**ametr** means out of proportion, and **-opia** means vision condition). Astigmatism, hyperopia, and myopia are all forms of ametropia.

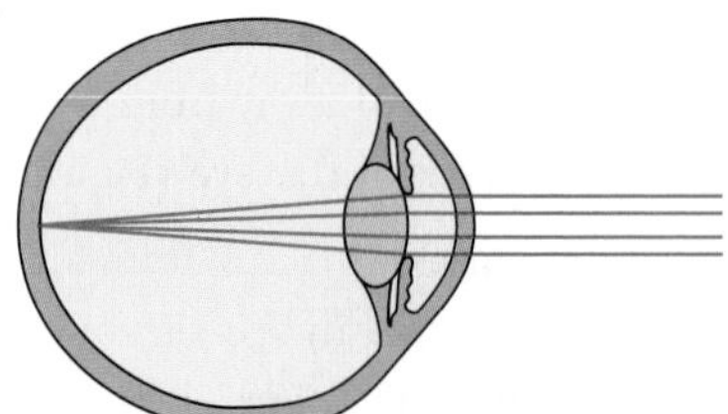

(A) Normal eye
Light rays focus on the retina.

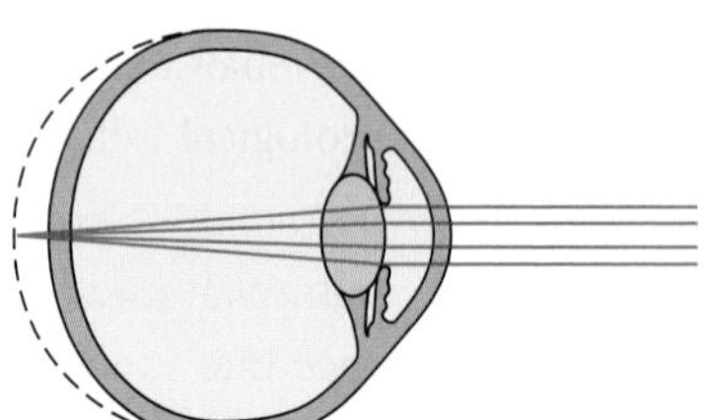

(B) Hyperopia (farsightedness)
Light rays focus beyond the retina.

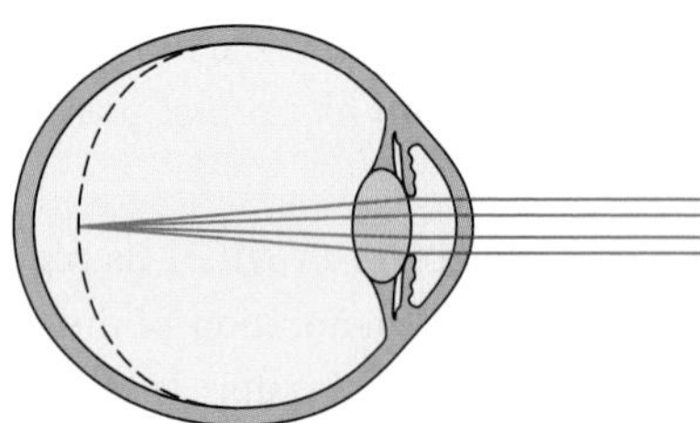

(C) Myopia (nearsightedness)
Light rays focus in front of the retina.

FIGURE 11.10 Refraction. (A) Normal eye. (B) Hyperopia. (C) Myopia.

- **Astigmatism** (ah-**STIG**-mah-tizm) is a condition in which the eye does not focus properly because of uneven curvatures of the cornea.
- **Hyperopia** (**high**-per-**OH**-pee-ah), also known as *farsightedness*, is a defect in which light rays focus beyond the retina (**hyper-** means excessive and **-opia** means vision condition). This condition can occur in childhood, but usually causes difficulty after age 40 (Figure 11.10B). Hyperopia is the opposite of *myopia.*
- **Myopia** (my-**OH**-pee-ah), also known as *nearsightedness*, is a defect in which light rays focus in front of the retina. This condition occurs most commonly around puberty (Figure 11.10C). Myopia is the opposite of *hyperopia.*

Blindness

Blindness is the inability to see. Although some sight remains, *legal blindness* is the point at which, under law, an individual is considered to be blind. A commonly used standard is that a person is legally blind when his or her best-corrected vision is reduced to 20/200 or less. See Normal Action of the Eyes earlier in this chapter.

- **Amblyopia** (**am**-blee-**OH**-pee-ah) is a dimness of vision or the partial loss of sight, especially in one eye, without detectable disease of the eye (**ambly** means dim or dull, and **-opia** means vision condition).
- **Scotoma** (skoh-**TOH**-mah), also known as *blind spot*, is an abnormal area of absent or depressed vision surrounded by an area of normal vision.

DIAGNOSTIC PROCEDURES OF THE EYES AND VISION

- A **Snellen chart** (SC) is used to measure visual acuity. The results for each eye are recorded as a fraction with 20/20 being considered normal (Figure 11.11). The *first number* indicates the standard distance from the chart, which is 20 feet. The *second number* indicates the deviation from the norm based on the ability to read progressively smaller lines of letters on the chart.
- **Refraction** is an examination procedure to determine an eye's refractive error so that the best corrective lenses to be prescribed.
- A **diopter** (dye-**AHP**-tur) is the unit of measurement of a lens' refractive power.
- **Ophthalmoscopy** (**ahf**-thal-**MOS**-koh-pee), also known as *funduscopy*, is the visual examination of the fundus (back part) of the eye with an ophthalmoscope (see Figure 15.8). This examination includes the retina, optic disk, choroid, and blood vessels.

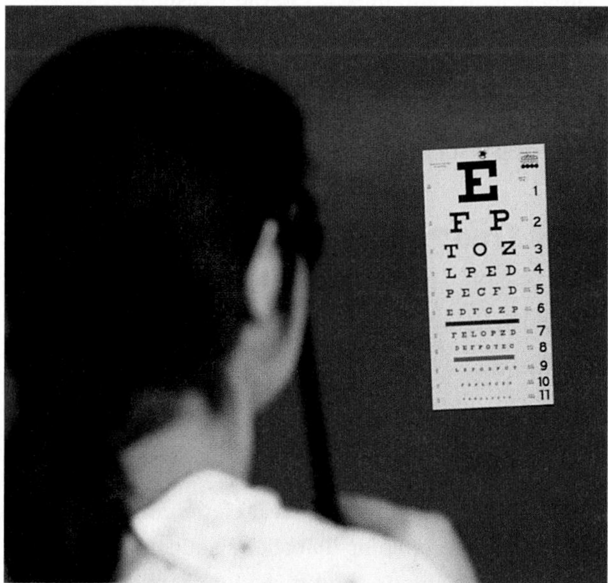

FIGURE 11.11 A Snellen chart is used to measure visual acuity.

- When ophthalmoscopy is performed as part of a complete eye examination, dilation is required. *Dilation* in preparation for an examination of the interior of the eye is the artificial enlargement of the pupil through the use of mydriatic drops.
- **Mydriatic drops** (**mid**-ree-**AT**-ick) are medicated drops placed into the eyes that produce temporary paralysis. This paralysis forces the pupils to remain dilated (wide open) even in the presence of bright light.
- **Slit-lamp ophthalmoscopy** (**ahf**-thal-**MOS**-koh-pee) is a diagnostic procedure in which a narrow beam of light is focused onto parts of the eye to permit the ophthalmologist to examine the structures at the front of the eye including the cornea, iris, and lens.
- **Tonometry** (toh-**NOM**-eh-tree) is the measurement of intraocular pressure (**ton/o** means tension, and **-metry** means to measure). Abnormally high pressure can be an indication of glaucoma.

Specialized Diagnostic Procedures

- **Fluorescein staining** (**flew**-oh-**RES**-ee-in) is the application of fluorescent dye to the surface of the eye. This dye causes a corneal abrasion to appear bright green.
- **Fluorescein angiography** (**flew**-oh-**RES**-ee-in **an**-jee-**OG**-rah-fee) is a radiographic study of the blood vessels in the retina of the eye following the intravenous injection of a fluorescein dye as a contrast me-dium. The resulting *angiograms* are used to determine whether there is proper circulation in the retinal vessels.
- **Visual field testing**, also known as *perimetry*, is performed to determine losses in peripheral vision. *Peripheral* means occurring away from the center. Blank sections in the visual field can be symptomatic of glaucoma or an optic nerve disorder.

TREATMENT PROCEDURES OF THE EYES AND VISION

The Orbit and Eyelids

- An **orbitotomy** (**or**-bih-**TOT**-oh-mee) is a surgical incision into the orbit (**orbit** means bony socket, and **-otomy** means surgical incision). This procedure is performed for biopsy, abscess drainage, or to remove a tumor or foreign object.

- **Tarsorrhaphy** (tahr-**SOR**-ah-fee) is the partial, or complete, suturing together of the upper and lower eyelids (**tars/o** means eyelid, and **-rrhaphy** means surgical suturing). This procedure is sometimes performed to protect the eye when the lids are paralyzed and unable to close normally.
- Cosmetic procedures relating to the eyelids are discussed in Chapter 12.

The Conjunctiva and Eyeball

- **Conjunctivoplasty** (**kon**-junk-**TYE**-voh-**plas**-tee) is the surgical repair of the conjunctiva (**conjunctiv** means conjunctiva, and **-plasty** means surgical repair).
- A **corneal transplant**, also known as *keratoplasty*, is the surgical replacement of a scarred or diseased cornea with clear corneal tissue from a donor.
- An **iridectomy** (**ir**-ih-**DECK**-toh-mee) is the surgical removal of a portion of the tissue of the iris (**irid** means iris, and **-ectomy** means surgical removal). This procedure is most frequently performed to treat closed-angle glaucoma.
- An **ocular prosthesis**, also known as an *artificial eye*, may be fitted to wear over a malformed eye or to replace an eyeball that is either congenitally missing or has been surgically removed. A *prosthesis* is an artificial substitute for a diseased or missing body replacement part.
- A **radial keratotomy** (**ker**-ah-**TOT**-oh-mee) is a surgical procedure to treat myopia (**kerat** means cornea, and **-otomy** means surgical incision). During the surgery, incisions are made in the cornea to cause it to flatten. These incisions allow the sides of the cornea to bulge outward and thereby flatten the central portion of the cornea. This brings the focal point of the eye closer to the retina and improves distance vision. Compare with *LASIK.*
- **Vitrectomy** (vih-**TRECK**-toh-mee) is the removal of the vitreous fluid and its replacement with a clear solution (**vitr** means vitreous fluid, and **-ectomy** means removal). This procedure is sometimes performed to treat a retinal detachment or when diabetic retinopathy causes blood to leak and cloud the vitreous fluid.

Cataract Surgery

- **Lensectomy** (len-**SECK**-toh-mee) is the general term used to describe the surgical removal of a cataract-clouded lens (**lens** means lens, and **-ectomy** means surgical removal).
- **Phacoemulsification** (**fack**-koh-ee-**mul**-sih-fih-**KAY**-shun) is the use of ultrasonic vibration to shatter and remove the lens clouded by a cataract. This is performed through a very small opening, and the same opening is used to slide the intraocular lens into place (**intra-** means within, **ocul** means eye, and **-ar** mean pertaining to).
- An **intraocular lens** (IOL) is a surgically implanted replacement for a natural lens that has been removed.
- **Pseudophakia** (**soo**-doh-**FAY**-kee-ah) is an eye in which the natural lens has been replaced with an intraocular lens (**pseudo/o** means false, **phak** means lens, and **-ia** means abnormal condition).

Corrective Lenses

Refractive errors in the eye can often be corrected with lenses that alter the angle of light rays before they reach the cornea. *Concave lenses* (curved inward) are used for myopia, or nearsightedness, and *convex lenses* (curved outward) for hyperopia (farsightedness).

- Corrective lenses can combine two or three different refractive powers, one above the other, to allow for better distance vision when looking up and near vision when looking down. *Bifocals* are lenses with two powers. *Trifocals* are lenses with three powers.
- Strabismus is sometimes treated with corrective lenses, or an eye patch, covering the stronger eye and thus strengthening the muscles in the weaker eye.
- *Contact lenses* are refractive lenses that float directly on the tear film in front of the eye. Rigid and gas-permeable lenses cover the central part of the cornea, and disposable soft lenses cover the entire cornea.

Laser Treatments of the Eyes

In the treatment of eye disorders, lasers are used for many reasons. For more details on how lasers work, see Chapter 12.

- A **laser iridotomy** (**ir**-ih-**DOT**-oh-mee) uses a focused beam of light to create a hole in the iris of the eye (**irid** means iris, and **-otomy** means surgical incision). This procedure is performed to treat closed-angle glaucoma by creating an opening that allows aqueous fluid to flow between the anterior and posterior chambers of the front part of the eye.

- **Laser trabeculoplasty** (trah-**BECK**-you-loh-**plas**-tee) is used to treat open-angle glaucoma by creating openings in the trabecular meshwork to allow fluid to drain properly.
- **LASIK** is the acronym for **L**aser-**A**ssisted in **Si**tu **K**eratomileusis (**kerat/o** means cornea, and **-mileusis** means carving). *In situ* means in its original place. LASIK is used to treat vision conditions, such as myopia, that are caused by the shape of the cornea. During this procedure, a flap is opened in the surface of the cornea and then a laser is used to change the shape of a deep corneal layer. Compare with *radial keratotomy.*
- **Photocoagulation** is the use of lasers to treat some forms of wet macular degeneration by sealing leaking or damaged blood vessels.
- **Retinopexy** (**RET**-ih-noh-**peck**-see) is used to reattach the detached area in a retinal detachment (**retin/o** means retina, and **-pexy** means surgical fixation).
- Lasers are used to treat retinal tears by sealing the torn portion.
- Lasers are used to remove clouded tissue that can have formed in the posterior portion of the lens capsule after cataract extraction.

FUNCTIONS OF THE EARS

The ears are the receptor organs of hearing, and their functions are to receive sound impulses and transmit them to the brain. The inner ear also helps to maintain balance. The abbreviations relating to the ears, with the Latin words from which they originated, are shown in Table 11.2.

- The term **auditory** (**AW**-dih-**tor**-ee) means pertaining to the sense of hearing (**audit** means hearing or sense of hearing, and **-ory** means pertaining to).
- **Acoustic** (ah-**KOOS**-tick) means relating to sound or hearing (**acous** means hearing or sound, and **-tic** means pertaining to).

TABLE 11.2

Abbreviations Relating to the Ears

AD	Right ear (*Auris Dexter*)
AS	Left ear (*Auris Sinister*)
AU	Each ear or both ears (*Auris Uterque*)

STRUCTURES OF THE EARS

The ear is divided into three separate regions: the outer ear, the middle ear, and the inner ear (Figure 11.12).

The Outer Ear

- The **pinna** (**PIN**-nah), also known as the *auricle*, is the external portion of the ear. This structure catches sound waves and transmits them into the external auditory canal.
- The **external auditory canal** transmits sound waves from the pinna to the tympanic membrane (eardrum) of the middle ear.
- **Cerumen** (seh-**ROO**-men), also known as *earwax*, is secreted by ceruminous glands that line the auditory canal. This sticky yellow-brown substance has protective functions because it traps small insects, dust, debris, and certain bacteria to prevent them from entering the middle ear.

The Middle Ear

The **middle ear**, which located between outer ear and the inner ear, transmits sound across this space (Figure 11.13).

- The **tympanic membrane** (tim-**PAN**-ick), also known as the *eardrum*, is located between the outer and middle ear (Figure 11.13). The word parts **myring/o** and **tympan/o** both mean tympanic membrane. When sound waves reach the eardrum, this membrane transmits the sound by vibrating.
- The middle ear is surrounded by the **mastoid bone cells**, which are hollow air spaces located in the mastoid process of the temporal bone.

The Auditory Ossicles

The **auditory ossicles** (**OSS**-ih-kulz) are three small bones found in the middle ear (see Figure 11.12). These bones transmit the sound waves from the eardrum to the inner ear by vibration. These bones, which are named for the Latin terms that describe their shapes, are the

- **Malleus** (**MAL**-ee-us), also known as the *hammer*.
- **Incus** (**ING**-kus), also known as the *anvil*.
- **Stapes** (**STAY**-peez), also known as the *stirrup*.

The Eustachian Tubes

The **eustachian tubes** (you-**STAY**-shun), also known as the *auditory tubes*, are narrow tubes that lead from the middle ear to the nasal cavity and the throat. These tubes

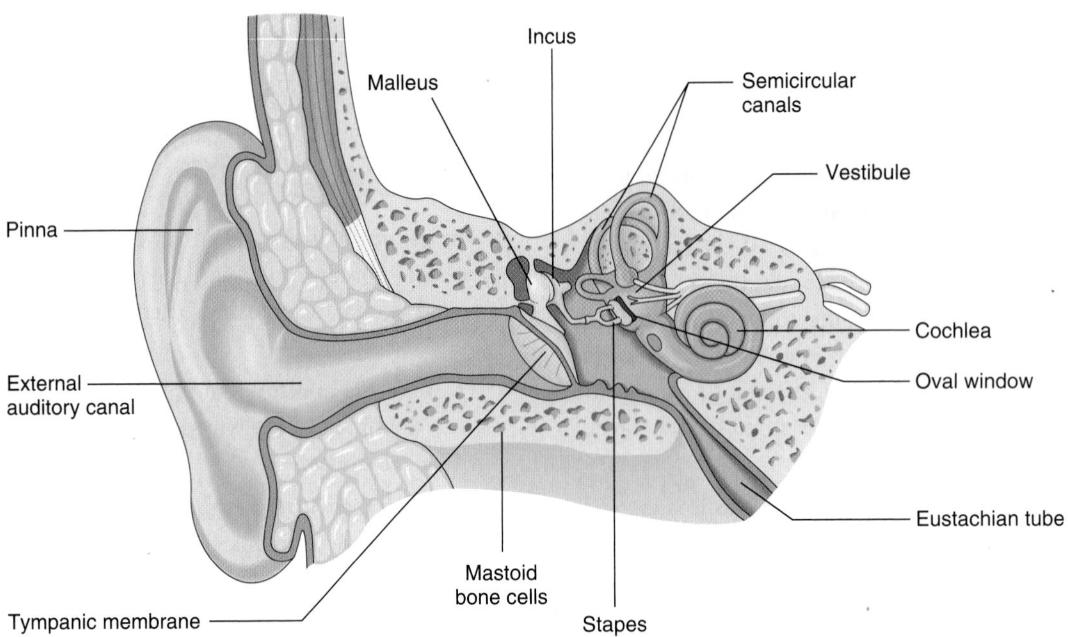

FIGURE 11.12 Structures of the ear shown in cross-section.

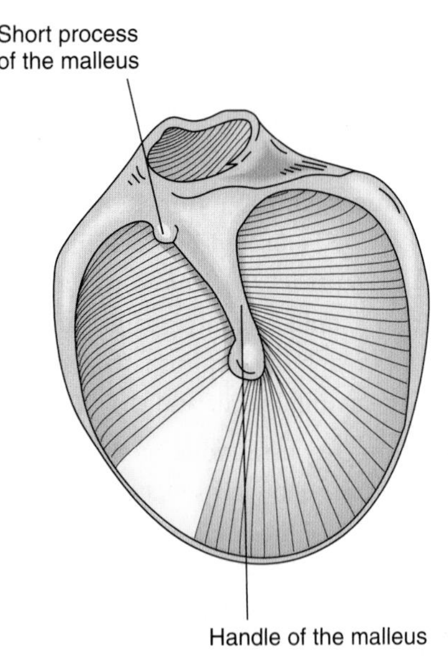

FIGURE 11.13 Schematic of the normal tympanic membrane as viewed from the auditory canal.

equalize the air pressure in the middle ear with that of the outside atmosphere.

The Inner Ear

The **inner ear**, also known as the *labyrinth*, contains the sensory receptors for hearing and balance (see Figure 11.12).

- The **oval window**, which is located under the base of the stapes, is the membrane that separates the middle ear from the inner ear. Vibrations enter the inner ear through this structure.
- The **cochlea** (**KOCK**-lee-ah) is the snail-shaped, fluid-filled structure that forms the inner ear. Located within the cochlea are the cochlear duct, the organ of Corti, the semicircular canals, and the acoustic nerves.
- The **cochlear duct** is a fluid filled cavity within the cochlea that vibrates when sound waves strike it.
- The **organ of Corti** receives the vibrations from the cochlear duct and relays them to the auditory nerve fibers. These fibers transmit them to the auditory center of the brain's cerebral cortex, where they are heard and interpreted.
- The three **semicircular canals** contain the liquid *endolymph* and sensitive hair-like cells. The bending of these hair-like cells in response to the movements of the head sets up impulses in nerve fibers to help maintain equilibrium. *Equilibrium* is the state of balance.
- The **acoustic nerves** (cranial nerve VIII) transmit this information to the brain, and the brain sends messages to muscles in all parts of the body to ensure that equilibrium is maintained.

Normal Action of the Ears

- **Air conduction** is the process by which sound waves enter the ear through the pinna. These waves then travel down the external auditory canal and strike the tympanic membrane between the outer and middle ear.

- **Bone conduction** occurs as the eardrum vibrates and moves the auditory ossicles. These bones conduct the sound waves through the middle ear to the oval window of the inner ear.
- **Sensorineural conduction** occurs when sound vibrations reach the inner ear. From here, the structures of the inner ear receive the sound waves and relay them to auditory nerve for transmission to the brain.

MEDICAL SPECIALTIES RELATED TO THE EARS

- An **audiologist** (**aw**-dee-**OL**-oh-jist) specializes in the measurement of hearing function and in the rehabilitation of persons with hearing impairments (**audi** means hearing, and **-ologist** means specialist).

PATHOLOGY OF THE EARS AND HEARING

The Outer Ear

- **Impacted cerumen** is an accumulation of earwax that forms a solid mass by adhering to the walls of the external auditory canal. *Impacted* means lodged or wedged firmly in place.
- **Otalgia** (oh-**TAL**-gee-ah), also known as an *earache*, is pain in the ear (**ot** means ear, and **-algia** means pain).
- **Otitis** (oh-**TYE**-tis) means any inflammation of the ear (**ot** means ear, and **-itis** means inflammation). The second part of the term gives the location of the inflammation: *otitis externa* is an inflammation of external auditory canal; *otitis media* is an inflammation of the middle ear; and *otitis interna* is an inflammation of the inner ear.
- **Otomycosis** (**oh**-toh-my-**KOH**-sis), also known as *swimmer's ear*, is a fungal infection of the external auditory canal (**ot/o** means ear, **myc** means fungus, and **-osis** means abnormal condition).
- **Otopyorrhea** (**oh**-toh-**pye**-oh-**REE**-ah) is the flow of pus from the ear (**ot/o** means ear, **py/o** means pus, and **-rrhea** means flow or discharge).
- **Otorrhagia** (**oh**-toh-**RAY**-jee-ah) is bleeding from the ear (**ot/o** means ear, and **-rrhagia** means bleeding).

The Middle Ear

- **Barotrauma** (**bar**-oh-**TRAW**-mah) is pressure-related ear discomfort that can be caused by pressure changes when flying, driving in the mountains, scuba diving, or when the eustachian tube is blocked (**bar/o** means pressure, and **-trauma** means injury).
- **Eustachitis** (**you**-stay-**KYE**-tis), also known as *salpingitis*, is inflammation of the eustachian tube (**eustach** means eustachian tube, and **-itis** means inflammation).
- **Mastoiditis** (**mas**-toy-**DYE**-tis) is an inflammation of any part of the mastoid bone cells (**mastoid** means mastoid process, and **-itis** means inflammation). This condition may develop when an infection in the middle ear that cannot be controlled with antibiotics spreads to the mastoid cells.
- **Infectious myringitis** (**mir**-in-**JIGH**-tis) is a contagious inflammation that causes painful blisters on the eardrum (**myring** means eardrum, and **-itis** means inflammation). This condition is associated with a middle ear infection.
- **Otosclerosis** (**oh**-toh-skleh-**ROH**-sis) is the ankylosis of the bones of the middle ear, resulting in a conductive hearing loss (**ot/o** means ear, and **-sclerosis** means abnormal hardening). *Ankylosis* means fused together. This condition is treated with a stapedectomy.
- **Patulous eustachian tube** (**PAT**-you-lus) is distention of the eustachian tube. *Patulous* means extended, spread wide open.

Otitis Media

Otitis media (oh-**TYE**-tis **MEE**-dee-ah) is an inflammation of the middle ear.

- **Acute otitis media** is usually associated with an upper respiratory infection and is most commonly seen in young children. This condition can lead to a *ruptured eardrum* due to the buildup of pus or fluid in the middle ear.
- **Serous otitis media** is a fluid buildup in the middle ear that can follow acute otitis media or can be caused by obstruction of the eustachian tube (Figure 11.14A).
- **Acute purulent otitis media** is a buildup of pus within the middle ear due to infection (Figure 11.14B). *Purulent* means producing or containing pus.

The Inner Ear

- **Labyrinthitis** (**lab**-ih-rin-**THIGH**-tis) is an inflammation of the labyrinth that can result in vertigo and deafness (**labyrinth** means labyrinth, and **-itis** means inflammation).

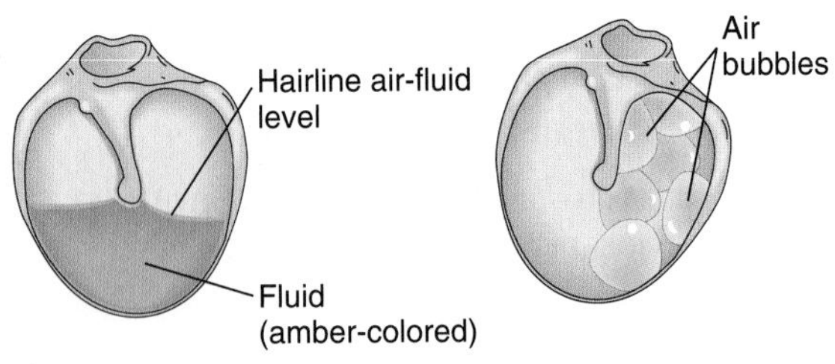

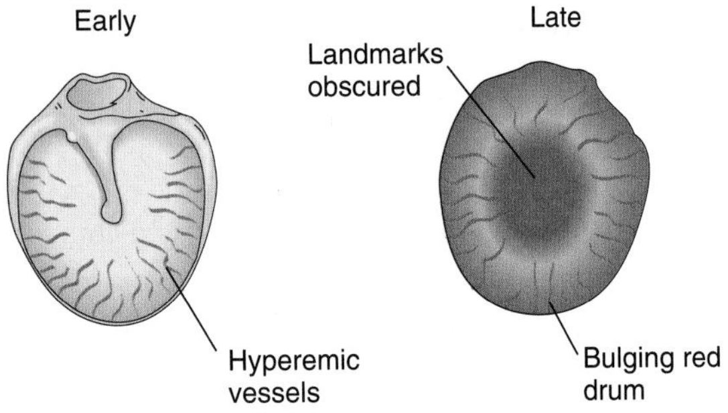

FIGURE 11.14 The tympanic membrane in the presence of otitis media. (A) Serous otitis media. (B) Acute purulent otitis media. *Hyperemic* means increased blood within these vessels.

- **Vertigo** (**VER**-tih-goh) is a sense of whirling, dizziness, and the loss of balance, that is often combined with nausea and vomiting. Although it is a symptom of many disorders, recurrent vertigo is sometimes associated with inner ear problems such as Ménière's syndrome.
- **Ménière's syndrome** is a rare chronic disease in which the amount of fluid in the inner ear increases intermittently, producing attacks of vertigo, a fluctuating hearing loss (usually in one ear), and tinnitus.
- **Tinnitus** (tih-**NIGH**-tus) is a ringing, buzzing, or roaring sound in one or both ears. It is often associated with hearing loss, and is more likely to occur when there has been prolonged exposure to loud noises.

Hearing Loss

- **Deafness** is the complete or partial loss of the ability to hear. It can range from the inability to hear sounds of a certain pitch or intensity, to a complete loss of hearing.
- **Presbycusis** (**pres**-beh-**KOO**-sis) is a gradual loss of sensorineural hearing that occurs as the body ages (**presby** means old age, and **-cusis** means hearing).
- A **conductive hearing loss** occurs when sound waves are prevented from passing from the air to the fluid-filled inner ear. Causes of this hearing loss include a buildup of earwax, infection, fluid in the middle ear, a punctured eardrum, otosclerosis, and scarring.
- A **sensorineural hearing loss**, also known as *nerve deafness*, develops when the auditory nerve or hair cells in the inner ear are damaged. The source of this hearing loss can be located in the inner ear, in the nerve from the inner ear to the brain, or in the brain.

Noise-Induced Hearing Loss

A **noise-induced hearing loss** (NIHL) is a type of nerve deafness caused by repeated exposure to extremely loud noises such as a gunshot, or to moderately loud noise that continues for long periods of time.

- These noises can permanently damage the hair cells in the cochlea, and at least partial hearing loss occurs. Unfortunately, this gradual hearing loss usually isn't noticed until some hearing has been permanently destroyed.
- Any sound above 90 decibels (db) can cause some hearing loss if the exposure is prolonged (Figure 11.15). Most portable music players can produce sounds up to 120 db which is louder than a lawn mower or a chain saw and is the equivalent to an ambulance siren.

DIAGNOSTIC PROCEDURES OF THE EARS AND HEARING

- An **audiological evaluation**, also known as *speech audiometry*, is the measurement of the ability to hear and understand speech sounds based on their pitch and loudness. This testing is best achieved in a sound-treated room with earphones. The resulting graph is an *audiogram* that represents the ability to hear a variety of sounds at various loudness levels.
- **Audiometry** (**aw**-dee-**OM**-eh-tree) is the use of an audiometer to measure hearing acuity (**audi/o** means hearing, and **-metry** means to measure). An *audiometer* is an electronic device that produces acoustic stimuli of a set frequency and intensity.
- Sound is measured in two different ways. A **hertz** (Hz) is a measure of sound frequency that determines how high or low a pitch is. A **decibel** is commonly used as the measurement of the loudness of sound.
- An *otoscope*, which is used to examine the external ear canal, is discussed in Chapter 15.

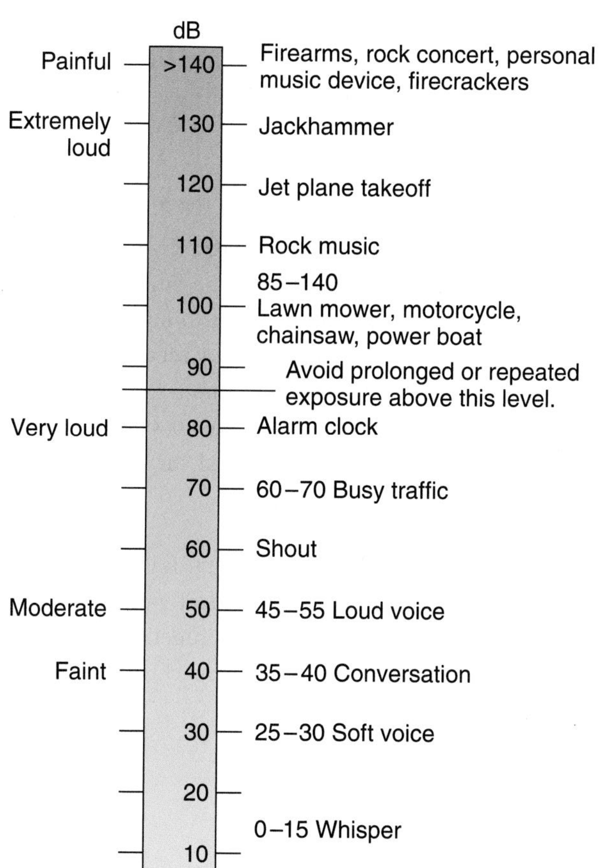

FIGURE 11.15 A decibel scale of frequently heard sounds.

- **Monaural testing** (mon-**AW**-rahl) involves one ear (**mon-** means one, **aur** means hearing, and **-al** means pertaining to). Compare with *binaural testing.*
- **Binaural testing** (bye-**NAW**-rul *or* bin-**AW**-rahl) involves both ears (**bi-** means two, **aur** means hearing, and **-al** means pertaining to). Compare with *monaural testing.*
- **Tympanometry** (**tim**-pah-**NOM**-eh-tree) is the use of air pressure in the ear canal to test for disorders of the middle ear (**tympan/o** means eardrum, and **-metry** means to measure). The resulting record is a *tympanogram*. This is used to test for middle ear fluid buildup or eustachian tube obstruction, or to evaluate a conductive hearing loss.

TREATMENT PROCEDURES OF THE EARS AND HEARING

The Outer Ear

- **Otoplasty** (**OH**-toh-**plas**-tee) is the surgical repair of the pinna of the ear (**ot/o** means ear, and **-plasty** means surgical repair).

The Middle Ear

- A **mastoidectomy** (**mas**-toy-**DECK**-toh-mee) is the surgical removal of mastoid cells (**mastoid** means mastoid process, and **-ectomy** means surgical removal). This procedure is used to treat a mastoiditis that cannot be controlled with antibiotics or in preparation for the placement of a cochlear implant.
- A **myringotomy** (**mir**-in-**GOT**-oh-mee) is the surgical incision in the eardrum to create an opening for the placement of tympanostomy tubes (**myring** means eardrum, and **-otomy** means surgical incision).
- **Tympanostomy tubes** (**tim**-pan-**OSS**-toh-mee), also known as *pediatric ear tubes*, are tiny ventilating tubes placed through the eardrum to provide ongoing drainage for fluids and to relieve pressure that can build up after childhood ear infections (Figure 11.16).
- **Tympanoplasty** (**tim**-pah-noh-**PLAS**-tee) is the surgical correction of a damaged middle ear, either to cure chronic inflammation or to restore function (**tympan/o** means eardrum, and **-plasty** means a surgical repair).

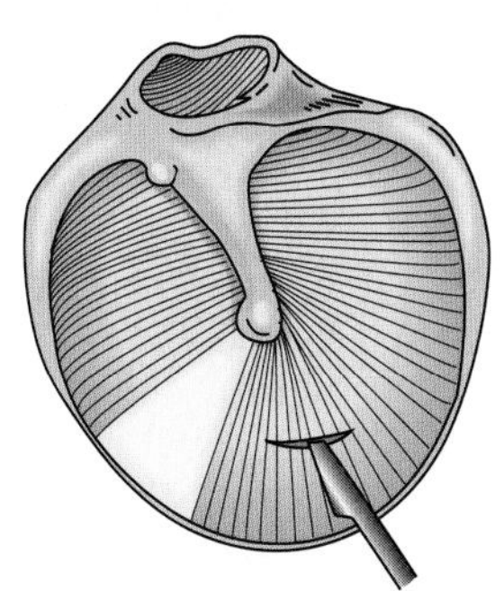

Tympanic membrane incision

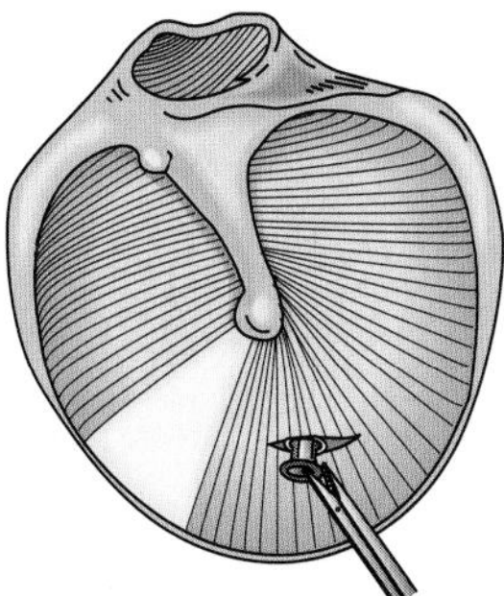

Tube placement

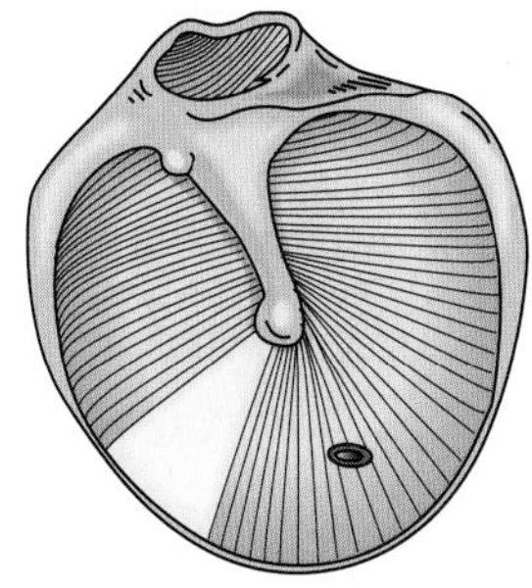

Tympanoplasty completed

FIGURE 11.16 Tympanoplasty and the placement of a pediatric ear tube.

- A **stapedectomy** (**stay**-peh-**DECK**-toh-mee) is the surgical removal of the top portion of the stapes bone and the insertion of a small prosthetic device known as a piston that conducts sound vibrations to the inner ear.

The Inner Ear

- **Fenestration** (**fen**-es-**TRAY**-shun) is a surgical procedure in which a new opening is created in the labyrinth to restore hearing (**fenestra** means window, and **-tion** means process).
- A **hearing aid** is an external electronic device that uses a microphone to detect sounds. The sounds may be coded into a digital representation and are filtered to best compensate for the hearing loss before being amplified into the ear canal. Sensorineural hearing loss can sometimes be corrected with a hearing aid.
- A **labyrinthectomy** (**lab**-ih-rin-**THECK**-toh-mee) is the surgical removal of all or a portion of the labyrinth (**labyrinth** means labyrinth, and **-ectomy** means surgical removal). This procedure is performed to relieve uncontrolled vertigo; however, this procedure causes a complete hearing loss in the affected ear.
- A **labyrinthotomy** (**lab**-ih-rin-**THOT**-oh-mee) is a surgical incision between two of the fluid chambers of the labyrinth to allow the pressure to equalize (**labyrinth** means labyrinth, and **-otomy** means a surgical incision). This procedure is performed to relieve severe vertigo; however, about half of patients suffer some loss of high tone hearing in the affected ear.

Cochlear Implant

A **cochlear implant** (**KOCK**-lee-ar) is an implanted electronic device that can give a deaf person a useful auditory understanding of the environment and/or hearing and help them to understand speech (Figure 11.17).

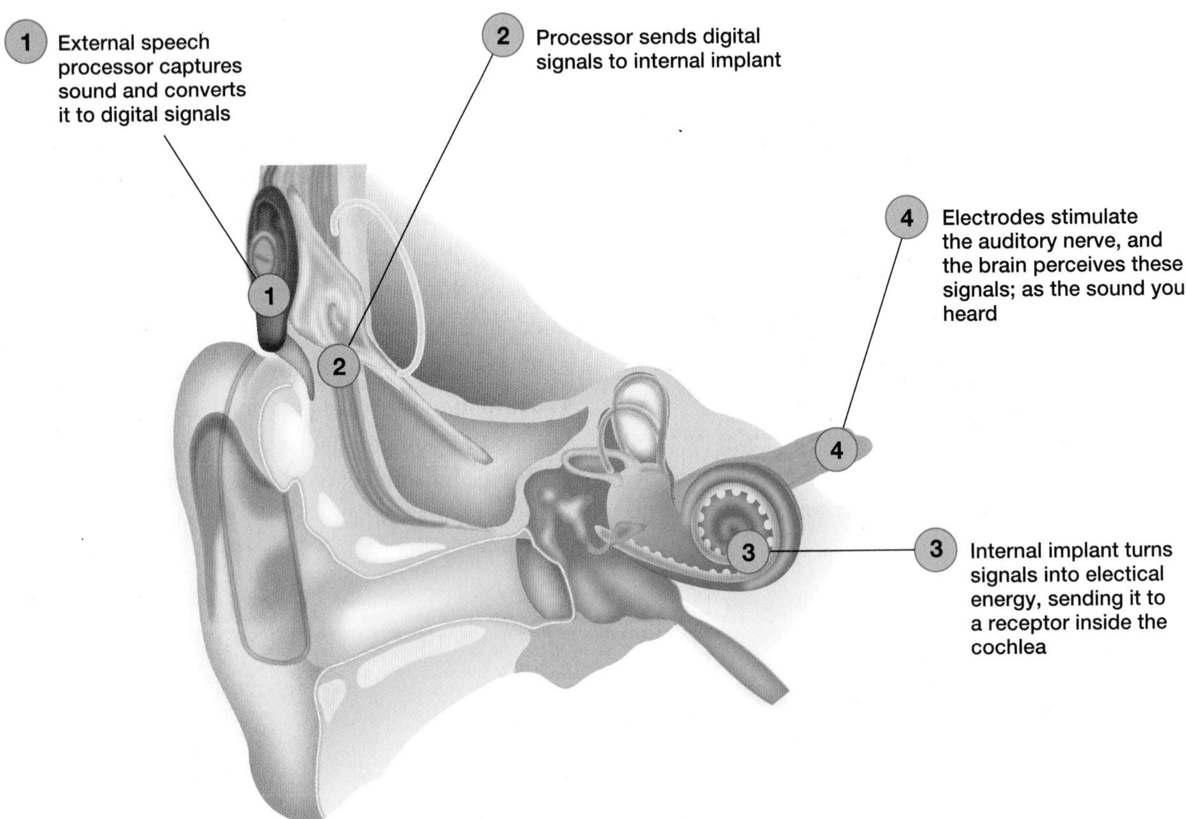
1 External speech processor captures sound and converts it to digital signals
2 Processor sends digital signals to internal implant
4 Electrodes stimulate the auditory nerve, and the brain perceives these signals; as the sound you heard
3 Internal implant turns signals into electical energy, sending it to a receptor inside the cochlea
1
2
3
4

FIGURE 11.17 A cochlear implant transmits signals to electrodes that are implanted in the cochlea. This provides limited hearing for an individual who has been deaf since birth.

The external speech processor captures sounds and converts them into digital signals. Electrodes implanted in the cochlea receive the signals and stimulate the auditory nerve. The brain receives these signals and perceives them as sound.

ABBREVIATIONS RELATED TO THE SPECIAL SENSES

Table 11.3 presents an overview of the abbreviations related to the terms introduced in this chapter. Note: To avoid errors or confusion, always be cautious when using abbreviations.

TABLE 11.3

ABBREVIATIONS RELATED TO THE SPECIAL SENSES

astigmatism = AS	**AS** = astigmatism
cataract = CAT	**CAT** = cataract
conjunctivitis = CI	**CI** = conjunctivitis
diopter = D, Dptr	**D, Dptr** = diopter
emmetropia = EM, em	**EM, em** = emmetropia
fluorescein angiography = FA, FAG	**FA, FAG** = fluorescein angiography
glaucoma = G, glc	**G, glc** = glaucoma
macular degeneration = MD	**MD** = macular degeneration
radial keratotomy = RK	**RK** = radial keratotomy
retinal detachment = RD	**RD** = retinal detachment
visual acuity = V, VA	**V, VA** = visual acuity

Career Opportunities

In addition to the medical specialties already discussed, some of the health occupations involving the treatment of the eyes and ears include:

- **Ophthalmic dispenser or dispensing optician:** places orders for prescribed ophthalmic laboratory work, helps patients select frames, adjusts finished glasses, and may fit patients for contact lenses
- **Ocularist:** a dispensing optician who specializes in fitting artificial eyes
- **Ophthalmic laboratory technician:** makes eyeglasses and contact lenses, cutting, grinding, and finishing them according to prescription specifications.
- **Optometric technician** (OpT) or **paraoptometric:** works under the supervision of an ophthalmologist (or optometrist) preparing patients for examinations, performing receptionist duties, helping patients with frame selection, and instructing patients on the care and use of their contact lenses. An OpT also administers basic vision tests and teaches eye exercises.
- **Optometric assistant:** performs the same duties as an OpT, with the exception of administering vision testing and teaching eye exercises
- **Orientation and mobility instructor:** teaches visually challenged individuals how to move about safely in a variety of environments
- **Audiologist:** provides care to individuals with hearing problems, tests, diagnoses, and prescribes treatment. Audiologists also conduct noise-level testing in workplaces and work to prevent hearing loss.
- **Speech/language therapist** or **pathologist:** identifies, evaluates, and treats patients with speech and language disorders; may work with elementary or preschool children, or in the rehabilitation of stroke patients

Health Occupation Profile

Audiologist

Perry C. Hanavan is an audiologist in Sioux Falls, South Dakota. *"As an audiologist, I identify, diagnose, treat, and manage individuals with communication disorders resulting from hearing loss. From diagnosing hearing problems in newborns to providing audiologic services to elderly persons who suffer a hearing loss, this profession provides challenging and stimulating career experiences across the life span.*

"Audiologists select, dispense, and fit hearing aids and assistive listening devices, and are a part of the cochlear implant team. Increasingly, audiologists rely on a variety of technologies to fit programmable and digital hearing aids, to assess auditory brain activity, and to assess middle ear and inner ear function.

"I was in search of a profession that included psychology, science, and technology when I discovered the fascinating field of audiology while in college. I am now an assistant professor, teaching audiology courses and supervising students providing audiologic services."

STUDY BREAK

Images seen through the *rods* and *cones* of the retina of the eye are converted into nerve impulses to be interpreted by the brain. Sometimes the brain gets confused by the images it receives, as is the case of an optical illusion. Try this famous Floating Finger optical illusion:

- **Hold your hands in front of you at eye level. Point your index fingers toward each other. Leave a little space (an inch or so) between your two index fingers. With your fingers at eye level, focus on a wall or an object a few feet away.**
- **You should see a finger with two ends floating between your two index fingers. If you have trouble seeing it, try moving your fingers closer to your eyes (still at eye level).**
- **For a different illusion, try this with your two index fingers actually touching each other.**

Optical illusions are part of our everyday vision. Newspaper illustrations and computer screens, for example, are made up of small colored dots that our brain merges into solid images. If the optic nerve could transmit only literal impulses to the brain, we would not be able to enjoy television, animation, and many other wonderful optical illusions.

REVIEW TIME

Write the answers to the following questions on a separate piece of paper or in your notebook. In addition, be prepared to take part in the classroom discussion.

1. ***Written Assignment:*** Using terms a physician would understand, describe the differences between **open-angle glaucoma** and **closed-angle glaucoma**.

   Discussion Assignment: What test is performed to detect open-angle glaucoma?

2. ***Written Assignment:*** Describe the differences between a **conductive hearing loss** and a **noise-induced hearing loss**.

   Discussion Assignment: What steps can be taken to prevent a noise-induced hearing loss, and at what age should one begin taking these precautions?

3. ***Written Assignment:*** Using terms a patient could understand, describe the difference in the vision loss associated with **cataracts** as contrasted with **macular degeneration**.

   Discussion Assignment: How would each of these vision losses affect the patient's quality of life?

4. ***Written Assignment:*** Describe the difference between **tinnitus** and **vertigo**.

   Discussion Assignment: How would each of these conditions affect the patient?

5. ***Written Assignment:*** Describe the difference between **hyperopia** and **myopia**.

   Discussion Assignment: How would you explain each of these conditions to a young patient and his or her family?

continues

Optional Internet Activity

The goal of this activity is to help you learn more about medical terminology as it applies to the "real world." Select **one** *of these two options and follow the instructions.*

1. Search for information about **cochlear implants**. Write a brief (one- or two-paragraph) report on something new you learned here and include the address of the web site where you found this information.
2. To learn more about **cataract symptoms and treatment**, go to the online MedlinePlus Medical Encyclopedia. Explore the site and then write a brief (one- or two-paragraph) report on something new you learned here.

THE HUMAN TOUCH: CRITICAL THINKING ACTIVITY

The following story and questions are designed to stimulate critical thinking through class discussion or as a brief essay response. There are no right or wrong answers to these questions.

Jose was thrilled that he'd won the radio station contest for four front-row tickets to a concert by his favorite band. Their music ranged from classic rock to heavy metal, and he knew the sound would be powerfully amplified as it blasted out of the speakers stacked at the corners of the stage and reverberated throughout the arena. His older sister had bugged him about taking earplugs, but he couldn't bring himself to wear the pair that she'd given him. Bright orange earplugs would look so dorky, and besides, he wouldn't be able to hear the music clearly if he had earplugs in.

The concert was great, and lasted for hours. By the time it ended, all of the sounds around him were muffled and Jose felt as if his ears had been stuffed with cotton. As he rode home with his friends, he realized that they all seemed to be having trouble hearing each other. Assuming that the ringing in his ears would go away by the morning, Jose wasn't worried when he went to bed.

In the morning, though, the ringing sound was still there and he had trouble figuring out what his sister was saying to him over breakfast. Jose didn't want her to know that he hadn't worn the earplugs she'd given him, so he didn't mention it. Surely the ringing would go away on its own. When he could still hear ringing in his ears in the late afternoon, he sat down at his computer to do some research. The results he found really worried him.

What if he had developed a permanent noise-induced hearing loss, accompanied by tinnitus, as the symptoms seemed to suggest? It was only one concert! Sure, it had been loud and he hadn't worn earplugs, but at 17, this sort of thing couldn't happen to him! Jose turned off his computer and went out for a walk to think things over.

continues

Suggested Discussion Topics

1. Jose's sister tried to get him to take appropriate protective steps, and he had refused. Discuss what, if anything, more she could have done. Also discuss Jose's responsibility in not using the earplugs.
2. Discuss the sounds Jose might encounter in his everyday activities, other than concerts, that might contribute to a noise-induced hearing loss. These could be anywhere, including in school, at home or at his part-time job.
3. Those who regularly work backstage, or perform in concerts such as the one Jose attended, are repeatedly exposed to damaging sound levels. What, if anything, do these individuals do to protect their hearing?
4. Jose's grandfather has a progressive hearing loss associated with aging, but he refuses to wear a hearing aid. Discuss how this affects the quality of life of his grandfather and other family members who care about him.

STUDENT WORKBOOK AND StudyWARE™ CD-ROM

1. Go to your **Student Workbook** and complete the Learning Exercises for this chapter.

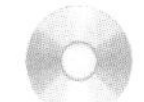

2. Go to the **StudyWARE™ CD-ROM** and have fun with the exercises and games for this chapter.

12

CHAPTER

SKIN: THE INTEGUMENTARY SYSTEM

OVERVIEW OF STRUCTURES, COMBINING FORMS, AND FUNCTIONS OF THE INTEGUMENTARY SYSTEM

MAJOR STRUCTURES	RELATED COMBINING FORMS	PRIMARY FUNCTIONS
Skin	cutane/o, dermat/o, derm/o	Intact skin is the first line of defense for the immune system. Waterproofs the body and is the major receptor for the sense of touch.
Sebaceous Glands	seb/o	Secrete sebum (oil) to lubricate the skin and discourage the growth of bacteria on the skin.
Sweat Glands	hidr/o	Secrete sweat to regulate body temperature and water content, and excrete some metabolic waste.
Hair	pil/i, pil/o	Aids in controlling the loss of body heat.
Nails	onych/o, ungu/o	Protect the dorsal surface of the last bone of each finger and toe.

Vocabulary Related to the Integumentary System

This list contains essential word parts and medical terms for this chapter. These terms are pronounced on the student StudyWARE™ CD-ROM and Audio CDs that are available for use with this text. These and the other important **primary terms** are shown in boldface throughout the chapter. *Secondary terms*, which appear in *orange* italics, clarify the meaning of primary terms.

Word Parts

- ☐ **bi/o**
- ☐ **derm/o, dermat/o**
- ☐ **erythr/o**
- ☐ **hidr/o**
- ☐ **hirsut/o**
- ☐ **kerat/o**
- ☐ **lip/o**
- ☐ **melan/o**
- ☐ **myc/o**
- ☐ **onych/o**
- ☐ **pedicul/o**
- ☐ **rhytid/o**
- ☐ **seb/o**
- ☐ **urtic/o**
- ☐ **xer/o**

Medical Terms

- ☐ **actinic keratosis** (ack-**TIN**-ick **kerr**-ah-**TOH**-sis)
- ☐ **albinism** (**AL**-bih-niz-um)
- ☐ **alopecia** (**al**-oh-**PEE**-shee-ah)
- ☐ **blepharoplasty** (**BLEF**-ah-roh-**plas**-tee)
- ☐ **bulla** (**BULL**-ah)
- ☐ **carbuncle** (**KAR**-bung-kul)
- ☐ **cellulitis** (**sell**-you-**LYE**-tis)
- ☐ **chloasma** (kloh-**AZ**-mah)
- ☐ **cicatrix** (sick-**AY**-tricks)
- ☐ **comedo** (**KOM**-eh-doh)
- ☐ **debridement** (day-breed-**MON**)
- ☐ **dermatitis** (**der**-mah-**TYE**-tis)
- ☐ **diaphoresis** (**dye**-ah-foh-**REE**-sis)
- ☐ **dysplastic nevi** (dis-**PLAS**-tick **NEE**-vye)
- ☐ **ecchymosis** (**eck**-ih-**MOH**-sis)
- ☐ **eczema** (**ECK**-zeh-mah)
- ☐ **erythema** (**er**-ih-**THEE**-mah)
- ☐ **erythroderma** (eh-**rith**-roh-**DER**-mah)
- ☐ **exfoliative dermatitis** (ecks-**FOH**-lee-**ay**-tiv eh-**rith**-roh-**DER**-mah)
- ☐ **folliculitis** (foh-**lick**-you-**LYE**-tis)
- ☐ **furuncles** (**FYOU**-rung-kulz)
- ☐ **granuloma** (**gran**-you-**LOH**-mah)
- ☐ **hematoma** (**hee**-mah-**TOH**-mah)
- ☐ **hirsutism** (**HER**-soot-izm)
- ☐ **ichthyosis** (**ick**-thee-**OH**-sis)
- ☐ **impetigo** (**im**-peh-**TYE**-go)
- ☐ **keloid** (**KEE**-loid)
- ☐ **keratosis** (**kerr**-ah-**TOH**-sis)
- ☐ **koilonychia** (**koy**-loh-**NICK**-ee-ah)
- ☐ **lipedema** (lip-eh-**DEE**-mah)
- ☐ **lipoma** (lih-**POH**-mah)
- ☐ **lupus erythematosus** (**LOO**-pus er-ih-**thee**-mah-**TOH**-sus)
- ☐ **macule** (**MACK**-youl)
- ☐ **malignant melanoma** (mel-ah-**NOH**-mah)
- ☐ **miliaria** (**mill**-ee-**AYR**-ee-ah)
- ☐ **necrotizing fasciitis** (**fas**-ee-**EYE**-tis)
- ☐ **onychocryptosis** (**on**-ih-koh-krip-**TOH**-sis)
- ☐ **onychomycosis** (**on**-ih-koh-my-**KOH**-sis)
- ☐ **papilloma** (**pap**-ih-**LOH**-mah)
- ☐ **papule** (**PAP**-youl)
- ☐ **paronychia** (**par**-oh-**NICK**-ee-ah)
- ☐ **pediculosis** (pee-**dick**-you-**LOH**-sis)
- ☐ **petechiae** (pee-**TEE**-kee-ee)
- ☐ **pruritus** (proo-**RYE**-tus)
- ☐ **psoriasis** (soh-**RYE**-uh-sis)
- ☐ **purpura** (**PUR**-pew-rah)
- ☐ **purulent** (**PYOU**-roo-lent)
- ☐ **rhytidectomy** (**rit**-ih-**DECK**-toh-mee)
- ☐ **rosacea** (roh-**ZAY**-shee-ah)
- ☐ **scabies** (**SKAY**-beez)
- ☐ **scleroderma** (**sklehr**-oh-**DER**-mah)
- ☐ **seborrhea** (**seb**-oh-**REE**-ah)
- ☐ **squamous cell carcinoma** (**SKWAY**-mus)
- ☐ **strawberry hemangioma** (hee-**man**-jee-**OH**-mah)
- ☐ **tinea** (**TIN**-ee-ah)
- ☐ **urticaria** (**ur**-tih-**KARE**-ree-ah)
- ☐ **verrucae** (veh-**ROO**-kee)
- ☐ **vitiligo** (**vit**-ih-**LYE**-goh)
- ☐ **wheal** (**WHEEL**)
- ☐ **xeroderma** (zee-roh-**DER**-mah)

OBJECTIVES

On completion of this chapter, you should be able to:

1. Identify and describe the functions and structures of the integumentary system.
2. Identify the medical specialists associated with the integumentary system.
3. Recognize, define, spell, and pronounce the terms used to describe the pathology and the diagnostic and treatment procedures related to the skin.
4. Recognize, define, spell, and pronounce terms used to describe the pathology and the diagnostic and treatment procedures related to hair, nails, and sebaceous glands.

FUNCTIONS OF THE INTEGUMENTARY SYSTEM

The **integumentary system** (in-**teg**-you-**MEN**-tah-ree), which is made up of the skin and its related structures, performs important functions in maintaining the health of the body.

Functions of the Skin

The skin forms the protective outer covering of the entire body.

- The skin waterproofs the body and prevents fluid loss.
- Intact (unbroken) skin plays an important role in the immune system by blocking the entrance of pathogens into the body (see Chapter 6).
- Skin is the major receptor for the sense of touch.
- Skin helps the body manufacture vitamin D, an essential nutrient, from the sun's ultraviolet light, while screening out some harmful ultraviolet radiation.

Functions of Related Structures

The related structures of the integumentary system are the sebaceous glands, sweat glands, hair, and nails (Figure 12.1).

- The **sebaceous glands** (seh-**BAY**-shus) secrete sebum (oil) that lubricates the skin and discourages the growth of bacteria on the skin.
- The **sweat glands** help regulate body temperature and water content by secreting sweat. A small amount of metabolic waste is also excreted through the sweat glands.
- **Hair** helps control the loss of body heat.
- **Nails** protect the dorsal surface of the last bone of each toe and finger.

THE STRUCTURES OF THE SKIN AND ITS RELATED STRUCTURES

The Skin

Skin covers the external surfaces of the body. The average adult has two square yards of skin, making it the largest bodily organ. The terms **cutaneous** (kyou-**TAY**-nee-us) means relating to the skin (**cutane** means skin, and **-ous** means pertaining to).

The skin is a complex system of specialized tissues and is made up of three basic layers: the epidermis, dermis, and the subcutaneous layer (see Figures 12.1 and 12.2).

The Epidermis

The **epidermis** (**ep**-ih-**DER**-mis), which is the outermost layer of the skin, is made up of several specialized epithelial tissues.

- **Epithelial tissues** (**ep**-ih-**THEE**-lee-al) form a protective covering for all of the internal *and* external surfaces of the body.
- **Squamous epithelial tissue** (**SKWAY**-mus) forms the upper layer of the epidermis. *Squamous* means scale-like. This layer consists of flat, scaly cells that are continuously shed.
- The epidermis, which does not contain any blood vessels or connective tissue, is dependent on lower layers for nourishment.
- The *basal layer* is the lowest layer of the epidermis. It is here that cells are produced and then pushed upward. When these cells reach the surface, they die and become filled with keratin.
- **Keratin** (**KER**-ah-tin) is a fibrous, water-repellent protein. Soft keratin is a primary component of the epidermis. Hard keratin is found in the hair and nails.

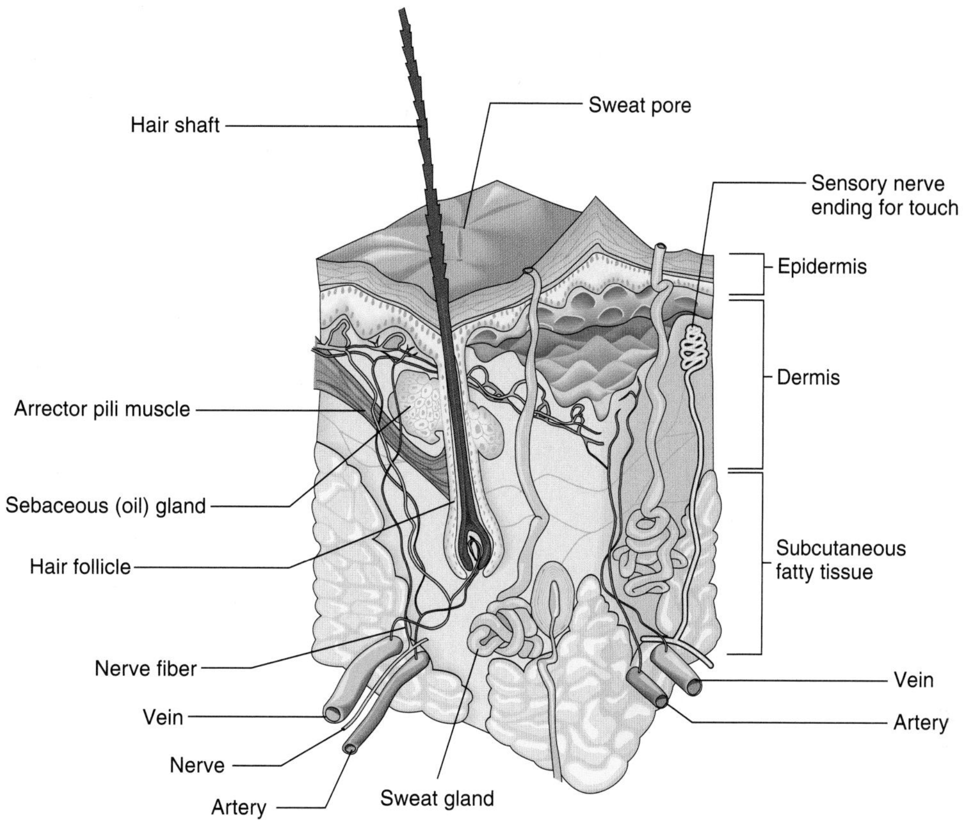

FIGURE 12.1 Structures of the skin.

- The basal cell layer also contains special cells called **melanocytes** (**MEL**-ah-noh-sights). These cells produce and contain a dark brown to black pigment called *melanin*. The type and amount of melanin pigment determines the color of the skin. It also produces spots of color such as freckles.
- Melanin has the important function of protecting the skin against some of the harmful ultraviolet rays of the sun. *Ultraviolet* (UV) refers to light that is beyond the visible spectrum at the violet end. Some UV rays help the skin produce vitamin D; however, other rays damage the skin.

The Dermis

The **dermis** (**DER**-mis), also known as the *corium*, is the thick layer of living tissue directly below the epidermis. It contains connective tissue, blood and lymph vessels, and nerve fibers. It also contains the associated structures of the skin, which are the hair follicles plus the sebaceous and sweat glands.

Sensory nerve endings in the dermis are the sensory receptors stimuli such as touch, temperature, pain, and pressure.

Tissues Within the Dermis

- **Collagen** (**KOL**-ah-jen), which means glue, is a tough, yet flexible, fibrous protein material found in the skin and in the bones, cartilage, tendons, and ligaments.
- **Mast cells**, which are found in the connective tissue of the dermis, respond to injury, infection, or allergy by producing and releasing substances, including heparin and histamine.
- **Heparin** (**HEP**-ah-rin), which is released in response to an injury, is an anticoagulant. An *anticoagulant* prevents blood clotting.
- **Histamine** (**HISS**-tah-meen), which is released in response to allergens, causes the signs of an allergic response, including itching and increased mucus secretion.

The Subcutaneous Layer

The **subcutaneous layer**, which is located just below the skin, connects the skin to the surface muscles.

- This layer is made up of loose connective tissue and **adipose tissue** (**AD**-ih-pohs). *Adipose* means fat.

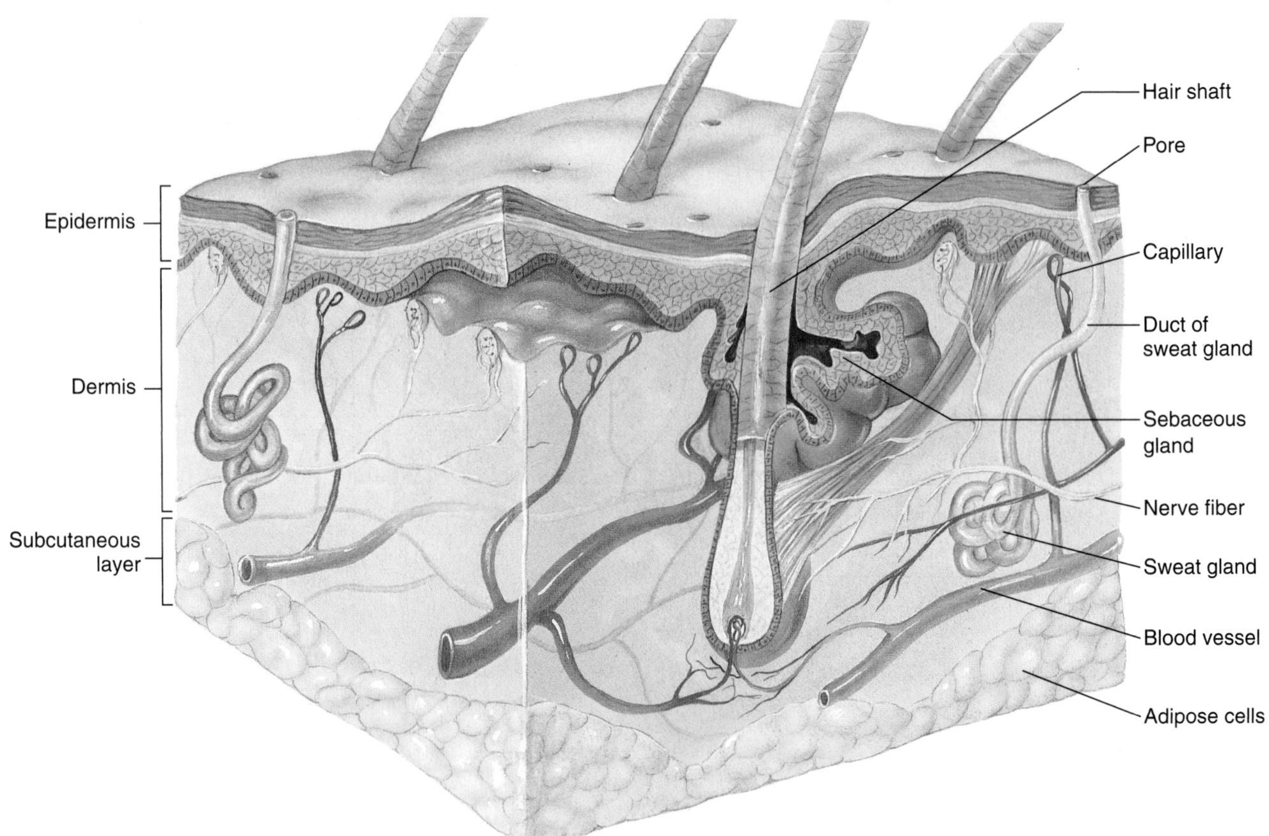

FIGURE 12.2 Sweat and sebaceous glands are associated structures of the skin.

- *Cellulite* is a term sometimes used to describe deposits of dimpled fat. This is not a medical term, and medical authorities agree that cellulite is simply ordinary fatty tissue. Note: Do not confuse cellulite with cellulitis, which is discussed later in this chapter.
- **Lipocytes** (**LIP**-oh-sights), also known as *fat cells*, are predominant in the subcutaneous layer where they manufacture and store large quantities of fat (**lip/o** means fat, and **-cytes** means cells).

The Sebaceous Glands

Sebaceous glands (seh-**BAY**-shus) are located in the dermis layer of the skin and are closely associated with hair follicles (see Figures 12.1 and 12.2).

- These glands secrete **sebum** (**SEE**-bum), which is released through ducts opening into the hair follicles. From here, the sebum moves onto the surface and lubricates the skin.
- Because sebum is slightly acidic, it discourages the growth of bacteria on the skin.
- The milk-producing **mammary glands**, which are modified sebaceous glands, are sometimes classified with the integumentary system. However, they also are part of the reproductive system and are discussed in Chapter 14.

The Sweat Glands

Sweat glands, also known as *sudoriferous glands*, are tiny, coiled glands found on almost all body surfaces. They are most numerous in the palms of the hands, the soles of the feet, the forehead, and the armpits.

- **Pores** are the openings on the surface of the skin for the ducts of the sweat glands.
- **Perspiration**, also known as *sweat*, is secreted by sweat glands and is made up of 99% water plus some salt and metabolic waste products.
- **Perspiring**, also known as *sweating*, is one way in which the body excretes excess water. As the sweat evaporates into the air it also cools the body. Body odor associated with sweat comes from the interaction of the perspiration with bacteria on the skin's surface.
- **Hidrosis** (high-**DROH**-sis) is the production and excretion of sweat.

The Hair

Hair fibers are rod-like structures composed of tightly fused, dead protein cells filled with hard keratin. The darkness and color of the hair is determined by the amount and type of melanin produced by the melanocytes that surround the core of the hair shaft.

- **Hair follicles** are the sacs that hold the root of the hair fibers. The shape of the follicle determines whether the hair is straight or curly.
- Although hair is dead tissue, it appears to grow because the cells at the base of the follicle divide rapidly and push the old cells upward. As these cells are pushed upward, they harden and undergo pigmentation.
- The **arrector pili** (ah-**RECK**-tor **PYE**-lye) are tiny muscle fibers attached to the hair follicles that cause the hair to stand erect. In response to cold or fright, these muscles contract, causing raised areas of skin known as goose bumps. This action reduces heat loss through the skin.

The Nails

An **unguis** (**UNG**-gwis), commonly known as a fingernail or toenail, is the keratin plate protecting the dorsal surface of the last bone of each finger and toe (plural, *ungues*). Each nail consists of these parts (Figure 12.3):

- The *nail body*, which is translucent, is closely molded to the surface of the underlying tissues. It is made up of hard, keratinized plates of epidermal cells.

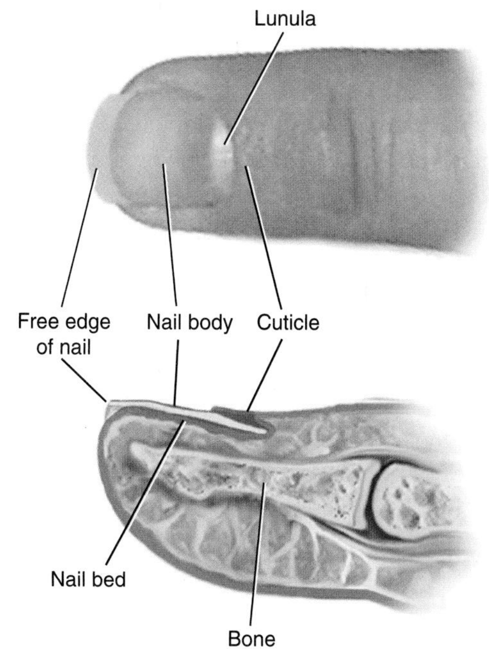

FIGURE 12.3 Structures of the fingernails and toenails.

- The *nail bed*, which joins the nail body to the underlying connective tissue, nourishes the nail. The blood vessels here give the nail its characteristic pink color.
- The *free edge*, which is the portion of the nail not attached to the nail bed, extends beyond the tip of the finger or toe.
- The **lunula** (**LOO**-new-lah) is a pale half-moon–shaped region at every nail root that is generally most easily seen in the thumbnail (plural, *lunulae*). This is the active area of the nail, where new keratin cells form. *Lunula* means little moon.
- The **cuticle** is a narrow band of epidermis attached to the surface of the nail just in front of the root, protecting the new keratin cells as they form. *Cuticle* means little skin.
- The **nail root** fastens the nail to the finger or toe by fitting into a groove in the skin.

MEDICAL SPECIALTIES RELATED TO THE INTEGUMENTARY SYSTEM

- A **dermatologist** (**der**-mah-**TOL**-oh-jist) is a physician who specializes in diagnosing and treating disorders of the skin (**dermat** means skin, and **-ologist** means specialist).
- A **cosmetic surgeon**, also known as a *plastic surgeon*, is a physician who specializes in the surgical restoration and reconstruction of body structures. As used here, *plastic* refers to the suffix **-plasty**, meaning surgical repair.

PATHOLOGY OF THE INTEGUMENTARY SYSTEM

The Sebaceous Glands

- **Acne vulgaris** (**ACK**-nee vul-**GAY**-ris), commonly known as *acne*, is a chronic inflammatory disease characterized by pustular eruptions of the skin caused by an overproduction of sebum. Although often triggered by hormones in puberty and adolescence, it also occurs in adults. *Vulgaris* is a Latin term meaning common.
- A **comedo** (**KOM**-eh-doh) is a noninfected lesion formed by the buildup of sebum and keratin in a hair follicle (plural, *comedones*). Comedones are often associated with acne vulgaris. When a sebum plug is exposed to air, it oxidizes and becomes a *blackhead*.

- A **sebaceous cyst** (seh-**BAY**-shus **SIST**) is a closed sac associated with a sebaceous gland that is found just under the skin. These cysts contain yellow, fatty material and are usually found on the face, neck, or trunk.
- **Seborrhea** (**seb**-oh-**REE**-ah) is overactivity of the sebaceous glands that results in the production of an excessive amount of sebum (**seb/o** means sebum, and **-rrhea** means flow or discharge).
- **Seborrheic dermatitis** (**seb**-oh-**REE**-ick **der**-mah-**TYE**-tis) is an inflammation that causes scaling and itching of the upper layers of the skin or scalp. Extensive *dandruff* is a form of seborrheic dermatitis, as is the scalp rash in infants known as *cradle cap*. In contrast, mild dandruff is usually caused by a yeast-like fungus on the scalp.
- A **seborrheic keratosis** (**seb**-oh-**REE**-ick **kerr**-ah-**TOH**-sis) is a benign skin growth that has a waxy or "pasted-on" look. These growths, which can vary in color from light tan to black, occur most commonly in the elderly.

The Sweat Glands

- **Anhidrosis** (**an**-high-**DROH**-sis) is the abnormal condition of lacking sweat in response to heat (**an-** means without, **hidr** means sweat, and **-osis** means abnormal condition).
- **Diaphoresis** (**dye**-ah-foh-**REE**-sis) is profuse sweating (**dia-** means through or complete, **phor** means movement, and **-esis** means abnormal condition). This is a normal condition when brought on by heat or exertion, but can also be the body's response to emotional or physical distress.
- **Hyperhidrosis** (**high**-per-high-**DROH**-sis) is a condition of sweating in one area or over the whole body (**hyper-** means excessive, **hidr** means sweat, and **-osis** means abnormal condition).
- **Miliaria** (**mill**-ee-**AYR**-ee-ah), also known as *heat rash* and *prickly heat*, is an intensely itchy rash caused by blockage of the sweat glands by bacteria and dead cells. Caution: Do not confuse this condition with the infectious disease *malaria*.
- **Sleep hyperhidrosis**, commonly known as *night sweats*, is the occurrence of excessive hyperhidrosis during sleep. There are many potential causes of this condition, including menopause, certain medications, and some infectious diseases.

The Hair

Folliculitis (foh-**lick**-you-**LYE**-tis) is an inflammation of the hair follicles (**follicul** means the hair follicle, and **-itis** means inflammation). This condition is especially common on the limbs and in the beard area of men.

Excessive Hairiness

Hirsutism (**HER**-soot-izm) is the presence of excessive body and facial hair in women, usually occurring in a male pattern (**hirsut** means hairy, and **-ism** means condition). This condition can be hereditary or caused by a hormonal imbalance.

Abnormal Hair Loss

- **Alopecia** (**al**-oh-**PEE**-shee-ah), also known as *baldness*, is the partial or complete loss of hair, most commonly on the scalp (**alopec** means baldness, and **-ia** means condition).
- **Alopecia areata** is an autoimmune disorder that attacks the hair follicles, causing well-defined bald areas on the scalp or elsewhere on the body. This condition often begins in childhood. *Areata* means occurring in patches.
- **Alopecia capitis totalis** is an uncommon condition characterized by the loss of all the hair on the scalp. *Capitis* means head.
- **Alopecia universalis** is the total loss of hair on all parts of the body. *Universalis* means total.
- **Female pattern baldness** is a condition in which the hair thins in the front and on the sides of the scalp and sometimes on the crown. This condition rarely leads to total hair loss.
- **Male pattern baldness** is a common hair-loss pattern in men, with the hairline receding from the front to the back until only a horseshoe-shaped area of hair remains in the back and at the temples.

The Nails

- **Clubbing** is abnormal curving of the nails that is often accompanied by enlargement of the fingertips. This condition can be hereditary, but usually is caused by changes associated with oxygen deficiencies related to coronary or pulmonary disease.
- **Koilonychia** (**koy**-loh-**NICK**-ee-ah), also known as *spoon nail*, is a malformation of the nails in which the outer surface is concave or scooped out like the bowl of a spoon (**koil** means hollow or concave, **onych** means

fingernail or toenail, and **-ia** means condition). Koilonychia is often an indication of iron-deficiency anemia.

- **Onychia** (oh-**NICK**-ee-ah), also known as *onychitis*, is an inflammation of the matrix of the nail that usually results in the loss of the nail (**onych** means fingernail or toenail, and **-ia** means condition).
- **Onychocryptosis** (**on**-ih-koh-krip-**TOH**-sis) is commonly known an *ingrown toenail* (**onych/o** means fingernail or toenail, **crypt** means hidden, and **-osis** means abnormal condition). The edges of a toenail, usually on the big toe, curve inward and cut into the skin. The affected area is prone to inflammation or infection.
- **Onychomycosis** (**on**-ih-koh-my-**KOH**-sis) is a fungal infection of the nail (**onych/o** means fingernail or toenail, **myc** means fungus, and **-osis** means abnormal condition). Depending on the type of fungus involved, this condition can cause the nails to turn white, yellow, green, or black and to become thick or brittle.
- **Onychophagia** (**on**-ih-koh-**FAY**-jee-ah) means nail biting or nail eating (**onych/o** means fingernail or toenail, and **-phagia** means eating or swallowing).
- **Paronychia** (**par**-oh-**NICK**-ee-ah) is an acute or chronic infection of the skin fold around a nail (**par-** means near, **onych** means fingernail or toenail, and **-ia** means condition).

Skin Pigmentation

- **Albinism** (**AL**-bih-niz-um) is a genetic condition characterized by a deficiency or the absence of pigment in the skin, hair, and irises of the eyes (**albin** means white, and **-ism** means condition). This condition is the result of a missing enzyme that is necessary for the production of melanin. A person with this condition is known as an *albino*.
- **Chloasma** (kloh-**AZ**-mah), also known as *melasma* or the *mask of pregnancy*, is a pigmentation disorder characterized by brownish spots on the face. This can occur during pregnancy, especially among women with dark hair and fair skin, and usually disappears after delivery.
- **Melanosis** (**mel**-ah-**NOH**-sis) is any condition of unusual deposits of black pigment in different parts of the body (**melan** means black, and **-osis** means abnormal condition).
- **Vitiligo** (**vit**-ih-**LYE**-goh) is a skin condition resulting from the destruction of the melanocytes due to unknown causes. Vitiligo is characterized by irregular patches of white skin. Hair growing in an affected area is also white.

Bleeding into the Skin

- A **contusion** (kon-**TOO**-zhun) is an injury to underlying tissues without breaking the skin and is characterized by discoloration and pain (**contus** means bruise, and **-ion** means condition). The discoloration is caused by an accumulation of blood within the skin.
- An **ecchymosis** (**eck**-ih-**MOH**-sis), also known as a *bruise*, is a large, irregular area of purplish discoloration due to bleeding under the skin (**ecchym** means pouring out of juice, and **-osis** means abnormal condition) (plural, *ecchymoses*).
- **Purpura** (**PUR**-pew-rah) is the appearance of multiple purple discolorations on the skin caused by bleeding underneath the skin (**purpur** means purple, and **-a** is a noun ending). These areas of discoloration are smaller than ecchymosis and larger than petechiae.
- **Petechiae** (pee-**TEE**-kee-ee) are very small, pinpoint hemorrhages that are less than 2 mm in diameter (singular, *petechia*). These hemorrhages sometimes result from high fevers.
- A **hematoma** (**hee**-mah-**TOH**-mah), which is usually caused by an injury, is a swelling of clotted blood trapped in the tissues (**hemat** means blood, and **-oma** means tumor). The body eventually resorbs this blood. A hematoma is often named for the area where it occurs. For example, a *subungual hematoma* is blood trapped under a finger or toenail.

Surface Lesions

A **lesion** (**LEE**-zhun) is a pathologic change of the tissues due to disease or injury. Skin lesions are described by their appearance, location, color, and size as measured in centimeters (cm) (Figure 12.4).

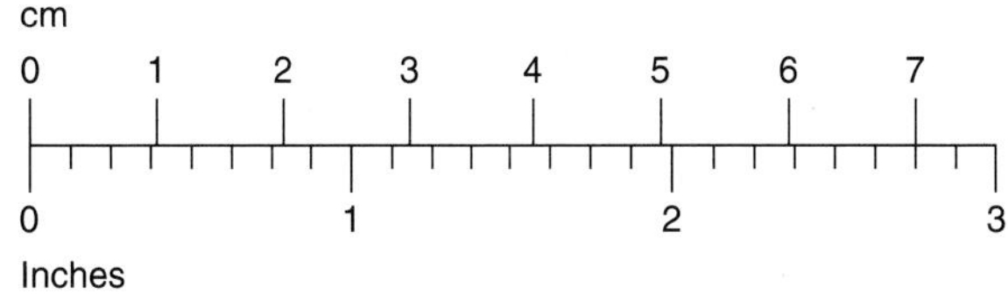

FIGURE 12.4 Lesions are described by length in centimeters. (Note: 2.5 cm equals 1 inch.)

- A **crust**, also known as *scab*, is a collection of dried serum and cellular debris (Figure 12.5A).
- A **macule** (**MACK**-youl), also known as a *macula*, is a discolored, flat spot that is less than 1 cm in diameter. Freckles, or flat moles, are examples of macules (Figure 12.5B).
- A **nodule** is a solid, raised skin lesion that is *larger than* 0.5 cm in diameter and deeper than a papule. In acne vulgaris, nodules can cause scarring.
- A **papule** (**PAP**-youl) is a small, raised red lesion that is *less than* 0.5 cm in diameter and does not contain pus. Small pimples and insect bites are types of papules (Figure 12.5C).
- A **plaque** (**PLACK**) is a scaly, solid raised area of closely spaced papules. For example, the lesions of psoriasis are plaques (see Figure 12.10). Note: The term *plaque* also means a fatty buildup in the arteries and a soft substance that forms on the teeth.
- **Scales** are flakes or dry patches made up of excess dead epidermal cells. Some shedding of scales is normal; however, excessive shedding is associated with skin disorders such as psoriasis (see Figure 12.10).
- **Verrucae** (veh-**ROO**-kee), also known as *warts*, are small, hard skin lesions caused by the human papilloma virus (singular, *verruca*). *Plantar warts* develop on the sole of the foot.
- A **wheal** (**WHEEL**), also known as a *welt*, is a small bump that itches. Wheals can appear as a symptom of an allergic reaction (Figure 12.5D).

Fluid-Filled Lesions

- An **abscess** (**AB**-sess) is a closed pocket containing pus that is caused by a bacterial infection. An abscess can appear on the skin or within other structures of the body. **Purulent** (**PYOU**-roo-lent) means producing or containing pus.
- A **cyst** (**SIST**) is an abnormal sac containing gas, fluid, or a semisolid material (see Figure 12.6A). The term *cyst* can also refer to a sac or vesicle elsewhere in the body. The most common type of skin cyst is a sebaceous cyst.
- A **pustule** (**PUS**-tyoul), also known as a *pimple*, is a small, circumscribed lesion containing pus (see Figure 12.6B). *Circumscribed* means contained within a limited area. Pustules can be cause by acne vulgaris, impetigo, or other infections.
- A **vesicle** (**VES**-ih-kul) is a small blister, *less than* 0.5 cm in diameter, containing watery fluid (see Figure 12.6C). For example, the rash of poison oak consists of vesicles (see Figure 12.9).
- A **bulla** (**BULL**-ah) is a large blister that is usually *more than* 0.5 cm in diameter (plural, *bullae*) (see Figure 12.6D).

Lesions Through the Skin

- An **abrasion** (ah-**BRAY**-zhun) is an injury in which superficial layers of skin are scraped or rubbed away. The term *abrasion* also describes a treatment that

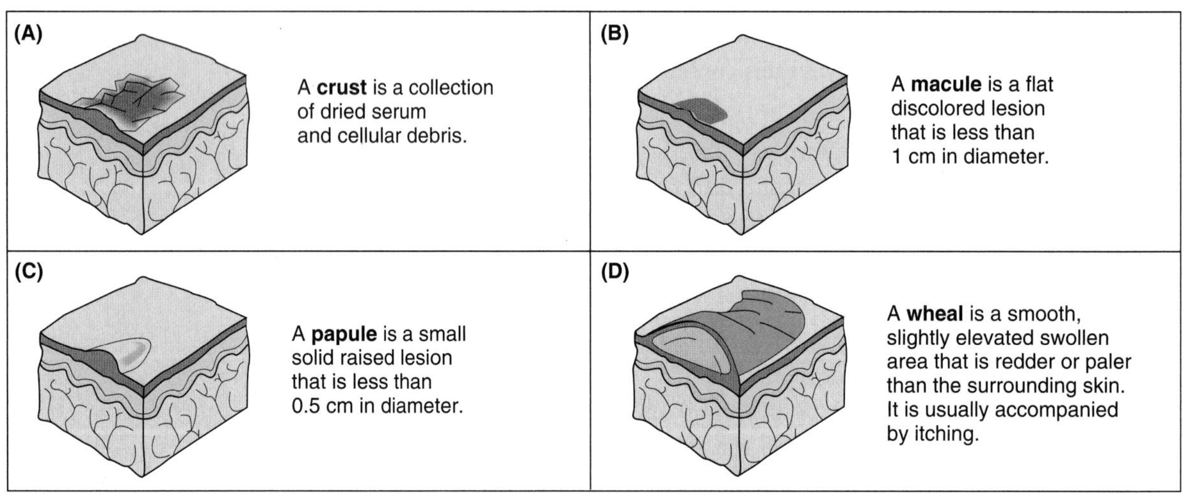

FIGURE 12.5 Surface lesions of the skin. (A) Crust. (B) Macule. (C) Papule. (D) Wheal.

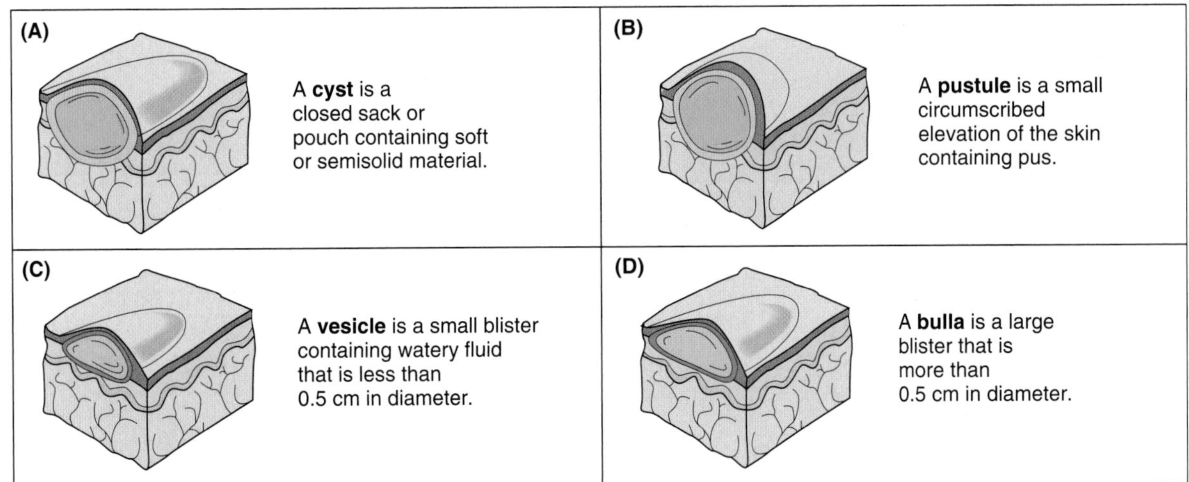

FIGURE 12.6 Fluid-filled lesions in the skin. (A) Cyst. (B) Pustule. (C) Vesicle. (D) Bulla.

involves scraping or rubbing away skin. See dermabrasion later in this chapter.

- A **pressure sore**, previously known as a *decubitus ulcer* or *bedsore*, is an ulcerated area in which prolonged pressure has caused tissue death. Without proper care, open sores quickly become infected.
- A **fissure** is a groove or crack-like break in the skin (Figure 12.7A). In tinea pedis (athlete's foot), fissures are commonly present between the toes. The term *fissure* also describes normal folds in the contours of the brain.
- A **laceration** (**lass**-er-**AY**-shun) is a torn or jagged wound, or an accidental cut wound.
- A **puncture wound** is a deep hole made by a sharp object such as a nail. The risk for infection, especially tetanus, is greater with this type of wound. A *needle-stick injury*, which can transmit infection, is an accidental puncture caused by a used hypodermic needle.
- An **ulcer** (**UL**-ser) is an open lesion of the skin or mucous membrane resulting in tissue loss around the edges (Figure 12.7B). Note: Ulcers also occur inside the body. Those associated with the digestive system are discussed in Chapter 8.

Birthmarks

- A **port-wine stain** is a large, reddish-purple discoloration of the face or neck. This discoloration will not resolve without treatment (Figure 12.8A). See Laser Treatment of Skin Conditions later in this chapter.
- A **strawberry hemangioma** (hee-**man**-jee-**OH**-mah) is a soft, raised, dark-reddish-purple birthmark (**hem** means blood, **angi/o** means blood or lymph vessels, and **-oma** means tumor). A *hemangioma* is a benign tumor made up of newly formed blood vessels. These birthmarks often, but not always, resolve by the age 5 without treatment (Figure 12.8B).

Dermatitis

The term **dermatitis** (**der**-mah-**TYE**-tis) means an inflammation of the skin (**dermat** means skin, and **-itis** means

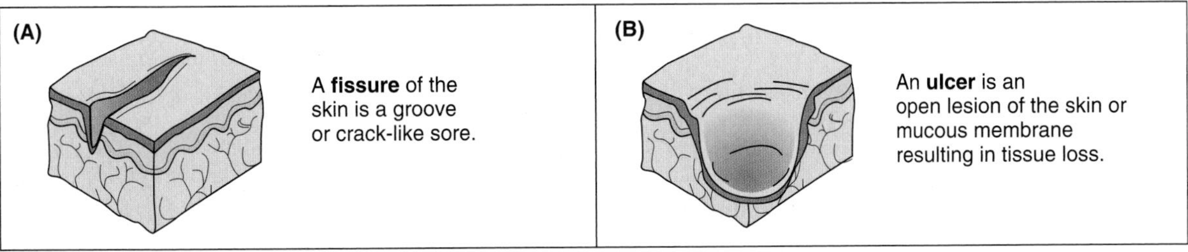

FIGURE 12.7 Lesions extending through the skin. (A) Fissure. (B) Ulcer.

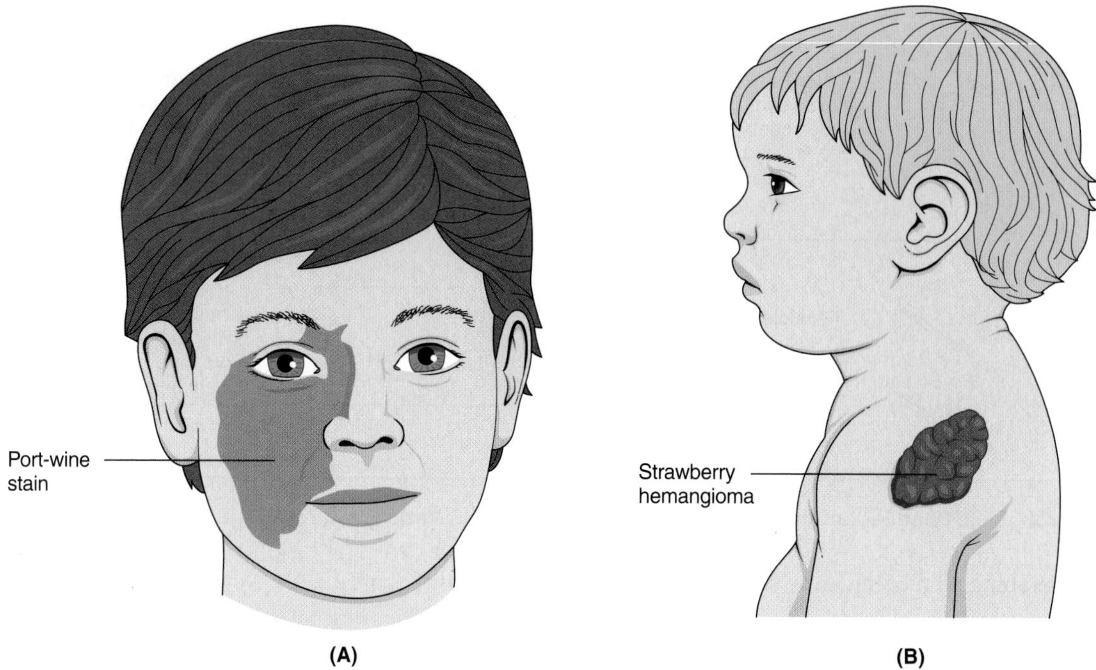

FIGURE 12.8 Types of birthmarks. (A) A port-wine stain is flat and consists of pigmented cells. (B) A strawberry hemangioma is raised and consists of blood vessels.

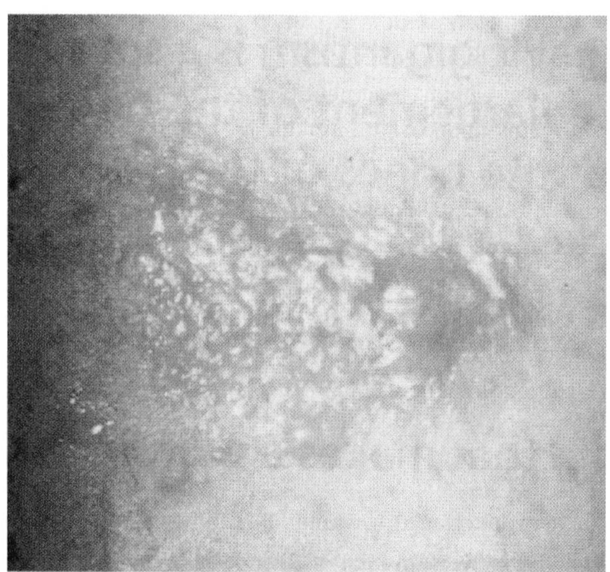

FIGURE 12.9 Contact dermatitis caused by poison oak. (Courtesy of Timothy Berger, MD, Associate Clinical Professor, Department of Dermatology, University of California, San Francisco, CA.)

inflammation). This condition, which takes many forms, usually includes redness, swelling, and itching.

- **Contact dermatitis** (CD) is a localized allergic response caused by contact with an irritant, for example, as seen with diaper rash. It is also caused by exposure to an allergen, such as an allergic reaction to latex gloves (Figure 12.9).
- **Eczema** (**ECK**-zeh-mah) is a form of persistent or recurring dermatitis that is usually characterized by redness, itching, and dryness, with possible blistering, cracking, oozing, or bleeding. This chronic condition appears to be an abnormal response of the body's immune system.
- **Pruritus** (proo-**RYE**-tus), also known as *itching*, is associated with most forms of dermatitis (**prurit** means itching, and **-us** is a singular noun ending).

Erythema

Erythema (**er**-ih-**THEE**-mah) is redness of the skin due to capillary dilation (**erythem** means flushed, and **-a** is a noun ending).

- *Erythema multiforme* is a skin disorder resulting from a generalized allergic reaction to an illness, infection, or medication. This reaction, which affects the skin and/or mucous membranes, is characterized by a rash that may appear as nodules or papules (raised red bumps), macules (flat discolored areas), or vesicles or bullae (blisters).
- *Erythema infectiosum*, also known as *fifth disease*, is a mildly contagious viral infection that is common in childhood. This infection produces a red, lace-like rash on the child's face that looks as if the child has been slapped.

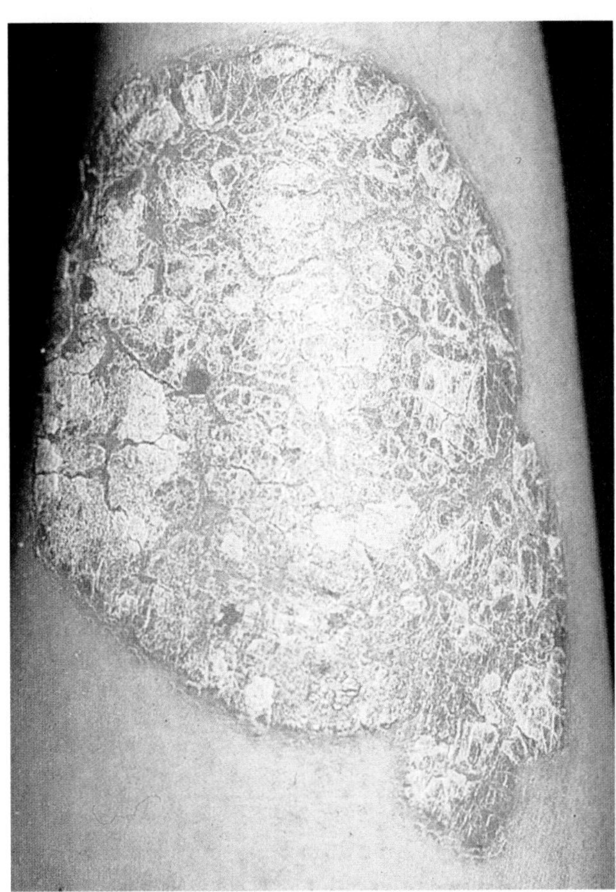

FIGURE 12.10 Psoriasis is characterized by plaques and silvery scales. (Courtesy of Robert A. Silverman, MD, Clinical Associate Professor, Department of Pediatrics, Georgetown University, Washington, DC.)

- *Erythema pernio*, also known as *chilblains*, is a purple-red inflammation that occurs when the small blood vessels below the skin are damaged, usually due to exposure to cold and damp weather. When warmth restores full circulation, the affected areas begin to itch; however, they usually heal without treatment.
- **Erythroderma** (eh-**rith**-roh-**DER**-mah) is abnormal redness of the entire skin surface (**erythr/o** means red, and **-derma** means skin).
- **Sunburn** is a form of erythema in which skin cells are damaged by exposure to the ultraviolet rays in sunlight. This damage increases the chances of later developing skin cancer.
- **Exfoliative dermatitis** (ecks-**FOH**-lee-**ay**-tiv eh-**rith**-roh-**DER**-mah) is a condition in which there is widespread scaling of the skin, often with pruritus, erythroderma, and hair loss. It may occur in severe cases of many common skin conditions, include eczema, psoriasis, and allergic reactions.

General Skin Conditions

- **Dermatosis** (**der**-mah-**TOH**-sis) is a general term used to denote skin lesions or eruptions of any type that are *not* associated with inflammation (**dermat** means skin, and **-osis** means abnormal condition).
- **Ichthyosis** (**ick**-thee-**OH**-sis) is a group of hereditary disorders characterized by dry, thickened, and scaly skin (**ichthy** means dry or scaly, and **-osis** means abnormal condition). These conditions are caused either by the slowing of the skin's natural shedding process or by a rapid increase in the production of the skin's cells.
- **Lipedema** (lip-eh-**DEE**-mah), also known as *painful fat syndrome*, is a chronic abnormal condition that is characterized by the accumulation of fat and fluid in the tissues just under the skin of the hips and legs (**lip** means fat, and **-edema** means swelling). This condition usually affects women and, even when weight is lost, this localized excess fat does not go away.
- **Lupus erythematosus** (**LOO**-pus er-ih-**thee**-mah-**TOH**-sus), also known as *lupus*, is an autoimmune disorder characterized by a red, scaly rash on the face and upper trunk. In addition to the skin, this condition also attacks the connective tissue in other body systems, especially in the joints.
- **Psoriasis** (soh-**RYE**-uh-sis) is a common skin disorder characterized by flare-ups in which red papules covered with silvery scales occur on the elbows, knees, scalp, back, or buttocks (Figure 12.10).
- **Rosacea** (roh-**ZAY**-shee-ah), which is also known as *adult acne*, is characterized by tiny red pimples and broken blood vessels. This chronic condition of unknown cause usually develops individuals with fair skin, between 30 and 60 years of ages.
- **Rhinophyma** (**rye**-noh-**FIGH**-muh), also known as *bulbous nose*, usually occurs in older men (**rhin/o** means nose, and **-phyma** means growth). This condition is characterized by hyperplasia (overgrowth) of the tissues of the nose and is associated with advanced rosacea (Figure 12.14).
- **Scleroderma** (**sklehr**-oh-**DER**-mah) is an autoimmune disorder in which the connective tissues become thickened and hardened, causing the skin to become hard and swollen (**scler/o** means hard, and **-derma** means skin). This condition can also affect the joints and internal organs.

- **Urticaria** (**ur**-tih-**KARE**-ree-ah), also known as *hives*, are itchy wheals caused by an allergic reaction (**urtic** means rash, and **-aria** means connected with).
- **Xeroderma** (zee-roh-**DER**-mah), also known as *xerosis*, is excessively dry skin (**xer/o** means dry, and **-derma** means skin).

Bacterial Skin Infections

- A **carbuncle** (**KAR**-bung-kul) is a cluster of connected furuncles (boils).
- **Cellulitis** (**sell**-you-**LYE**-tis) is an acute, rapidly spreading infection within the connective tissues that is characterized by malaise, swelling, warmth, and red streaks. *Malaise* is a feeling of general discomfort or uneasiness that is often the first indication of an infection or other disease.
- **Furuncles** (**FYOU**-rung-kulz), also known as *boils*, are large, tender, swollen areas caused by a staphylococcal infection around hair follicles or sebaceous glands.
- **Gangrene** (**GANG**-green), which is tissue necrosis (death), is most commonly caused by a loss of circulation to the affected tissues. The tissue death is followed by bacterial invasion that causes putrefaction, and if this infection enters the bloodstream, it can be fatal. *Putrefaction* is decay that produces foul-smelling odors.
- **Impetigo** (**im**-peh-**TYE**-goh) is a highly contagious bacterial skin infection that commonly occurs in children. This condition is characterized by isolated pustules that become crusted and rupture.
- **Necrotizing fasciitis** (**fas**-ee-**EYE**-tis) is a severe infection caused by Group A strep bacteria (also known as *flesh-eating bacteria*). *Necrotizing* means causing tissue death, and *fasciitis* is inflammation of fascia. These bacteria normally live harmlessly on the skin; however, if they enter the body through a skin wound, this serious infection can result. If untreated, the infected body tissue is destroyed, and the illness can be fatal.
- **Pyoderma** (**pye**-oh-**DER**-mah) is any acute, inflammatory, pus-forming bacterial skin infection such as impetigo (**py/o** means pus, and **-derma** means skin).

Fungal Skin Infections

- **Tinea** (**TIN**-ee-ah) is a fungal infection that can grow on the skin, hair, or nails. This condition is also known as *ringworm*, not because a worm is involved, but because as the fungus grows, it spreads out in a worm-like circle leaving normal-looking skin in the middle.
- **Tinea capitis** is found on the scalps of children. *Capitis* means head.
- **Tinea corporis** is a fungal infection of the skin on the body. *Corporis* means body.
- **Tinea cruris**, also known as *jock itch*, is found in the genital area.
- **Tinea pedis**, also known as *athlete's foot*, is found between the toes and on the feet. *Pedis* means feet.
- **Tinea versicolor**, also known as *pityriasis versicolor*, is a fungal infection that causes painless, discolored areas on the skin. *Versicolor* means a variety of color.

Parasitic Skin Infestations

An **infestation** is the dwelling of microscopic parasites on external surface tissue. Some parasites live temporarily on the skin. Others lay eggs and reproduce there.

- **Pediculosis** (pee-**dick**-you-**LOH**-sis) is an infestation with *lice* (**pedicul** means lice, and **-osis** means abnormal condition). The lice eggs, known as *nits*, must be destroyed in order to get rid of the infestation. There are three types of lice, each attracted to a specific part of the body:
    - **Pediculosis capitis** is an infestation with head lice.
    - **Pediculosis corporis** is an infestation with body lice.
    - **Pediculosis pubis** is an infestation with lice in the pubic hair and pubic region.
- **Scabies** (**SKAY**-beez) is a skin infection caused by an infestation with the *itch mite*, which causes small, itchy bumps and blisters due to tiny mites that burrow into the top layer of human skin to lay their eggs. Medications applied to the skin kill the mites; however, itching may persist for several weeks.

Skin Growths

- A **callus** (**KAL**-us) is a thickening of part of the skin on the hands or feet caused by repeated rubbing. Compare with *callus* in Chapter 3. A *clavus*, or *corn*, is a callus in the keratin layer of the skin covering the joints of the toes, usually caused by ill-fitting shoes.
- A **cicatrix** (sick-**AY**-tricks) is a normal scar resulting from the healing of a wound (plural, *cicatrices*).
- **Granulation tissue** is the tissue that normally forms during the healing of a wound. This tissue eventually forms the scar.

- **Granuloma** (**gran**-you-**LOH**-mah) is a general term used to describe small, knot-like swellings of granulation tissue in the epidermis (**granul** meaning granular, and **-oma** means tumor). Granulomas can result from inflammation, injury, or infection.
- A **keloid** (**KEE**-loid) is an abnormally raised or thickened scar that expands beyond the boundaries of the incision (**kel** means growth or tumor, and **-oid** means resembling). A tendency to form keloids is often inherited, and is more common among people with dark-pigmented skin.
- A **keratosis** (**kerr**-ah-**TOH**-sis) is any skin growth, such as a wart or a callus, in which there is overgrowth and thickening of the skin (**kerat** means hard or horny, and **-osis** means abnormal condition). Note: **kerat/o** also refers to the cornea of the eye (plural, *keratoses*).
- A **lipoma** (lih-**POH**-mah) is a benign, slow-growing fatty tumor located between the skin and the muscle layer (**lip** means fatty, and **-oma** means tumor). This fatty tumor is usually harmless, and treatment is rarely necessary unless the tumor is in a bothersome location, is painful, or is growing rapidly.
- **Nevi** (**NEE**-vye), also known as *moles*, are small, dark, skin growths that develop from melanocytes in the skin (singular, *nevus*). Normally, these growths are benign. In contrast, **dysplastic nevi** (dis-**PLAS**-tick **NEE**-vye) are atypical moles that can develop into skin cancer.
- A **papilloma** (**pap**-ih-**LOH**-mah) is a benign, superficial wart-like growth on the epithelial tissue or elsewhere in the body, such as in the bladder (**papill** means resembling a nipple, and **-oma** means tumor.)
- **Polyp** (**POL**-ip) is a general term used most commonly to describe a mushroom-like growth from the surface of a mucous membrane, such as a polyp in the nose. These growths have many causes and are not necessarily malignant.
- **Skin tags** are small, flesh-colored or light-brown polyps that hang from the body by fine stalks. Skin tags are benign and tend to enlarge with age.

Skin Cancer

Skin cancer is a harmful, malignant growth on the skin, which can have many causes, including repeated severe sunburns or long-term exposure to the sun. There are three main types of skin cancer: basal cell carcinoma, squamous cell carcinoma, and melanoma.

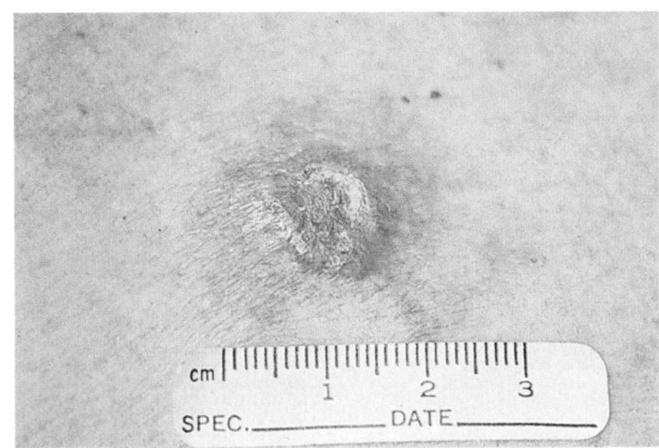

FIGURE 12.11 Basal cell carcinoma. (Courtesy of Robert A. Silverman, MD, Clinical Associate Professor, Department of Pediatrics, Georgetown University, Washington, DC.)

- An **actinic keratosis** (ack-**TIN**-ick **kerr**-ah-**TOH**-sis) is a precancerous skin growth that occurs on sun-damaged skin. It often looks like a red scaly patch and feels like sandpaper. *Precancerous* describes a growth that is not yet malignant; however, if not treated, it is likely to become malignant.
- A **basal cell carcinoma** is a malignant tumor of the basal cell layer of the epidermis. This is the most common, and least harmful, type of skin cancer because it is slow growing and rarely spreads to other parts of the body. The lesions, which occur mainly on the face or neck and tend to bleed easily, are usually pink, smooth, and are raised with a depression in the center (see Figure 12.11).
- **Squamous cell carcinoma** (**SKWAY**-mus) originates as a malignant tumor of the scaly squamous cells of the epithelium; however, it can quickly spread to other body systems. These cancers begin as skin lesions that appear to be sores that will not heal or that have a crusted look (see Figure 12.12).
- **Malignant melanoma** (mel-ah-**NOH**-mah), also known as *melanoma*, is a type of skin cancer that occurs in the melanocytes (**melan** means black, and **-oma** means tumor). This is the most serious type of skin cancer and often the first signs are changes in the size, shape, or color of a mole (see Figure 12.13).

Burns

A **burn** is an injury to body tissues caused by heat, flame, electricity, sun, chemicals, or radiation. The severity of a burn is described according to the percentage of the total body skin surface affected (more than 15% is considered

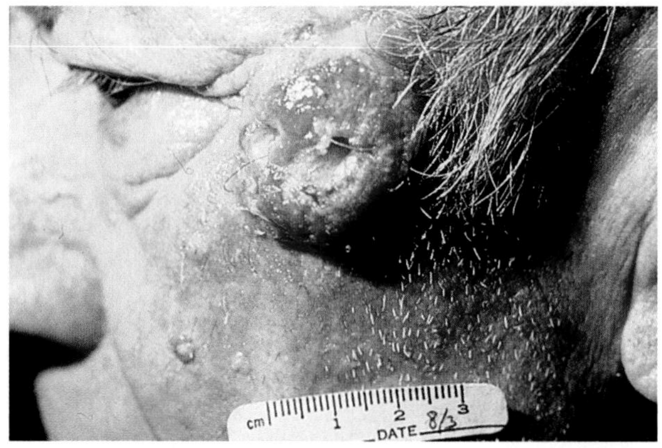

FIGURE 12.12 Squamous cell carcinoma. (Courtesy of Robert A. Silverman, MD, Clinical Associate Professor, Department of Pediatrics, Georgetown University. Washington, DC.)

serious). It is also described according to the depth or layers of skin involved (Table 12.1 and Figure 12.14).

DIAGNOSTIC PROCEDURES OF THE INTEGUMENTARY SYSTEM

A **biopsy** (**BYE**-op-see) is the removal of a small piece of living tissue for examination to confirm or establish a diagnosis (**bi** means pertaining to life, and **-opsy** means view of).

- In an *incisional biopsy*, a piece, but not all, of the tumor or lesion is removed. The term *incision* means to cut into.
- In an *excisional biopsy*, the entire tumor or lesion and a margin of surrounding tissue are removed. *Excision* means the complete removal of a lesion or organ.
- In a *needle biopsy*, a hollow needle is used to remove a core of tissue for examination.
- **Exfoliative cytology** is a technique in which cells are scraped from the tissue and examined under a microscope. To *exfoliate* means to remove a specimen in flakes or scales.

TREATMENT PROCEDURES OF THE INTEGUMENTARY SYSTEM

Preventive Measures

Sunscreen that blocks out the harmful ultraviolet B (UVB) rays is sometimes measured in terms of the strength of the *sun protection factor*. Some sunscreens also give protection against ultraviolet A (UVA rays).

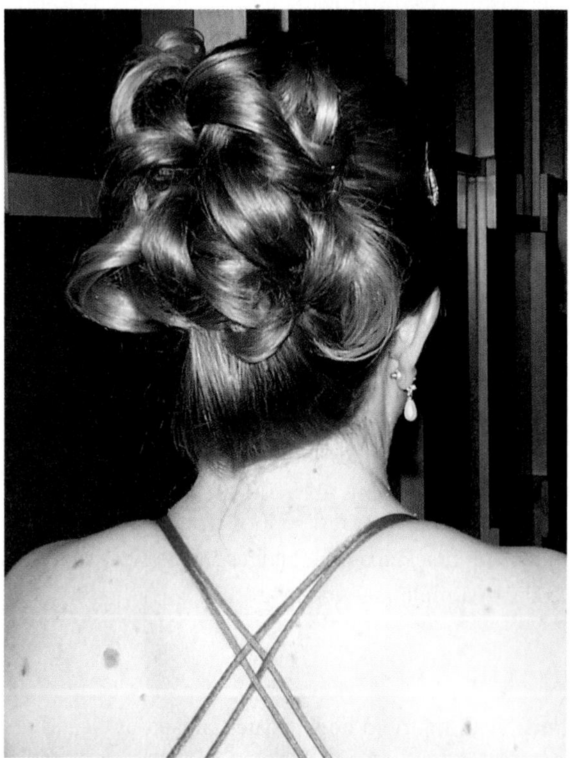

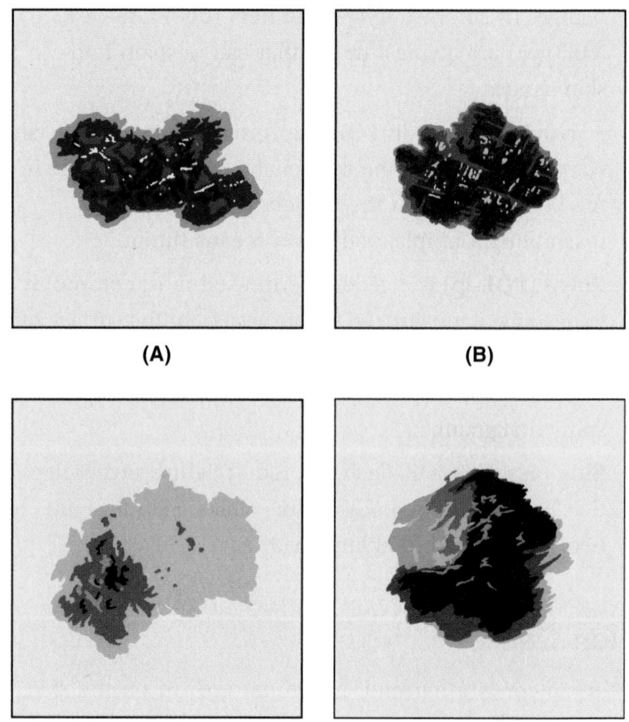

FIGURE 12.13 Left: Melanoma in situ visible on the left shoulder blade. (Photo courtesy of Sherry Morris.) Right: The A-B-C-D signs of melanoma are (A) asymmetry, (B) border irregularity, (C) color variation, and (D) diameter larger than a pencil eraser.

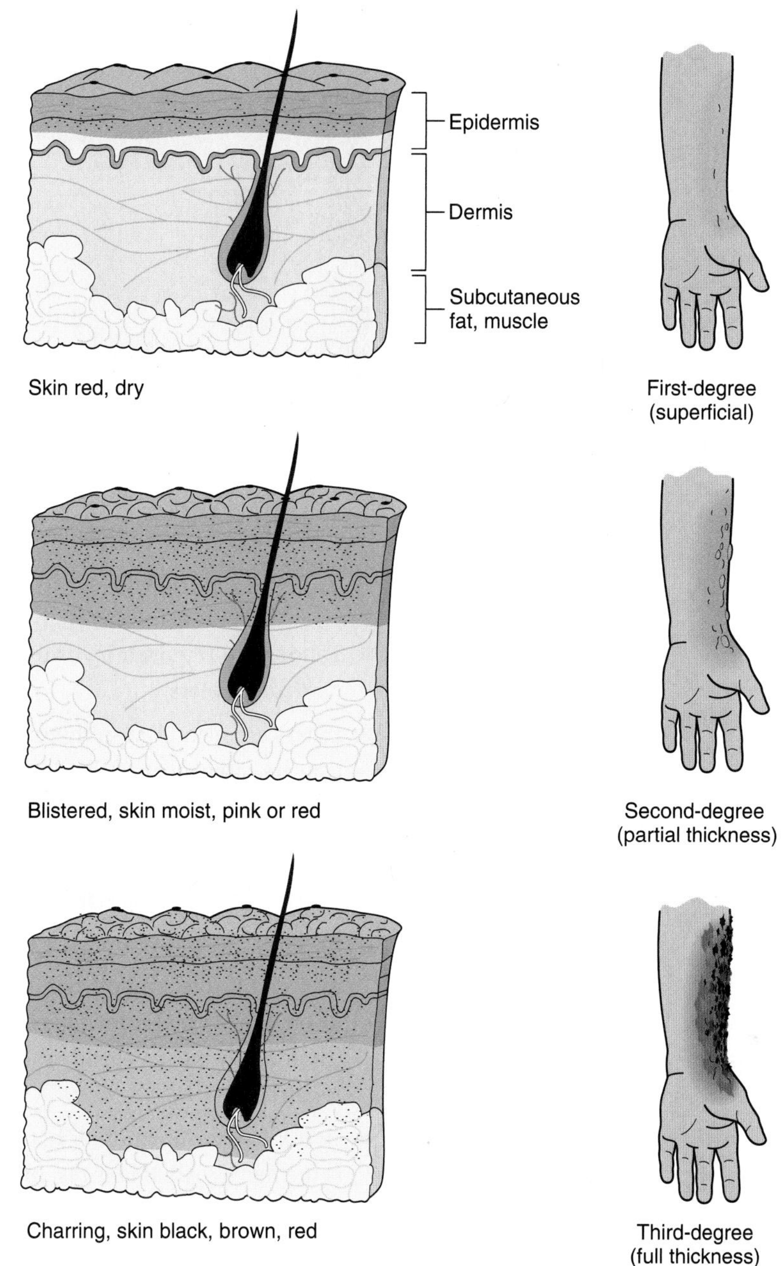

FIGURE 12.14 The degree of a burn is determined by the layers of skin involved.

TABLE 12.1

CLASSIFICATION OF BURN SEVERITY

Type of Burn	Also Known As	Layers of Skin Involved
First-degree burn	*Superficial burn*	No blisters, superficial damage to the epidermis
Second-degree burn	*Partial thickness burn*	Blisters, damage to the epidermis, and dermis.
Third-degree burn	*Full thickness burn*	Damage to the epidermis, dermis, and subcutaneous layers, and possibly also the muscle below.

Tissue Removal

- **Cauterization** (**kaw**-ter-eye-**ZAY**-zhun) is the destruction of tissue by burning.
- **Chemabrasion**, also known as *chemical peel*, is the use of chemicals to remove the outer layers of skin to treat acne scaring, fine wrinkling, and keratoses.
- **Cryosurgery** (**krye**-oh-**SIR**-jur-ee) is the destruction or elimination of abnormal tissue cells, such as warts or tumors, through the application of extreme cold by using liquid nitrogen (**cry/o** means cold, and **-surgery** means operative procedure).
- **Curettage** (**kyou**-reh-**TAHZH**) is the removal of material from the surface by scraping. One use of this technique is to remove basal cell tumors.
- **Debridement** (day-breed-**MON**) is the removal of dirt, foreign objects, damaged tissue, and cellular debris from a wound to prevent infection and to promote healing.
- **Dermabrasion** (**der**-mah-**BRAY**-zhun) is a form of abrasion involving the use of a revolving wire brush or sandpaper. It is used to remove acne and chickenpox scars as well as for facial skin rejuvenation.
- **Incision and drainage** (I & D) involves incision (cutting open) of a lesion, such as an abscess, and draining the contents.
- **Mohs surgery** is a technique used to treat skin cancer. Individual layers of cancerous tissue are removed and examined under a microscope one at a time until all cancerous tissue has been removed.

Laser Treatment of Skin Conditions

The term **laser** is an acronym. The letters stand for *light amplification by stimulated emission of radiation*. Lasers are used to treat skin conditions and other disorders of the body.

A laser tube can be filled with a solid, liquid, or gas substance that is stimulated to emit light at a specific wavelength. Some wavelengths are capable of destroying all skin tissue; others target tissue of a particular color.

- Port-wine stain is treated using short pulses of laser light to remove the birthmark (Figure 12.9A). Treatment can require many sessions, because only a small section is treated at a time.
- Rhinophyma is treated by using a laser to reshape the nose by vaporizing the excess tissue (see Figure 12.15).

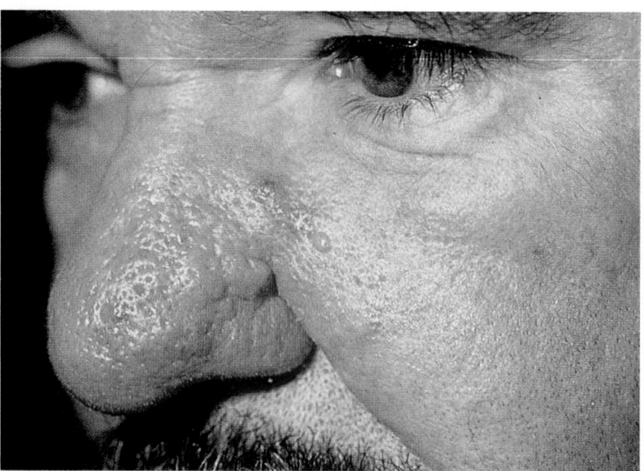

FIGURE 12.15 Rhinophyma before laser treatment. (Courtesy of Robert A. Silverman, MD, Clinical Associate Professor, Department of Pediatrics, Georgetown University, Washington, DC.)

- Tattoos are removed by using lasers that target particular colors.
- Lasers are also used in the treatment of some skin cancers, precancer of the lip, and warts that recur around nails and on the soles of feet.

Cosmetic Procedures

- **Blepharoplasty** (**BLEF**-ah-roh-**plas**-tee), also known as a *lid lift*, is the surgical reduction of the upper and lower eyelids by removing excess fat, skin, and muscle (**blephar/o** means eyelid, and **-plasty** means surgical repair).
- **Botox** is a formulation of botulinum toxin type A. This is the neurotoxin that is responsible for the form of food poisoning known as botulism. Botox injections, which temporarily block the nerve signals to the injected muscle, reduce moderate to severe frown lines for up to 3–4 months. *Frown lines* are located between the eyebrows.
- **Collagen replacement therapy** is a form of soft-tissue augmentation used to soften facial lines or scars or to make lips appear fuller. Tiny quantities of collagen are injected under a line or scar to boost the skin's natural supply of collagen. The effect usually lasts for 3–12 months.
- **Dermatoplasty** (**DER**-mah-toh-**plas**-tee), also known as a *skin graft*, is the replacement of damaged skin with healthy tissue taken from a donor site on the patient's body (**dermat/o** means skin, and **-plasty** means surgical repair).

- **Electrolysis** is the use of electric current to destroy hair follicles in order to produce the relatively permanent removal of undesired hair (**electr/o** means electric, and **-lysis** means destruction).
- **Lipectomy** (lih-**PECK**-toh-mee) is the surgical removal of fat beneath the skin (**lip** means fat, and **-ectomy** means surgical removal).
- **Liposuction** (**LIP**-oh-**suck**-shun), also known as *suction-assisted lipectomy*, is the surgical removal of fat beneath the skin with the aid of suction.
- **Rhytidectomy** (**rit**-ih-**DECK**-toh-mee), also known as a *facelift*, is the surgical removal of excess skin and fat around the face to eliminate wrinkles (**rhytid** means wrinkle, and **-ectomy** means surgical removal).
- **Sclerotherapy** (**sklehr**-oh-**THER**-ah-pee) is used in the treatment of spider veins. *Spider veins* are small, nonessential veins that can be seen through the skin. This treatment involves injecting a sclerosing solution (saline solution) into the vein being treated. This solution irritates the tissue, causing the veins to collapse and disappear.

ABBREVIATIONS RELATED TO THE INTEGUMENTARY SYSTEM

Table 12.2 presents an overview of the abbreviations related to the terms introduced in this chapter. Note: To avoid errors or confusion, always be cautious when using abbreviations.

TABLE 12.2
Abbreviations Related to the Integumentary System

alopecia areata = AA	**AA** = alopecia areata
basal cell carcinoma = BCC, BCCA	**BCC, BCCA** = basal cell carcinoma
cauterization = caut	**caut** = cauterization
cryosurgery = CRYO	**CRYO** = cryosurgery
debridement = debm	**debm** = debridement
eczema = Ecz, Ez	**Ecz, Ez** = eczema
lupus erythematosus = LE	**LE** = lupus erythematosus
malignant melanoma = MM, mm	**MM, mm** = malignant melanoma
necrotizing fasciitis = NF	**NF** = necrotizing fasciitis
psoriasis = PS, Ps	**PS, Ps** = psoriasis
sclerotherapy = ST	**ST** = sclerotherapy
squamous cell carcinoma = SCC	**SCC** = squamous cell carcinoma

Career Opportunities

In addition to the medical specialties already discussed, some of the health occupations involving the treatment of skin include:

- **Esthetician** (also spelled **aesthetician**): professionally trained to treat the skin to maintain and improve its appearance through facials, massage, hair removal, and cosmetics
- **Paramedical esthetician:** has medical training and works under the guidance of a plastic surgeon or dermatologist in pre- and postoperative skin care
- **Dermatology nurse certified (DNC):** an RN specially trained to provide care and information to dermatology patients
- **Burn care nurse:** an RN specializing in the treatment of burn patients

Health Occupation Profile

Dermatologist

Dr. Diane Thaler, M.D., is a dermatologist and an assistant clinical professor in dermatology. ***"For me, medicine is a way of life. Not only do I see patients during the day, but I am also continuously reading and learning. The more one learns, the more one realizes how much more there is to know, and I'm always looking for new ideas to help my patients.***

"It's a great feeling to help patients feel better when they leave my office than when they came in. Dermatology requires a trained eye and a passion for details and the 'trivia' of medicine, such as the Latin names of diseases. An understanding of infectious, inflammatory, and oncologic disease and of skin manifestations of internal disease, as well as surgery and photobiology, is also needed. I love the sleuthing involved in 'reading' these signs on the skin in order to help bring a patient to wellness."

STUDY BREAK

Despite the fact that about a million Americans develop skin cancer each year, many Caucasian Americans still considered a suntan to be a sign of good health and being able to afford a beach vacation. Thousands of people die each year from *malignant melanoma*, yet we ignore the fact that skin cancer can often be directly linked to sun exposure or tanning salons.

In early times, a tan was considered a sign of outdoor labor, so it was a status symbol to be as "white" as possible. Yet some of the ways of looking pale were as dangerous as getting a suntan:

- **Greek and Roman women whitened their faces with chalks and lead paints, a practice that sometimes caused a slow death by lead poisoning.**
- **In France, both men and women wore fake beauty marks to emphasize the contrast with their light skin. Frequently these beauty marks were made of lead and eventually caused death by lead poisoning.**
- **In the 900s, some of the nobility bleached their skin with arsenic compounds. Unfortunately, this poison occasionally brought about a *truly* deadly pallor.**

REVIEW TIME

Write the answers to the following questions on a separate piece of paper or in your notebook. In addition, be prepared to take part in the classroom discussion.

1. ***Written Assignment:*** Using your own words, describe **acne vulgaris**.

   Discussion Assignment: Tiffany's severe acne has never been treated. What physical and psychological impact do you think having acne might have on her?

2. ***Written Assignment:*** Describe **lipedema** in terms a layperson can understand.

   Discussion Assignment: Since dieting doesn't cure lipedema, discuss how a patient with this condition must feel when a well-meaning friend recommends yet another diet.

3. ***Written Assignment:*** Using terms a physician would understand, describe the difference between **eczema** and **psoriasis**.

   Discussion Assignment: Contrast the characteristics of these two conditions in terms that the patient would understand.

4. ***Written Assignment:*** Describe the difference between a **port-wine stain** and a **strawberry hemangioma**.

   Discussion Assignment: Trisha Nelson was born with a small strawberry hemangioma on her face. How would you explain this condition and the prognosis to her parents?

5. ***Written Assignment:*** Using terms a patient would understand, describe the difference between **blepharoplasty** and **rhytidectomy**.

   Discussion Assignment: Be prepared to discuss in class some of the reasons why a patient might want to have either of these procedures performed.

continues

Optional Internet Activity

The goal of this activity is to help you learn more about medical terminology as it applies to the "real world." Select **one** *of these two options and follow the instructions.*

1. Search for information about **skin cancer**. Write a brief (one- or two-paragraph) report on something new you learned here and include the address of the web site where you found this information.
2. To learn more about **birthmarks**, go to the web site of the Vascular Birthmarks Foundation. Explore the site and then write a brief (one- or two-paragraph) report on something new you learned here.

THE HUMAN TOUCH: CRITICAL THINKING ACTIVITY

The following story and questions are designed to stimulate critical thinking through class discussion or as a brief essay response. There are no right or wrong answers to these questions.

"C'mon, Chad, stop slathering on that girly lotion and get to work!"

Installing decks and railings for his Uncle Ben's construction company was not exactly Chad's dream job for the summer, but he loved being outside all day, and he couldn't argue with the pay. He was also learning new things about his uncle, like the fact that when it came to construction, he was all business. Chad finished rubbing the sunscreen onto his legs and ran over to meet up with the rest of the crew. He didn't like the fact that his uncle was always ribbing him in front of the others about wanting to keep from getting sunburned.

Chad knew that they had a family history of skin cancer, and he didn't want to take any risks. And with a job like his, his uncle was exposed to the sun's rays almost every single day, so Chad thought that he should take precautions, too. Chad's mom had tried explaining that when they grew up, sunscreen was not readily available; the only products were suntan lotions, used to enhance tanning, and they were used mostly by girls. As the times changed and studies came out showing how harmful sun rays can be, Uncle Ben had not changed his attitude toward using lotions, and he certainly did not appreciate being lectured by his sister or nephew about it.

One morning, as Uncle Ben was getting dressed for work, he noticed a change in a spot he had always assumed was a mole. It looked like the color had gotten mottled without him really noticing, and the shape didn't look like his other freckles and moles anymore. He remembered his nagging sister telling him about the signs of skin cancer, and this spot sure fit that description. As he finished dressing, he resolved to make an appointment to get the mole looked at, just to get some peace of mind. And maybe he should ask his nephew Chad about that sunscreen stuff he was always slathering on himself.

continues

Suggested Discussion Topics

1. Discuss why Uncle Ben may not have wanted to use sunscreen.
2. What other precautions might someone working outdoors take to prevent sun exposure?
3. Uncle Ben prides himself on running a construction site with a "safety first" motto. Does he have any responsibility to make sure his workers do not come down with skin cancer?
4. How would Chad know what type of sunscreen to use, and how often to apply it?

STUDENT WORKBOOK AND StudyWARE™ CD-ROM

1. Go to your **Student Workbook** and complete the Learning Exercises for this chapter.

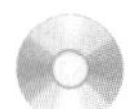

2. Go to the **StudyWARE™ CD-ROM** and have fun with the exercises and games for this chapter.

13

CHAPTER

The Endocrine System

Overview of Structures, Combining Forms, and Functions of the Endocrine System

Major Structures	Related Combining Forms	Primary Functions
Adrenal Glands	adren/o	Regulate electrolyte levels, influence metabolism, and respond to stress.
Gonads Male: testicles Female: ovaries	gonad/o	Regulate development and maintenance of secondary sex characteristics.
Pancreatic Islets	pancreat/o	Control blood sugar levels and glucose metabolism.
Parathyroid Glands	parathyroid/o	Regulate calcium levels throughout the body.
Pineal Gland	pineal/o	Influences the sleep-wakefulness cycle.
Pituitary Gland	pituit/o, pituitar/o	Secretes hormones that control the activity of the other endocrine glands.
Thymus	thym/o	Plays a major role in the immune reaction.
Thyroid Gland	thyr/o, thyroid/o	Stimulates metabolism, growth, and the activity of the nervous system.

VOCABULARY RELATED TO THE ENDOCRINE SYSTEM

This list contains essential word parts and medical terms for this chapter. These terms are pronounced on the student StudyWARE™ CD-ROM and Audio CDs that are available for use with this text. These and the other important **primary terms** are shown in boldface throughout the chapter. *Secondary terms*, which appear in *orange* italics, clarify the meaning of primary terms.

Word Parts

- ☐ **acr/o**
- ☐ **adren/o**
- ☐ **crin/o**
- ☐ **-dipsia**
- ☐ **glyc/o**
- ☐ **gonad/o**
- ☐ **-ism**
- ☐ **pancreat/o**
- ☐ **parathyroid/o**
- ☐ **pineal/o**
- ☐ **pituitar/o**
- ☐ **poly-**
- ☐ **somat/o**
- ☐ **thym/o**
- ☐ **thyr/o, thyroid/o**

Medical Terms

- ☐ **acromegaly** (**ack**-roh-**MEG**-ah-lee)
- ☐ **Addison's disease** (**AD**-ih-sonz)
- ☐ **adrenalitis** (ah-**dree**-nal-**EYE**-tis)
- ☐ **aldosteronism** (al-**DOSS**-teh-roh-**niz**-em)
- ☐ **antidiuretic hormone (an**-tih-dye-you-**RET**-ick)
- ☐ **calcitonin** (**kal**-sih-**TOH**-nin)
- ☐ **chemical thyroidectomy** (**thigh**-roi-**DECK**-toh-mee)
- ☐ **Conn's syndrome**
- ☐ **cortisol** (**KOR**-tih-sol)
- ☐ **cretinism** (**CREE**-tin-izm)
- ☐ **Cushing's syndrome** (**KUSH**-ingz)
- ☐ **diabetes insipidus** (**dye**-ah-**BEE**-teez in-**SIP**-ih-dus)
- ☐ **diabetes mellitus** (**dye**-ah-**BEE**-teez mel-**EYE**-tus)
- ☐ **diabetic retinopathy** (**ret**-ih-**NOP**-ah-thee)
- ☐ **electrolytes** (ee-**LECK**-troh-lytes)
- ☐ **epinephrine** (**ep**-ih-**NEF**-rin)
- ☐ **estrogen** (**ES**-troh-jen)
- ☐ **exophthalmos** (**eck**-sof-**THAL**-mos)
- ☐ **follicle-stimulating hormone follicle** (**FOL**-lick-kul)
- ☐ **fructosamine test** (fruck-**TOHS**-ah-meen)
- ☐ **gestational diabetes** (jes-**TAY**-shun-al **dye**-ah-**BEE**-teez)
- ☐ **gigantism** (jigh-**GAN**-tiz-em)
- ☐ **glucagon** (**GLOO**-kah-gon)
- ☐ **glucose** (**GLOO**-kohs)
- ☐ **glycogen** (**GLYE**-koh-jen)
- ☐ **Graves' disease** (**GRAYVZ** dih-**ZEEZ**)
- ☐ **gynecomastia** (**guy**-neh-koh-**MAS**-tee-ah)
- ☐ **Hashimoto's thyroiditis** (hah-shee-**MOH**-tohz **thigh**-roi-**DYE**-tis)
- ☐ **hypercalcemia** (**high**-per-kal-**SEE**-mee-ah)
- ☐ **hypercrinism** (**high**-per-**KRY**-nism)
- ☐ **hyperglycemia** (**high**-per-glye-**SEE**-mee-ah)
- ☐ **hyperinsulinism** (**high**-per-**IN**-suh-lin-izm)
- ☐ **hyperpituitarism** (**high**-per-pih-**TOO**-ih-tah-rizm)
- ☐ **hyperthyroidism** (**high**-per-**THIGH**-roid-izm)
- ☐ **hypoglycemia** (**high**-poh-gly-**SEE**-mee-ah)
- ☐ **hypothyroidism** (**high**-poh-**THIGH**-roid-izm)
- ☐ **insulinoma** (**in**-suh-lin-**OH**-mah)
- ☐ **interstitial cell-stimulating hormone**
- ☐ **laparoscopic adrenalectomy** (ah-**dree**-nal-**ECK**-toh-mee)
- ☐ **leptin** (**LEP**-tin)
- ☐ **luteinizing hormone (LOO**-tee-in-eye-zing)
- ☐ **myxedema** (**mick**-seh-**DEE**-mah)
- ☐ **norepinephrine** (**nor**-ep-ih-**NEF**-rin)
- ☐ **oxytocin** (**ock**-sih-**TOH**-sin)
- ☐ **pancreatalgia** (**pan**-kree-ah-**TAL**-jee-ah)
- ☐ **pancreatitis** (**pan**-kree-ah-**TYE**-tis)
- ☐ **pheochromocytoma** (fee-oh-**kroh**-moh-sigh-**TOH**-mah)
- ☐ **pinealoma** (pin-ee-ah-**LOH**-mah)
- ☐ **pituitarism** (pih-**TOO**-ih-tar-izm)
- ☐ **pituitary adenoma** (pih-**TOO**-ih-**tair**-ee **ad**-eh-**NOH**-mah)
- ☐ **polydipsia** (**pol**-ee-**DIP**-see-ah)
- ☐ **polyphagia** (**pol**-ee-**FAY**-jee-ah)
- ☐ **polyuria** (**pol**-ee-**YOU**-ree-ah)
- ☐ **progesterone** (proh-**JES**-ter-ohn)
- ☐ **prolactinoma** (proh-**lack**-tih-**NOH**-mah)
- ☐ **testosterone** (tes-**TOS**-teh-rohn)
- ☐ **thymectomy** (thigh-**MECK**-toh-mee)
- ☐ **thymitis** (thigh-**MY**-tis)
- ☐ **thymosin** (**THIGH**-moh-sin)
- ☐ **thyroxine** (thigh-**ROCK**-sin)

OBJECTIVES

On completion of this chapter, you should be able to:

1. Describe the role of the endocrine glands in maintaining homeostasis.
2. Name and describe the functions of the primary hormones secreted by each of the endocrine glands.
3. Recognize, define, spell, and pronounce terms relating to the pathology and the diagnostic and treatment procedures of the endocrine glands.

FUNCTIONS OF THE ENDOCRINE SYSTEM

The primary function of the endocrine system is to produce hormones that work together to maintain *homeostasis* (constant internal environment) throughout the body systems.

- **Hormones** are chemical messengers that are secreted by endocrine glands and have specialized functions in regulating the activities of specific cells, organs, or both.
- Because the hormones are secreted directly into the bloodstream, they are able to reach cells and organs throughout the body. Blood, or urine, tests are used to measure hormone levels. These tests are discussed in Chapter 15.
- The major hormones, their sources, and functions are described in Table 13.1.

STRUCTURES OF THE ENDOCRINE SYSTEM

There are 13 major glands of the endocrine system (Figure 13.1):

- One **pituitary gland** (divided into two lobes)
- One **pineal gland**

TABLE 13.1

HORMONES FROM A TO T

Hormone	Source	Functions
Aldosterone (ALD)	Adrenal cortex	Aids in regulating the levels of salt and water in the body.
Androgens	Adrenal cortex and gonads	Influence sex-related characteristics.
Adrenocorticotropic hormone (ACTH)	Pituitary gland	Stimulates the growth and secretions of the adrenal cortex.
Antidiuretic hormone (ADH)	Secreted by the hypothalamus, then stored and released from the pituitary gland.	Helps control blood pressure by reducing the amount of water that is excreted.
Calcitonin (CAL)	Thyroid gland	Works with the parathyroid hormone to regulate calcium levels in the blood and tissues.
Cortisol	Adrenal cortex	Regulates the metabolism of carbohydrates, fats, and proteins in the body. Also has an anti-inflammatory action.
Epinephrine (Epi, EPI)	Adrenal medulla	Stimulates the sympathetic nervous system.
Estrogen (E)	Ovaries	Develops and maintains the female secondary sex characteristics and regulates the menstrual cycle.

continues

TABLE 13.1

HORMONES FROM A TO T (Continued)

Hormone	Source	Functions
Follicle-stimulating hormone (FSH)	Pituitary gland	In the female, stimulates the secretion of estrogen and the growth of ova (eggs). In the male, stimulates the production of sperm.
Glucagon (GCG)	Pancreatic islets (alpha cells)	Increases the level of glucose in the bloodstream.
Growth hormone (GH)	Pituitary gland	Regulates the growth of bone, muscle, and other body tissues.
Human chorionic gonadotropin (HCG)	Placenta	Stimulates the secretion of the hormones required to maintain pregnancy.
Insulin	Pancreatic islets (beta cells)	Regulates the transport of glucose to body cells and stimulates the conversion of excess glucose to glycogen for storage.
Interstitial cell-stimulating hormone (ICSH)	Pituitary gland	Stimulates ovulation in the female. Stimulates the secretion of testosterone in the male.
Lactogenic hormone (LTH)	Pituitary gland	Stimulates and maintains the secretion of breast milk.
Luteinizing hormone (LH)	Pituitary gland	In the female, stimulates ovulation. In the male, stimulates testosterone secretion.
Melanocyte-stimulating hormone (MSH)	Pituitary gland	Increases the production of melanin in melanocytes of the skin.
Melatonin	Pineal gland	Influences the sleep-wakefulness cycles.
Norepinephrine	Adrenal medulla	Stimulates the sympathetic nervous system.
Oxytocin (OXT)	Pituitary gland	Stimulates uterine contractions during childbirth. It also causes milk to flow from the mammary glands after childbirth.
Parathyroid hormone (PTH)	Parathyroid glands	Works with calcitonin to regulate calcium levels in the blood and tissues.
Progesterone	Ovaries	Completes preparation of the uterus for possible pregnancy.
Testosterone	Testicles	Stimulates the development of male secondary sex characteristics.
Thymosin	Thymus	Plays an important role in the immune system.
Thyroxine (T_4) **and triiodothyronine** (T_3)	Thyroid gland	Regulate the rate of metabolism.
Thyroid-stimulating hormone (TSH)	Pituitary gland	Stimulates the secretion of hormones by the thyroid gland.

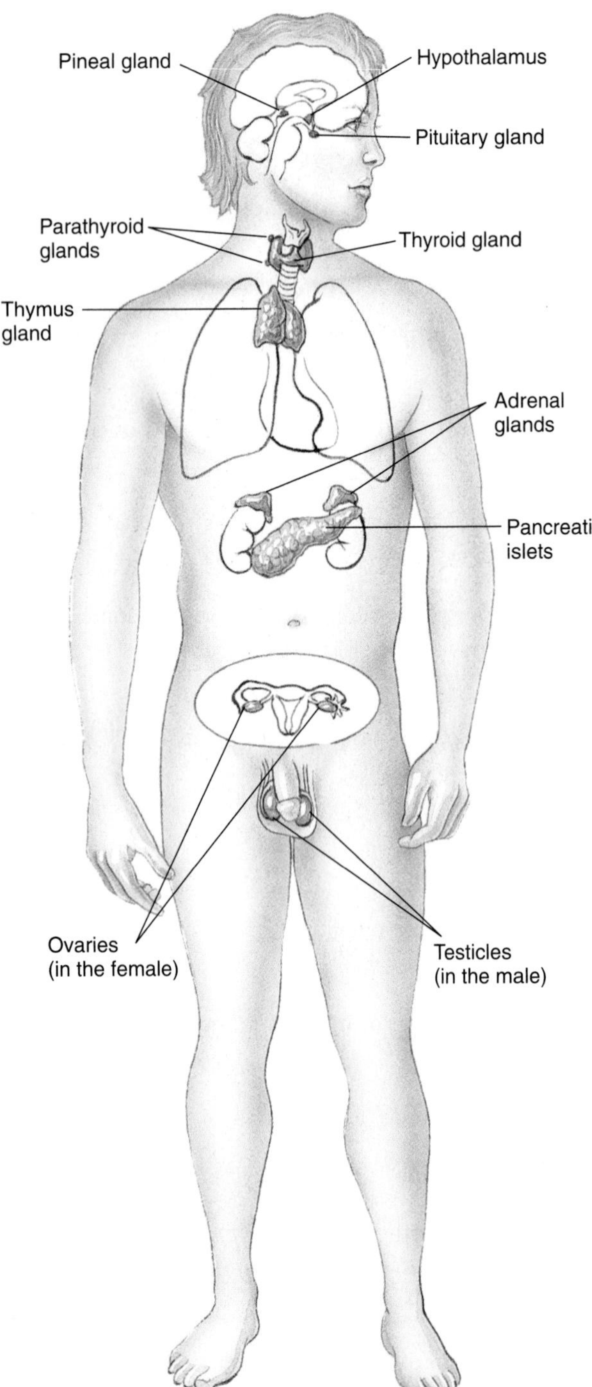

FIGURE 13.1 Structures of the endocrine system.

- One **thyroid gland**
- Four **parathyroid glands**
- One **thymus**
- One **pancreas (pancreatic islets)**
- Two **adrenal glands**
- Two **gonads** (ovaries in females, testes in males)

Specialized Types of Hormones

There are several specialized types of hormones that do not fit the tradition hormone definition.

Steroids

A **steroid** (**STEHR**-oid) is any one of a large number of hormone-like substances secreted by endocrine glands or artificially produced as medications to relieve swelling and inflammation in conditions such as asthma.

- **Anabolic steroids** (**an**-ah-**BOL**-ick **STEHR**-oidz) are chemically related to the male sex hormone testosterone. These have been used illegally by athletes to increase strength and muscle mass. Serious side effects of anabolic steroid use include liver damage, altered body chemistry, testicular shrinkage, and breast development in males, plus unpredictable mood swings and violence.

Hormones Secreted by Fat Cells

Fat is not commonly thought of as an endocrine gland; however, research has revealed that fat cells do secrete at least one, and possibly more, hormones that play an important role in the balance and health of the body.

- **Leptin** (**LEP**-tin) is a hormone secreted by *adipocytes* (fat cells).
- Leptin leaves the fat cells and travels in the bloodstream to brain centers. Here, it acts to control the balance of food intake and energy expenditure.
- Leptin also affects female reproduction, immune function, and the function of many other hormones, including insulin.

Neurohormones

Unlike the hormones, which are secreted by endocrine glands, **neurohormones** (**new**-roh-**HOR**-mohnz) are secreted by specialized cells of the brain. Although produced in the brain, they are able to affect cells throughout distant parts of the body (see Figure 13.2).

MEDICAL SPECIALTIES RELATED TO THE ENDOCRINE SYSTEM

- An **endocrinologist** (**en**-doh-krih-**NOL**-oh-jist) is a physician who specializes in diagnosing and treating diseases and malfunctions of the endocrine glands (**endocrin** means to secrete within, and **-ologist** means specialist).

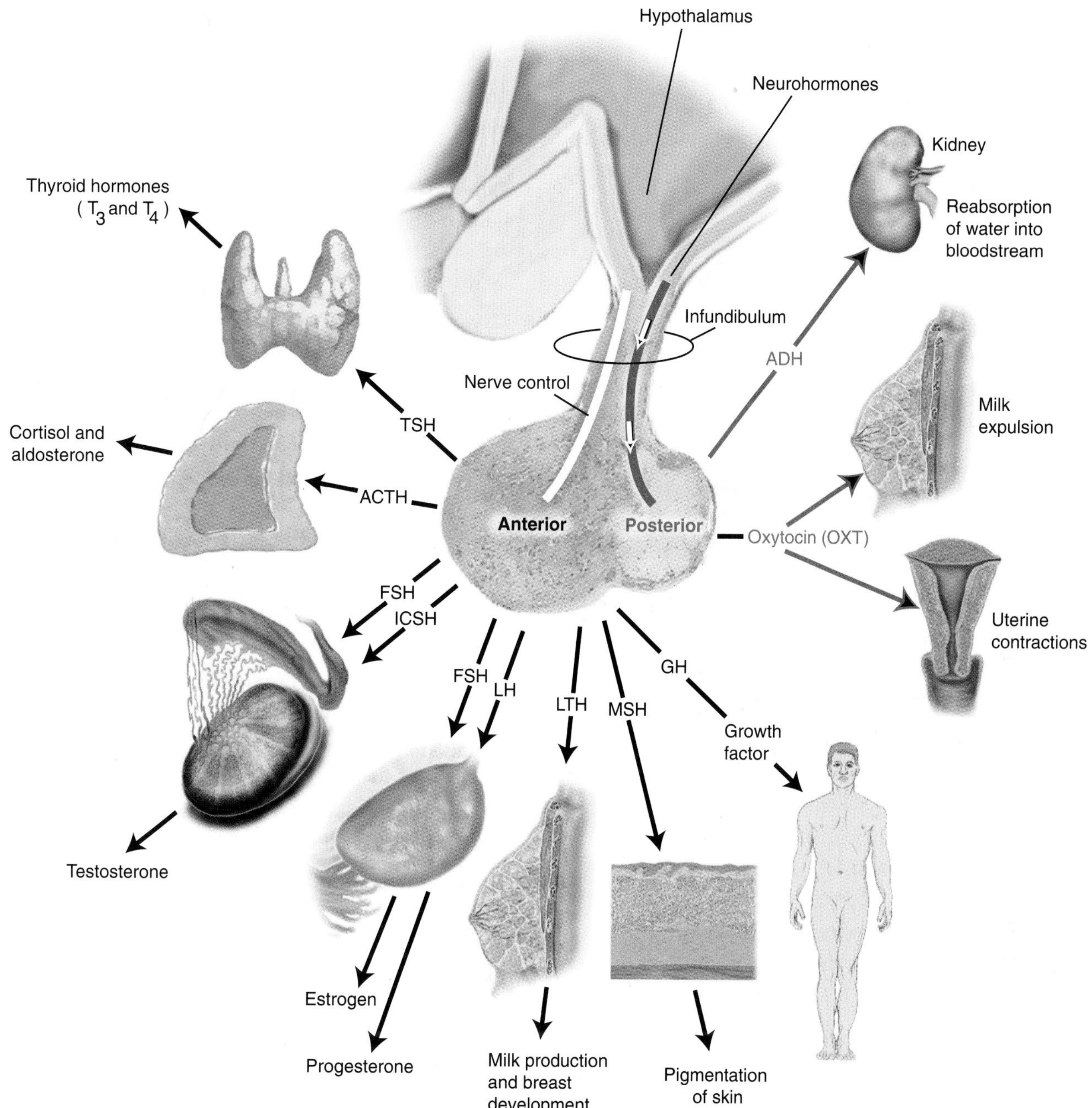

FIGURE 13.2 The pituitary gland secretes hormones that control the activities of other endocrine glands.

PATHOLOGY OF THE ENDOCRINE SYSTEM

- **Endocrinopathy** (**en**-doh-krih-**NOP**-ah-thee) is any disease caused by a disorder of the endocrine system (**endo-** means within, **crin/o** means to secrete, and **-pathy** means disease).
- **Hypercrinism** (**high**-per-**KRY**-nism) is a condition due to excessive secretion of any gland, especially an endocrine gland (**hyper-** means excessive, **crin** means to secrete, and **-ism** means condition). Hypercrinism is the opposite of *hypocrinism.*
- **Hypocrinism** (**high**-poh-**KRY**-nism) is a condition caused by deficient secretion of any gland, especially an endocrine gland (**hypo-** means deficient, **crin** means to secrete, and **-ism** means condition). Hypocrinism is the opposite of *hypercrinism.*

THE PITUITARY GLAND

The pea-sized **pituitary gland** (pih-**TOO**-ih-**tair**-ee), which is composed of anterior and posterior lobes, hangs from the infundibulum below the hypothalamus, which is part of the brain (Figure 13.2). An *infundibulum* is a stalk-like structure.

Functions of the Pituitary Gland

The primary function of the pituitary gland is to secrete hormones that control the activity of other endocrine glands (see Figure 13.2). The pituitary acts in response to stimuli from the hypothalamus. This creates a system of checks and balances to maintain an appropriate blood level of each hormone.

Secretions of the Pituitary Gland: Anterior Lobe

- The **adrenocorticotropic hormone** (ACTH) stimulates the adrenal cortex to secrete cortisol.
- The **follicle-stimulating hormone** (FSH) stimulates the secretion of estrogen and the growth of ova (eggs) in the ovaries of the female. In the male, it stimulates the production of sperm in the testicles.
- The **growth hormone** (GH), also known as a *somatotropic hormone*, regulates the growth of bone, muscle, and other body tissues (**somat/o** means body and **-tropic** means having an affinity for).
- The **interstitial cell-stimulating hormone** (ICSH) stimulates ovulation in the female. In the male, it stimulates the secretion of testosterone.
- The **lactogenic hormone** (LTH), also known as *prolactin*, stimulates and maintains the secretion of breast milk in the mother after childbirth.
- The **luteinizing hormone (LOO**-tee-in-**eye**-zing) stimulates ovulation in the female and production of the female sex hormone progesterone. In the male, LH it stimulates the secretion of testosterone.
- The **melanocyte-stimulating hormone** (MSH) increases the production of melanin in melanocytes, thereby causing darkening the pigmentation of the skin (see Chapter 12).
- The **thyroid-stimulating hormone** (TSH) stimulates the growth and secretions of the thyroid gland.

Secretions of the Pituitary Gland: Posterior Lobe

- The **antidiuretic hormone (an**-tih-dye-you-**RET**-ick) maintains the water balance within the body by promoting the reabsorption of water through the kidneys (see Chapter 9). When more antidiuretic hormone is secreted, less urine is produced. In contrast, a *diuretic* is a medication that is administered to increase urine secretion.
- **Oxytocin** (**ock**-sih-**TOH**-sin) (OXT) stimulates uterine contractions during childbirth (**oxy-** means swift, and **-tocin** means labor). After childbirth, oxytocin stimulates the flow of milk from the mammary glands. *Pitocin* is a synthetic form of oxytocin that is administered to induce or speed up labor.

Pathology of the Pituitary Gland

- **Acromegaly** (**ack**-roh-**MEG**-ah-lee) is abnormal enlargement of the extremities (hands and feet) that is caused by excessive secretion of growth hormone *after* puberty (**acr/o** means extremities, and **-megaly** means abnormal enlargement). Contrast with *gigantism*.
- **Gigantism** (jigh-**GAN**-tiz-em), also known as *giantism*, is abnormal overgrowth of the entire body that is caused by excessive secretion of the growth hormone *before* puberty. Contrast with *acromegaly*.
- **Hyperpituitarism** (**high**-per-pih-**TOO**-ih-tah-rizm) is pathology resulting in the excessive secretion by the anterior lobe of the pituitary gland (**hyper-** means excessive, **pituitar** means pituitary, and **-ism** means condition). Hyperpituitarism is the opposite of *hypopituitarism*.
- **Hypopituitarism** (**high**-poh-pih-**TOO**-ih-tah-rizm) is a condition of reduced secretion due to the partial, or complete, loss of the function of the anterior lobe of the pituitary gland (**hypo-** means deficient, **pituitar** means pituitary, and **-ism** means condition). Hypopituitarism is the opposite of *hyperpituitarism*.
- **Pituitarism** (pih-**TOO**-ih-tar-izm) is any disorder of pituitary function (**pituitar** means pituitary, and **-ism** means condition).
- A **pituitary adenoma** (pih-**TOO**-ih-**tair**-ee **ad**-eh-**NOH**-mah), also known as a *pituitary tumor*, is a slow-growing, benign tumor of the pituitary gland. The two types of these tumors are functioning and nonfunctioning pituitary tumors. *Functioning pituitary tumors* often produce hormones in large and unregulated

amounts. *Nonfunctioning pituitary tumors* do not produce significant amounts of hormones.

- A **prolactinoma** (proh-**lack**-tih-**NOH**-mah), also known as a *prolactin-producing adenoma*, is a benign tumor of the pituitary gland that causes it to produce too much prolactin. In females, this overproduction causes infertility and changes in menstruation. In males, it causes impotence (see Chapter 14).

Diabetes Insipidus

Diabetes insipidus (**dye**-ah-**BEE**-teez in-**SIP**-ih-dus) is caused by insufficient production of the antidiuretic hormone or by the inability of the kidneys to respond appropriately to this hormone.

When there is an insufficient quantity of ADH, too much fluid to be excreted by the kidneys. This causes extreme polydipsia (excessive thirst) and polyuria (excessive urination). If this problem is not controlled, it can become a very serious condition due to dehydration.

Treatment Procedures of the Pituitary Gland

The **human growth hormone**, also known as *recombinant GH*, is a synthetic version of the growth hormone that is administered to stimulate growth when the natural supply of growth hormone is insufficient for normal development.

THE PINEAL GLAND

The **pineal gland** (**PIN**-ee-al) is very small endocrine gland that is located in the central portion of the brain (Figure 13.3)

Functions of the Pineal Gland

The pineal gland, also known as the *pineal body*, influences the sleep-wakefulness cycle.

Secretion of the Pineal Gland

The pineal gland secretes the hormone **melatonin** (**mel**-ah-**TOH**-nin), which influences the sleep and wakefulness portions of the circadian cycle. The term *circadian cycle* refers to the biological functions that occur within a 24-hour period.

Pathology and Treatment of the Pineal Gland

- A **pinealoma** (pin-ee-ah-**LOH**-mah) is a tumor of the pineal gland that can disrupt the production of melatonin (**pineal** means pineal gland, and **-oma** means tumor). This tumor can also cause insomnia by disrupting the circadian cycle.
- A **pinealectomy** (**pin**-ee-al-**ECK**-toh-mee) is the surgical removal of the pineal gland (**pineal** means pineal gland, and **-ectomy** means surgical removal).

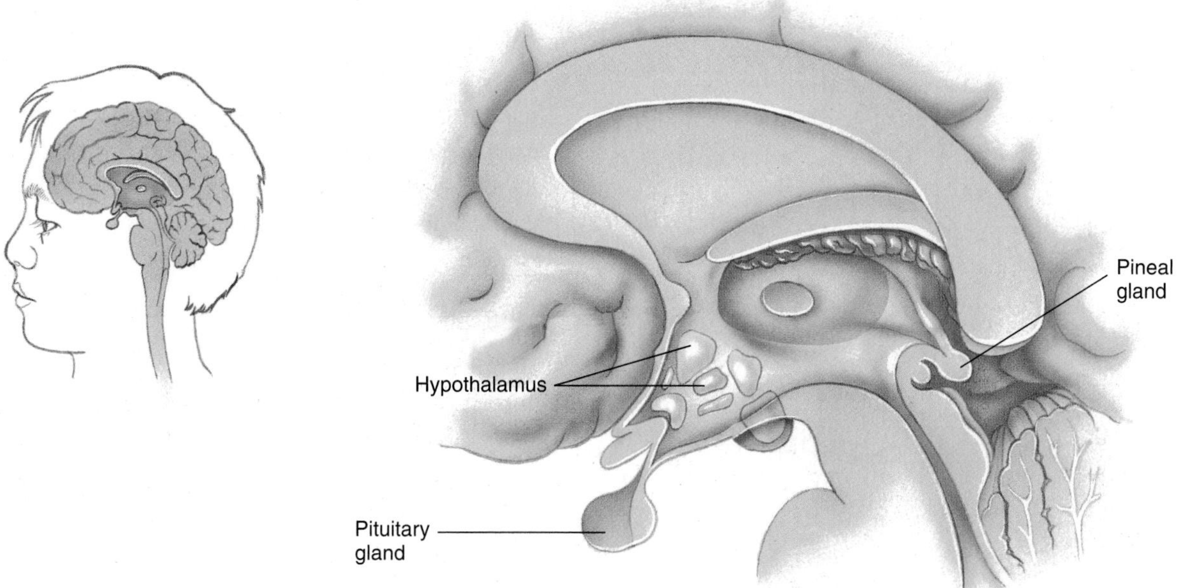

FIGURE 13.3 The pineal gland is located within the brain.

THE THYROID GLAND

The butterfly-shaped **thyroid gland** lies on either side of the larynx, just below the thyroid cartilage (Figure 13.4).

Functions of the Thyroid Gland

- One of the primary functions of the thyroid gland is to regulate the body's metabolism. The term *metabolism* describes all of the processes involved in the body's use of nutrients, including the rate at which they are utilized.
- Thyroid secretions also influence growth and the functioning of the nervous system.

Secretions of the Thyroid Gland

- The two primary thyroid hormones are **thyroxine** (thigh-**ROCK**-sin) and **triiodothyronine** (try-**eye**-oh-doh-**THIGH**-roh-neen). The rate of metabolism is influenced by these hormones. The rate of secretion of these hormones is controlled by the thyroid-stimulating hormone produced by the anterior lobe of the pituitary gland.
- **Calcitonin** (**kal**-sih-**TOH**-nin), which is secreted by cells of the thyroid gland, works with the parathyroid hormone to regulate the calcium levels in the blood and tissues. Calcitonin *decreases* blood levels by moving calcium into storage in the bones and teeth. Compare with the function of the *parathyroid hormone*.

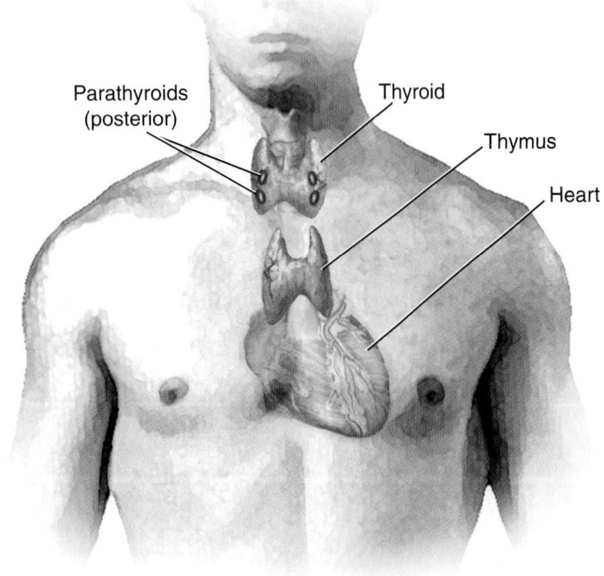

FIGURE 13.4 The thyroid, parathyroids, and thymus glands.

Pathology of the Thyroid Gland

Insufficient Thyroid Secretion

- **Hashimoto's thyroiditis** (hah-shee-**MOH**-tohz **thigh**-roi-**DYE**-tis), also known as *chronic lymphocytic thyroiditis*, is an autoimmune disease in which the body's own antibodies attack and destroy the cells of the thyroid gland.
- **Hypothyroidism** (**high**-poh-**THIGH**-roid-izm), also known as an *underactive thyroid*, is caused by a deficiency of thyroid secretion (**hypo**- means deficient, **thyroid** means thyroid, and **-ism** means condition). Symptoms include fatigue, depression, sensitivity to cold, and a decreased metabolic rate.
- **Cretinism** (**CREE**-tin-izm) is a congenital form of hypothyroidism. If treatment is not started soon after birth, cretinism causes arrested physical and mental development.
- **Myxedema** (**mick**-seh-**DEE**-mah), which is also known as *adult hypothyroidism*, is caused by extreme deficiency of thyroid secretion. Symptoms include swelling, particularly around the eyes and cheeks, fatigue, and a subnormal temperature.

Excessive Thyroid Secretion

- **Hyperthyroidism** (**high**-per-**THIGH**-roid-izm), also known as *thyrotoxicosis*, is an imbalance of metabolism caused by the overproduction of thyroid hormones (**hyper**- means excessive, **thyroid** means thyroid, and **-ism** means condition). Symptoms include an increased metabolic rate, sweating, nervousness, and weight loss.
- A **thyroid storm**, also known as a *thyrotoxic crisis*, is a relatively rare, life-threatening condition caused by exaggerated hyperthyroidism. Patients experiencing a thyroid storm may complain of fever, chest pain, palpitations, shortness of breath, tremors, increased sweating, disorientation, and fatigue.

Graves' Disease

Graves' disease (**GRAYVZ** dih-**ZEEZ**), which is an autoimmune disorder that is caused by hyperthyroidism, is characterized by goiter and/or exophthalmos.

- **Goiter** (**GOI**-ter), also known as *thyromegaly*, is an abnormal nonmalignant enlargement of the thyroid gland (**thyr/o** means thyroid, and **-megaly** means abnormal enlargement). This enlargement produces a swelling in the front of the neck. A simple goiter usually occurs when the thyroid gland is not able to produce enough thyroid hormone to meet the body's needs.

- **Exophthalmos** (**eck**-sof-**THAL**-mos) is an abnormal protrusion of the eyeball out of the orbit.

Diagnostic and Treatment Procedures Related to the Thyroid Gland

- A **thyroid-stimulating hormone assay** is a diagnostic test to measure the circulating blood level of thyroid-stimulating hormone. This test is used to detect abnormal thyroid activity resulting from excessive pituitary stimulation.
- A **thyroid scan**, which measures thyroid function, is a form of nuclear medicine that is discussed in Chapter 15.
- An **antithyroid drug** is a medication administered to slow the ability of the thyroid gland to produce thyroid hormones.
- A **chemical thyroidectomy** (**thigh**-roi-**DECK**-toh-mee), also known as *radioactive iodine therapy*, is the administration of radioactive iodine to destroy thyroid cells. This procedure, which disables at least part of the thyroid gland, is used to treat chronic hyperthyroid disorders such as Graves' disease.
- A **lobectomy** (loh-**BECK**-toh-mee) is the surgical removal of one lobe of the thyroid gland. This term is also used to describe the removal of a lobe of the liver, brain, or lung.
- **Synthetic thyroid hormones** are administered to replace lost thyroid function.

THE PARATHYROID GLANDS

The four **parathyroid glands**, each of which is about the size of a grain of rice, are embedded in the posterior surface of the thyroid gland (see Figure 13.4).

Functions of the Parathyroid Glands

The primary function of the parathyroid glands is to regulate calcium levels throughout the body. These calcium levels are important to the smooth functioning of the muscular and nervous systems.

Secretions of the Parathyroid Glands

The **parathyroid hormone** works with the hormone calcitonin that is secreted by the thyroid gland. Together, they regulate the calcium levels in the blood and tissues. The parathyroid hormone *increases* calcium levels in the blood by mobilizing the release of calcium from storage in the bones and teeth. Compare with the function of the *calcitonin.*

Pathology and Treatment of the Parathyroid Glands

- **Hyperparathyroidism** (**high**-per-**par**-ah-**THIGH**-roid-izm) is the overproduction of the parathyroid hormone (**hyper**- means excessive, **parathyroid** means parathyroid, and **-ism** means condition). *Primary hyperparathyroidism* is caused to a disorder of the parathyroid gland and it can lead to weakened bones and the formation of kidney stones. (See *hypercalcemia* below). In 85 percent of people with primary hyperparathyroidism, a benign tumor known as an adenoma has formed on one of the parathyroid glands, causing it to become overactive. An *adenoma* is a small slow growing benign growth of glandular origin *Secondary hyperparathyroidism* is due to a disorder elsewhere in the body, such as kidney failure. Hyperparathyroidism is the opposite of *hypoparathyroidism.* When symptoms do appear, they are often mild and nonspecific, such as a feeling of weakness and fatigue, depression, or aches and pains. With more severe disease, a person may have a loss of appetite, nausea, vomiting, constipation, confusion or impaired thinking and memory, and increased thirst and urination.
- **Hypercalcemia** (**high**-per-kal-**SEE**-mee-ah) is characterized by abnormally *high* concentrations of calcium circulating in the blood instead of being stored in the bones (**hyper**- means excessive, **calc** means calcium, and **-emia** means blood condition). This can lead to weakened bones and the formation of kidney stones. Hypercalcemia is the opposite of *hypocalcemia.*
- **Hypocalcemia** (**high**-poh-kal-**SEE**-mee-ah) is characterized by abnormally *low* levels of calcium in the blood (**hypo**- means deficient, **calc** means calcium, and **-emia** means blood condition). Hypocalcemia is the opposite of *hypercalcemia.*
- **Osteitis fibrosa** is a complication of hyperparathyroidism in which bone becomes softened and deformed, and may develop cysts. This condition can be caused by overproduction of parathyroid hormone or by parathyroid cancer.
- **Hypoparathyroidism** (**high**-poh-**par**-ah-**THIGH**-roid-izm) is caused by an insufficient or absent secretion of the parathyroid hormone (**hypo**- means deficient, **parathyroid** means parathyroid, and **-ism** means condition). This condition causes hypocalcemia, and in severe cases, it leads to tetany. *Tetany* is the condition of periodic, painful muscle spasms and tremors. Hypoparathyroidism is the opposite of *hyperparathyroidism.*
- A **parathyroidectomy** (**par**-ah-**thigh**-roi-**DECK**-toh-mee), which is the surgical removal of one or more of the parathyroid glands, is performed to control hyperparathyroidism.

THE THYMUS

The **thymus** (**THIGH**-mus) is located near the midline in the anterior portion of the thoracic cavity. It is posterior to (behind) the sternum and slightly superior to (above) the heart (see Figure 13.4).

Functions of the Thymus

The thymus functions as part of the endocrine system by secreting a hormone that functions as part of the immune system.

Secretions of the Thymus

- **Thymosin** (**THIGH**-moh-sin) stimulates the maturation of lymphocytes into T cells of the immune system. These mature cells are important in coordinating immune defenses (see Chapter 6).

Pathology and Treatment of the Thymus

- **Thymitis** (thigh-**MY**-tis) is an inflammation of the thymus gland (**thym** means thymus, and **-itis** means inflammation).
- A **thymectomy** (thigh-**MECK**-toh-mee) is the surgical removal of the thymus gland (**thym** means thymus, and **-ectomy** means surgical removal).

THE PANCREATIC ISLETS

The **pancreas** (**PAN**-kree-as) is a feather-shaped organ located posterior to the stomach that functions as part of both the digestive and the endocrine systems (see Figure 13.1).

The **pancreatic islets** (**pan**-kree-**AT**-ick **EYE**-lets) are those parts of the pancreas that have endocrine functions.

Functions of the Pancreatic Islets

The endocrine functions of these islets are to control blood sugar levels and glucose metabolism throughout the body.

- **Glucose** (**GLOO**-kohs), also known as *blood sugar*, is the basic form of energy used by the body.
- **Glycogen** (**GLYE**-koh-jen) is the form in which the liver stores the excess glucose.

Secretions of the Pancreatic Islets

- **Glucagon** (**GLOO**-kah-gon) is the hormone secreted by the *alpha cells* of the pancreatic islets in response to low blood sugar levels. Glucagon increases the glucose level by stimulating the liver to convert glycogen into glucose for release into the bloodstream.
- **Insulin** (**IN**-suh-lin) is the hormone secreted by the *beta cells* of the pancreatic islets in response to high blood sugar levels. It functions in two ways. First, insulin allows glucose to enter the cells for use as energy. When additional glucose is *not* needed, insulin stimulates the liver to convert glucose into glycogen for storage.

Pathology and Treatment of the Pancreas

- An **insulinoma** (**in**-suh-lin-**OH**-mah) is a benign tumor of the pancreas that causes hypoglycemia by secreting additional insulin (**insulin** means insulin, and **-oma** means tumor).
- **Pancreatalgia** (**pan**-kree-ah-**TAL**-jee-ah) is pain in the pancreas (**pancreat** means pancreas, and **-algia** means pain).
- **Pancreatitis** (**pan**-kree-ah-**TYE**-tis) is an inflammation of the pancreas (**pancreat** means pancreas, and **-itis** means inflammation). Long-term alcohol abuse is a leading cause of pancreatitis.
- A **pancreatectomy** (**pan**-kree-ah-**TECK**-toh-mee) is the surgical removal all or part of the pancreas (**pancreat** means pancreas, and **-ectomy** means surgical removal). A *total pancreatectomy* is performed to treat pancreatic cancer, and this procedure involves the spleen, gallbladder, common bile duct, and portions of the small intestine and stomach.

Abnormal Blood Sugar Levels

- **Hyperglycemia** (**high**-per-glye-**SEE**-mee-ah) is an abnormally high concentration of glucose in the blood (**hyper-** means excessive, **glyc** means sugar, and **-emia** means blood condition). Hyperglycemia is seen primarily in patients with diabetes mellitus. The symptoms include polydipsia, polyphagia, and polyuria. Hyperglycemia is the opposite of *hypoglycemia*.
- **Polydipsia** (**pol**-ee-**DIP**-see-ah) is excessive thirst (**poly-** means many, and **-dipsia** means thirst).
- **Polyphagia** (**pol**-ee-**FAY**-jee-ah) is excessive hunger (**poly-** means many, and **-phagia** means eating).
- **Polyuria** (**pol**-ee-**YOU**-ree-ah) is excessive urination (**poly-** means many, and **-uria** means urination).

- **Hyperinsulinism** (**high**-per-**IN**-suh-lin-izm) is the condition of excessive secretion of insulin in the bloodstream (**hyper-** means excessive, **insulin** means insulin, and **-ism** means condition). Hyperinsulinism can cause hypoglycemia.
- **Hypoglycemia** (**high**-poh-glye-**SEE**-mee-ah) is an abnormally low concentration of glucose in the blood (**hypo-** means deficient, **glyc** means sugar, and **-emia** means blood condition). Symptoms include nervousness and shakiness, confusion, perspiration, or feeling anxious or weak. Hypoglycemia is the opposite of *hyperglycemia*.

Diabetes Mellitus

Diabetes mellitus (**dye**-ah-**BEE**-teez **MEL**-ih-tus) is a group of metabolic disorders characterized by hyperglycemia resulting from defects in insulin secretion, insulin action, or both.

- This condition is described as type 1 and type 2.
- Many patients present with symptoms of both types of diabetes, and their treatment must be modified accordingly.
- In the past, when a child developed diabetes, this condition was referred to as *juvenile diabetes*; however, the condition in children in now described as being type 1 or type 2.
- The treatment goals for all types of diabetes are to most effectively control the blood sugar levels and prevent complications.

Type 1 Diabetes

Type 1 diabetes is an autoimmune insulin deficiency disorder caused by the destruction of pancreatic islet beta cells. *Insulin deficiency* means that the pancreatic beta cells do not secrete enough insulin.

- Symptoms of type 1 diabetes include polydipsia, polyphagia, polyuria, weight loss, blurred vision, extreme fatigue, and slow healing.
- Type 1 diabetes is treated with diet and exercise as well as carefully regulated insulin replacement therapy administered by injection or pump.

Type 2 Diabetes

Type 2 diabetes is an insulin resistance disorder. *Insulin resistance* means that insulin is being produced, but the body does not use it effectively. In an attempt to compensate for this lack of response, the body secretes more insulin.

- With the rise of childhood obesity, type 2 diabetes is increasingly common in children and young adults. Obese adults are also at high risk for this condition.
- *Prediabetes* is a condition in which the blood sugar level is higher than normal, but not high enough to be classified as type 2 diabetes. However, this condition indicates an increased risk of developing type 2 diabetes, heart disease, and stroke.
- Type 2 diabetes can have no symptoms for years. When symptoms do occur, they include those of type 1 diabetes plus recurring infections, irritability, and a tingling sensation in the hands or feet.
- Type 2 diabetes is usually treated with diet, exercise, and oral medications.
- *Oral hypoglycemics* lower blood sugar by causing the body to release more insulin.
- *Glucophage* (metformin hydrochloride) and similar medications work within the cells to combat insulin resistance and to help insulin let blood sugar into the cells.

Gestational Diabetes

Gestational diabetes (jes-**TAY**-shun-al **dye**-ah-**BEE**-teez) is a form of diabetes mellitus that occurs during some pregnancies. This condition usually disappears after delivery; however, many of these women later develop type 2 diabetes.

Diabetes Mellitus Diagnostic Procedures

- A **fasting blood sugar test** measures the glucose (blood sugar) levels after the patient has not eaten for 8–12 hours. This test is used to screen for diabetes. This test is also used to monitor treatment of this condition.
- An **oral glucose tolerance test** is performed to confirm a diagnosis of diabetes mellitus and to aid in diagnosing hypoglycemia.
- **Home blood glucose monitoring** measures the current blood sugar level. This test, which requires a drop of blood, is performed by the patient.
- The **fructosamine test** (fruck-**TOHS**-ah-meen) measures average glucose levels over the past 3 weeks. The fructosamine test is able to detect changes more rapidly than the HbA1c test.
- **Hemoglobin A1c testing**, also known as *HbA1c* and pronounced as *"H-B A-one-C,"* is a blood test that measures the average blood glucose level over the previous 3–4 months.

Diabetic Emergencies

Diabetic emergencies are due to either too much or too little blood sugar. Treatment depends on accurately diagnosing the cause of the emergency (Figure 13.5).

- **Insulin shock** is caused by very low blood sugar (hypoglycemia). *Oral glucose*, which is a sugary substance that can quickly be absorbed into the bloodstream, is administered orally to rapidly raise the blood sugar level.
- A **diabetic coma** is caused by very high blood sugar (hyperglycemia). Also known as *diabetic ketoacidosis*, this condition is treated by the prompt administration of insulin.

Diabetic Complications

Most diabetic complications result from the damage to capillaries and other blood vessels due to long-term exposure to excessive blood sugar.

- **Diabetic retinopathy** (**ret**-ih-**NOP**-ah-thee) occurs when diabetes damages the tiny blood vessels in the retina, causing blood to leak into the posterior segment of the eyeball. This can cause the loss of vision.
- *Heart disease* occurs because excess blood sugar makes the walls of the blood vessels sticky and rigid. This encourages hypertension and atherosclerosis (see Chapter 5).

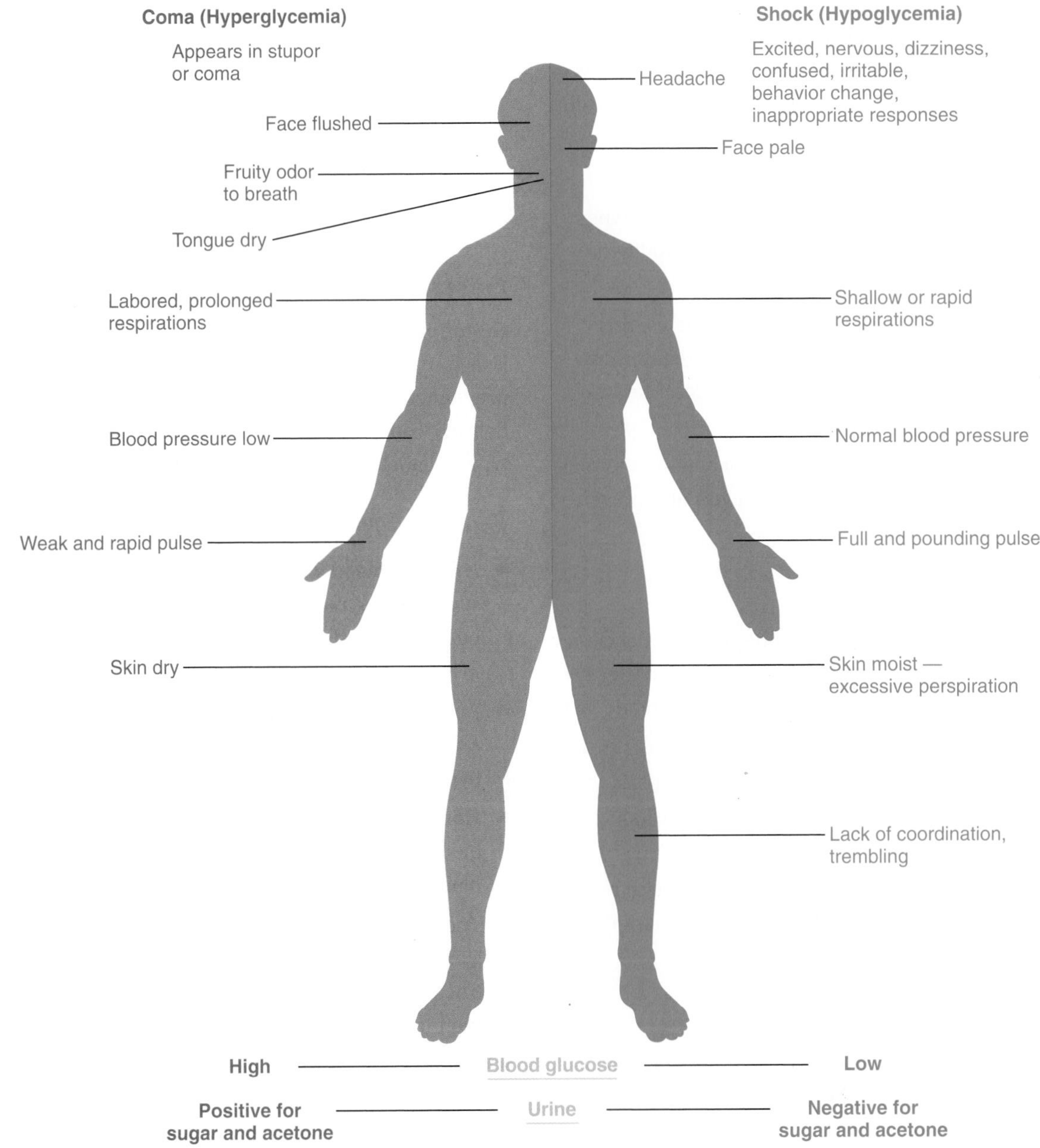

FIGURE 13.5 Left: Diabetic coma (hyperglycemia). Right: Insulin shock (hypoglycemia).

- *Kidney disease* can lead to renal failure because damage to the blood vessels reduces blood flow through the kidneys (see Chapter 9).
- *Peripheral neuropathy* is damage to the nerves affecting the hands and feet (see Chapter 10).

THE ADRENAL GLANDS

The **adrenal glands** are also known as the *suprarenals* because they are located with one on top of each kidney. Each of these glands consists of an outer portion, known as the *adrenal cortex*, and the middle portion, which is the *adrenal medulla*. Each of these parts has a specialized role, and the entire gland is surrounded by an *adrenal capsule* (Figure 13.6).

Functions of the Adrenal Glands

One of the primary functions of the adrenal glands is to control electrolyte levels within the body.

- **Electrolytes** (ee-**LECK**-troh-lytes) are mineral substances, such as sodium and potassium, that are normally found in the blood.
- Other important functions of the adrenal glands include helping to regulate metabolism and interacting with the sympathetic nervous system in response to stress.

Secretions of the Adrenal Cortex

Corticosteroids (**kor**-tih-koh-**STEHR**-oidz) are the steroid hormones produced by the adrenal cortex. The same term describes synthetically produced equivalents that are administered as medications.

- **Aldosterone** (al-**DOSS**-ter-ohn) regulates the salt and water levels in the body by increasing sodium reabsorption and potassium excretion by the kidneys. *Reabsorption* means returning a substance to the bloodstream.
- **Androgens** (**AN**-droh-jenz) are hormones that influence sex-related characteristics. Normally, in adults the production of androgens in the adrenal cortex is minimal; instead, these hormones are produced in the male and female gonads.
- **Cortisol** (**KOR**-tih-sol), also known as *hydrocortisone*, has an anti-inflammatory action, and it regulates the metabolism of carbohydrates, fats, and proteins in the body.

Secretions of the Adrenal Medulla

- **Epinephrine** (**ep**-ih-**NEF**-rin), also known as *adrenaline*, stimulates the sympathetic nervous system in response to stress or other stimuli. It makes the heart beat faster and can raise blood pressure. It also helps the liver release glucose (sugar) and limits the release of insulin.
- **Norepinephrine** (**nor**-ep-ih-**NEF**-rin) is both a hormone and a neurohormone. It is released as a neurohormone by the sympathetic nervous system and as a hormone by the adrenal medulla. It plays an important role in the "fight-or-flight response" by raising blood pressure, strengthening the heartbeat, and stimulating muscle contractions.

Pathology of the Adrenal Glands

- **Addison's disease** (**AD**-ih-sonz) occurs when the adrenal glands do not produce enough of the hormones cortisol or aldosterone. This condition is characterized by chronic, worsening fatigue and muscle weakness, loss of appetite, and weight loss.

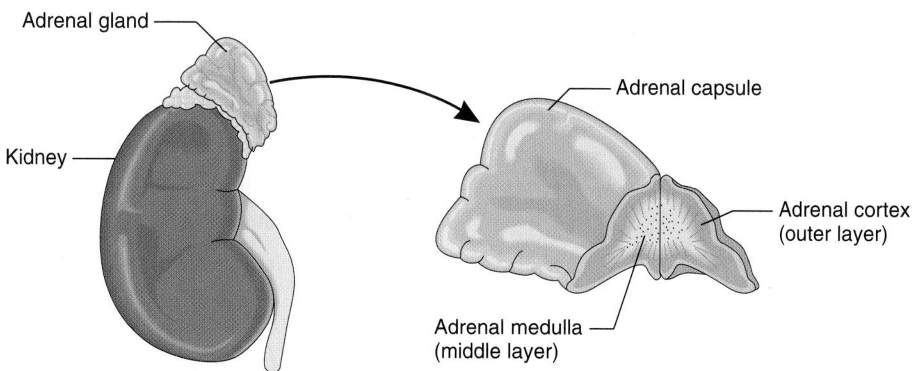

FIGURE 13.6 One adrenal gland is located on top of each kidney. Each adrenal gland consists of the adrenal cortex and adrenal medulla, and the entire gland is surrounded by the adrenal capsule.

- **Adrenalitis** (ah-**dree**-nal-**EYE**-tis) is inflammation of the adrenal glands (**adrenal** means adrenal glands, and **-itis** means inflammation).
- **Aldosteronism** (al-**DOSS**-teh-roh-**niz**-em) is an abnormality of electrolyte balance caused by the excessive secretion of aldosterone.
- **Conn's syndrome** is a disorder of the adrenal glands due to excessive production of aldosterone.
- A **pheochromocytoma** (fee-oh-**kroh**-moh-sigh-**TOH**-mah) is a benign tumor of the adrenal medulla that causes the gland to produce excess epinephrine (**phe/o** means dusky, **chrom/o** means color, **cyt** means cell, and **-oma** means tumor).

Cushing's Syndrome

Cushing's syndrome (**KUSH**-ingz **SIN**-drohm), also known as *hypercortisolism*, is caused by prolonged exposure to high levels of cortisol. The symptoms include a rounded or "moon face" (Figure 13.7).

This condition can be caused by overproduction of cortisol by the body or by taking glucocorticoid hormone medications to treat inflammatory diseases such as asthma and rheumatoid arthritis.

Treatment Procedures of the Adrenal Glands

- A **laparoscopic adrenalectomy** (ah-**dree**-nal-**ECK**-toh-mee) is a minimally invasive procedure to surgically remove one or both adrenal glands (**adrenal** means adrenal gland, and **-ectomy** means surgical removal).
- **Cortisone** (**KOR**-tih-sohn), also known as *hydrocortisone*, is the synthetic equivalent of corticosteroids produced by the body. Cortisone is administered to suppress inflammation and as an immunosuppressant.
- **Epinephrine** is a synthetic hormone used as a vasoconstrictor to treat conditions such as heart dysrhythmias and asthma attacks. A *vasoconstrictor* causes the blood vessels to contract.

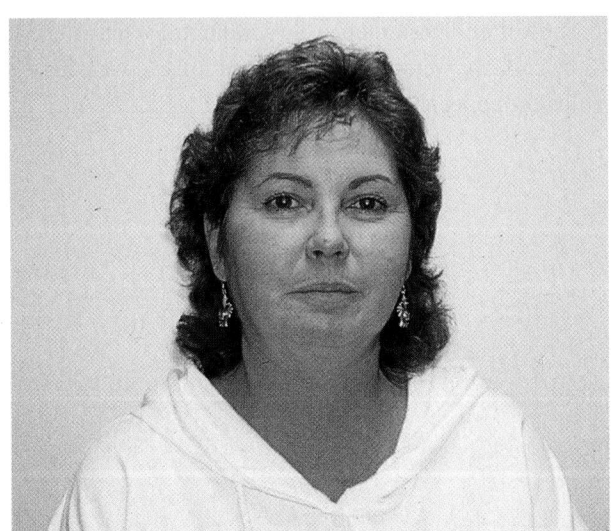

FIGURE 13.7 Cushing's syndrome causes a characteristic "moon" face. (Courtesy of Matthew C. Leinung, MD, Acting head, Division of Endocrinology Albany Medical College, Albany, NY.)

THE GONADS

The **gonads** (**GOH**-nadz), which are ovaries in females and testicles in males, are gamete-producing glands.

- A **gamete** (**GAM**-eet) is a reproductive cell. These are sperm in the male and ova (eggs) in the female.
- **Gonadotropin** is any hormone that stimulates the gonads (**gonad/o** means gonad, and **-tropin** means to simulate).

Functions of the Gonads

The gonads secrete the hormones that are responsible for the development and maintenance of the secondary sex characteristics that develop during puberty. The additional functions of these glands are discussed in Chapter 14.

- **Puberty** is the condition of first being capable of reproducing sexually. It is marked by maturing of the genital organs, development of secondary sex characteristics, and by the first occurrence of menstruation in the female. The average age at which puberty occurs is 12 years in females and 14 in males.
- *Precocious puberty* is the early onset of the changes of puberty. This is before age 9 years in females and before age 10 in males.

Secretions of the Testicles

- **Testosterone** (tes-**TOS**-teh-rohn), which is secreted by the testicles, stimulates the development of male secondary sex characteristics (Figure 13.8).
- The term **virile** (**VIR**-ill) means having the nature, properties, or qualities of an adult male.

Secretions of the Ovaries

- **Estrogen** (**ES**-troh-jen) is important in the development and maintenance of the female secondary sex

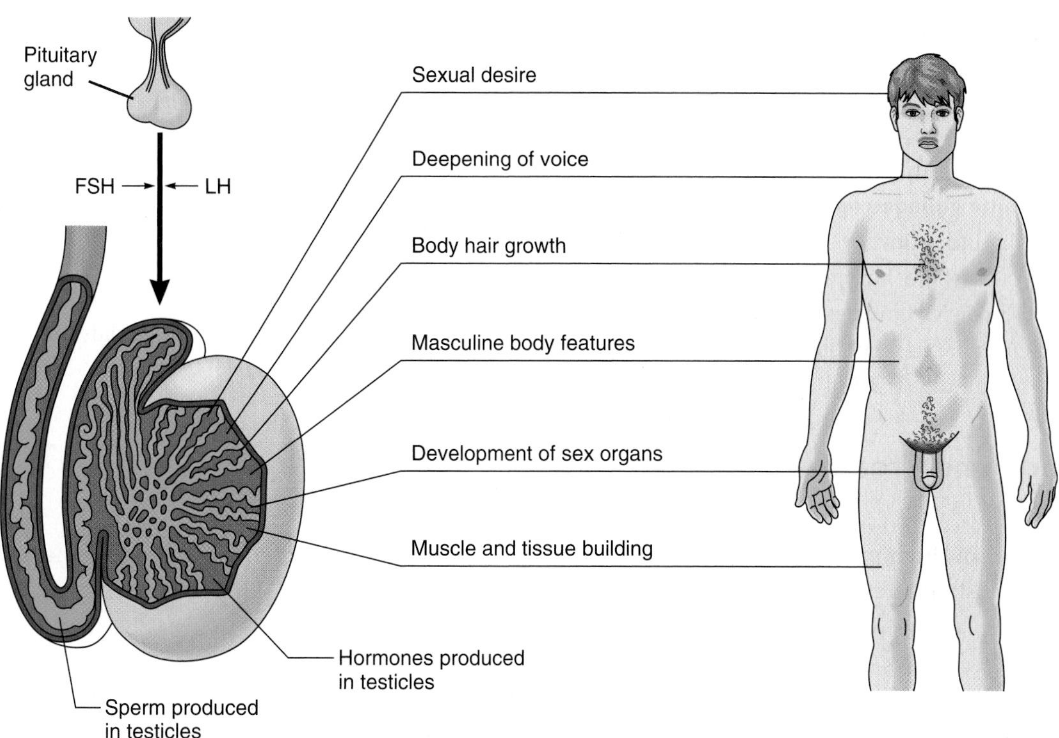

FIGURE 13.8 In the male, the luteinizing hormone, which is secreted by the pituitary gland, stimulates the testicles to secrete testosterone. Testosterone then stimulates the development of the secondary sex characteristics of the male.

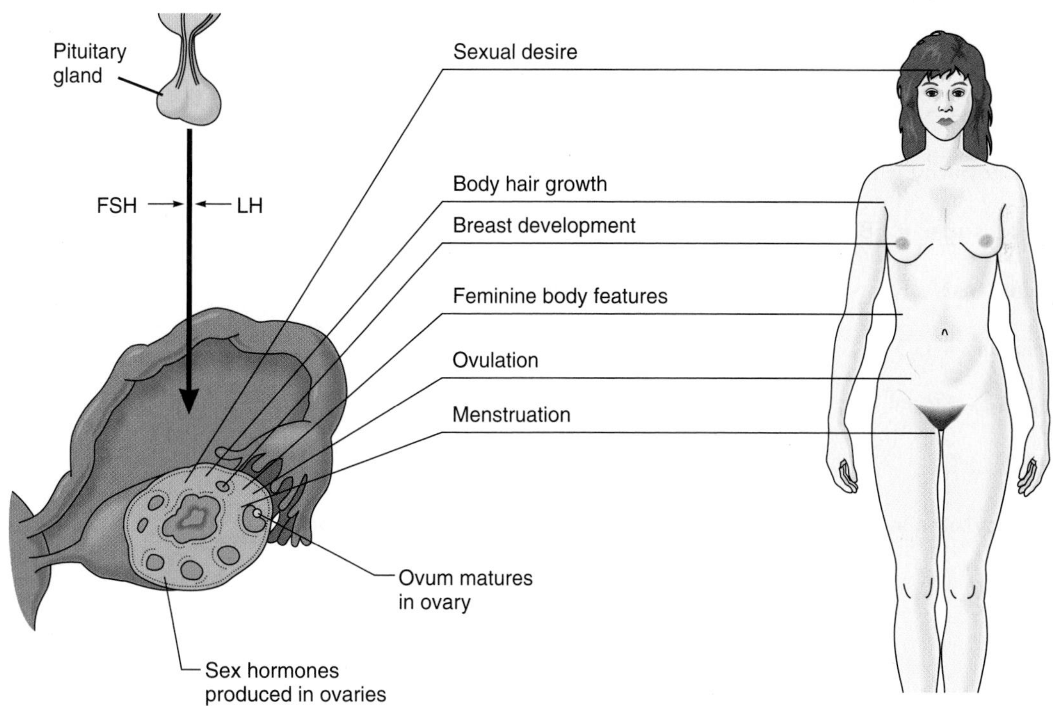

FIGURE 13.9 In the female, the luteinizing hormone, which is secreted by the pituitary gland, stimulates the secretion of estrogen by the ovaries. Estrogen then stimulates the development of the secondary sex characteristics of the female.

characteristics and in regulation of the menstrual cycle (Figure 13.9).

- **Progesterone** (proh-**JES**-ter-ohn) is the hormone released during the second half of the menstrual cycle by the corpus luteum in the ovary. Its function is to complete the preparations for pregnancy.
- If pregnancy occurs, the placenta takes over the production of progesterone.

- If pregnancy does not occur, secretion of the hormone stops and is followed by the menstrual period.

The Placenta

During pregnancy, the placenta secretes the hormone **human chorionic gonadotropin** (**kor**-ee-**ON**-ick **gon**-ah-doh-**TROH**-pin) to stimulate the corpus luteum to continue producing the hormones required to maintain the pregnancy. It also stimulates the hormones required to stimulate lactation after childbirth. The *placenta* and *corpus luteum* are discussed in Chapter 14.

Pathology and Treatment of the Gonads

- **Hypergonadism** (**high**-per-**GOH**-nad-izm) is the condition of excessive secretion of hormones by the sex glands (**hyper-** means excessive, **gonad** means sex gland, and **-ism** means condition).
- **Hypogonadism** (**high**-poh-**GOH**-nad-izm) is the condition of deficient secretion of hormones by the sex glands (**hypo-** means deficient, **gonad** means sex gland, and **-ism** means condition).
- **Gynecomastia** (**guy**-neh-koh-**MAS**-tee-ah) is the condition of excessive mammary development in the male (**gynec/o** means female, **mast** means breast, and **-ia** means abnormal condition).
- Treatment procedures of the gonads are discussed in Chapter 14.

ABBREVIATIONS RELATED TO THE ENDOCRINE SYSTEM

Table 13.2 presents an overview of the abbreviations related to the terms introduced in this chapter. Note: To avoid errors or confusion, always be cautious when using abbreviations.

TABLE 13.2

ABBREVIATIONS RELATED TO THE ENDOCRINE SYSTEM

diabetes insipidus = DI	**DI** = diabetes insipidus
diabetes mellitus = DM	**DM** = diabetes mellitus
diabetic retinopathy = DR, DRP	**DR, DRP** = diabetic retinopathy
fasting blood sugar = FBS	**FBS** = fasting blood sugar
fructosamine test = FA	**FA** = fructosamine test
Graves' disease = GD	**GD** = Graves' disease
hypoglycemia = HG	**HG** = hypoglycemia
leptin = LEP, LPT	**LEP, LPT** = leptin
pheochromocytoma = PC, PCC, Pheo	**PC, PCC, Pheo** = pheochromocytoma

CAREER OPPORTUNITIES

In addition to the medical specialties already discussed, some of the health occupations involving the treatment of the endocrine system include:

- **Diabetes dietitian:** a clinical dietitian specializing in nutritional counseling and therapy for diabetic patients
- **Diabetes management nurse:** an RN who helps diabetics manage their disease by teaching them proper self-care and showing them how to test blood sugar levels and administer insulin injections
- **Pediatric endocrine nurse:** specializes in the treatment of children with conditions such as thyroid disease and diabetes

HEALTH OCCUPATION PROFILE

CLINICAL INSTRUCTOR

Hyacinth C. Martin, RN, is a lecturer/clinical instructor with a focus on treating patients with endocrine problems. *"Patients with diabetes mellitus and other endocrine problems often come to the hospital with presenting symptoms of fluid and electrolyte alterations. Nurses need to be able to identify these symptoms immediately and dependably administer the care prescribed by a physician or a nurse practitioner in order to prevent these patients from going into a crisis.*

"During my years of working in the hospital setting, I loved seeing the patients we cared for return home in a state of wellness. As an educator in the field of nursing, I enjoy imparting to students the knowledge I gained from nursing school and the new information I have acquired through experience and research. I want to share with them the fact that nursing is not only a challenging career, but also a rewarding one financially and emotionally."

STUDY BREAK

What makes teenage boys' voices change? One of the rites of passage for young men going through puberty is the voice changing, or getting deeper. Somewhere between the ages of 12 and 15, most boys experience a lengthening of the vocal chords caused by the secretion of testosterone by the testicles. These hormones stimulate the growth of the vocal cords and of muscles in the throat. As the vocal cords, which are mucous membranes, lengthen and thicken, they produce lower notes. Meanwhile, the muscles around the throat are also getting bigger. They are supposed to control the sounds a boy's voice makes, but until they are fully developed, they do not always do their job. Instead, they allow a boy's voice to jump from pitch to pitch, producing a squeaking or cracking sound when the boy is speaking or singing.

Many prepubescent boys can sing in a high range similar to that of a female soprano, but most (not all) lose that ability when the vocal chords lengthen. In 16th to 18th century Italy, certain talented boys were castrated to prevent their vocal chords from lengthening, thereby maintaining their pure, high singing voice. These men, called *castrati*, were prized as solo performers, especially for religious music.

REVIEW TIME

Write the answers to the following questions on a separate piece of paper or in your notebook. In addition, be prepared to take part in the classroom discussion.

1. ***Written Assignment:*** Using your own words, describe **acromegaly** and **gigantism**.

   Discussion Assignment: At what age does each of these conditions occur, and what parts of the body are primarily affected?

2. ***Written Assignment:*** Report on your research about the person for whom **Cushing's syndrome** was named. Include in your report his or her full name and dates.

   Discussion Assignment: Use terms a physician would understand to describe the signs, symptoms, and causes of Cushing's syndrome.

3. ***Written Assignment:*** Describe the primary differences between **type 1 diabetes** and **type 2 diabetes**.

   Discussion Assignment: Lizzy, who is 79 years of age and overweight, has just been diagnosed with type 2 diabetes. How would you explain this condition and the necessary treatment to her?

4. ***Written Assignment:*** Using terms a layperson would understand, explain the symptoms of **Graves' disease**.

   Discussion Assignment: What are the causes and treatment of Graves' disease?

5. ***Written Assignment:*** Using your own words, describe **anabolic steroids** and why they are used illegally by some athletes.

   Discussion Assignment: What are the dangerous side-effects of using anabolic steroids?

Optional Internet Activity

The goal of this activity is to help you learn more about medical terminology as it applies to the "real world." Select **one** *of these two options and follow the instructions.*

1. Search for information about **diabetes**. Write a brief (one- or two-paragraph) report on something new you learned here and include the address of the web site where you found this information.
2. To learn more about **pituitary disorders**, go to the web site of the Pituitary Network Association. Explore the site and then write a brief (one- or two-paragraph) report on something new you learned here.

THE HUMAN TOUCH: CRITICAL THINKING ACTIVITY

The following story and questions are designed to stimulate critical thinking through class discussion or as a brief essay response. There are no right or wrong answers to these questions.

Josh Stanton, 18, had almost finished high school and was looking forward to college. He'd been accepted by both his first-choice school across the country and his backup school, a small college close to home. As a type 1 diabetic, Josh had worries that weren't factors for most kids. Keeping himself healthy wasn't easy. He needed to track his blood sugar, eat well, remember to take his insulin, and exercise regularly.

continues

He led a fairly structured life at home, so it would be a big change to be completely on his own at college. Before his diagnosis, which came just as he'd finished his college applications, he'd eaten fast food several times a week, and usually had one or more sodas every day. He was still overweight, though he'd lost some weight since his family changed their eating habits after the initial shock of his diagnosis. He'd never quite gotten the hang of exercising every day without his Mom reminding him, but he ate the healthy meals she served at home.

Sitting down, he listed all the issues he worried about facing on his own at a distant school. Exercise: he'd have to figure out how to remember to exercise every day despite an irregular schedule of classes and homework. Diet: with buffet dining hall food, it would be hard to figure out exactly what he was eating or control his portions, and with food only available at certain times of the day, he'd have to keep food on hand in case he experienced an episode of hypoglycemia. Drinking: his doctor had mentioned that alcohol could lower his blood glucose, that sugary mixers could raise it, and that drinking might impair his ability to recognize the signs of hypoglycemia. Medicine: he'd have to remember to take his insulin regularly, since Mom wouldn't be there to remind him.

With a frustrated sigh, he put the pen down and looked at his list. If he went away to the college that he really wanted to attend, there would be so many things to remember, worry about, and take care of. Diabetes had messed up his life, and now it was messing up his future. It was all so overwhelming. Maybe he'd be better off not going to college at all.

Suggested Discussion Topics

1. Josh is well into his senior year of high school. Discuss how he might go about assuming responsibility for managing his own diabetes care before school opens in the fall.
2. Discuss ways in which Josh can master the social challenges associated with college, including irregular eating, beer parties, and the lack of exercise.
3. If Josh goes away to school, should he make sure that his roommates can identify a diabetic emergency and know how it is treated?
4. Do you think Josh would be better off attending a nearby college and living at home—or going to his first choice college despite the fact that it is not near his parents and his doctor?

STUDENT WORKBOOK AND StudyWARE™ CD-ROM

1. Go to your **Student Workbook** and complete the Learning Exercises for this chapter.

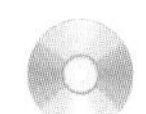

2. Go to the **StudyWARE™ CD-ROM** and have fun with the exercises and games for this chapter.

14

CHAPTER

The Reproductive Systems

Overview of Structures, Combining Forms, and Functions of the Reproductive Systems

Major Structures	Related Combining Forms	Primary Functions
Male		
Penis	pen/i, phall/i	Used for sexual intercourse and urination.
Testicles, Testes	orch/o, orchid/o, test/i, test/o	Produce sperm and the hormone testosterone.
Female		
Ovaries	oophor/o, ovari/o	Produce ova (eggs) and female hormones.
Fallopian Tubes	salping/o	Catch the mature ovum (egg) and transport it to the uterus. Also the site of fertilization.
Uterus	hyster/o, metr/o, metri/o, uter/o	Protects and supports the developing child.
Vagina	vagin/o, colp/o	Used for sexual intercourse, acts as channel for menstrual flow, and functions as the birth canal.
Placenta	placent/o	Exchanges nutrients and waste between the mother and fetus during pregnancy.

VOCABULARY RELATED TO THE REPRODUCTIVE SYSTEMS

This list contains essential word parts and medical terms for this chapter. These terms are pronounced on the student StudyWARE™ CD-ROM and Audio CDs that are available for use with this text. These and the other important **primary terms** are shown in boldface throughout the chapter. *Secondary terms*, which appear in *orange* italics, clarify the meaning of primary terms.

Word Parts

- ☐ **cervic/o**
- ☐ **colp/o**
- ☐ **-gravida**
- ☐ **gynec/o**
- ☐ **hyster/o**
- ☐ **mast/o**
- ☐ **men/o**
- ☐ **nulli-**
- ☐ **ov/o**
- ☐ **ovari/o**
- ☐ **-para**
- ☐ **-pexy**
- ☐ **salping/o**
- ☐ **test/i, test/o**
- ☐ **vagin/o**

Medical Terms

- ☐ **amenorrhea** (ah-**men**-oh-**REE**-ah)
- ☐ **amniocentesis** (**am**-nee-oh-sen-**TEE**-sis)
- ☐ **andropause** (**AN**-droh-pawz)
- ☐ **Apgar score**
- ☐ **azoospermia** (ay-**zoh**-oh-**SPER**-mee-ah)
- ☐ **cervical dysplasia** (**SER**-vih-kal dis-**PLAY**-see-ah)
- ☐ **cervicitis** (**ser**-vih-**SIGH**-tis)
- ☐ **chlamydia** (klah-**MID**-ee-ah)
- ☐ **chorionic villus sampling (kor-ee-ON-ick VIL-us)**
- ☐ **colostrum** (kuh-**LOS**-trum)
- ☐ **colpopexy** (**KOL**-poh-**peck**-see)
- ☐ **colporrhaphy** (kol-**POR**-ah-fee)
- ☐ **colposcopy** (kol-**POS**-koh-pee)
- ☐ **dysmenorrhea** (**dis**-men-oh-**REE**-ah)
- ☐ **eclampsia** (eh-**KLAMP**-see-ah)
- ☐ **ectopic pregnancy** (eck-**TOP**-ick)
- ☐ **endocervicitis** (**en**-doh-**ser**-vih-**SIGH**-tis)
- ☐ **endometriosis** (**en**-doh-**mee**-tree-**OH**-sis)
- ☐ **epididymitis** (**ep**-ih-did-ih-**MY**-tis)
- ☐ **episiotomy** (eh-**piz**-ee-**OT**-oh-mee)
- ☐ **fibroadenoma** (**figh**-broh-**ad**-eh-**NOH**-mah)
- ☐ **fibrocystic breast disease** (**figh**-broh-**SIS**-tick)
- ☐ **galactorrhea** (gah-**lack**-toh-**REE**-ah)
- ☐ **gonorrhea** (**gon**-oh-**REE**-ah)
- ☐ **hemospermia** (**hee**-moh-**SPER**-mee-ah)
- ☐ **hydrocele** (**HIGH**-droh-seel)
- ☐ **hypomenorrhea** (**high**-poh-men-oh-**REE**-ah)
- ☐ **hysterectomy** (**hiss**-teh-**RECK**-toh-mee)
- ☐ **hysterosalpingography** (**hiss**-ter-oh-**sal**-pin-**GOG**-rah-fee)
- ☐ **hysteroscopy** (**hiss**-ter-**OSS**-koh-pee)
- ☐ **leukorrhea** (**loo**-koh-**REE**-ah)
- ☐ **mastalgia** (mass-**TAL**-jee-ah)
- ☐ **mastopexy** (**MAS**-toh-**peck**-see)
- ☐ **menarche** (meh-**NAR**-kee)
- ☐ **menometrorrhagia** (**men**-oh-**met**-roh-**RAY**-jee-ah)
- ☐ **metrorrhea** (**mee**-troh-**REE**-ah)
- ☐ **neonate** (**NEE**-oh-nayt)
- ☐ **nulligravida** (**null**-ih-**GRAV**-ih-dah)
- ☐ **nullipara** (nuh-**LIP**-ah-rah)
- ☐ **obstetrician** (**ob**-steh-**TRISH**-un)
- ☐ **oligomenorrhea** (**ol**-ih-goh-**men**-oh-**REE**-ah)
- ☐ **orchidectomy** (**or**-kih-**DECK**-toh-mee)
- ☐ **orchiopexy** (**or**-keeoh-**PECK**-see)
- ☐ **ovariectomy** (**oh**-vay-ree-**ECK**-toh-mee)
- ☐ **ovariorrhexis** (oh-**vay**-ree-oh-**RECK**-sis)
- ☐ **perimenopause** (pehr-ih-**MEN**-oh-pawz)
- ☐ **Peyronie's disease** (pay-roh-**NEEZ**)
- ☐ **placenta previa** (plah-**SEN**-tah **PREE**-vee-ah)
- ☐ **polycystic ovary syndrome** (**pol**-ee-**SIS**-tick)
- ☐ **preeclampsia** (**pree**-ee-**KLAMP**-see-ah)
- ☐ **priapism** (**PRYE**-ah-**piz**-em)
- ☐ **primigravida** (**prye**-mih-**GRAV**-ih-dah)
- ☐ **primipara** (prye-**MIP**-ah-rah)
- ☐ **pruritus vulvae** (proo-**RYE**-tus **VUL**-vee)
- ☐ **salpingo-oophorectomy** (sal-**ping**-goh oh-**ahf**-oh-**RECK**-toh-mee)
- ☐ **syphilis** (**SIF**-ih-lis)
- ☐ **trichomoniasis** (**trick**-oh-moh-**NYE**-ah-sis)
- ☐ **uterine prolapse** (proh-**LAPS**)
- ☐ **varicocele** (**VAR**-ih-koh-**seel**)
- ☐ **vasovasostomy** (**vay**-soh-vah-**ZOS**-toh-mee)

OBJECTIVES

On completion of this chapter, you should be able to:

1. Identify and describe the major functions and structures of the male reproductive system.
2. Recognize, define, spell, and pronounce the terms related to the pathology and the diagnostic and treatment procedures of the male reproductive system.
3. Name at least six sexually transmitted diseases.
4. Identify and describe the major functions and structures of the female reproductive system.
5. Recognize, define, spell, and pronounce the terms related to the pathology and the diagnostic and treatment procedures of the female reproductive system.
6. Recognize, define, spell, and pronounce the terms related to the pathology and the diagnostic and treatment procedures of the female during pregnancy, childbirth, and the postpartum period.

TERMS RELATED TO THE REPRODUCTIVE SYSTEMS OF BOTH SEXES

The **genitalia** (**jen**-ih-**TAY**-lee-ah) are the organs of reproduction and their associated structures. *External genitalia* are reproductive organs located outside of the body cavity. *Internal genitalia* are reproductive organs protected within the body.

The **perineum** (pehr-ih-**NEE**-um) is the external surface region in both males and females between the pubic symphysis and the coccyx.

- The *male perineum* extends from the scrotum to the anus.
- The *female perineum* extends from the vaginal orifice to the anus (see Figure 14.6).

FUNCTIONS OF THE MALE REPRODUCTIVE SYSTEM

- The primary function of the male reproductive system is to produce millions of sperm and deliver them into the female body where one sperm can unite with a single ovum (egg) to create a new life. The structures of the male reproductive system that also function as part of the urinary system are discussed in Chapter 9.

STRUCTURES OF THE MALE REPRODUCTIVE SYSTEM

- The *external male genitalia* are the penis and the scrotum, which contains two testicles.
- The *internal male genitalia* includes the remaining structures of the male reproductive system (Figures 14.1 and 14.2).

The Scrotum and Testicles

The **scrotum** (**SKROH**-tum) is the saclike structure that surrounds, protects, and supports the testicles. This scrotum is suspended from the pubic arch behind the penis and lies between the thighs.

The **testicles**, also known as *testes*, are the two small, egg-shaped glands that produce the sperm (singular, *testis*). These glands develop within the abdomen of the male fetus and normally descend into the scrotum before, or soon after, birth.

- Sperm are formed within the **seminiferous tubules** (**see**-mih-**NIF**-er-us **TOO-byouls**) of each testicle (see Figure 14.2).
- The **epididymis** (**ep**-ih-**DID**-ih-mis) is a coiled tube at the upper part of each testicle. This tube runs down the length of the testicle then turns upward toward the body. Here, it narrows to form the tube known as the *vas deferens.*
- The **spermatic cord** extends upward from the epididymis and is attached to each testicle. Each cord contains a vas deferens plus the arteries, veins, nerves, and lymphatic vessels required by each testicle.

The Penis

The **penis** (**PEE**-nis) is the male sex organ that transports the sperm into the female vagina. The penis is composed of three columns of erectile tissue (see Figures 14.1 and 14.2).

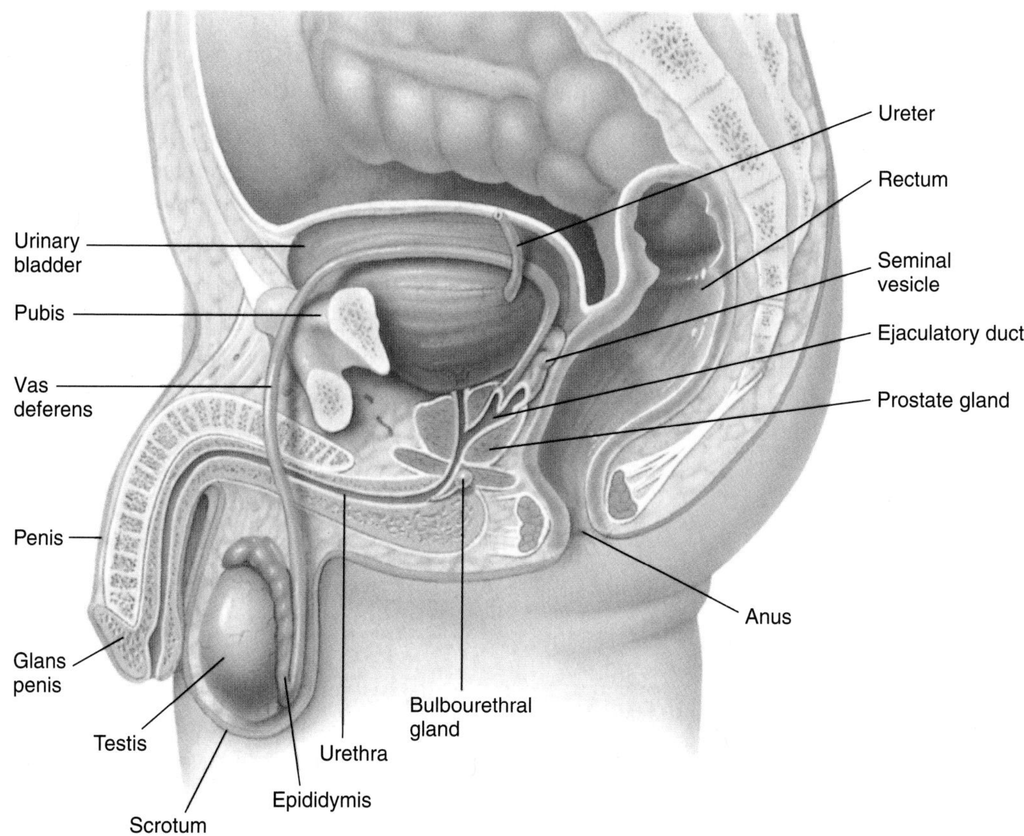

FIGURE 14.1 Organs and ducts of the male reproductive system shown in a lateral cross-section.

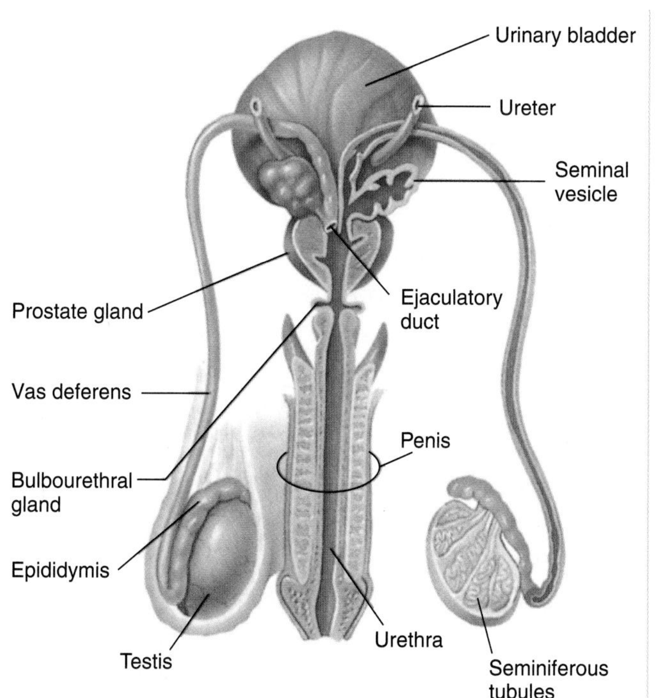

FIGURE 14.2 Structures of the male reproductive system as shown in an anterior cross-section view.

- During sexual stimulation, the erectile tissue fills with blood under high pressure. This causes the swelling, hardness, and stiffness known an *erection*.
- The adjectives *penile* and *phallic* both mean relating to the penis (both **pen/i** and **phall/i** mean penis).
- The **glans penis** (glanz **PEE**-nis), also known as the *head of the penis*, is the sensitive region located at the tip of the penis (see Figure 14.1).
- The **foreskin,** also known as the *prepuce*, is a retractable double-layered fold of skin and mucous membrane that covers and protects the glans penis.

The Vas Deferens, Seminal Vesicles, and the Ejaculatory Duct

- The **vas deferens** (vas **DEF**-er-enz), also known as the *ductus deferens*, are the long, narrow continuations of each epididymis. These structures lead upward, eventually join the urethra (see Figures 14.1 and 14.2).
- The **seminal vesicles** (**SEM**-ih-nal) are glands that secrete a thick, yellow substance to nourish the sperm

cells. This secretion forms 60% of the volume of semen. These glands are located at the base of the urinary bladder and open into the vas deferens as it joins the urethra.

- The **ejaculatory duct**, which begins at the vas deferens, passes through the prostate gland, and empties into the urethra. During ejaculation, a reflex action caused by these ducts, semen passes into the urethra, which exits the body via the penis.
- **Semen** (**SEE**-men) is the whitish fluid containing sperm that is ejaculated through the urethra at the peak of male sexual excitement. The term *ejaculate* means to expel suddenly.

The Prostate Gland

The **prostate gland** (**PROS**-tayt) lies under the bladder and surrounds the end of the urethra in the region where the vas deferens enters the urethra (see Figures 14.1 and 14.2).

During ejaculation, the prostate gland secretes a thick, alkaline fluid into the semen that aids the motility of the sperm. *Motility* means ability to move. Disorders and treatment of the prostate gland are discussed in Chapter 9.

The Bulbourethral Glands

The two **bulbourethral glands** (**bul**-boh-you-**REE**-thral), also known as *Cowper's glands*, are located just below the prostate gland. One of these glands is located on either side of the urethra, and they open into the urethra (see Figures 14.1 and 14.2).

During sexual arousal, these glands secrete a fluid known as *pre-ejaculate*. This fluid helps flush out any residual urine or foreign matter in the urethra. It also lubricates the urethra for sperm to pass through. This fluid can contain sperm and is able to cause pregnancy even if ejaculation does not occur.

The Urethra

The **urethra** passes through the penis to the outside of the body. In the male, the urethra serves both the reproductive and the urinary systems. Disorders of the urethra are discussed in Chapter 9.

Semen Formation

- **Spermatogenesis** (**sper**-mah-toh-**JEN**-eh-sis) is the process of sperm formation (**spermat/o** means sperm, and **-genesis** means creation).
- The ideal temperature for sperm formation is 93.2°F. The scrotum aids in maintaining this temperature by adjusting how closely it holds the testicles to the body.
- **Sperm** are the male gametes (reproductive cells). Also known as *spermatozoa*, these gametes are formed in the seminiferous tubules of the testicles.
- From here, the sperm move into the epididymis where they become motile and are temporarily stored. *Motile* means capable of spontaneous motion.
- From the epididymis, the sperm travel upward into the body and enter the vas deferens. Here, the seminal vesicles and the prostate gland add their secretions to form semen.

MEDICAL SPECIALTIES RELATED TO THE MALE REPRODUCTIVE SYSTEM

A **urologist** (you-**ROL**-oh-jist) is a physician who specializes in diagnosing and treating diseases and disorders of the urinary system of females and the genitourinary system of males (**ur** means urine, and **-ologist** means specialist). The term *genitourinary* refers to both the genital and urinary organs.

PATHOLOGY OF THE MALE REPRODUCTIVE SYSTEM

The Penis

- **Balanitis** (**bal**-ah-**NIGH**-tis) is an inflammation of the glans penis that is usually caused by poor hygiene in men who have not had the foreskin removed by circumcision (**balan** means glans penis, and **-itis** means inflammation).
- **Phimosis** (figh-**MOH**-sis) is a narrowing of the opening of the foreskin so it cannot be retracted (pulled back) to expose the glans penis. This condition can be present at birth or become apparent during childhood.
- **Impotence** (**IM**-poh-tens), also known as *erectile dysfunction*, is the inability of the male to achieve or maintain a penile erection. A penis that is not erect is referred to as being *flaccid* (limp).
- **Peyronie's disease** (pay-roh-**NEEZ**), also known as *penile curvature*, is a form of sexual dysfunction in which the penis is bent or curved during erection.
- **Premature ejaculation** is a condition in which the male reaches climax too soon, usually before, or shortly after, penetration of the female.

The Testicles and Related Structures

- **Andropause** (**AN**-droh-pawz), which is often referred to as *male menopause*, is marked by the decrease of the male hormone testosterone (**andr/o** means male or masculine, and **-pause** means stopping). This change is also referred to as *ADAM* (***A****ndrogen* ***D****ecline in the* ***A****ging* ***M****ale*). It usually begins in the late 40s and progresses very gradually over several decades.
- **Anorchism** (an-**OR**-kizm) is the absence of one or both testicles (**an-** means without, **orch** means testicle, and **-ism** means abnormal condition). This condition can be congenital or caused by trauma or surgery (Figure 14.3A).
- **Cryptorchidism** (krip-**TOR**-kih-dizm), also known as an *undescended testicle*, is a developmental defect in which one or both of the testicles fail to descend into their normal position in the scrotum (**crypt/o** means hidden, **orchid** means testicle, and **-ism** means abnormal condition).
- **Epididymitis** (**ep**-ih-did-ih-**MY**-tis) is inflammation of the epididymis that is frequently caused by the spread of infection from the urethra or the bladder (**epididym** means epididymis, and **-itis** means inflammation) (Figure 14.3B).
- A **hydrocele** (**HIGH**-droh-seel) is a fluid-filled sac in the scrotum along the spermatic cord leading from the testicles (**hydr/o** means relating to water, and **-cele** means a hernia or swelling). Note: The term *hydrocele* is also used to describe the accumulation of fluid in any body cavity.
- **Priapism** (**PRYE**-ah-**piz**-em) is a painful erection that lasts 4 hours or more but is not accompanied by sexual excitement. The condition can be caused by

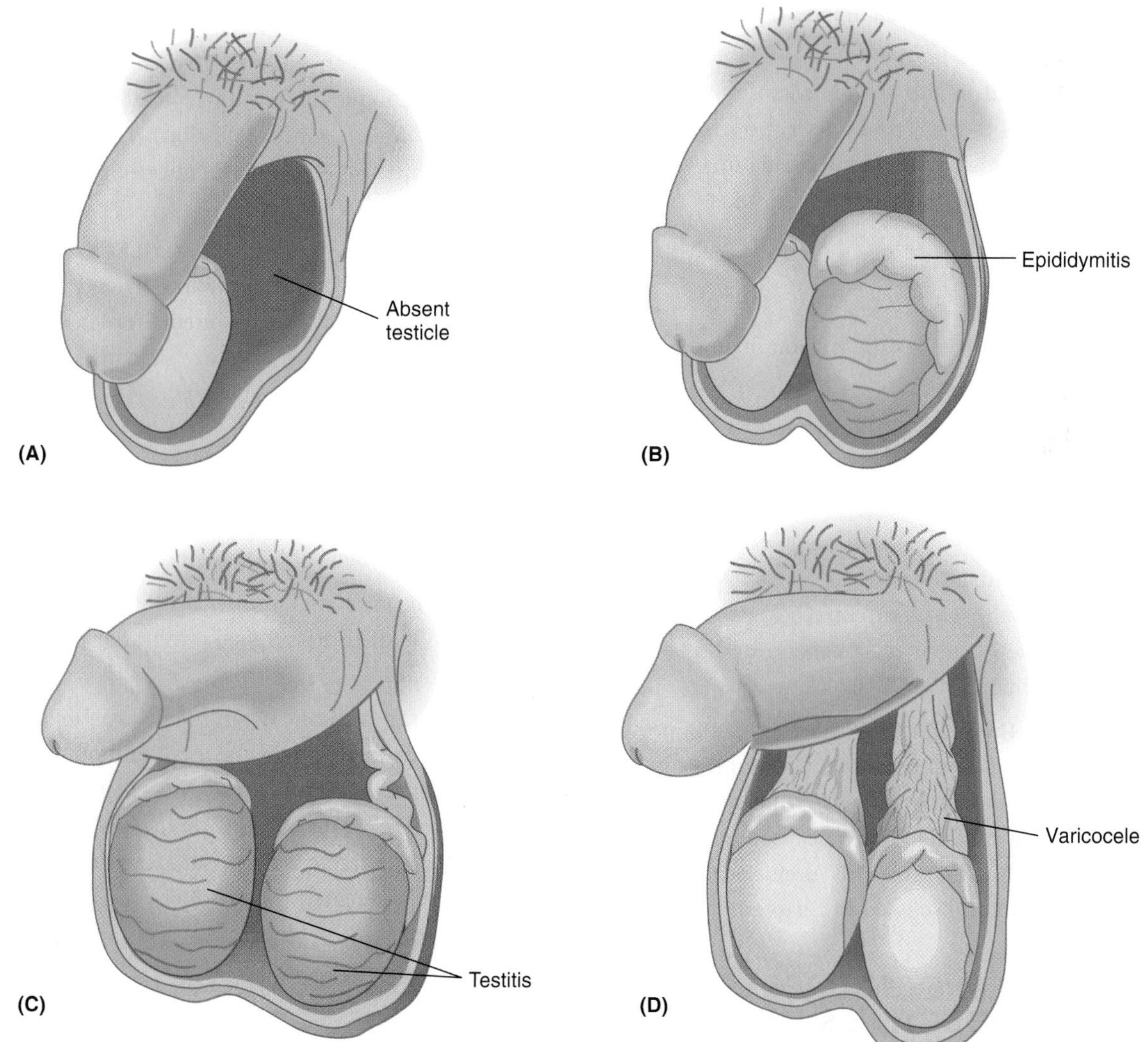

FIGURE 14.3 Pathology of the testicles. (A) Anorchism in which one testicle is absent. (B) Epididymitis of the left testicle. (C) Testitis of both testicles. (D) A varicocele affecting the left testicle.

medications or by blood-related diseases such as sickle cell anemia or leukemia.

- A **spermatocele** (sper-**MAH**-toh-seel) is a cyst that develops in the epididymis and is filled with a milky fluid containing sperm (**spermat/o** means sperm, and **-cele** means hernia, tumor, or swelling).
- **Testicular cancer** is the most common cancer in American males between the ages of 15 and 34 years. This cancer is highly treatable when diagnosed early.
- **Testicular pain**, also known as *orchalgia*, is pain in one or both testicles. This pain can be due to an injury, testicular torsion, epididymitis, or a spermatocele.
- **Testicular torsion** is a sharp pain in the scrotum caused by twisting of the vas deferens and blood vessels leading into the testicle. *Torsion* means twisting.
- **Testitis** (test-**TYE**-tis), also known as *orchitis*, is inflammation of one or both testicles (**test** means testicle, and **-itis** means inflammation) (Figure 14.3C).
- A **varicocele** (**VAR**-ih-koh-**seel**) is a knot of varicose veins in one side of the scrotum (**varic/o** means varicose veins, and **-cele** means a hernia or swelling). *Varicose veins* are abnormally swollen veins (Figure 14.3D).

Sperm Count

A **normal sperm count** is 20–120 million or more sperm per milliliter (ml) of semen.

- **Azoospermia** (ay-**zoh**-oh-**SPER**-mee-ah) is the absence of sperm in the semen (**a-** means without, **zoo** means life, **sperm** means sperm, and **-ia** means abnormal condition).
- A **low sperm count**, also known as *oligospermia* (**ol**-ih-goh-**SPER**-mee-ah), is a sperm count below 20 million/ml (**olig/o** means few, **sperm** means sperm, and **-ia** means abnormal condition).
- **Hemospermia** (**hee**-moh-**SPER**-mee-ah) is the presence of blood in the seminal fluid (**hem/o** means blood, **sperm** means sperm, and **-ia** means abnormal condition). This condition can be caused by infections of the seminal vesicles, prostatitis, urethritis, or urethral strictures which are discussed in Chapter 9.

DIAGNOSTIC PROCEDURES OF THE MALE REPRODUCTIVE SYSTEM

- **Sperm count**, also known as a *sperm analysis*, is the testing of freshly ejaculated semen to determine the volume plus the number, shape, size, and motility of the sperm.
- **Testicular self-examination** is a self-help step in early detection of testicular cancer by detecting lumps, swelling, or changes in the skin of the scrotum.

TREATMENT PROCEDURES OF THE MALE REPRODUCTIVE SYSTEM

General Treatment Procedures

- **Circumcision** (**ser**-kum-**SIZH**-un) is the surgical removal of the foreskin of the penis. This procedure is usually performed within a few days of birth.
- An **orchidectomy** (**or**-kih-**DECK**-toh-mee), also spelled as *orchiectomy*, is the surgical removal of one or both testicles (**orchid** means testicle, and **-ectomy** means surgical removal).
- **Orchiopexy** (**or**-kee-oh-**PECK**-see) is endoscopic surgery to move an undescended testicle into its normal position in the scrotum (**orchi/o** means testicle, and **-pexy** means surgical fixation). This procedure is usually performed on infants before the age of 1 year.
- A **varicocelectomy** (**var**-ih-koh-sih-**LECK**-toh-mee) is the removal of a portion of an enlarged vein to relieve a varicocele (**varic/o** means varicose vein, **cel** means swelling, and **-ectomy** means surgical removal).

Male Sterilization

Sterilization is any procedure rendering an individual (male or female) incapable of reproduction.

- **Castration** (kas-**TRAY**-shun), also known as *bilateral orchidectomy*, is the surgical removal or destruction of both testicles.
- A **vasectomy** (vah-**SECK**-toh-mee) is the male sterilization procedure in which a small portion of the vas deferens is surgically removed (**vas** means vas deferens, and **-ectomy** means surgical removal). This prevents sperm from entering the ejaculate, but does not change the volume of semen (Figure 14.4).
- A **vasovasostomy** (**vay**-soh-vah-**ZOS**-toh-mee), also known as a *vasectomy reversal*, is a procedure performed as an attempt to restore fertility to a vasectomized male (**vas/o** means blood vessel, **vas** means the vas deferens, and **-ostomy** means surgically creating an opening).

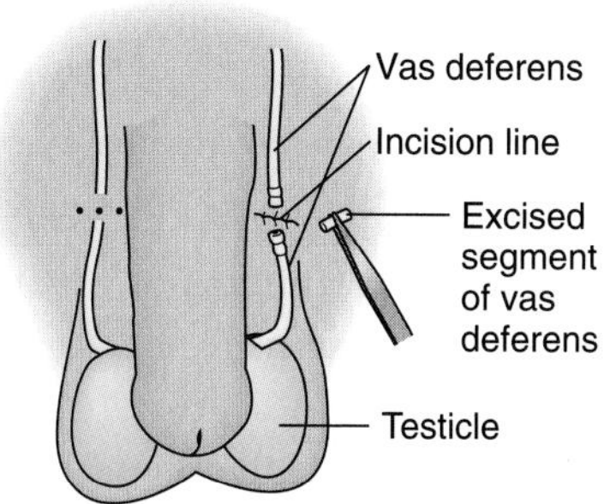

FIGURE 14.4 In a vasectomy, a portion of the vas deferens is removed to prevent sperm from entering the semen.

SEXUALLY TRANSMITTED DISEASES

Sexually transmitted diseases (STDs), also known as *venereal diseases* (VD), are infections that affect both males and females. These conditions are commonly spread through sexual intercourse or other genital contact.

- A pregnant woman who is infected with one of these diseases can transmit it to her baby during birth. For this reason, all newborns receive one drop of silver nitrate or an antibiotic ointment in each eye immediately after birth to prevent *ophthalmia neonatorum*. This condition is a form of conjunctivitis that is caused by the bacteria responsible for chlamydia or gonorrhea.

Chlamydia

Chlamydia (klah-**MID**-ee-ah), which is caused by the bacterium *Chlamydia trachomatis*, is the most commonly reported STD in the US. It is highly contagious and requires early treatment with antibiotics.

- In females, chlamydia can damage the reproductive organs. Even though symptoms are usually mild or absent, serious complications can cause irreversible damage, including infertility.
- In males, chlamydia is one of the causes of urethritis (see Chapter 9).

Other Sexually Transmitted Diseases

- **Bacterial vaginosis** (**vaj**-ih-**NOH**-sis) is a condition in women in which there is an abnormal overgrowth of certain bacteria in the vagina (**vagin** means vagina, and **-osis** means abnormal condition or disease). This condition can cause complications during pregnancy and an increased risk of HIV infection. Symptoms sometimes include a discharge, odor, pain, itching, or burning.
- **Genital herpes** (**HER**-peez) is caused by the herpes simplex virus type 2. Symptoms include itching or burning before the appearance of lesions (sores). This condition is highly contagious at all times, including when visible lesions are not present. Antiviral drugs ease symptoms and can suppress future outbreaks; however, currently there is no cure. Note: The herpes simplex virus type 1, which causes cold sores, is discussed in Chapter 8.
- **Genital warts**, which are caused by the *human papilloma virus* (HPV), are highly contagious. In the male, this virus infects the urethra. In the female, it infects the external genitalia, cervix, and vagina. It also increases the risk of cervical cancer.
- A **human papilloma virus** vaccine is available to prevent the spread of this disease. It is recommended that it be administered to girls between the ages 11 and 12 or before they become sexually active.
- **Gonorrhea** (**gon**-oh-**REE**-ah) is a highly contagious condition caused by the bacterium *Neisseria gonorrhoeae*. In women, this condition affects the cervix, uterus, and fallopian tubes. In men, it affects the urethra by causing painful urination and an abnormal discharge. It can also affect the mouth, throat, and anus of both men and women.
- The **human immunodeficiency virus** (HIV) is transmitted through exposure to infected body fluids, particularly through sexual intercourse with an infected partner. HIV and AIDS are discussed in Chapter 6.
- **Syphilis** (**SIF**-ih-lis), which is caused by the bacterium *Treponema pallidum*, has many symptoms that are difficult to distinguish from other STDs. Syphilis is highly contagious and is passed from person to person through direct contact with a *chancre*, which is a sore caused by syphilis. This condition can be detected through the VDRL (**V**enereal **D**isease **R**esearch **L**aboratory) blood test before the lesions appear. The RPR test (**R**apid **p**lasma **r**eagin) is another blood test for syphilis.
- **Trichomoniasis** (**trick**-oh-moh-**NYE**-ah-sis), also known as *trich*, is an infection caused by the protozoan parasite *Trichomonas vaginalis*. One of the most common symptoms in infected women is a thin, frothy, yellow-green, foul-smelling vaginal discharge. Infected men often do not have symptoms; however, when symptoms are present, they include painful urination or a clear discharge from the penis.

FUNCTIONS OF THE FEMALE REPRODUCTIVE SYSTEM

The primary function of the female reproductive system is the creation and support of new life.

- The ovaries produce mature eggs to be fertilized by the sperm.
- The uterus provides the environment and support for the developing child.
- After birth, the breasts produce milk to feed the child.

STRUCTURES OF THE FEMALE REPRODUCTIVE SYSTEM

The structures of the female reproductive system are described as being the external female genitalia and the internal female reproductive organs (Figure 14.5).

The External Female Genitalia

The external female genitalia are located posterior to the **mons pubis** (monz **PYOU**-bis), which is a rounded, fleshy prominence located over the pubic symphysis (Figure 14.6). These structures are known collectively as the **vulva** (**VUL**-vah) or the *pudendum*. The vulva consists of the labia, clitoris, Bartholin's glands, and vaginal orifice.

- The **labia majora** and **labia minora** are the vaginal lips that protect the other external genitalia and the urethral meatus (singular, *labium*). The *urethral meatus*, which is the external opening of the urethra, is discussed in Chapter 9.
- The **clitoris** (**KLIT**-oh-ris) is an organ of sensitive, erectile tissue located anterior to the urethral meatus and the vaginal orifice.
- **Bartholin's glands** produce a mucus secretion to lubricate the vagina. These two small, round glands are located on either side of the vaginal orifice.
- The **vaginal orifice** is the exterior opening of the vagina. *Orifice* means opening. The **hymen** (**HIGH**-men) is a mucous membrane that partially covers this opening before a woman has had intercourse. However, this tissue can be absent in a woman who has not been sexually active.

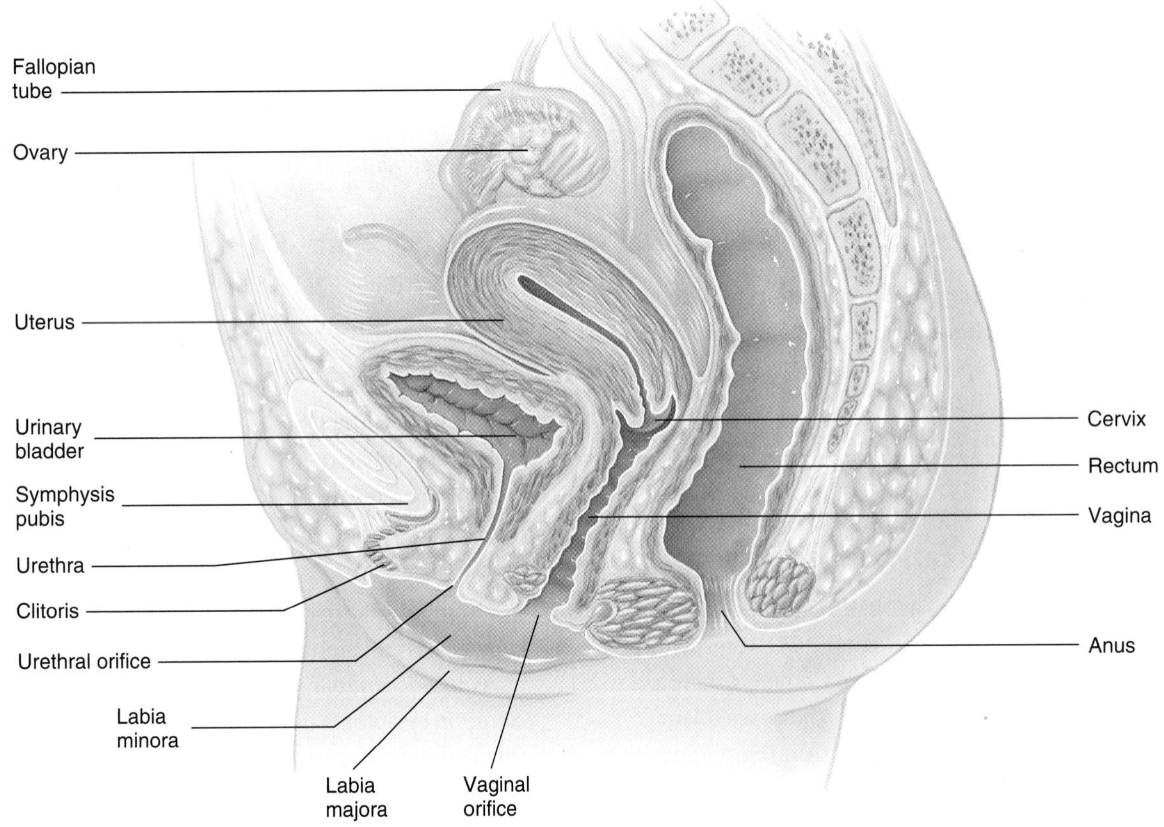

FIGURE 14.5 Structures of the female reproductive system shown in a lateral cross-section.

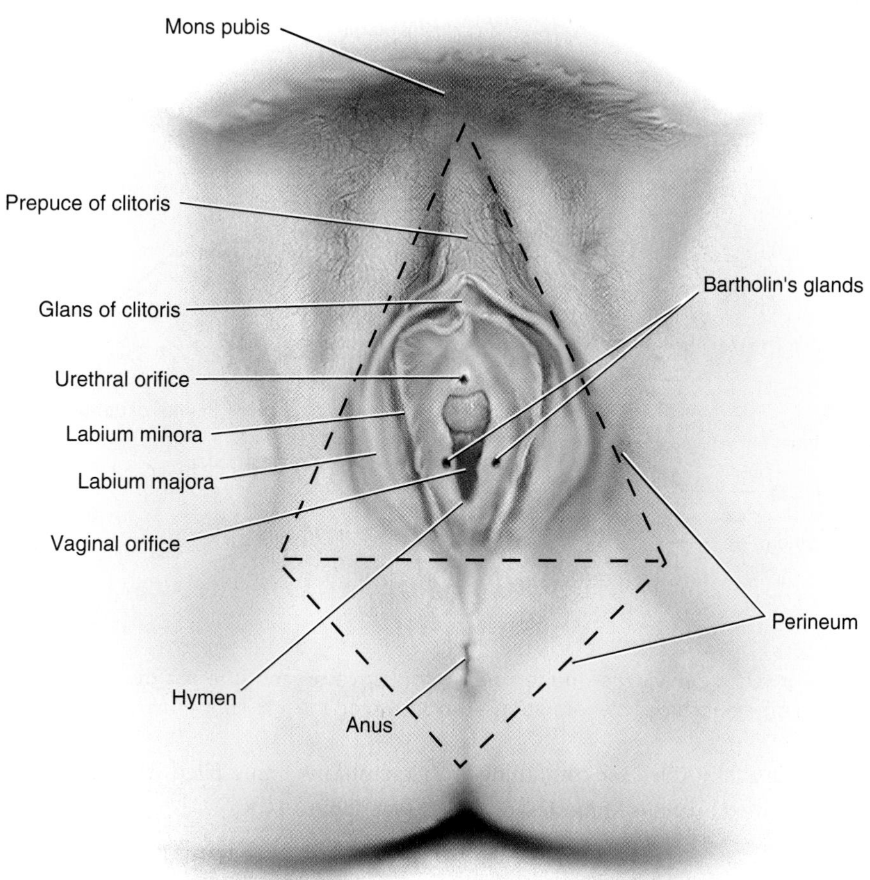

FIGURE 14.6 Female external genitalia.

The Mammary Glands

Breasts are made up of fat, connective tissue, and the mammary glands (the word parts **mamm/o** and **mast/o** both mean breast). Each breast is fixed to the overlying skin and the underlying pectoral muscles by suspensory ligaments (Figure 14.7). Breast cancer, its diagnosis and treatment, are discussed in Chapter 6.

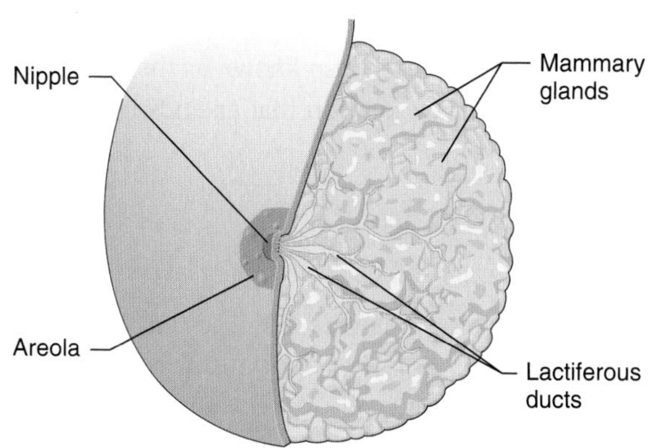

FIGURE 14.7 Structures of the breast.

- **Mammary glands**, also known as the *lactiferous glands*, are the milk-producing glands that develop during puberty.
- The **lactiferous ducts** (lack-**TIF**-er-us), also known as *milk ducts*, carry milk from the mammary glands to the nipple (**lact** means milk, and **-iferous** means carrying or producing).
- Breast milk flows through the **nipple**, which is surrounded by the dark-pigmented area known as the **areola** (ah-**REE**-oh-lah).

The Internal Female Genitalia

The internal female genitalia are located within the pelvic cavity where they are protected by the bony pelvis. These structures include two ovaries, two fallopian tubes, one uterus, and the vagina (see Figures 14.5 and 14.8).

The Ovaries

The **ovaries** (**OH**-vah-rees) are a pair of small, almond-shaped organs located in the lower abdomen, one on either side of the uterus.

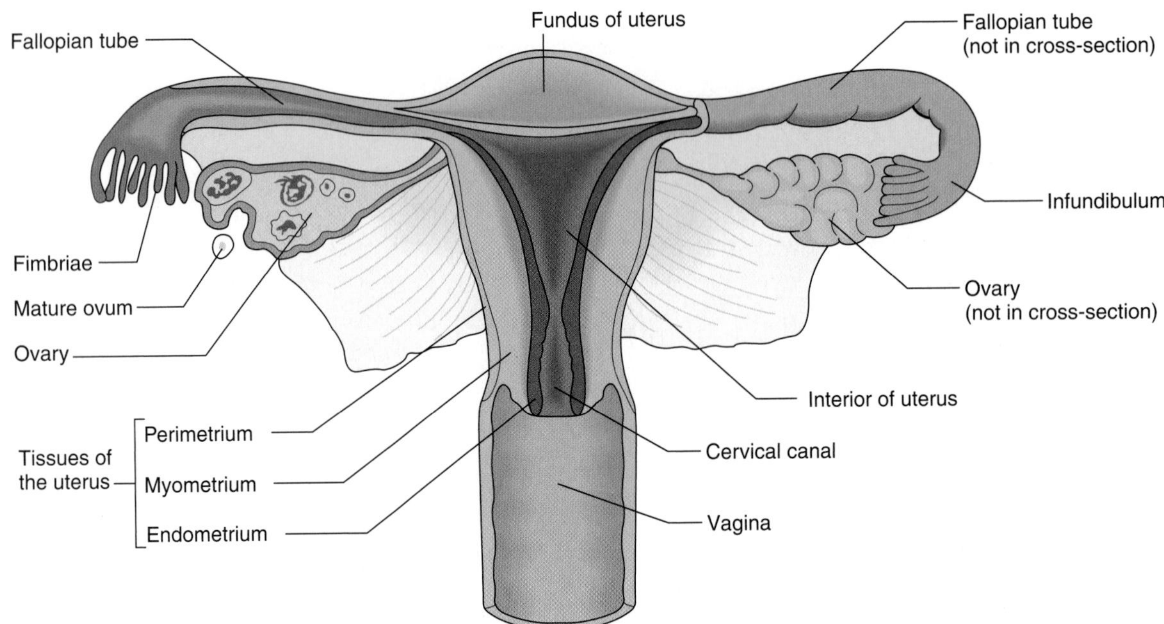

FIGURE 14.8 An anterior schematic view of the female reproductive organs. The left ovary, shown in cross-section, contains developing ova in different stages of maturation. Also shown on the left is a mature ovum that has just been released.

- A **follicle** (**FOL**-lick-kul) is a fluid-filled sac containing a single ovum (egg). There are thousands of these sacs on the inside surface of the ovaries.
- The **ova** (**OH**-vah), also known as *eggs*, are the female gametes (singular, *ovum*). These immature ova are present at birth. Normally, after puberty, one ovum matures and is released each month.
- The ovaries also produce the sex hormones estrogen and progesterone, which are discussed in Chapter 13.

The Fallopian Tubes

There are two **fallopian tubes** (fal-**LOH**-pee-an), which are also known as *uterine tubes*. These tubes extend from the upper end of the uterus to a point near, but not attached to, an ovary.

- The **infundibulum** (**in**-fun-**DIB**-you-lum) is the funnel-shaped opening into the fallopian tube near the ovary.
- The **fimbriae** (**FIM**-bree-ee) are the fringed, finger-like extensions of this opening. Their role is to catch the mature ovum when it leaves the ovary (singular, *fimbria*).
- Each month, one of these tubes carries a mature ovum from the ovary to the uterus (see Figure 14.8). These tubes also carry sperm upward from the uterus toward the descending mature ovum so that fertilization can occur.

The Uterus

The **uterus** (**YOU**-ter-us), formerly known as the *womb*, is a pear-shaped organ with muscular walls and a mucous membrane lining filled with a rich supply of blood vessels (see Figure 14.8).

- The uterus is located between the urinary bladder and the rectum and midway between the sacrum and the pubic bone.
- In its normal position, which is known as **anteflexion** (**an**-tee-**FLECK**-shun), the body of the uterus is bent forward (**ante-** means forward, **flex** means bend, and **-ion** means condition) (see Figure 14.5).

The Parts of the Uterus

The body of the uterus consists of three major anatomic areas.

- The **fundus** (**FUN**-dus) is the bulging, rounded part above the entrance of the fallopian tubes.
- The **corpus** (**KOR**-pus), also known as the *body of the uterus*, is the middle portion.
- The **cervix** (**SER**-vicks), also known as the *cervix uteri*, is the lower, narrow portion that extends into the vagina.

The Tissues of the Uterus

The uterus is composed of three major layers of tissue.

- The **perimetrium** (pehr-ih-**MEE**-tree-um) is the tough, membranous outer layer (**peri-** means surrounding, **metri** means uterus, and **-um** is a singular noun ending). *Membranous* means pertaining to a thin layer of tissue.

- The **myometrium** (my-oh-**MEE**-tree-um) is the muscular middle layer (**my/o** means muscle, **metri** means uterus, and **-um** is a singular noun ending).
- The **endometrium** (en-doh-**MEE**-tree-um), which is the inner layer of the uterus, consists of specialized epithelial mucosa that is rich in blood vessels (**endo-** means within, **metri** means uterus, and **-um** is a singular noun ending). *Mucosa* means referring to mucous membrane.

Vagina

The **vagina** (vah-**JIGH**-nah) is the muscular tube lined with mucosa that extends from the cervix to the outside of the body. The word parts **colp/o** and **vagin/o** both mean vagina (see Figures 14.7 and 14.8).

Menstruation

Menstruation (**men**-stroo-**AY**-shun), also known as *menses*, is the normal periodic discharge of the endometrial lining and unfertilized egg from uterus.

- **Menarche** (meh-**NAR**-kee) is the beginning of the menstrual function (**men** means menstruation, and **-arche** means beginning). This function begins after the maturation that occurs during puberty.
- The average *menstrual cycle* consists of 28 days. These days are grouped into four phases and are summarized in Table 14.1.
- **Menopause** (**MEN**-oh-pawz) is the normal termination of the menstrual function (**men/o** means menstruation and **-pause** means stopping). Menopause is considered to be confirmed when a woman has gone 1 year without having a period.
- **Perimenopause** (pehr-ih-**MEN**-oh-pawz) is the term used to designate the transition phase between regular menstrual periods and no periods at all (**peri-** means surrounding, **men/o** means menstruation, and **-pause** means stopping). During this phase, which can last as long as 10 years, changes in hormone production can cause symptoms including irregular menstrual cycles, hot flashes, mood swings, and disturbed sleep.

MEDICAL SPECIALTIES RELATED TO THE FEMALE REPRODUCTIVE SYSTEM AND CHILDBIRTH

- A **gynecologist** (**guy**-neh-**KOL**-oh-jist) is a physician who specializes in diagnosing and treating diseases and disorders of the female reproductive system (**gynec** means female, and **-ologist** means specialist).
- An **obstetrician** (**ob**-steh-**TRISH**-un) is a physician who specializes in providing medical care to women during pregnancy, childbirth, and immediately thereafter. This specialty is referred to as *obstetrics*.

TABLE 14.1

Phases of the Menstrual Cycle

Approximately Days 1–5	*Menstrual phase*. These are the days when the endometrial lining of the uterus is sloughed off and discharged through the vagina as the menstrual flow.
Approximately Days 6–12	*Postmenstrual phase*. After the menstrual period, the pituitary gland secretes follicle-stimulating hormone (FSH), causing an ovum to mature. Estrogen, which is secreted by the ovaries, stimulates the lining of the uterus to prepare itself to receive a zygote (fertilized egg).
Approximately Days 13–14	*Ovulatory phase*. On, or about, the 13th or 14th day of the cycle ovulation occurs. Ovulation is the release of a mature ovum. The mature egg leaves the ovary and travels slowly down the fallopian tube toward the uterus. During this time, the female is fertile and can become pregnant.
Approximately Days 15–28	*Premenstrual phase*. If fertilization does not occur, hormone levels change to cause the breakdown of the uterine endometrium and the beginning of a new menstrual cycle.

- A **neonatologist** (**nee**-oh-nay-**TOL**-oh-jist) is a physician who in diagnosing and treating disorders of the newborn (**neo-** means new, **nat** means born, and **-ologist** means specialist).
- A **pediatrician** (**pee**-dee-ah-**TRISH**-un) is a physician who specializes in diagnosing, treating, and preventing disorders and diseases of children. This specialty is known as *pediatrics*.

PATHOLOGY OF THE FEMALE REPRODUCTIVE SYSTEM

The Ovaries, Fallopian Tubes, and Ovulation

- **Anovulation** (**an**-ov-you-**LAY**-shun) is the absence of ovulation when it would be normally expected (**an-** means without, and **ovulation** means the release of a mature egg). This condition can be caused by stress, inadequate nutrition, or hormonal imbalances. Menstruation can continue, although ovulation does not occur.
- **Oophoritis** (**oh**-ahf-oh-**RYE**-tis) is inflammation of an ovary (**oophor** means ovary, and **-itis** means inflammation). This condition frequently occurs when salpingitis or pelvic inflammatory disease are present.
- **Ovarian cancer** originates within the cells of the ovaries. These cancer cells can break away from the ovary and spread (metastasize) to other tissues and organs within the abdomen or travel through the blood stream to other parts of the body.
- **Ovariorrhexis** (oh-**vay**-ree-oh-**RECK**-sis) is the rupture of an ovary (**ovari/o** means ovary, and **-rrhexis** means to rupture).
- **Pelvic inflammatory disease** (PID) is any inflammation of the female reproductive organs that is not associated with surgery or pregnancy. This condition occurs most frequently as a complication of a sexually transmitted disease and can lead to infertility, ectopic pregnancy, and other serious disorders.
- **Polycystic ovary syndrome** (**pol**-ee-**SIS**-tick), also known as *Stein-Leventhal syndrome*, is a condition caused by a hormonal imbalance in which the ovaries are enlarged by the presence of many cysts formed by incompletely developed follicles.
- **Pyosalpinx** (**pye**-oh-**SAL**-pinks) is an accumulation of pus in the fallopian tube (**py/o** means pus, and **-salpinx** means fallopian tube).
- **Salpingitis** (**sal**-pin-**JIGH**-tis) is an inflammation of a fallopian tube (**salping** means fallopian or eustachian tube, and **-itis** means inflammation).

The Uterus

- **Endometriosis** (**en**-doh-**mee**-tree-**OH**-sis) is a condition in which patches of endometrial tissue escape the uterus and become attached to other structures in the pelvic cavity (**endo-** means within, **metri** means uterus, and **-osis** means abnormal condition). It is a leading cause of infertility.
- **Metrorrhea** (**mee**-troh-**REE**-ah) is an abnormal discharge, such as mucus or pus, from the uterus (**metr/o** means uterus, and **-rrhea** means flow or discharge).
- **Uterine cancer** involves cancerous growth on the lining of the uterus. One of the earliest symptoms of this cancer that frequently occurs after menopause is abnormal bleeding from the uterus.
- A **uterine fibroid**, also known as a *myoma*, is a benign tumor composed of muscle and fibrous tissue that occurs in the wall of the uterus.
- A **uterine prolapse** (proh-**LAPS**), also known as a *pelvic floor hernia*, is the condition in which the uterus slides from its normal position in the pelvic cavity and sags into the vagina (see Figure 14.9). *Prolapse* means the falling or dropping down of an organ or internal part.

The Cervix

- **Cervical cancer** is the second-most common cancer in women and usually affects women between the ages of 45 and 65 years. It can be detected early through routine Pap tests.
- **Cervical dysplasia** (**SER**-vih-kal dis-**PLAY**-see-ah), also known as *precancerous lesions*, is the growth of abnormal cells in the cervix, which can be detected by a

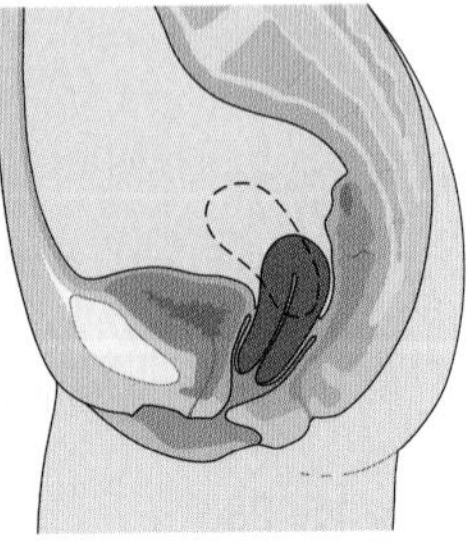

FIGURE 14.9 Uterine prolapse.

Pap smear. Without early detection and treatment, these cells can become malignant.

- **Cervicitis** (**ser**-vih-**SIGH**-tis) is an inflammation of the cervix that is usually caused by an infection (**cervic** means cervix, and **-itis** means inflammation).
- **Endocervicitis** (**en**-doh-**ser**-vih-**SIGH**-tis) is an inflammation of the mucous membrane lining of the cervix (**endo-** means within, **cervic** means cervix, and **-itis** means inflammation).

The Vagina

- **Colporrhexis** (**kol**-poh-**RECK**-sis) means tearing or laceration of the vaginal wall (**colp/o** means vagina, and **-rrhexis** means to rupture). A *laceration* is a torn, ragged wound or an accidental cut.
- **Leukorrhea** (**loo**-koh-**REE**-ah) is a profuse, whitish mucus discharge from the uterus and vagina (**leuk/o** means white, and **-rrhea** means flow or discharge). Women normally have a vaginal discharge; however, leukorrhea describes a change and increase in this discharge that can be due to an infection, malignancy, or hormonal changes.
- **Vaginal candidiasis** (**kan**-dih-**DYE**-ah-sis), also known as *vaginal thrush* or a *yeast infection*, is a vaginal infection caused by the yeast-like fungus *Candida albicans*. The growth of this fungus in the vagina is usually controlled by the bacteria normally present there. When these bacteria are not able to control the fungal growth, symptoms occur that include burning, itching, and a "cottage cheese-like" vaginal discharge.
- **Vaginitis** (**vaj**-ih-**NIGH**-tis), also known as *colpitis*, is an inflammation of the lining of the vagina (**vagin** and **colp** both mean vagina, and **-itis** means inflammation). The most common causes of a vaginal inflammation are bacterial vaginosis, trichomoniasis, and vaginal candidiasis.

The External Genitalia

- **Pruritus vulvae** (proo-**RYE**-tus **VUL**-vee) is a condition of severe itching of the external female genitalia. *Pruritus* means itching.
- **Vulvodynia** (vul-voh-**DIN**-ee-ah) is a syndrome of unknown cause that is characterized by chronic burning, pain during sexual intercourse, itching, or stinging irritation of the vulva (**vulv/o** means vulva, and **-dynia** means pain).
- **Vulvitis** (vul-**VYE**-tis) is an inflammation of the vulva (**vulv** means vulva, and **-itis** means inflammation). Possible causes include fungal or bacterial infections, chafing, skin conditions, or allergies to products such as soaps and bubble bath.

Breast Diseases

- **Breast cancer**, its diagnosis and treatment, are discussed in Chapter 6.
- A **fibroadenoma** (**figh**-broh-**ad**-eh-**NOH**-mah) is a round, firm, rubbery mass that arises from excess growth of glandular and connective tissue in the breast (see Figure 14.10). These masses, which can grow to the size of a small plum, are benign and usually painless. Fibroadenomas often enlarge during pregnancy and shrink during menopause.
- **Fibrocystic breast disease** (**figh**-broh-**SIS**-tick) is the presence of single or multiple benign cysts in the breasts. This condition occurs more frequently in older women. A *cyst* is a closed sac containing fluid or semisolid material.
- **Galactorrhea** (gah-**lack**-toh-**REE**-ah) is the production of breast milk in a woman who is not breastfeeding (**galact/o** means milk, and **-rrhea** means flow or discharge). This condition is caused by a malfunction of the thyroid or pituitary gland.
- **Mastalgia** (mass-**TAL**-jee-ah), also known as *mastodynia*, is pain in the breast (**mast** means breast, and **-algia** means pain).
- **Mastitis** (mas-**TYE**-tis) is a breast infection that is most frequently caused by bacteria that enter the breast tissue during breastfeeding (**mast** means breast, and **-itis** means inflammation).

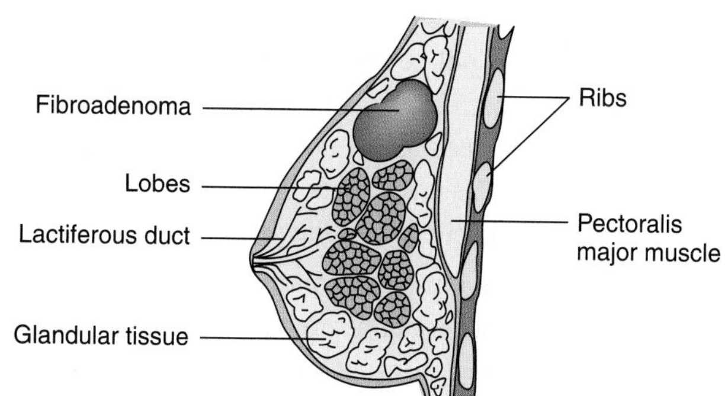

FIGURE 14.10 A fibroadenoma of the breast.

Menstrual Disorders

- **Amenorrhea** (ah-**men**-oh-**REE**-ah) is an abnormal absence of menstrual periods for 3 or more months (**a-** means without, **men/o** means menstruation, and **-rrhea** means flow or discharge). This condition is normal only before puberty, during pregnancy, while breastfeeding, and after menopause.
- **Dysmenorrhea** (**dis**-men-oh-**REE**-ah) is pain caused by uterine cramps during a menstrual period (**dys-** means bad, **men/o** means menstruation, and **-rrhea** means flow or discharge). This pain, which occurs in the lower abdomen, can be sharp, intermittent, dull, or aching.
- **Hypermenorrhea** (**high**-poh-men-oh-**REE**-ah), also known as *menorrhagia*, is an excessive amount of menstrual flow over a period of more than 7 days (**hyer-** means excessive, **men/o** means menstruation, and **-rrhea** means flow or discharge). Hypermenorrhea is the opposite of *hypomenorrhea.*
- **Hypomenorrhea** (**high**-poh-men-oh-**REE**-ah) is an unsually small amount of menstrual flow during a shortened regular menstrual period (**hypo-** means deficient, **men/o** means menstruation, and **-rrhea** means flow or discharge). Hypomenorrhea is the opposite of *hypermenorrhea.*
- **Menometrorrhagia** (**men**-oh-**met**-roh-**RAY**-jee-ah), also known as *intermenstrual bleeding*, is excessive uterine bleeding at both the usual time of menstrual periods and at other irregular intervals (**men/o** means menstruation, **metr/o** means uterus, and **-rrhagia** means abnormal bleeding).
- **Oligomenorrhea** (**ol**-ih-goh-**men**-oh-**REE**-ah) is the term used to describe infrequent or very light menstruation in a woman with previously normal periods (**olig/o** means scanty, **men/o** means menstruation, and **-rrhea** means flow or discharge). Oligomenorrhea is the opposite of *polymenorrhea.*
- **Polymenorrhea** (**pol**-ee-**men**-oh-**REE**-ah) is the occurrence of menstrual cycles more frequently than is normal (**poly-** means many, **men/o** means menstruation, and **-rrhea** means flow or discharge). Polymenorrhea is the opposite of *oligomenorrhea.*
- **Premature menopause** is a condition in which the ovaries cease functioning before age 40 years due to disease, a hormonal disorder, or surgical removal. This causes infertility and often bringing on menopausal symptoms.
- **Premenstrual syndrome** (PMS) is a group of symptoms experienced by some women within the 2-week period before menstruation. These symptoms can include bloating, swelling, headaches, mood swings, and breast discomfort.
- **Premenstrual dysphoric disorder** (PMDD) is a condition associated with severe emotional and physical problems that are closely linked to the menstrual cycle. Symptoms occur regularly in the second half of the cycle and end when menstruation begins or shortly thereafter.

DIAGNOSTIC PROCEDURES OF THE FEMALE REPRODUCTIVE SYSTEM

- **Colposcopy** (kol-**POS**-koh-pee) is the direct visual examination of the tissues of the cervix and vagina (**colp/o** means vagina, and **-scopy** means direct visual examination). This examination is performed using a binocular magnifier known as a *colposcope.*
- In an **endometrial biopsy**, a small amount of the tissue from the lining the uterus is removed for microscopic examination. This test is most often used to determine the cause of abnormal vaginal bleeding.
- **Endovaginal ultrasound** (**en**-doh-**VAJ**-ih-nal) is performed to determine the cause of abnormal vaginal bleeding. This test is performed by placing an ultrasound transducer in the vagina so that the sound waves can create images of the uterus and ovaries.
- **Hysterosalpingography** (**hiss**-ter-oh-**sal**-pin-**GOG**-rah-fee) is a radiographic examination of the uterus and fallopian tubes (**hyster/o** means uterus, **salping/o** means tube, and **-graphy** means the process of producing a picture or record). This test requires the instillation of radiopaque contrast material into the uterine cavity and fallopian tubes to make them visible. *Instillation* means slowly pouring a liquid onto a body part or into a body cavity.
- **Hysteroscopy** (**hiss**-ter-**OSS**-koh-pee) is the direct visual examination of the interior of the uterus and fallopian tubes (**hyster/o** means uterus, and **-scopy** means direct visual examination). This examination is performed by using the magnification of a *hysteroscope* (see Figure 15.19).
- A **Papanicolaou test** (**pap**-ah-**nick**-oh-**LAY**-ooh), also known as a *Pap smear*, is an exfoliative biopsy for the detection of conditions that can be early indicators of cervical cancer (Figure 14.11). As used here, *exfoliative*

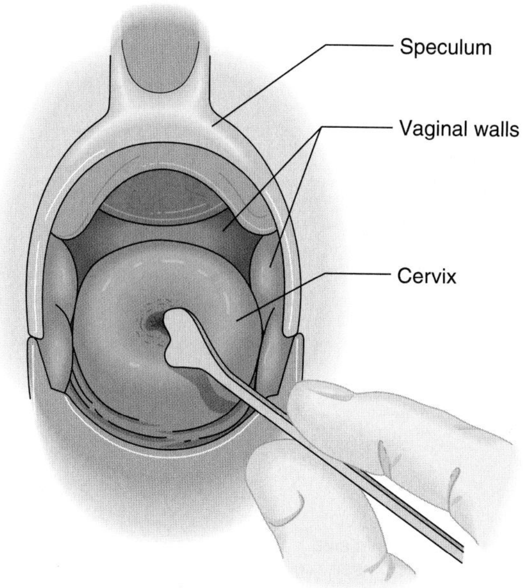

FIGURE 14.11 A Pap smear involves the removal of a few cervical cells for microscopic examination.

means that cells are scraped from the tissue and examined under a microscope.

- *Ultrasound* and *laparoscopy*, which are also used to diagnose disorders of the reproductive system, are discussed further in Chapter 15.

TREATMENT PROCEDURES OF THE FEMALE REPRODUCTIVE SYSTEM

Medications

- A **contraceptive** is a measure taken, or device used, to lessen the likelihood of conception and pregnancy. *Birth control pills* are a form of hormones that are administered as a contraceptive.
- An **intrauterine device** is a molded plastic contraceptive inserted through the cervix into the uterus (**intra-** means within, and **uterine** means uterus).
- **Hormone replacement therapy** is the use of the female hormones estrogen and progestin to replace those the body no longer produces during and after perimenopause. *Progestin* is a synthetic form of the female hormone progesterone.

The Ovaries and Fallopian Tubes

- An **ovariectomy** (**oh**-vay-ree-**ECK**-toh-mee), also known as an *oophorectomy*, is the surgical removal of one or both ovaries (**ovari** mean ovary, and **-ectomy** means surgical removal). If both ovaries are removed in a premenopausal woman, the patient experiences *surgical menopause*.
- A **salpingectomy** (**sal**-pin-**JECK**-toh-mee) is the surgical removal of one or both fallopian tubes (**salping** means tube, and **-ectomy** means surgical removal).
- A **salpingo-oophorectomy** (sal-**ping**-goh oh-**ahf**-oh-**RECK**-toh-mee) (SO) is the surgical removal of a fallopian tube and ovary (**salping/o** means tube, **oophor** means ovary, and **-ectomy** means surgical removal). A *bilateral salpingo-oophorectomy* is the removal of both of the fallopian tubes and ovaries.
- **Tubal ligation** is a surgical sterilization procedure in which the fallopian tubes are sealed or cut to prevent sperm from reaching a mature ovum.

The Uterus, Cervix, and Vagina

- A **colpopexy** (**KOL**-poh-**peck**-see), also known as *vaginofixation*, is the surgical fixation of a prolapsed vagina to a surrounding structure such as the abdominal wall (**colp/o** means vagina, and **-pexy** means surgical fixation in place).
- **Conization** (**kon**-ih-**ZAY**-shun), also known as a *cone biopsy*, is the surgical removal of a cone-shaped specimen of tissue from the cervix. This is performed as a diagnostic procedure or to remove abnormal tissue.
- **Colporrhaphy** (kol-**POR**-ah-fee) is the surgical suturing of a tear in the vagina (**colp/o** means vagina, and **-rrhaphy** means surgical suturing).
- **Dilation and curettage** (dye-**LAY**-shun and **kyou**-reh-**TAHZH**), commonly known as a *D & C*, is a surgical procedure in which the cervix is dilated and the endometrium of the uterus is scraped away. This can be performed as a diagnostic or a treatment procedure (Figure 14.12). *Dilation* means the expansion of an opening. *Curettage* is the removal of material from the surface by scraping with an instrument known as a curette.
- A **myomectomy** (**my**-oh-**MECK**-toh-mee) is the surgical removal of uterine fibroids (**myom** means muscle tumor, and **-ectomy** means surgical removal).

Hysterectomies

A **hysterectomy** (**hiss**-teh-**RECK**-toh-mee) is the surgical removal of the uterus (**hyster** means uterus, and **-ectomy** means surgical removal). The procedure is further described depending upon the structures that are removed (Figure 14.13).

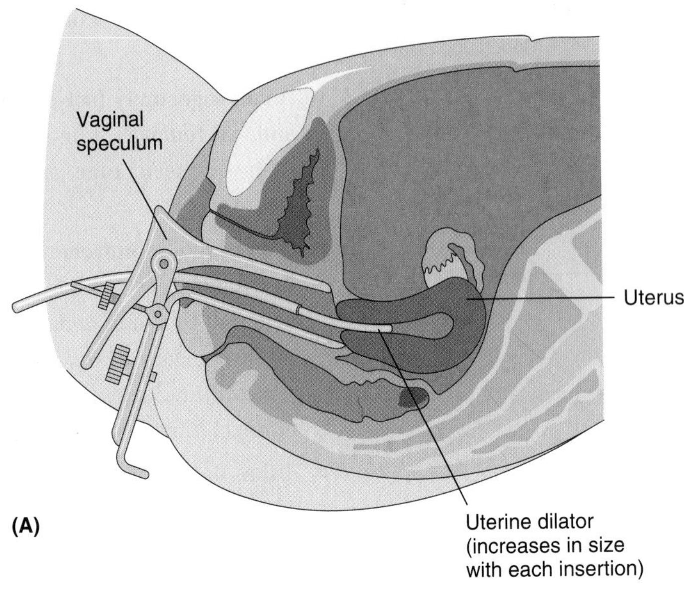

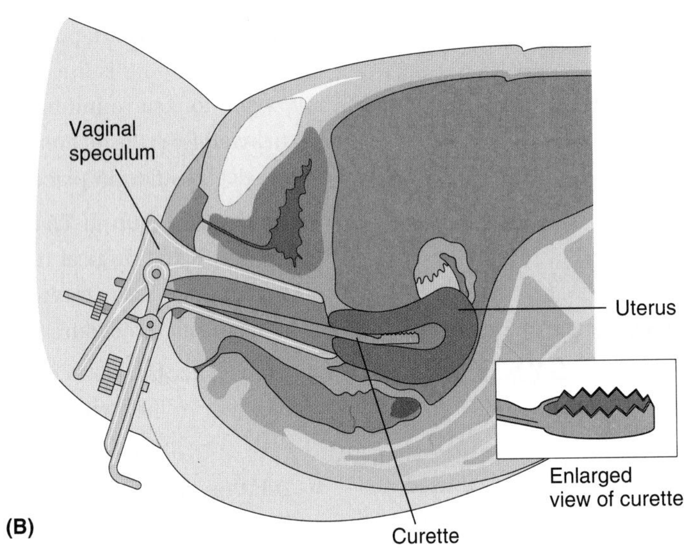

FIGURE 14.12 Dilation and curettage (D & C). (A) Dilation is the expansion of the cervical opening. (B) Curettage is the removal of material from the surface of the uterus.

- In a **total hysterectomy**, also known as a *complete hysterectomy*, the uterus and cervix are removed. This procedure can be performed through the vagina or laparoscopically through the abdomen.
- In a *partial* or *subtotal hysterectomy*, the uterus is removed and the cervix is left in place.
- A **radical hysterectomy**, also known as a *bilateral hysterosalpingo-oophorectomy*, is most commonly performed to treat uterine cancer (Figure 14.13B). This procedure includes the surgical removal of the ovaries and fallopian tubes, the uterus and cervix, plus nearby lymph nodes. If this surgery is performed before natural menopause, the patient immediately experiences *surgical menopause*.

Mammoplasty

Mammoplasty (**MAM**-oh-**plas**-tee), also spelled *mammaplasty*, is a general term for a cosmetic operation on the breasts (**mamm/o** means breast, and **-plasty** means surgical repair).

- **Breast augmentation** is mammoplasty performed to increase breast size. *Augmentation* means the process of adding to make larger. Breast augmentation is the opposite of *breast reduction*.

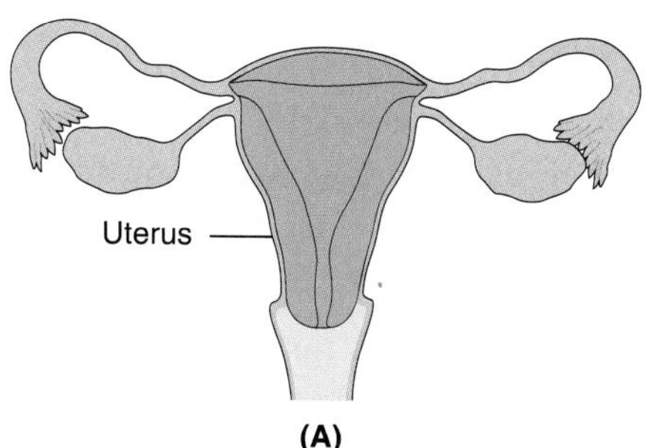

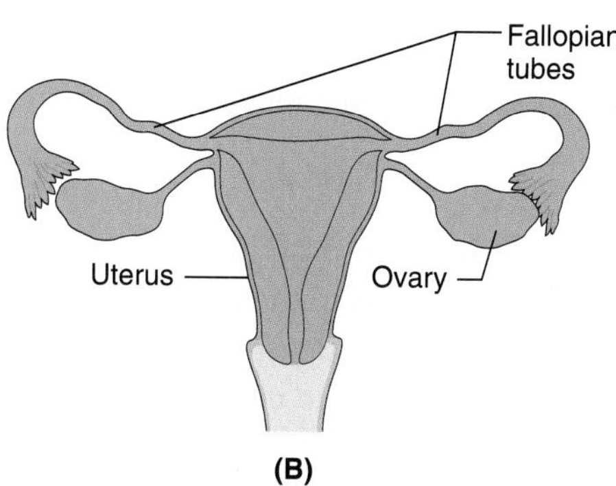

FIGURE 14.13 Types of hysterectomy. (A) In a total hysterectomy, the uterus and cervix are removed. (B) In a radical hysterectomy, the ovaries, fallopian tubes, uterus, and cervix are removed.

- **Breast reduction** is mammoplasty performed to decrease and reshape excessively large, heavy breasts. Breast reduction is the opposite of *breast augmentation*.
- **Mastopexy** (**MAS**-toh-**peck**-see) is mammoplasty to affix sagging breasts in a more elevated position (**mast/o** means breast, and **-pexy** means surgical fixation).
- *Breast reconstruction* following a mastectomy is discussed in Chapter 6.

PREGNANCY AND CHILDBIRTH

Ovulation

Ovulation (**ov**-you-**LAY**-shun) is the release of a mature egg from a follicle on the surface of the ovary.

- After the ovum is released, it is caught up by the fimbriae of the fallopian tube. Wave-like peristaltic actions move the ovum down the fallopian tube toward the uterus.
- It usually takes an ovum about 5 days to pass through the fallopian tube. If sperm are present, fertilization occurs within the fallopian tube.
- After the ovum has been released, the ruptured follicle enlarges, takes on a yellow fatty substance, and becomes the corpus luteum.
- The **corpus luteum** (**KOR**-pus **LOO**-tee-um) secretes the hormone progesterone during the second half of the menstrual cycle. This maintains the growth of the uterine lining in preparation for the fertilized egg.
- If the ovum is not fertilized, the corpus luteum dies, and the endometrium lining of the uterus sloughs off as the menstrual flow occurs.
- If the ovum is fertilized, the corpus luteum continues to secrete the hormones required to maintain the pregnancy.

Fertilization

- During **coitus** (**KOH**-ih-tus), also known as *copulation* or *sexual intercourse*, the male ejaculates approximately 100 million sperm into the female's vagina. The sperm travel upward through the vagina, into the uterus, and on into the fallopian tubes.
- **Conception** occurs when a sperm penetrates and fertilizes the descending ovum. This union, which is the beginning of a new life, forms a single cell known as a **zygote** (**ZYE**-goht).
- After fertilization occurs in the fallopian tube, the zygote travels to the uterus where it is implanted. *Implantation* is the embedding of the zygote into the lining of the uterus.
- From implantation through the 8th week of pregnancy, the developing child is known as an **embryo** (**EM**-bree-oh).
- From the 9th week of pregnancy, to the time of birth, the developing child in utero is known as a **fetus** (**fet** means unborn child, and **-us** is a singular noun ending). *In utero* means within the uterus (Figure 14.14).

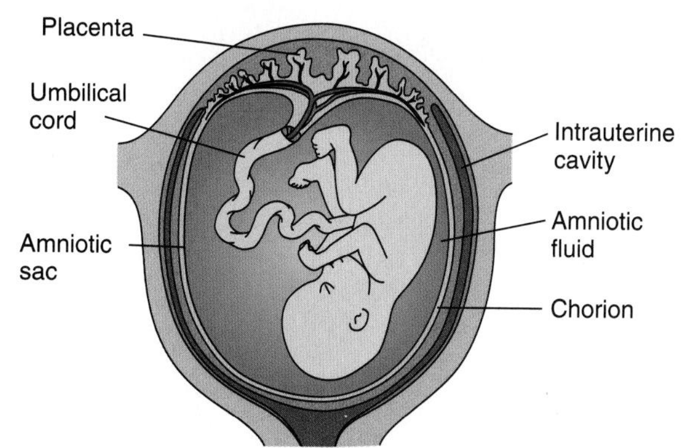

FIGURE 14.14 A normal pregnant uterus viewed in cross-section.

Multiple Births

If more than one egg is passing down the fallopian tube when sperm are present, the fertilization of more than one egg is possible.

- **Fraternal twins** result from the fertilization of separate ova by separate sperm cells. These develop into two separate embryos.
- **Identical twins** are formed by the fertilization of a single egg cell by a single sperm that divides to from two embryos. Each of these twins receives exactly the same genetic information from the parents.
- The term **multiples** is used to describe a birth involving more than two infants.

The Chorion and Placenta

- The **chorion** (**KOR**-ee-on) is the thin outer membrane that encloses the embryo. It contributes to the formation of the placenta (see Figure 14.14).
- The **placenta** (plah-**SEN**-tah) is a temporary organ that forms within the uterus to allow the exchange of nutrients, oxygen, and waste products between the mother and fetus without allowing maternal blood and fetal blood to mix (Figure 14.15). The placenta also produces hormones necessary to maintain the pregnancy. These hormones are discussed in Chapter 13.
- After delivery of the newborn, the placenta is expelled as the **afterbirth**.

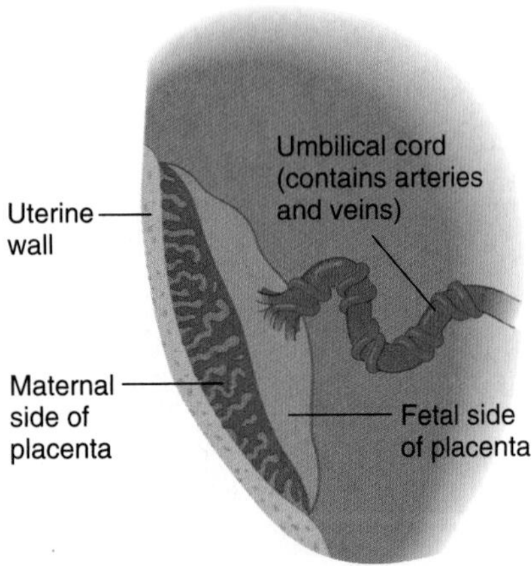

FIGURE 14.15 The placenta allows the exchange of nutrients and waste materials between mother and child without intermingling blood.

The Amniotic Sac

The **amniotic sac** (**am**-nee-**OT**-ick), which is also known as the *amnion*, is the innermost membrane that surrounds the embryo in the uterus (see Figure 14.14). The common name for this structure is the *bag of waters*.

- The developing embryo is surrounded by the **amniotic cavity**. This is the fluid-filled space between the embryo and the amniotic sac.
- **Amnionic fluid** (**am**-nee-**ON**-ick), also known as *amniotic fluid*, is the liquid that protects the fetus and makes possible its floating movements.

The Umbilical Cord

The **umbilical cord** (um-**BILL**-ih-kal) is the tube that carries blood, oxygen, and nutrients from the placenta to the developing child. It also transports waste from the fetus to be disposed of through the mother's excretory system. This cord is cut soon after the birth of the infant and before the delivery of the placenta.

- After birth, the **navel**, also known as the *belly button*, is formed where the umbilical cord was attached to the fetus.

Gestation

Gestation (jes-**TAY**-shun), which lasts approximately 280 days, is the period of development of the child in the mother's uterus. Upon completion of this developmental time, the fetus is described as being *at term* and should be ready for birth (see Figure 14.16).

- The term **pregnancy**, which is often used interchangeably with *gestation*, means the condition of having a developing child in the uterus.
- The length of pregnancy is described according to the number of weeks of gestation (usually 40 weeks total). For descriptive purposes, pregnancy can also be divided into three **trimesters** of about 13 weeks each
- The **due date**, or *estimated date of confinement*, is calculated from the first day of the last menstrual period (LMP). *Confinement* is an old-fashioned term describing the period of rest for the mother that followed childbirth.
- **Quickening** is the first movement of the fetus in the uterus that can be felt by the mother. This usually occurs during the 16th to 20th week of pregnancy.
- **Braxton Hicks contractions** are intermittent painless uterine contractions that occur with increasing

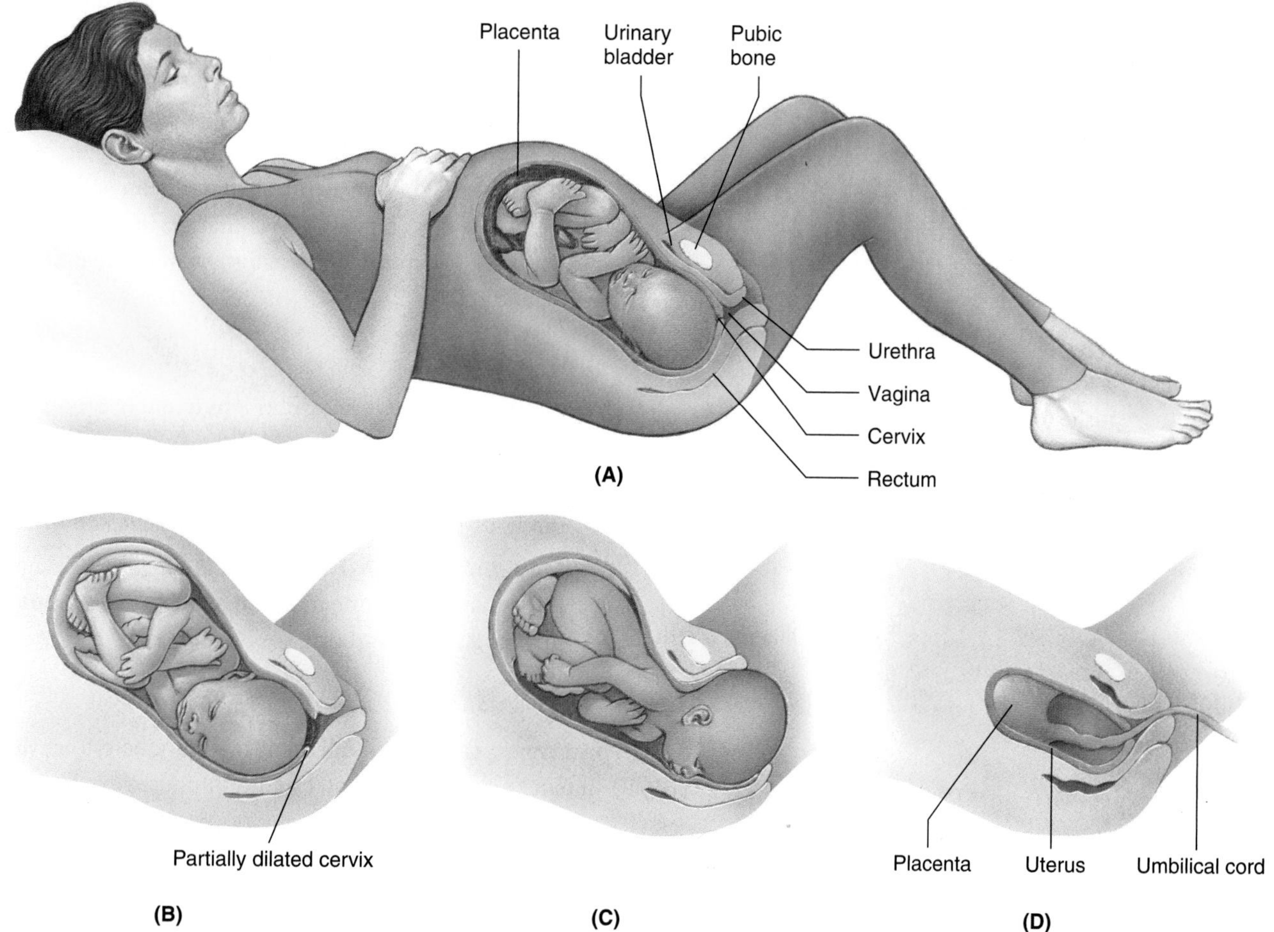

FIGURE 14.16 The stages of labor. (A) Position of the fetus before labor. (B) First state of labor, cervical dilation. (C) Second stage of labor, fetal delivery. (D) Third stage of labor, delivery of the placenta.

frequently as the pregnancy progresses. These contractions are not true labor pains and are usually infrequent, irregular, and essentially painless.

- The fetus is described as being **viable** when it is capable of living outside the uterus. Viability depends on the developmental age, birth weight, and developmental stage of the lungs of the fetus.
- The term **antepartum** (**an**-tee-**PAHR**-tum) refers to the final stage of pregnancy just before the onset of labor.

The Mother

- A **nulligravida** (**null**-ih-**GRAV**-ih-dah) is a woman who has never been pregnant (**nulli-** means none, and **-gravida** means pregnant). Compare with *nullipara.*
- A **nullipara** (nuh-**LIP**-ah-rah) is a woman who has never borne a viable child (**nulli-** means none, and **-para** means to bring forth). Compare with *nulligravida.*
- A **primigravida** (**prye**-mih-**GRAV**-ih-dah) is a woman during her first pregnancy (**primi-** means first, and **-gravida** means pregnant). Compare with *primipara.*
- A **primipara** (prye-**MIP**-ah-rah) is a woman who has borne one viable child (**primi-** means first, and **-para** means to bring forth). Compare with *primigravida.*
- **Multiparous** (mul-**TIP**-ah-rus) means a woman who has given birth two or more times (**multi-** means many, and **-parous** means having borne one or more children).

Childbirth

Labor and delivery, also known as *childbirth* or *parturition*, occurs in three stages. These are dilation, delivery of the baby, and expulsion of the afterbirth (Figure 14.16).

The First Stage

During the first, and longest, stage of labor, the changes that occur include the gradual dilatation and effacement of the cervix and the rupture of the amniotic sac. *Effacement* is the process by which the cervix prepares for delivery as it gradually softens, shortens, and becomes thinner (see Figure 14.16B).

- **Fetal monitoring** is the use of an electronic device to record the fetal heart rate and the maternal uterine contractions during labor.

The Second Stage

The second stage is the delivery of the infant. As the uterine contractions become stronger and more frequent, the mother pushes to help expel the child through the *birth canal* (vagina). Normally, the baby's head presents first. *Crowning* describes when the head can be seen at the vaginal opening (see Figure 14.16C).

The Third Stage

The third stage is the expulsion of the placenta as the *afterbirth* (see Figure 14.16D).

Postpartum

The term **postpartum** (pohst-**PAR**-tum) means after childbirth.

The Mother

- **Puerperium** (**pyou**-er-**PEE**-ree-um) is the time from the delivery of the placenta through approximately the first 6 weeks after the delivery. By the end of this period, most of the changes in the mother's body due to pregnancy have resolved, and the body has reverted to the nonpregnant state.
- **Lochia** (**LOH**-kee-ah) is the postpartum vaginal discharge that typically continues for 4–6 weeks after childbirth (**loch** means childbirth, and **-ia** means pertaining to). It consists of blood, mucus, and placental tissue.
- **Uterine involution** is the return of the uterus to its normal size and former condition after delivery. *Involution* means the return of an enlarged organ to its normal size.
- **Colostrum** (kuh-**LOS**-trum) is a specialized form of milk that delivers essential nutrients and antibodies in a form that the newborn can digest. Colostrum is produced by the mammary glands in late pregnancy and during the first few days after giving birth.
- **Lactation** (lack-**TAY**-shun) is the process of forming and secreting milk from the breasts as nourishment for the infant. The breast milk develops a few days after giving birth to replace the colostrum.
- **Postpartum depression** is a mood disorder characterized by feelings of sadness and the loss of pleasure in normal activities that can occur shortly after giving birth. One cause of this depression is the rapid change in the hormone levels that occurs after giving birth. When the depression is severe, treatment is required.

The Baby

The newborn infant is known as a **neonate** (**NEE**-oh-nayt) during the first 4 weeks after birth.

- **Vernix** (**VER**-nicks) is a greasy substance that protects the fetus in utero and can still be present at birth.
- **Meconium** (meh-**KOH**-nee-um) is the greenish material that collects in the intestine of a fetus and forms the first stools of a newborn.

Apgar Scores

An **Apgar score** is a scale of 1–10 to evaluate a newborn infant's physical status at 1 and 5 minutes after birth.

- The newborn is evaluated by assigning numerical values (0–2) to each of five criteria: (1) heart rate, (2) respiratory effort, (3) muscle tone, (4) response stimulation, and (5) skin color.
- A total score of 8–10 indicates the best possible condition.

PATHOLOGY OF PREGNANCY AND CHILDBIRTH

Pregnancy

- An **abortion** (ah-**BOR**-shun) is the interruption or termination of pregnancy before the fetus is viable. A *spontaneous abortion*, also known as a *miscarriage*, usually occurs early in the pregnancy and is due to an abnormality or genetic disorder.
- An *induced abortion*, caused by human intervention, is achieved through the use of drugs or suctioning. When done for medical purposes, it is known as known as a *therapeutic abortion*.
- An **ectopic pregnancy** (eck-**TOP**-ick), also known as an *extrauterine pregnancy*, is a potentially dangerous condition in which a fertilized egg is implanted and begins to develop outside of the uterus. *Ectopic* means out of place, and Figure 14.17 illustrates three of these potential locations.

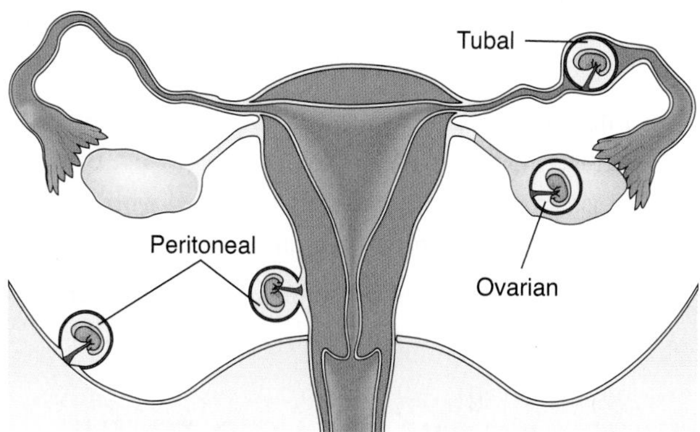

FIGURE 14.17 Potential sites of an ectopic pregnancy.

- **Preeclampsia** (**pree**-ee-**KLAMP**-see-ah), also known as *pregnancy-induced hypertension* or *toxemia*, is a complication of pregnancy characterized by hypertension (high blood pressure), edema (swelling), and proteinuria (an abnormally high level of protein in the urine).
- **Eclampsia** (eh-**KLAMP**-see-ah), which is a more serious form of preeclampsia, is characterized by convulsions and sometimes coma. Treatment for this condition is delivery of the fetus.

The Rh Factor

When the mother's blood is Rh-negative (Rh–), and the father's is Rh-positive (Rh+), the baby can inherit the Rh+ factor from the father. The Rh factor is discussed further in Chapter 5.

- During labor or a miscarriage of a first pregnancy, some of the baby's Rh+ blood can enter the mother's Rh– blood circulation. This can cause the mother's body to develop Rh+ antibodies, and these antibodies can cause problems during subsequent pregnancies.
- Blood tests of the parents can identify this potential problem. If it exists, the mother is vaccinated with Rh immune globulin to prevent the development of these antibodies.

Childbirth

- **Abruptio placentae** (ab-**RUP**-shee-oh plah-**SEN**-tee) is an abnormal disorder in which the placenta separates from the uterine wall before the birth of the fetus.
- **Breech presentation** is one in which the buttocks or feet of the fetus are positioned to enter the birth canal first instead of the head.
- **Placenta previa** (plah-**SEN**-tah **PREE**-vee-ah) is the abnormal implantation of the placenta in the lower portion of the uterus. *Previa* means appearing before or in front of. Symptoms include painless, sudden-onset bleeding during the third trimester.
- A **premature infant**, also known as a *preemie*, is a fetus born before the 37th week of gestation.
- A **stillbirth** is the birth of a fetus that died before, or during, the delivery.

Diagnostic Procedures Related to Pregnancy and Childbirth

- A **pregnancy test** is performed to detect an unusually high level of the human chorionic gonadotropin hormone in either a blood or urine specimen, which is usually an indication of pregnancy. A "home pregnancy test" uses a urine specimen. A pregnancy test based on a blood specimen usually provides more reliable results.
- **Fetal ultrasound** is discussed in Chapter 15.
- **First trimester screening**, also known as *combined screening*, is performed between 11 and 13 weeks of pregnancy and involves an ultrasound and a fingerstick blood test. The combined results of these two measurements, plus the mother's age, detect most of the fetuses at risk for Down syndrome. Diagnostic tests, such as amniocentesis or chorionic villus sampling, are recommended for those at increased risk for this condition.
- **Chorionic villus sampling** (**kor**-ee-**ON**-ick **VIL**-us) is the examination of cells retrieved from the chorionic villi, which are minute, vascular projections on the chorion. This test is performed between the 8th and 10th weeks of pregnancy to search for genetic abnormalities in the developing fetus.
- **Amniocentesis** (**am**-nee-oh-sen-**TEE**-sis) is a surgical puncture with a needle to obtain a specimen of amniotic fluid (**amnio** means amnion and fetal membrane, and **-centesis** means a surgical puncture to remove fluid). This specimen, which is obtained after the 14th week of pregnancy, is used to evaluate fetal health and to diagnose certain congenital disorders.
- **Pelvimetry** (pel-**VIM**-eh-tree) is a radiographic study to measure the dimensions of the pelvis to evaluate its capacity to allow passage of the fetus through the birth canal (**pelvi** means pelvis, and **-metry** means to measure).

Treatment Procedures Related to Pregnancy and Childbirth

- A **cesarean section** (seh-**ZEHR**-ee-un **SECK**-shun), also known as a *C-section*, is the delivery of the child through an incision in the maternal abdominal and uterine walls. This is usually performed when a vaginal birth would be unsafe for either the mother or baby.

- *VBAC* is the acronym used to describe **V**aginal **B**irth **A**fter a **C**esarean.
- An **episiotomy** (eh-**piz**-ee-**OT**-oh-mee) is a surgical incision made through the perineum to enlarge the vaginal orifice to prevent tearing of the tissues as the infant moves out of the birth canal (**episi** means vulva, and **-otomy** means a surgical incision).
- An **episiorrhaphy** (eh-**piz**-ee-**OR**-ah-fee) is the surgical suturing to repair an episiotomy (**episi/o** means vulva, and **-rrhaphy** means surgical suturing).

ASSISTED REPRODUCTION

Infertility is the inability of a couple to achieve pregnancy after 1 year of regular, unprotected intercourse, or the inability of a woman to carry a pregnancy to a live birth.

- An infertile couple may seek the help of an **infertility specialist**, also known as a *fertility specialist*, who diagnoses and treats problems associated with conception and maintaining pregnancy.
- Table 14.2 summarizes the abbreviations and terms commonly associated with assisted reproduction.

ABBREVIATIONS RELATED TO THE REPRODUCTIVE SYSTEMS

Table 14.3 presents an overview of the abbreviations related to the terms introduced in this chapter. Note: To avoid errors or confusion, always be cautious when using abbreviations.

TABLE 14.2

ABBREVIATIONS AND TERMS RELATED TO ASSISTED FERTILIZATION

AMA	**Advanced maternal age** is the term is applied to women in their late thirties to late forties. As the woman ages, the possibility of her becoming pregnant frequently decreases.
AI	**Artificial insemination** is a technique in which sperm from a woman's partner, or from a donor, are introduced into the vagina or uterus during the ovulatory phase of her menstrual cycle.
ART	The term **assisted reproductive technology** describes techniques used to aid an infertile couple in achieving a viable pregnancy.
IVF	**In vitro fertilization** is a procedure in which mature ova are removed from the mother to be fertilized. The resulting embryos are transferred into the uterus with the hope that they will implant and continue to develop as in a normal pregnancy. *In vitro* means in an artificial environment such as a test tube.

TABLE 14.3

ABBREVIATIONS RELATED TO THE REPRODUCTIVE SYSTEMS

amniocentesis = AMN	**AMN** = amniocentesis
bacterial vaginosis = BV	**BV** = bacterial vaginosis
chorionic villus sampling = CVS	**CVS** = chorionic villus sampling
circumcision = CIRC, circum	**CIRC, circum** = circumcision
digital rectal examination = DRE	**DRE** = digital rectal examination
erectile dysfunction = ED	**ED** = erectile dysfunction
hormone replacement therapy = HRT	**HRT** = hormone replacement therapy
human papilloma virus = HPV	**HPV** = human papilloma virus
hysterosalpingography = HSG	**HSG** = hysterosalpingography
hysteroscopy = HYS	**HYS** = hysteroscopy
intrauterine device = IUD	**IUD** = intrauterine device
labor and delivery = L & D	**L & D** = labor and delivery
pelvic inflammatory disease = PID	**PID** = pelvic inflammatory disease
trichomoniasis = Trich	**Trich** = trichomoniasis

Career Opportunities

In addition to the medical specialties already discussed, some of the health occupations involving the treatment of the reproductive systems include:

- **Midwife:** assists in labor and delivery. A certified nurse midwife (CNM) is an RN with specialized training in obstetrics and gynecology who provides primary care in normal pregnancies and deliveries.
- **Doula:** provides emotional, physical, and informational support to the mother before and during labor and delivery
- **Lactation consultant:** a health care professional specializing in breastfeeding management, employed in hospitals, physician's offices, public health clinics, corporate lactation centers, and in private practice
- **Registered nurse mother/baby unit (RN-MBU):** an RN who specializes in maternity and newborn care
- **Childbirth educator:** teaches expectant parents about prenatal care, the experience of childbirth, and infant care

Health Occupation Profile

Certified Nurse Midwife

Maureen Darcey is a certified nurse midwife. ***"I started out as a nurse in orthopedics at a small hospital. When I became the night supervisor, I was often needed in labor and delivery. Doctors sometimes couldn't get to the hospital in time, so I would help women in labor and even "catch" their babies. I loved supporting these women through their labor and being present with them at such a defining moment in their lives. I decided to enroll in the SUNY Downstate Medical Center midwifery program and became a certified nurse midwife.***

"Midwives believe that women deserve to have both a choice and a voice in their health care. Midwives are able to function independently and to offer complete well-woman health care throughout a woman's life—from a young girl's first menses through and beyond menopause. The primary focus is on obstetrical care: prenatal, labor and delivery, and postpartum. Midwives approach birth as a natural process and invite a woman to trust her own body. Midwives do not independently handle high-risk birth situations requiring medical intervention, but for a birth without complications, we help create a home-like environment where birth is honored as a special family event."

STUDY BREAK

The period of *gestation* for the development of a human fetus in the uterus is usually around 9 months (253–300 days). The fact that women are limited to about one pregnancy a year is an important factor in determining human population growth.

Imagine how many people there might be on the planet if the human gestation period were that of a:

- **Wolf (60–63 days)**
- **Rabbit (30–35 days)**
- **Mouse (19–30 days)**

Another factor limiting human population is the relatively low number of children born to most mothers. Our population would truly explode if every mother matched the record set by Mrs. Feodor Vassilyev of Russia in the 18th century: 69 children, consisting of 16 pairs of twins, 7 sets of triplets and 4 sets of quadruplets!

REVIEW TIME

Write the answers to the following questions on a separate piece of paper or in your notebook. In addition, be prepared to take part in the classroom discussion.

1. ***Written Assignment:*** Describe five common **sexually transmitted diseases.**

   Discussion Assignment: What measures are effective in preventing the transmission of STDs?

2. ***Written Assignment:*** Using terms a physician would understand, describe the **male** and **female sterilization procedures.**

   Discussion Assignment: How would you explain each of these procedures to a patient?

3. ***Written Assignment:*** Identify the phase of the menstrual cycle during which the female is capable of **becoming pregnant.**

   Discussion Assignment: How would you explain this concept to a couple who want this information to help with birth control planning?

4. ***Written Assignment:*** Using terms a patient would understand, describe the difference between **preeclampsia** and **eclampsia.**

   Discussion Assignment: Why is prenatal care so important in detecting and preventing these conditions?

5. ***Written Assignment:*** Report on your research about the person for whom **Apgar scores** were named. Include in your report his or her full name and dates.

   Discussion Assignment: How are these scores used to evaluate the physical status of a newborn?

continues

Optional Internet Activity

The goal of this activity is to help you learn more about medical terminology as it applies to the "real world." Select **one** *of these two options and follow the instructions.*

1. Search for information about **premenstrual dysphoric disorder** Write a brief (one- or two-paragraph) report on something new you learned here and include the address of the web site where you found this information.
2. To learn more about **childbirth classes**, go to the web site of Parenthood.com and search on "childbirth preparation." Write a brief (one- or two-paragraph) report on something new you learned here, including the names of at least two commonly used childbirth preparation training methods.

THE HUMAN TOUCH: CRITICAL THINKING ACITVITY

The following story and questions are designed to stimulate critical thinking through class discussion or as a brief essay response. There are no right or wrong answers to these questions.

"Amniocentesis: Friday @ 3:30." ***Julia read the note on the refrigerator with a puzzled look. What was an amniocentesis and why was her stepmother scheduled to have one? She assumed it had something to do with Sylvia's pregnancy. At first, Julia had been 100% opposed to her father and his new (very young) wife having a baby: how could Julia compete with a cute newborn? But as Sylvia had started to show a little bulge, and included Julia in shopping for baby clothes and planning the nursery, she had gotten excited.***

Now she wanted to know all that she could about the pregnancy. She had ooohed and aaahed at the ultrasound pictures, and was now helping search for cute names on the Internet. As far as she was concerned, the perfect name could make all the difference in a child's life. Her current favorites were Owen for a boy and Cassidy for a girl. But when she read the term **"amniocentesis,"** ***she started to worry, and all of the frivolous decisions like names and clothes were the furthest thing from her mind.***

Julia typed Amniocentesis ***into her computer's search engine to find out what it might be.*** **"Amniocentesis: a test sometimes done after the 14th week of pregnancy to check for genetic and chromosomal disorders."** ***Birth defects? chromosomal disorders? Why would Sylvia need to be tested for any of that? Julia began getting worried as she read on about the disorders that this procedure tests for: Down syndrome, spina bifida ... the list went on. Was her new little brother or sister going to be OK?***

continues

Suggested Discussion Topics

1. Discuss the options that are open to Julia's father and stepmother if they learn that their baby has a serious developmental disorder.
2. Talk about why parents might decide not to have this test done, even if a doctor recommends it.
3. Discuss the ethical questions that the results of this test could raise.
4. Discuss why you think Julia's dad and Sylvia have not told Julia about the need for this test. Do you think that Julia, as a member of the family, should have a voice in any decision that is made?

STUDENT WORKBOOK AND StudyWARE™ CD-ROM

1. Go to your **Student Workbook** and complete the Learning Exercises for this chapter.

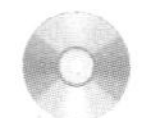

2. Go to the **StudyWARE™ CD-ROM** and have fun with the exercises and games for this chapter.

15

CHAPTER

Diagnostic Procedures and Pharmacology

Overview of Diagnostic Procedures and Pharmacology

Major Headings	**Including**
Basic Diagnostic Procedures	Vital signs Auscultation Palpation and percussion Basic examination instruments
Examination Positions	Recumbent positions Sims' position Knee-chest position Lithotomy position
Laboratory Tests	Blood tests Urinalysis
Endoscopy	Endoscopes
Centesis	Diagnostic procedures involving the removal of body fluids
Imaging Techniques	Radiography Computed tomography Magnetic resonance imaging Fluoroscopy Ultrasonography
Nuclear Medicine	Nuclear medicine
Pharmacology	Prescription and over-the-counter drugs Generic and brand-name drugs Terminology related to pharmacology Medications for pain management Methods of drug administration

Vocabulary Related to Diagnostic Procedures and Pharmacology

This list contains essential word parts and medical terms for this chapter. These terms are pronounced on the student StudyWARE™ CD-ROM and Audio CDs that are available for use with this text. These and the other important **primary terms** are shown in boldface throughout the chapter. *Secondary terms*, which appear in *orange* italics, clarify the meaning of primary terms.

Word Parts

- ☐ albumin/o
- ☐ calc/i
- ☐ -centesis
- ☐ creatin/o
- ☐ glycos/o
- ☐ -graphy
- ☐ hemat/o
- ☐ lapar/o
- ☐ -otomy
- ☐ phleb/o
- ☐ radi/o
- ☐ -scope
- ☐ -scopy
- ☐ son/o
- ☐ -uria

Medical Terms

- ☐ **acetaminophen** (ah-**seet**-ah-**MIN**-oh-fen)
- ☐ **albuminuria** (**al**-byou-mih-**NEW**-ree-ah)
- ☐ **analgesic** (**an**-al-**JEE**-zick)
- ☐ **antipyretic** (**an**-tih-pye-**RET**-ick)
- ☐ **arthrocentesis** (**ar**-throh-sen-**TEE**-sis)
- ☐ **auscultation** (**aws**-kul-**TAY**-shun)
- ☐ **bacteriuria** (back-**tee**-ree-**YOU**-ree-ah)
- ☐ **bruit** (**BREW**-ee)
- ☐ **calciuria** (**kal**-sih-**YOU**-ree-ah)
- ☐ **compliance**
- ☐ **computed tomography** (toh-**MOG**-rah-fee)
- ☐ **contraindication**
- ☐ **creatinuria** (kree-**at**-ih-**NEW**-ree-ah)
- ☐ **echocardiography** (**eck**-oh-**kar**-dee-**OG**-rah-fee)
- ☐ **endoscope** (**EN**-doh-**skope**)
- ☐ **fluoroscopy** (**floo**-or-**OS**-koh-pee)
- ☐ **glycosuria** (**glye**-koh-**SOO**-ree-ah)
- ☐ **hematocrit** (hee-**MAT**-oh-krit)
- ☐ **hematuria** (**hee**-mah-**TOO**-ree-ah)
- ☐ **hyperthermia** (**high**-per-**THER**-mee-ah)
- ☐ **hypothermia** (**high**-poh-**THER**-mee-ah)
- ☐ **idiosyncratic reaction** (**id**-ee-oh-sin-**KRAT**-ick)
- ☐ **intradermal injection**
- ☐ **intramuscular injection**
- ☐ **intravenous injection**
- ☐ **ketonuria** (**kee**-toh-**NEW**-ree-ah)
- ☐ **laparoscopy** (**lap**-ah-**ROS**-koh-pee)
- ☐ **lithotomy position** (lih-**THOT**-oh-mee)
- ☐ **magnetic resonance imaging**
- ☐ **ophthalmoscope** (ahf-**THAL**-moh-skope)
- ☐ **otoscope** (**OH**-toh-skope)
- ☐ **palliative** (**PAL**-ee-**ay**-tiv)
- ☐ **parenteral** (pah-**REN**-ter-al)
- ☐ **percussion** (per-**KUSH**-un)
- ☐ **perfusion** (per-**FYOU**-zuhn)
- ☐ **pericardiocentesis** (**pehr**-ih-**kar**-dee-oh-sen-**TEE**-sis)
- ☐ **phlebotomist** (fleh-**BOT**-oh-mist)
- ☐ **phlebotomy** (fleh-**BOT**-oh-mee)
- ☐ **placebo** (plah-**SEE**-boh)
- ☐ **positron emission tomography**
- ☐ **potentiation** (poh-**ten**-shee-**AY**-shun)
- ☐ **prone position**
- ☐ **proteinuria** (**proh**-tee-in-**YOU**-ree-ah)
- ☐ **pyuria** (pye-**YOU**-ree-ah)
- ☐ **radiolucent** (**ray**-dee-oh-**LOO**-sent)
- ☐ **radiopaque** (**ray**-dee-oh-**PAYK**)
- ☐ **rale** (**RAHL**)
- ☐ **recumbent** (ree-**KUM**-bent)
- ☐ **rhonchus** (**RONG**-kus)
- ☐ **Sims' position**
- ☐ **single photon emission computed tomography**
- ☐ **speculum** (**SPECK**-you-lum)
- ☐ **sphygmomanometer** (**sfig**-moh-mah-**NOM**-eh-ter)
- ☐ **stethoscope** (**STETH**-oh-skope)
- ☐ **stridor** (**STRYE**-dor)
- ☐ **subcutaneous injection**
- ☐ **transdermal**
- ☐ **transesophageal echocardiography** (**trans**-eh-**sof**-ah-**JEE**-al **eck**-oh-**kar**-dee-**OG**-rah-fee)
- ☐ **ultrasonography** (**ul**-trah-son-**OG**-rah-fee)
- ☐ **urinalysis** (**you**-rih-**NAL**-ih-sis)

OBJECTIVES

On completion of this chapter, you should be able to:

1. Describe the vital signs recorded for most patients.
2. Recognize, define, spell, and pronounce the terms associated with basic examination procedures.
3. Identify and describe the basic examination positions.
4. Recognize, define, spell, and pronounce terms associated with frequently performed blood and urinalysis laboratory tests.
5. Recognize, define, spell, and pronounce terms associated with radiography and other imaging techniques.
6. Differentiate between projection and position, and describe basic radiographic projections.
7. Recognize, define, spell, and pronounce the pharmacology terms introduced in this chapter.

BASIC EXAMINATION PROCEDURES

Basic examination procedures are performed during the assessment of the patient's condition. As used in medicine, the term **assessment** means the evaluation or appraisal of a condition. This information is used in reaching a diagnosis and in formulating a patient care plan.

Vital Signs

Vital signs are the four key indications that the body systems are functioning. These signs, which are recorded for most patient visits, include temperature, pulse, respiration, and blood pressure.

Temperature

An average normal **temperature** is 98.6°F (Fahrenheit) or 37.0°C (Celsius) (Figure 15.1).

- Temperature readings are named for the location in which they are taken: *oral* (in the mouth), *aural* (in the ear), *axillary* (under the arm), and *rectal* (in the rectum). Caution: *oral* and *aural* sound alike; however, they require different equipment and are taken in different locations.
- Temperature readings vary slightly depending upon the location where they are taken (Figure 15.2).
- **Hypothermia** (**high**-poh-**THER**-mee-ah) is an abnormally low body temperature (**hypo-** means deficient, **therm** means heat, and **-ia** means pertaining to).
- **Hyperthermia** (**high**-per-**THER**-mee-ah) is an extremely high fever (**hyper-** means excessive, **therm** means heat, and **-ia** means pertaining to).

Pulse

The **pulse** is the rhythmic pressure against the walls of an artery caused by the contraction of the heart. The pulse rate reflects the number of times the heart beats each minute and is recorded as *bpm* (beats per minute). As shown in Figure 15.3, the pulse can be measured at different points on the body.

- Normal resting pulse rates differ by age group. In adults, a normal resting pulse is from 50 to 80 bpm. Generally pulse rates are higher in younger people and for a newborn the pulse rate ranges from 100 to 160 bpm.

Respiration

Respiration, also known as the **respiratory rate** (RR), is the number of complete respirations per minute. One

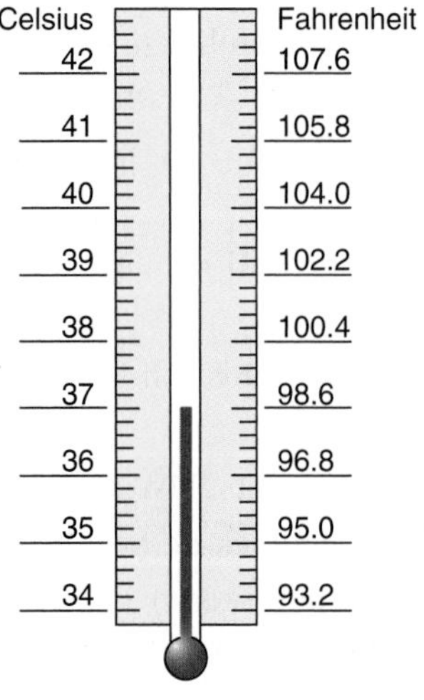

FIGURE 15.1 The average normal body temperature is 37.0°C (Celsius) or 98.6°F (Fahrenheit).

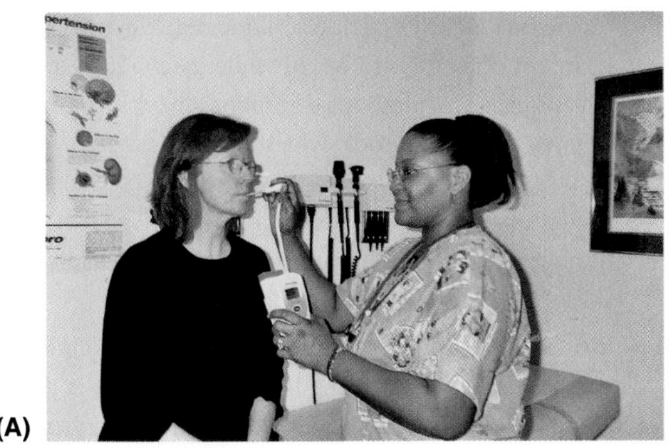
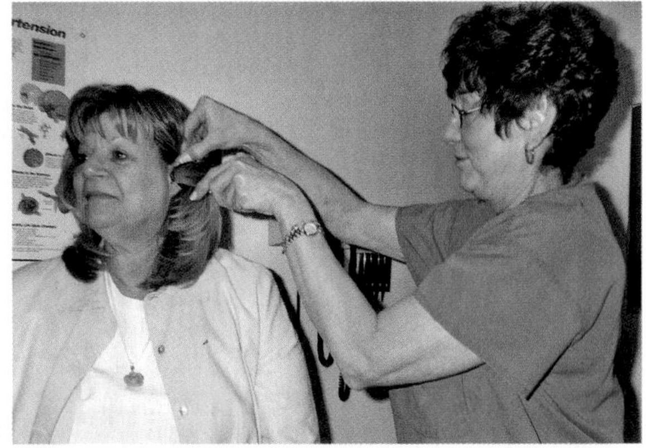

FIGURE 15.2 (A) An oral temperature reading is taken in the mouth. (B) An aural temperature reading is taken in the ear.

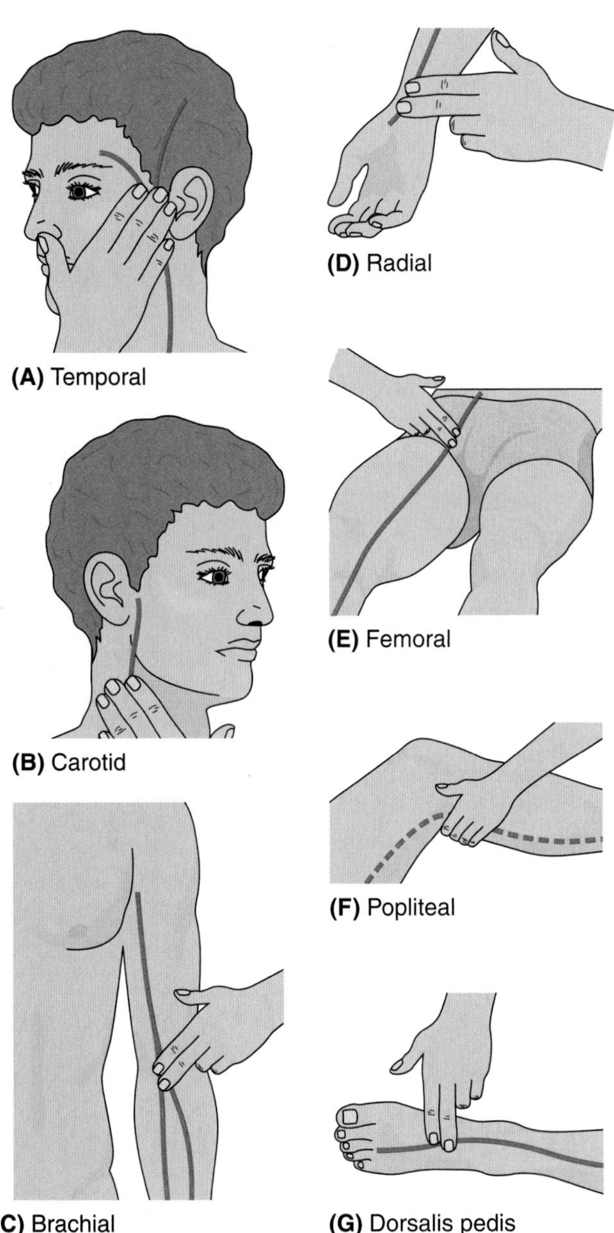

FIGURE 15.3 Pulse points of the body.

inhalation and one exhalation are counted as a single respiration (see Chapter 7). The normal respiratory rate for adults ranges from 12 to 20 respirations per minute.

Blood Pressure

Blood pressure is the force of the blood against the walls of the arteries. This force is measured using a **sphygmomanometer** (**sfig**-moh-mah-**NOM**-eh-ter). When using manual style, as shown in Figure 15.4, a stethoscope is required to listen to the blood sounds. A digital sphygmomanometer is automated and does not require the use of a stethoscope.

- Blood pressure is recorded as a ratio with the **systolic** over the **diastolic** reading. For example, 120/80. Systolic (the first beat heard) and diastolic (the last beat heard) are explained in Chapter 5. Memory aid: *SSSS-systolic* is like steam going up. *DDDD-diastolic* as in going down (Figure 15.5).

Pain

In certain settings, such as a hospital, **pain** is considered to be the fifth vital sign. Since this is a subjective symptom that cannot be measured objectively, it must be determined as reported by the patient.

- Using a *pain rating scale*, the patient is asked to describe his or her level of pain.
- *Acute pain*, which comes on quickly, can be severe and lasts only a relatively short time.
- *Chronic pain*, which can be mild or severe, persists over a long period of time.

Auscultation

The term **auscultation** (**aws**-kul-**TAY**-shun) means listening for sounds within the body and is usually performed

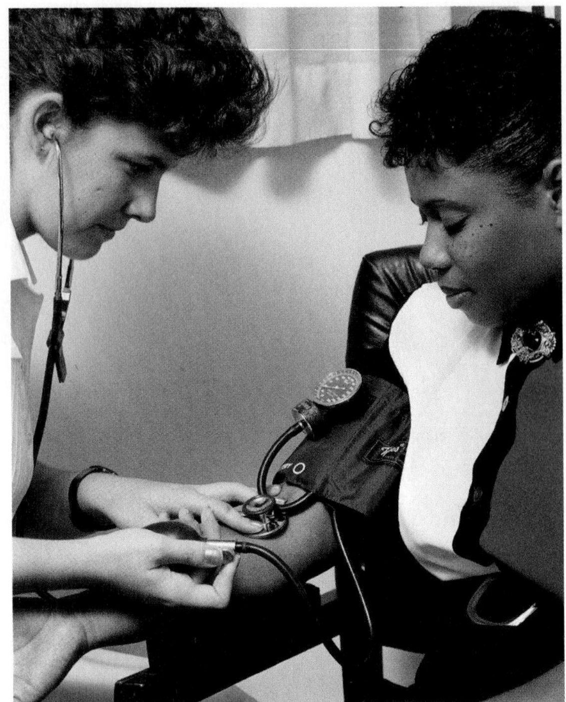

FIGURE 15.4 A manual sphygmomanometer being used with a stethoscope to measure blood pressure.

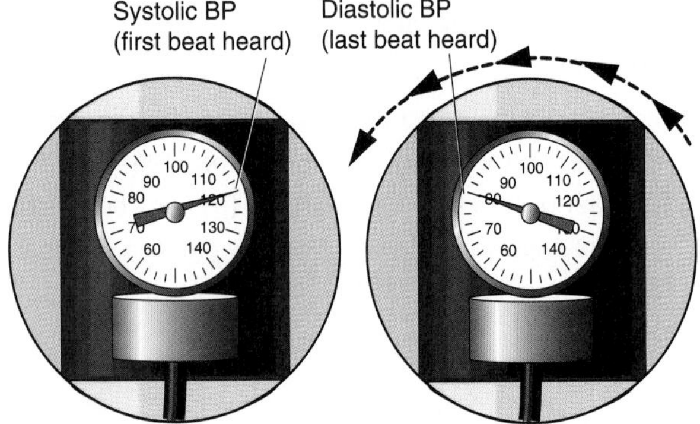

FIGURE 15.5 Using a stethoscope, the systolic pressure is the first sound heard and the diastolic pressure is the last beat heard.

through a stethoscope (**auscult/a** means to listen, and **-tion** means the process of) (Figure 15.6).

Respiratory Sounds

Respiratory sounds heard through a stethoscope provide information about the condition of the lungs and pleura (see Chapter 7).

- A **rale** (**RAHL**), also known as a *crackle*, is an abnormal rattle or crackle-like respiratory sound heard during inspiration (breathing in). Memory aid: Rale is a "rattley" sound.
- **Rhonchus** (**RONG**-kus), also known as *wheezing*, is an abnormal sound heard while listening to the chest during inspiration, expiration or both (plural, *rhonchi*). These sounds, which are low-pitched, whistle-like, or similar to snoring, are caused are partial obstruction of the airway. *Memory aid*: Rhonchus occurs in a partially blocked bronchus. Compare rhonchus with *stridor*.
- **Stridor** (**STRYE**-dor) is an abnormal high-pitched harsh sound heard during inhalation. Stridor is the result of a partial blockage of the pharynx, larynx, and trachea. Memory aid: Stridor is a harsh sound. Compare stridor with *rhonchus*.

Heart Sounds

The heartbeat heard through a stethoscope has two distinct sounds. These are known as the "lubb dupp" or "lub dub" sounds.

- The *lubb sound* is heard first. This is caused by the tricuspid and mitral valves closing between the atria and the ventricles.
- The *dupp sound*, which is shorter and higher pitched, is heard next. It is caused by the closing of the semilunar valves in the aorta and pulmonary arteries as blood is pumped out of the heart.
- A **bruit** (**BREW**-ee) is an abnormal sound heard during auscultation of an artery. These sounds are usually due to a partially blocked, narrowed, or diseased artery. These sounds are also produced by the blood flowing though a graft, fistula, or shunt.
- A **heart murmur** is an abnormal heart sound that is most commonly a sign of abnormal function of the heart valves.

Abdominal Sounds

Abdominal sounds, also known as *bowel sounds*, are normal noises made by the intestines. Auscultation of the abdomen is performed to evaluate these sounds and to detect abnormalities. For example, increased bowel sounds can indicate a bowel obstruction. The absence of these sounds can indicate ileus, which is the stopping of intestinal peristalsis (see Chapter 8).

Palpation and Percussion

- **Palpation** (pal-**PAY**-shun) is an examination technique in which the examiner's hands are used to feel the texture, size, consistency, and location of certain body parts (Figure 15.7).

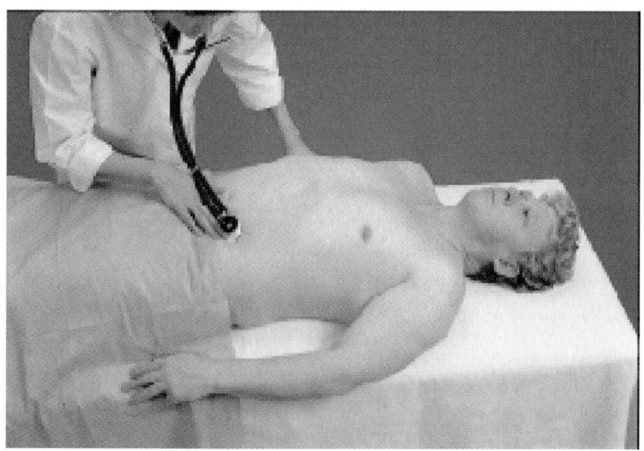

FIGURE 15.6 Auscultation is listening through a stethoscope to sounds within the body.

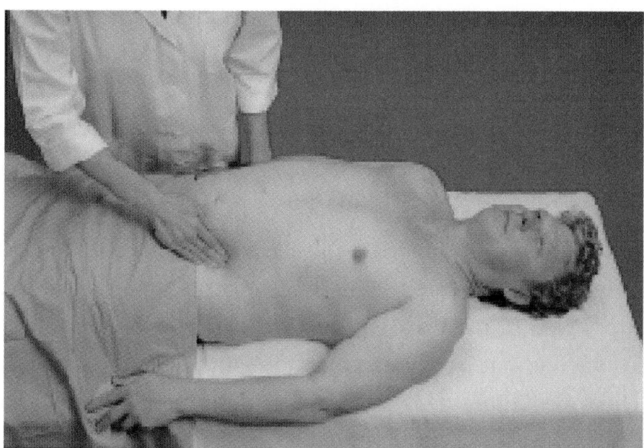

FIGURE 15.7 Palpation is an examination technique in which the examiner's hands are used to feel the texture, size, consistency, and location of certain body parts.

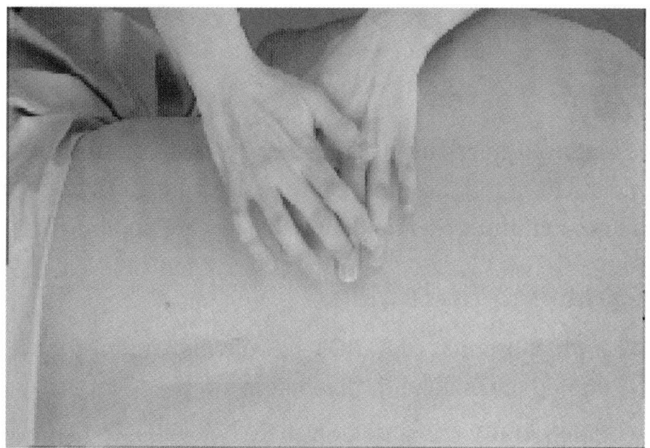

FIGURE 15.8 Percussion is a diagnostic procedure in which the examiner's hands are used to determine the density of a body area.

- **Percussion** (per-**KUSH**-un) is a diagnostic procedure designed to determine the density of a body part by the sound produced by tapping the surface with the fingers. As shown in Figure 15.8, this is performed over the chest to determine the presence of normal air content in the lungs.

Basic Examination Instruments

- An **ophthalmoscope** (ahf-**THAL**-moh-skope) is an instrument used to examine the interior of the eye (**ophthalm/o** means eye, and **-scope** means instrument for visual examination) (Figure 15.9).
- An **otoscope** (**OH**-toh-skope) is an instrument used to visually examine the external ear canal and tympanic membrane (**ot/o** means ear, and **-scope** means instrument for visual examination) (Figure 15.10).
- A **speculum** (**SPECK**-you-lum) is an instrument used to enlarge the opening of any canal or cavity to facilitate inspection of its interior (Figure 15.11).
- A **stethoscope** (**STETH**-oh-skope) is an instrument used to listen to sounds within the body (see Figures 15.4 and 15.6).

BASIC EXAMINATION POSITIONS

Specific positions are used to examine different areas of the body.

Recumbent Positions

The term **recumbent** (ree-**KUM**-bent) describes any position in which the patient is lying down. This can be on the back, front, or side. In radiography the term *decubitus* is used to describe the patient lying in a recumbent position.

Prone Position

In a **prone position**, the patient is lying on the belly with the *face down*. The arms may be placed under the head for comfort (Figure 15.12). This position is used for the examination and treatment of the back and buttocks.

Horizontal Recumbent Position

In the **horizontal recumbent position**, also known as the *supine position*, the patient is lying on the back with the *face up* (Figure 15.13). This position is used for examination and treatment of the anterior surface of the body and for x-rays.

Dorsal Recumbent Position

In the **dorsal recumbent position**, the patient is lying on the back with the knees bent (Figure 15.14). This position

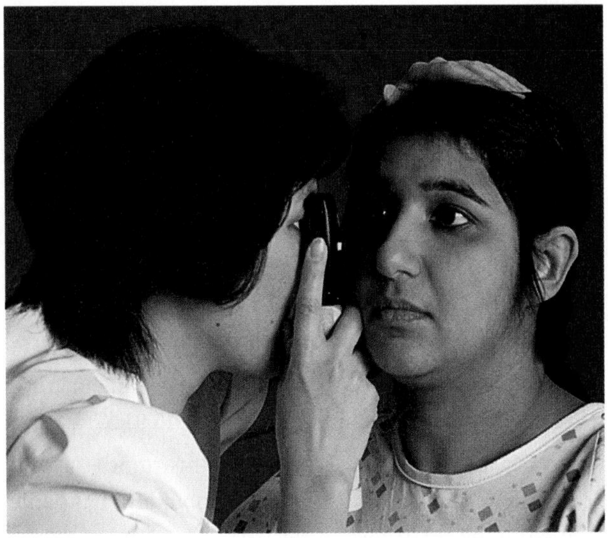

FIGURE 15.9 An ophthalmoscope is used to examine the interior of the eye.

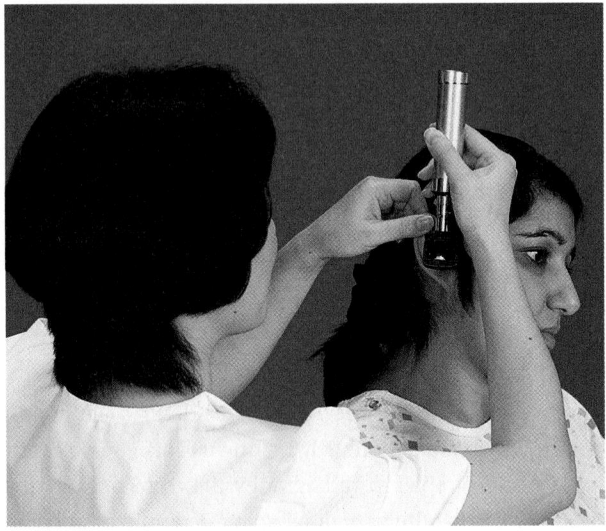

FIGURE 15.10 An otoscope is used to examine the external ear canal and the tympanic membrane.

is used for the examination and treatment of the abdominal area and for vaginal or rectal examinations.

Sims' Position

In the **Sims' position**, the patient is lying on the left side with the right knee and thigh drawn up with the left arm placed along the back (Figure 15.15). This position is used in the examination and treatment of the rectal area. The name of this position is also spelled as *Sims position*.

Knee-Chest Position

In the **knee-chest position**, the patient is lying face down with the hips bent so that the knees and chest rest on

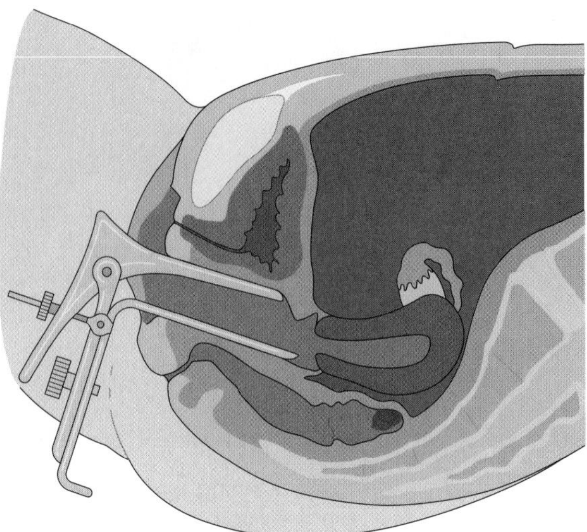

FIGURE 15.11 A speculum is used to enlarge the opening of the vagina during the examination of the cervix and vagina.

the table (Figure 15.16). This position is used for rectal examinations.

Lithotomy Position

In the **lithotomy position** (lih-**THOT**-oh-mee) the patient is lying on the back with the feet and legs raised and supported in stirrups (Figure 15.17). This position is used for vaginal and rectal examinations and during childbirth. The term *lithotomy* is also used to describe the removal of a stone from the urinary bladder (see Chapter 9).

LABORATORY TESTS

When a laboratory test is ordered **stat**, the results are needed immediately, and the tests have top priority in the laboratory. *Stat* comes from the Latin word meaning immediately.

Blood Tests

When used in regard to laboratory tests, the term **profile** means tests that are frequently performed as a group on automated multichannel laboratory testing equipment.

Obtaining Specimens

- A **phlebotomist** (fleh-**BOT**-oh-mist) is an individual trained and skilled in phlebotomy.
- **Phlebotomy** (fleh-**BOT**-oh-mee), which is also known as *venipuncture*, is the puncture of a vein for the purpose of drawing blood (**phleb** means vein, and **-otomy** means a surgical incision).

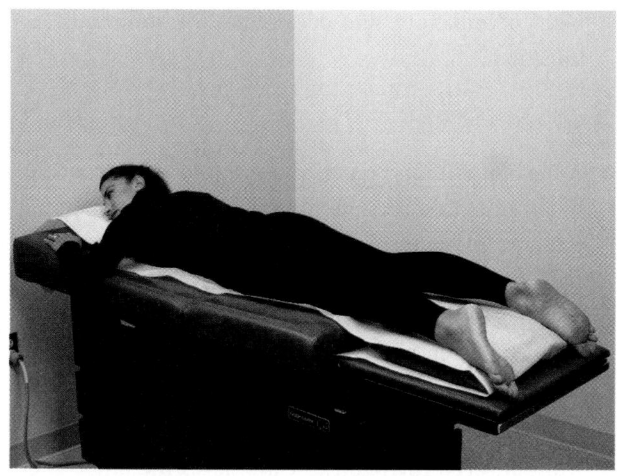

FIGURE 15.12 In the prone position, this patient is lying flat on her belly.

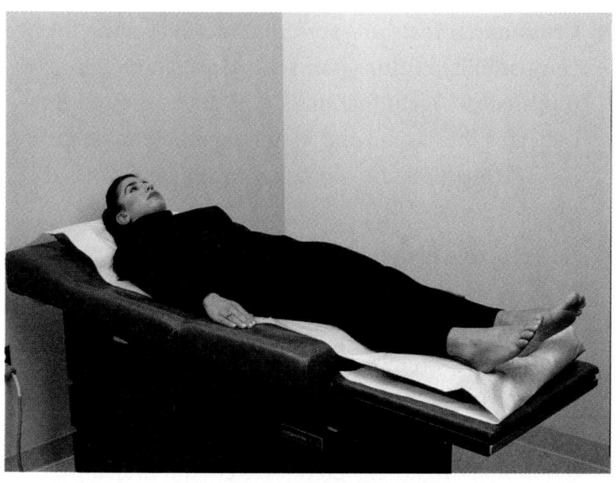

FIGURE 15.13 In the horizontal recumbent position, this patient is lying flat on her back.

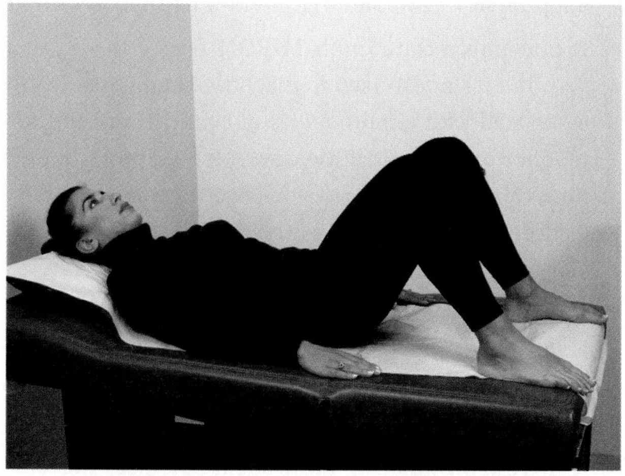

FIGURE 15.14 In the dorsal recumbent position, this patient is lying on her back with the knees drawn up.

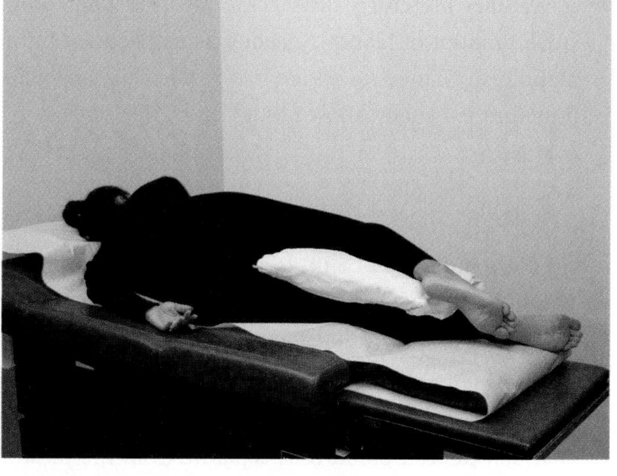

FIGURE 15.15 In the Sims' position, this patient is lying on her left side with the right knee and thigh drawn up with the left arm placed along the back.

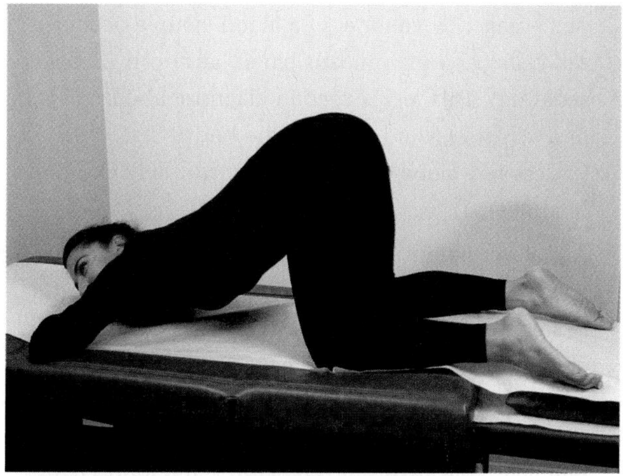

FIGURE 15.16 In the knee-chest position, this patient is lying face down with the hips bent so that the knees and chest rest on the table.

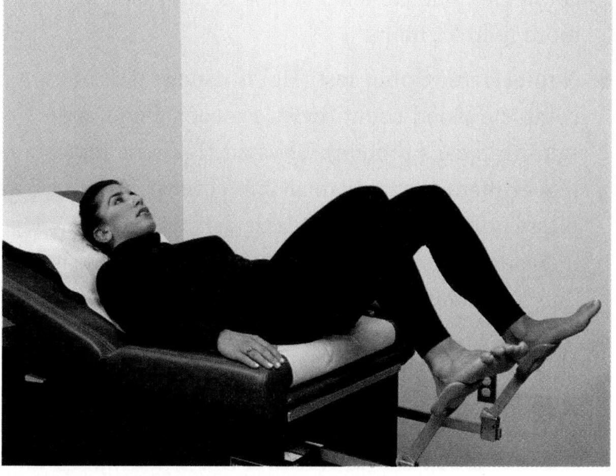

FIGURE 15.17 In the lithotomy position, this patient is lying on her back with the feet and legs raised and supported in stirrups.

- A **capillary puncture** is the technique used when only a small amount of blood is needed as a specimen for a blood test. Named for where it is performed, a capillary puncture is usually known as a *finger*, *heel*, or an *earlobe stick*.

Complete Blood Cell Counts

A **complete blood cell count** is a series of tests performed as a group to evaluate several blood conditions. Blood disorders are discussed in Chapter 5.

- **Erythrocyte sedimentation rate** (eh-**RITH**-roh-site), also known as a *sed rate*, is a test based on the speed at which the red blood cells separate from the plasma and settle to the bottom of the container. An elevated sed rate indicates the presence of inflammation in the body.
- The term **hematocrit** (hee-**MAT**-oh-krit) describes the percentage, by volume, of a blood sample occupied by red cells (**hemat/o** means blood, and **-crit** means to separate). This test is used to diagnose abnormal states of *hydration* (fluid levels in the body), *polycythemia* (excess red blood cells), and *anemia* (deficient red blood cells).
- A **platelet count** measures the number of platelets in a specified amount of blood and is a screening test to evaluate platelet function. It is also used to monitor changes in the blood associated with chemotherapy and radiation therapy. These changes include *thrombocytosis* (an abnormal increase in the number of platelets) and *thrombocytopenia* (an abnormal decrease in the number of platelets).
- A **red blood cell count** is a determination of the number of erythrocytes in the blood. A depressed count can indicate anemia or a hemorrhage lasting more than 24 hours.
- A **total hemoglobin test** (Hg) is usually part of a complete blood count (**hem/o** means blood, and **-globin** means protein). Elevated Hg levels indicate a higher than normal hemoglobin concentration in the plasma due to polycythemia or dehydration. Low Hg indicates lower then normal hemoglobin concentration due to anemia, recent hemorrhage, or fluid retention.
- A **white blood cell count** is a determination of the number of leukocytes in the blood. An elevated count can be an indication of infection or inflammation.
- A **white blood cell differential test** determines what percentage of the total count is composed of each of the five types of leukocyte. This test provides information about the patient's immune system, detects certain types of leukemia, and determines the severity of infection.

Additional Blood Tests

- A **basic metabolic panel** is a group of eight specific blood tests that provide important information about the current status of the patient's kidneys, electrolyte balance, blood sugar, and calcium levels. Significant changes in these test results can indicate acute problems such as kidney failure, insulin shock or diabetic coma, respiratory distress, or heart rhythm changes.
- A **blood urea nitrogen test** measures the amount of nitrogen in the blood due to the waste product urea. This test is performed to obtain an indication of kidney function. **Urea** (you-**REE**-ah) is the major end product of protein metabolism found in urine and blood.
- **Crossmatch tests** are performed to determine the compatibility of donor and recipient blood before a transfusion. Agglutination is a positive reaction that indicates the donor unit is not a suitable match. *Agglutination* is the clumping together of the red blood cells.
- A **C-reactive protein test** (CRP) is performed to identify high levels of inflammation within the body. The information is obtained by the presence of the C-reactive protein, which is produced by the liver only during episodes of acute inflammation. Although this test does not identify the specific cause of the inflammation, an elevated level can be indicative of a heart attack or coronary artery disease.
- A **lipid panel** measures the amounts of total cholesterol, high-density lipoprotein (HDL), low-density lipoprotein (LDL), and triglycerides in a blood sample.
- **Prothrombin time** (proh-**THROM**-bin), also known as *pro time*, is a test used to diagnose conditions associated with abnormalities of clotting time and to monitor anticoagulant therapy. A longer prothrombin time can be caused by serious liver disease, bleeding disorders, blood-thinning medicines or a lack of vitamin K.
- A **serum bilirubin test** measures the ability of the liver ability to take up, process, and secrete bilirubin into the bile. This test is useful in determining whether a patient has liver disease or a blocked bile duct.
- A **thyroid-stimulating hormone assay** measures circulating blood levels of thyroid-stimulating hormone that can indicate abnormal thyroid activity (see Chapter 13).

Urinalysis

Urinalysis (**you**-rih-**NAL**-ih-sis) is the examination of the physical and chemical properties of urine to determine the presence of abnormal elements.

- *Routine urinalysis* is performed to screen for urinary and systemic disorders. This test utilizes a dipstick. This is a plastic strip impregnated with chemicals that react with substances in the urine and change color when abnormalities are present (Figure 15.18).
- *Microscopic examination* of the specimen is performed when more-detailed testing of the specimen is necessary, for example to identify casts. **Casts** are fibrous or protein materials, such as pus and fats, that are thrown off into the urine in kidney disease.

pH Values of Urine

The average normal **pH** range of urine is from 4.5 to 8.0. The abbreviation pH describes the degree of acidity or alkalinity of a substance.

- A pH value *below* 7 indicates acid urine and is an indication of acidosis. *Acidosis* is excessive acid in the body fluids.
- A pH value *above* 7 indicates alkaline urine and can indicate conditions such as a urinary tract infection.

Specific Gravity

The **specific gravity** of urine reflects the amount of wastes, minerals, and solids that are present.

- *Low specific gravity* (dilute urine) is characteristic of diabetes insipidus, which is discussed in Chapter 13.
- *High specific gravity* (concentrated urine) occurs in conditions such as dehydration, liver failure, or shock.

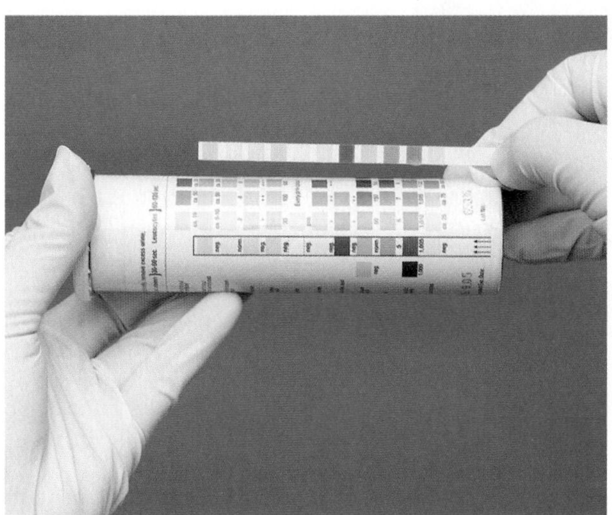

FIGURE 15.18 A dipstick is used for routine urinalysis.

Conditions Identified through Urinalysis

- **Acetone** (**ASS**-eh-tohn), which has a sweet, fruity odor, is found in small quantities in normal urine and in larger amounts in the urine of a diabetic.
- **Albuminuria** (**al**-byou-mih-**NEW**-ree-ah) is the presence of the protein albumin in the urine and is a sign of impaired kidney function (**albumin** means albumin or protein, and **-uria** means urine). *Albumin* is a form of protein found in most body tissues.
- **Bacteriuria** (back-**tee**-ree-**YOU**-ree-ah) is the presence of bacteria in the urine (**bacteri** means bacteria, and **-uria** means urine).
- **Calciuria** (**kal**-sih-**YOU**-ree-ah) is the presence of calcium in the urine (**calci** means calcium, and **-uria** means urine). Abnormally high levels can be diagnostic for hyperparathyroidism as described in Chapter 13. Lower-than-normal levels can indicate osteomalacia, which is discussed in Chapter 3.
- **Creatinuria** (kree-**at**-ih-**NEW**-ree-ah) is an increased concentration of creatine in the urine (**creatin** means creatinine, and **-uria** means urine). *Creatinine* is a waste product of muscle metabolism that is normally removed by the kidneys. The presence of excess creatinine is an indication of increased muscle breakdown or a disruption of kidney function.
- A **drug-screening** urine test is a rapid method of identifying the presence in the body of one or more drugs of abuse such as cocaine, heroin, and marijuana. These tests are also used to detect the use of performance-enhancing drugs by athletes.
- **Glycosuria** (**glye**-koh-**SOO**-ree-ah), which is the presence of glucose in the urine, is most commonly caused by diabetes (**glycos** means glucose, and **-uria** means urine).
- **Hematuria** (**hee**-mah-**TOO**-ree-ah) is the presence of blood in the urine (**hemat** means blood, and **-uria** means urine). This condition can be caused by kidney stones, infection, damage to the kidney, or bladder cancer.
- In *gross hematuria*, the presence of blood can be detected without magnification because the urine is pink, brown, or bright red in color. In *microscopic hematuria*, the urine is clear; however, the blood cells can be seen under a microscope.
- **Ketonuria** (**kee**-toh-**NEW**-ree-ah) is the presence of ketones in the urine (**keton** means ketones, and **-uria**

means urine). *Ketones* are formed when the body breaks down fat. Their presence in urine can indicate starvation or uncontrolled diabetes.

- **Proteinuria** (**proh**-tee-in-**YOU**-ree-ah) is the presence of an abnormal amount of protein in the urine (**protein** means protein, and **-uria** means urine). This condition is usually a sign of kidney disease.
- **Pyuria** (pye-**YOU**-ree-ah) is the presence of pus in the urine (**py** means pus, and **-uria** means urine). When pus is present, the urine has a turbid appearance. *Turbid* means a cloudy or smoky appearance.
- **Urine culture and sensitivity tests** are laboratory tests that are used to identify the cause of a urinary tract infection and to determine which antibiotic would be the most effective treatment.

ENDOSCOPY

Endoscopy (en-**DOS**-koh-pee) is the visual examination of the interior of a body cavity (**endo-** means within, and **-scopy** means visual examination). These procedures are usually named for the organs involved.

The term **endoscopic surgery** describes a surgical procedure performed through very small incisions with the use of an endoscope and specialized instruments. These procedures are named for the body parts involved, for example, arthroscopic surgery, which is discussed in Chapter 3.

Endoscopes

An **endoscope** (**EN**-doh-**skope**) is a small flexible tube with a light and a lens on the end. These fiber optic instruments are named for the body parts they are designed to examine. For example, a hysteroscope is used to examine the interior of the uterus while a laparoscope is used to examine the interior of the abdomen (Figure 15.19).

Laparoscopic Procedures

Laparoscopy (**lap**-ah-**ROS**-koh-pee) is the visual examination of the interior of the abdomen with the use of a laparoscope that is passed through a small incision in the abdominal wall (**lapar/o** means abdomen, and **-scopy** means visual examination).

Laparoscopic surgery involves the use of a laparoscope plus specialized instruments inserted into the abdomen

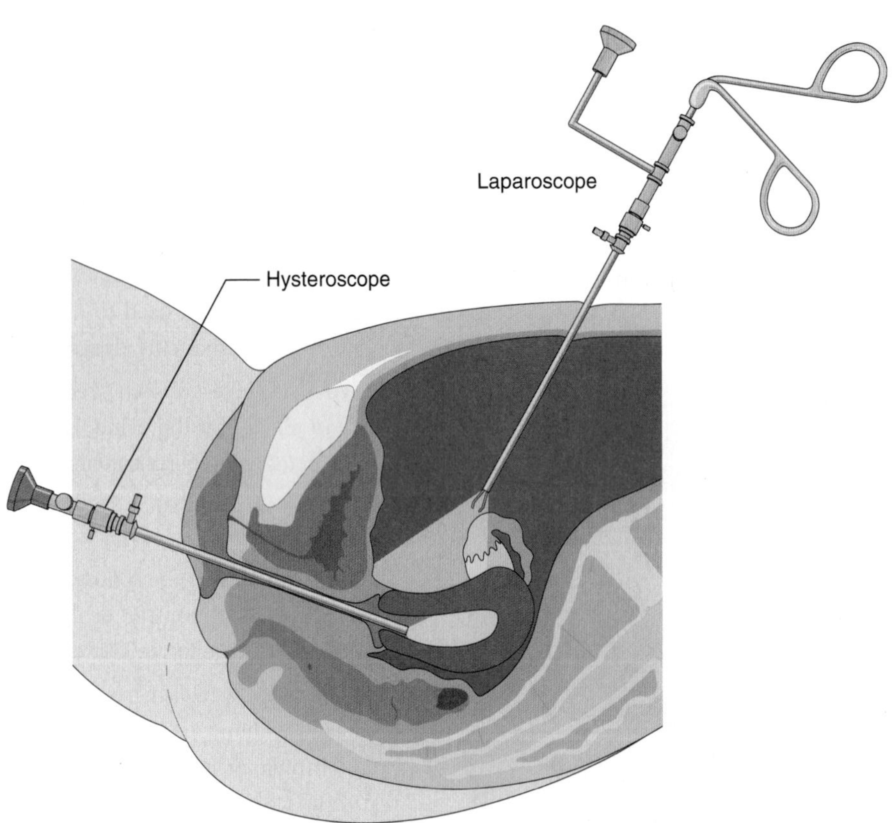

FIGURE 15.19 A laparoscope is used to examine the interior of the abdomen. A hysteroscope is used to examine the interior of the uterus.

through small incisions (see Figure 15.19). A laparoscope is used to:

- Explore and examine the interior of the abdomen.
- Take specimens to be biopsied.
- Perform surgical procedures.

CENTESIS

Centesis (sen-**TEE**-sis) is a surgical puncture to remove fluid for diagnostic purposes or to remove excess fluid. Note: Centesis is used alone as a noun or as a suffix in conjunction with the combining form describing the body part being treated.

- **Abdominocentesis** (ab-**dom**-ih-noh-sen-**TEE**-sis) is the surgical puncture of the abdominal cavity to remove fluid (**abdomin/o** means abdomen, and **-centesis** means a surgical puncture to remove fluid).
- *Amniocentesis*, which is a diagnostic test performed during pregnancy, is discussed in Chapter 14.
- **Arthrocentesis** (**ar**-throh-sen-**TEE**-sis) is a surgical puncture of the joint space to remove synovial fluid for analysis to determine the cause of pain or swelling in a joint (**arthr/o** means joint, and **-centesis** means a surgical puncture to remove fluid).
- **Cardiocentesis** (**kar**-dee-oh-sen-**TEE**-sis), also known as *cardiopuncture*, is the puncture of a chamber of the heart for diagnosis or therapy (**cardi/o** means heart, and **-centesis** means a surgical puncture to remove fluid).
- **Pericardiocentesis** (**pehr**-ih-**kar**-dee-oh-sen-**TEE**-sis) is the puncture of the pericardial sac for the purpose of removing fluid (**peri-** means surrounding, **cardi/o** means heart, and **-centesis** means a surgical puncture to remove fluid). This procedure is performed to treat pericarditis (see Chapter 5).
- **Tympanocentesis** (**tim**-pah-noh-sen-**TEE**-sis) is the surgical puncture of the tympanic membrane with a needle to remove fluid or pus from an infected the middle ear (**tympan/o** means eardrum, and **-centesis** means a surgical puncture to remove fluid).

IMAGING TECHNIQUES

Imaging techniques are used to visualize and examine internal body structures. The three most commonly used techniques are compared in Table 15.1. Two of these techniques are compared in Figure 15.20.

Contrast Medium

A **contrast medium** is administered by swallowing, via an enema, or intravenously to make specific body structures visible. Specialized substances are used depending upon the imaging systems and the body parts to be enhanced. These media are either radiopaque or radiolucent.

- **Radiopaque** (**ray**-dee-oh-**PAYK**) means that the substance *does not allow* x-rays to pass through and appears white or light gray on the resulting film. Radiopaque is the opposite of *radiolucent*.
- **Radiolucent** (**ray**-dee-oh-**LOO**-sent) means that the substance, such as air or nitrogen gas, *does allow* x-rays to pass through and appears black or dark gray on the resulting film. Radiolucent is the opposite of *radiopaque*.

TABLE 15.1

IMAGING SYSTEMS COMPARED

Method	How It Works
Radiography (x-ray)	Uses x-radiation (x-rays) passing through the patient to expose a film or create a digital image that shows the body in profile. In the resulting film, hard tissues are light, soft tissues are shades of gray, and air is black.
Computed tomography (CT)	Uses x-radiation (x-rays) with computer assistance to produce multiple cross-sectional views of the body. Hard tissues are light, and soft tissues appear as shades of gray.
Magnetic resonance imaging (MRI)	Uses a combination of radio waves and a strong magnetic field to produce images. Hard tissues are dark, and soft tissues appear as shades of gray.

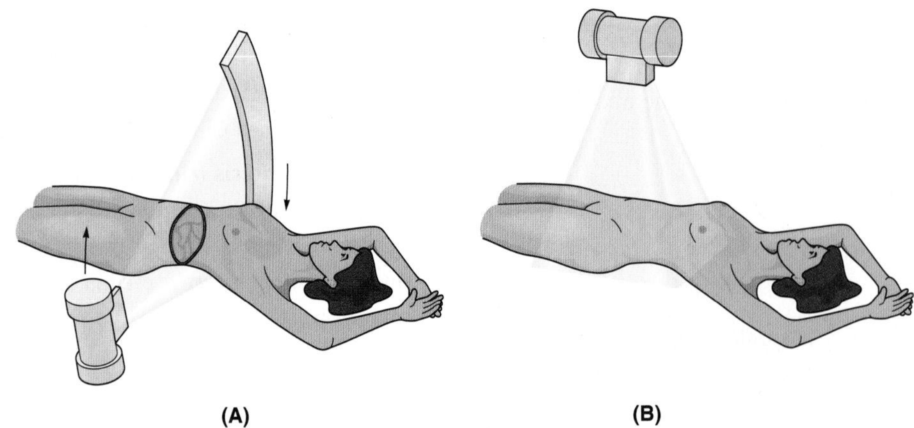

FIGURE 15.20 (A) Computed tomography provides cross-sectional images. (B) Conventional radiographs are able to capture images in only one plane and can superimpose anatomy.

- An **intravenous contrast medium** is injected into a vein to make the flow of blood through blood vessels and organs visible. This technique, which is usually named for the vessels or organs involved, is illustrated in Figure 5.22.

Barium

Barium (Ba) is a radiopaque contrast medium used primarily to visualize the gastrointestinal tract (Figure 15.21). It is administered orally as a *barium swallow* for an upper GI study. It is administered rectally as a *barium enema* for a lower GI study. Radiography and fluoroscopy are used to trace the flow of the barium.

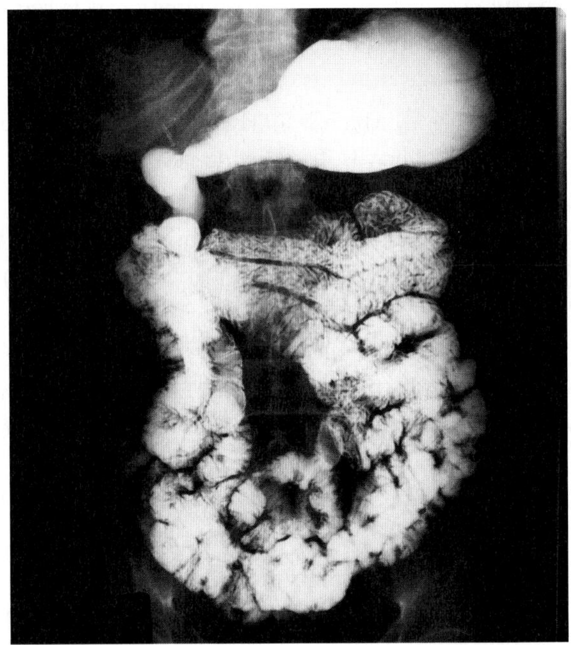

FIGURE 15.21 A radiograph after a barium swallow. The stomach and a portion of the small intestine are visible.

Radiology

In conventional **radiology**, also known as *x-rays*, an image of hard-tissue internal structures is created by the exposure of sensitized film to x-radiation (**radi/o** means radiation, and **-graphy** means the process of producing a picture or record). The resulting film is known as a *radiograph* or *radiogram*; however, it is commonly referred to as an *x-ray*.

- X-radiation, which is also referred to as *ionizing radiation*, is beneficial in producing diagnostic images and in treating cancer; however, excess exposure to this radiation is dangerous, and the effects are cumulative. Because x-radiation is invisible, has no odor, and cannot be felt, appropriate precautions must always be taken to protect the technician and the patient.
- Radiographs are made up of shades of gray. Radiopaque hard tissues, such as bone and tooth enamel, appear white or light gray on the radiograph. Radiolucent soft tissues appear as shades of gray to black on the radiograph (Figure 15.22).
- A **radiologist** (**ray**-dee-**OL**-oh-jist) is a physician who specializes in diagnosing and treating diseases and disorders with x-rays and other forms of radiant energy (**radi** means radiation, and **-ologist** means specialist).

Radiographic Positioning

The term **radiographic positioning** describes the body placement and the part of the body closest to the x-ray film. For example, in a left lateral position, the left side of the body is placed nearest the film.

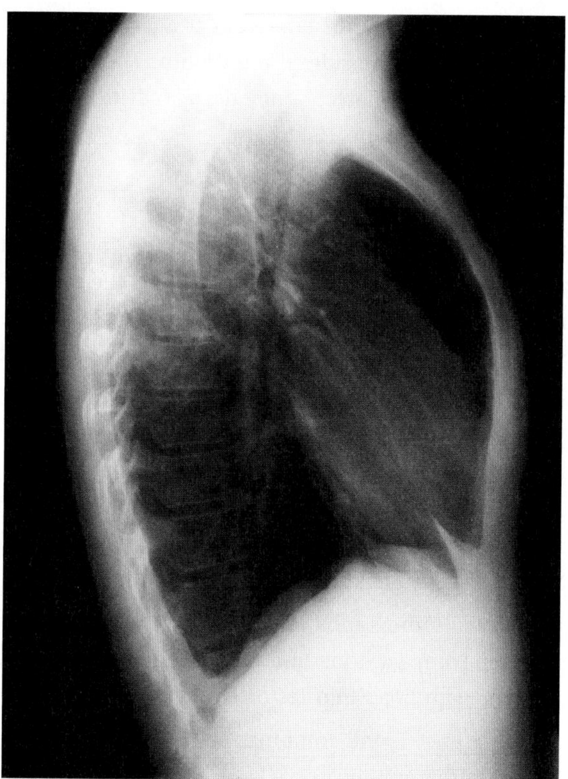

FIGURE 15.22 A lateral chest x-ray. Bones of the spine are white, and the soft tissues are shades of gray. The surrounding air is black.

Radiographic Projections

The term **radiographic projection** describes the path that the x-ray beam follows through the body from entrance to exit.

- When the name of the projection combines two terms into a single word, the term listed first is the one that the x-ray penetrates first.
- The basic projections described in the next section can be used for most body parts (Figure 15.23). These projections can be exposed with the patient in a standing or recumbent position.

Basic Radiographic Projections

- An **anteroposterior projection** (AP) has the patient positioned with the back parallel to the film (**anter/o** means front, **poster** means back, and **-ior** means pertaining to). The x-ray beam travels from anterior (front) to posterior (back).
- A **posteroanterior projection** (PA) has the patient positioned facing the film and parallel to it (**poster/o** means back, **anter** means front, and **-ior** means pertaining to). The x-ray beam travels through the body from posterior to anterior.
- A **lateral projection** (LAT) has the patient positioned at right angles to the film. This view is named for the side of the body nearest the film.

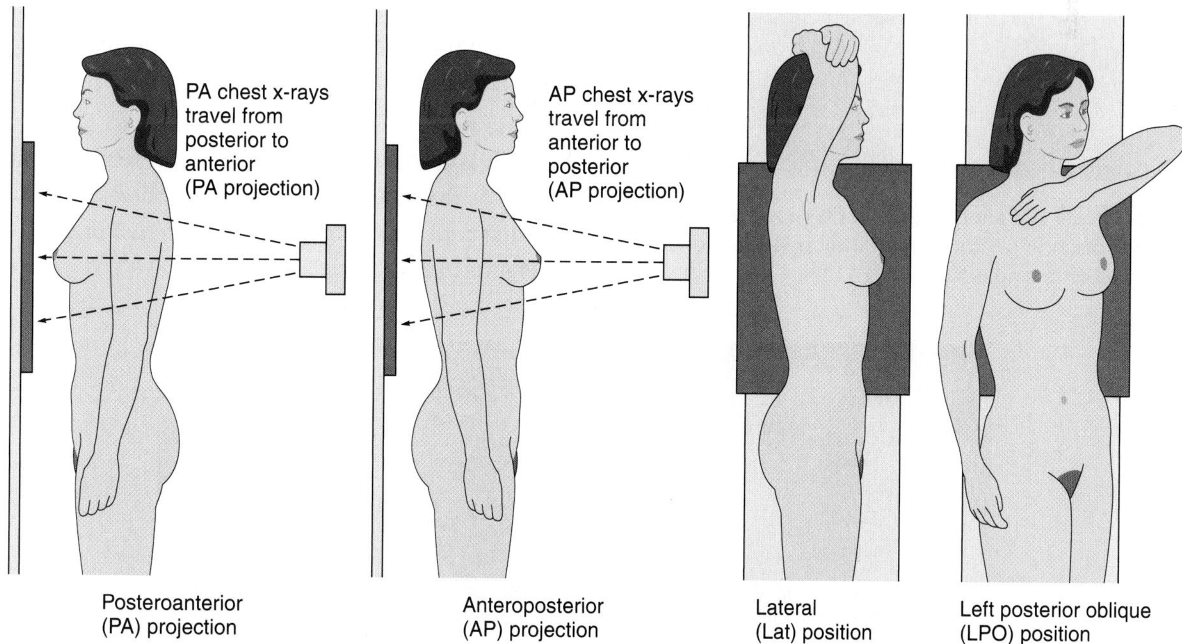

FIGURE 15.23 Radiographic projection positions: posteroanterior, anteroposterior. lateral. and left posterior oblique.

- An **oblique projection** (OBL) has the patient positioned so the body is slanted sideways to the film. This is halfway between a parallel and a right angle position. This view is named for the side of the body nearest the film. *Oblique* means slanted sideways.

Dental Radiography

Specialized techniques and equipment are used in obtaining dental radiographs.

- The term **extraoral radiography** means that the film is placed and exposed outside of the mouth. Figure 15.24 is a **panoramic radiograph**, which is commonly known as a *Panorex*, which shows all of the structures in both dental arches in a single film.
- **Intraoral radiography** means that the film is placed within the mouth and exposed by a camera positioned next to the exterior of the cheek (Figure 15.25).
- **Periapical radiographs** show the entire tooth and some surrounding tissue (**peri-** means surrounding, **apic** means apex, and **-al** means pertaining to). These films are used to detect abnormalities, such as an abscess at the tip of the root (see Figure 15.25A).

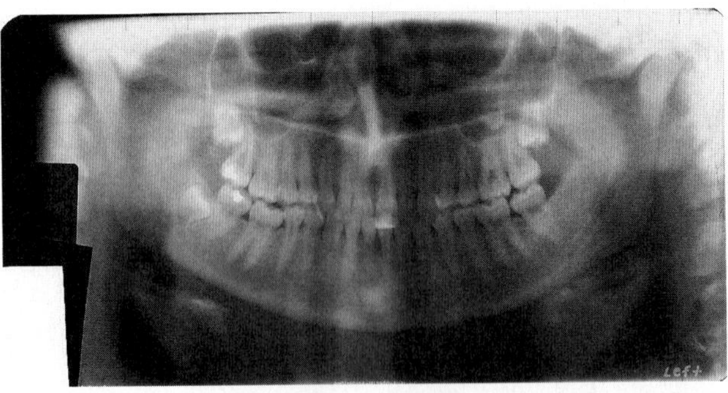

FIGURE 15.24 A Panorex radiograph shows all of the teeth and surrounding structures of the upper and lower dental arches on a single film.

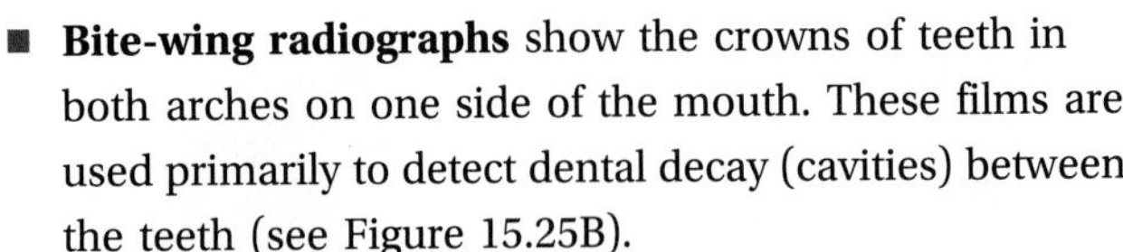

- **Bite-wing radiographs** show the crowns of teeth in both arches on one side of the mouth. These films are used primarily to detect dental decay (cavities) between the teeth (see Figure 15.25B).

Computed Tomography

Computed tomography (toh-**MOG**-rah-fee) uses a thin, fan-shaped x-ray beam that rotates around the patient to produce multiple cross-sectional views of the body (**tom/o** means to cut, section, or slice, and **-graphy** means the process of recording a picture or record) (Figure 15.26).

- Information gathered by radiation detectors is downloaded to a computer, analyzed, and converted into gray-scale images corresponding to anatomic slices of the body (Figure 15.27). These images are viewed on a monitor, stored as digital files, or printed as films.
- Computed tomography is more effective than MRI at imaging compact bone and is frequently preferred for patients with head injuries or strokes.
- *Tomotherapy* is the combination of tomography with radiation therapy to precisely target the tumor being treated, avoiding healthy tissue.

Magnetic Resonance Imaging

Magnetic resonance imaging, also known as *MRI*, uses a combination of radio waves and a strong magnetic field to create signals that are sent to a computer and converted into images of any plane through the body.

- These images can be produced in coronal, sagittal, or oblique planes and are created without the use of ionizing radiation (x-rays).
- These images have excellent low-contrast resolution, which is useful for differentiating soft tissue densities such as the tissues of the heart, blood vessels, brain, spinal cord, joints, muscles, and internal organs (Figure 15.28).

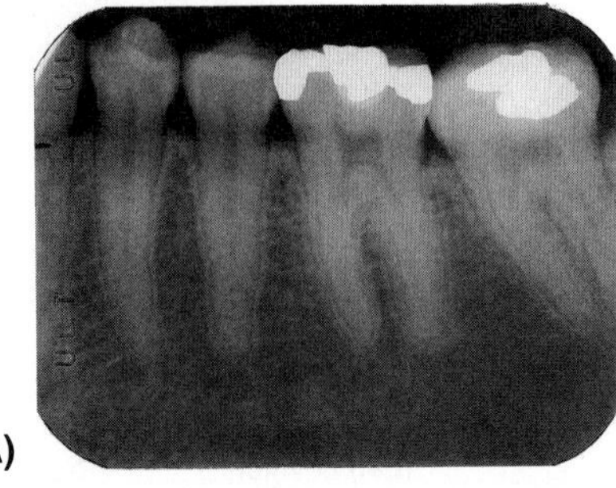

(A)

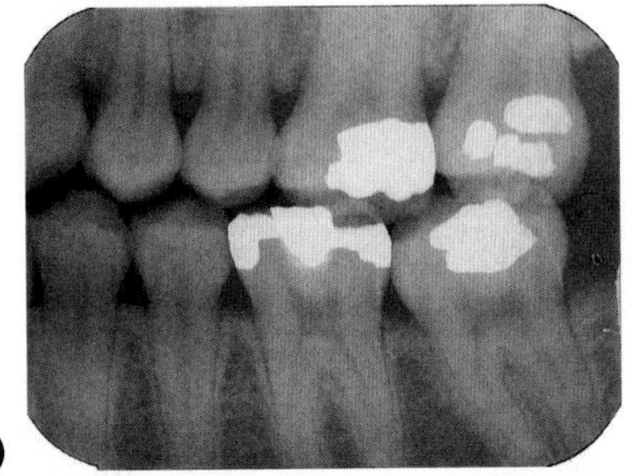

(B)

FIGURE 15.25 Intraoral dental radiographs. (A) A periapical film shows the entire length of a tooth and some of the tissues surrounding the root. (B) A bite-wing film shows the crowns of the upper and lower teeth in one area of both jaws. The white areas on these teeth are amalgam (silver) fillings.

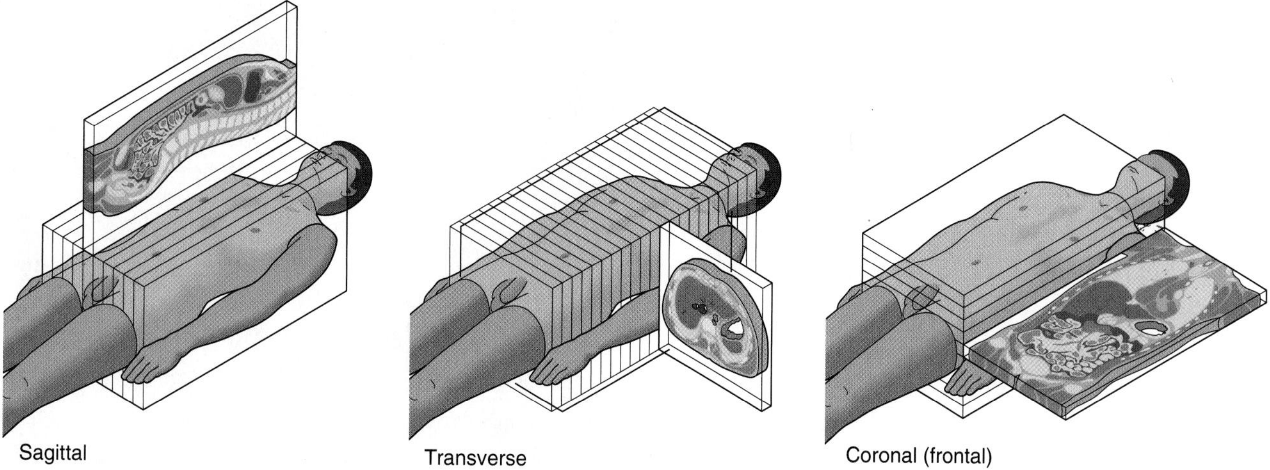

FIGURE 15.26 Computed tomography provides cross-sectional views of different body planes.

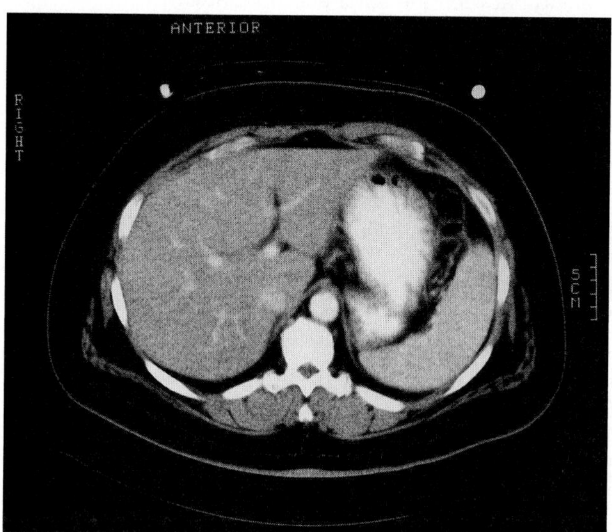

FIGURE 15.27 An abdominal CT scan in which the liver is predominant in the upper left and the stomach is visible in the upper right.

- Because of the use of powerful magnets, the presence of metal implants such as a knee replacement, an artificial pacemaker, or metal stents can be contraindications for using an MRI on a patient.
- *Closed architecture MRI*, which is the most commonly used type of equipment, produces the most accurate images; however, patients can be uncomfortable because of the noise generated by the machine and the feeling of being closed in. As an alternative *open architecture MRI* is designed to be less confining and is more comfortable for some patients.
- **Magnetic resonance angiography** (MRA), also known as *magnetic resonance angio*, combines MRI with the use of a contrast medium to locate problems within blood vessels throughout the body. This diagnostic imaging is frequently used as an alternative to conventional angiography, which is discussed in Chapter 5.

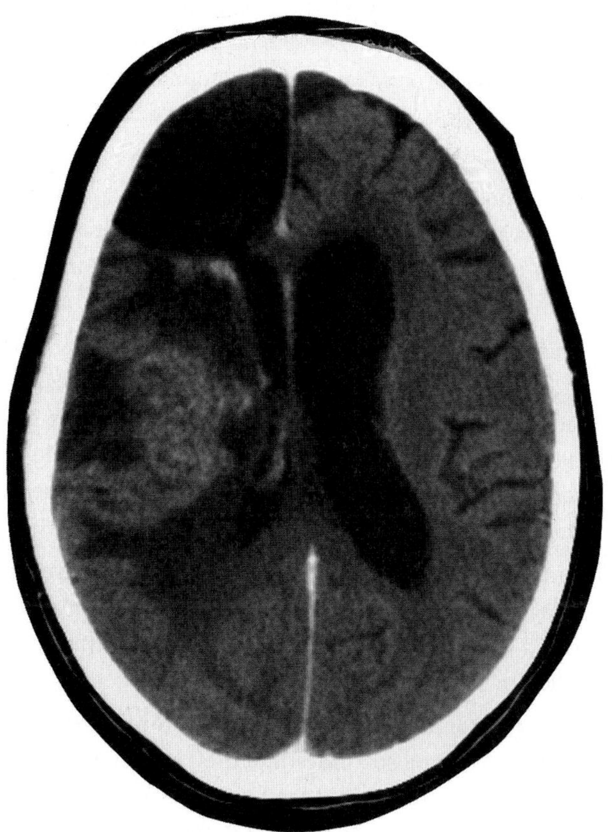

FIGURE 15.28 An MRI of the brain with a tumor visible in the upper left.

Fluoroscopy

Fluoroscopy (**floo**-or-**OS**-koh-pee) is the visualization of body parts in motion by projecting x-ray images on a luminous fluorescent screen (**fluor/o** means glowing, and **-scopy** means visual examination). *Luminous* means glowing.

- **Cineradiography** (**sin**-eh-**ray**-dee-**OG**-rah-fee) is the recording of images as they appear in motion on a fluorescent screen (**cine-** means relationship to movement, **radi/o** means radiation, and **-graphy** means process of recording a picture or record).
- Fluoroscopy can also be used in conjunction with conventional x-ray techniques to capture a record of parts of the examination.

Ultrasonography

Ultrasonography (**ul**-trah-son-**OG**-rah-fee), commonly referred to as *ultrasound* or *diagnostic ultrasound*, is imaging of deep body structures by recording the echoes of pulses of sound waves that are above the range of human hearing (**ultra-** means beyond, **son/o** means sound, and **-graphy** means the process of recording a picture or record).

- A **sonogram** (**SOH**-noh-gram) is the image created by ultrasonography (**son/o** means sound, and **-gram** means a picture or record). These images are created by a *sonographer* who is a technician specifically trained in this technique.
- This technique is most effective for viewing solid organs of the abdomen and soft tissues where the signal is not stopped by intervening bone or air. Common uses of ultrasound include evaluating fetal development, detecting the presence of gallstones, or confirming the presence of a mass found on a mammogram.
- *Carotid ultrasonography* is the use of sound waves to image the carotid artery to detect an obstruction that could cause an ischemic stroke, which is described in Chapter 10.
- **Echocardiography** (**eck**-oh-**kar**-dee-**OG**-rah-fee) is an ultrasonic diagnostic procedure used to evaluate the structures and motion of the heart (**ech/o** means sound, **cardi/o** means heart, and **-graphy** means the process of recording a picture or record). The resulting record is an *echocardiogram*.
- A **Doppler echocardiogram** is performed in the same way as an echocardiogram; however, this procedure measures the speed and direction of the blood flow within the heart. Shown in Figure 15.29 is a Doppler echocardiogram computer-enhanced with color.

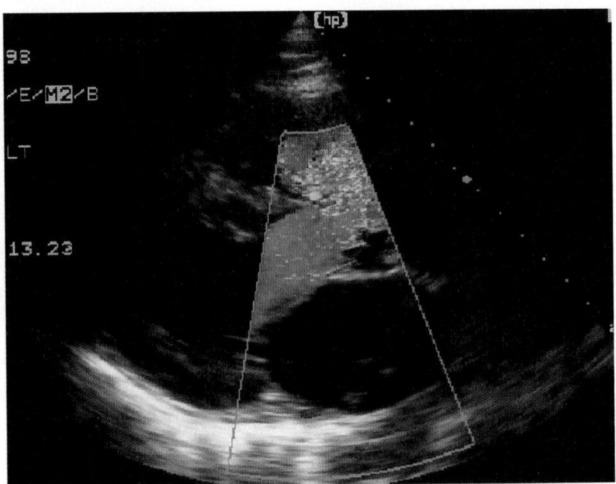

FIGURE 15.29 A Doppler echocardiogram. The large area of red shows the flow of blood through an abnormal opening between the aorta and right atrium.

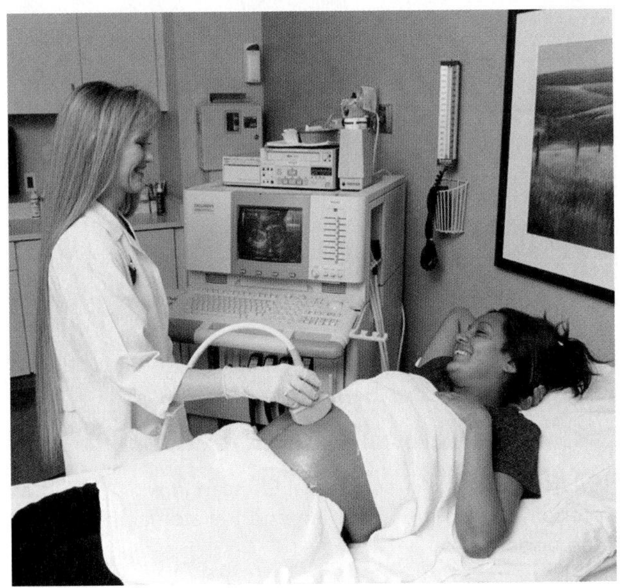
FIGURE 15.30 Fetal ultrasound is a noninvasive procedure used to image and evaluate fetal before birth.

- **Fetal ultrasound** is a noninvasive procedure used to image and evaluate fetal development during pregnancy (Figure 15.30). *3D/4D ultrasound* is a technique that uses specialized equipment to create photograph-like images of the developing child.
- **Transesophageal echocardiography** (**trans**-eh-**sof**-ah-**JEE**-al **eck**-oh-**kar**-dee-**OG**-rah-fee), also known as *TEE*, is an ultrasonic imaging technique used to evaluate heart structures. This diagnostic test is performed from inside the esophagus, and because the esophagus is so close to the heart, this technique produces clearer images than those obtained with echocardiography.

Nuclear Medicine

In **nuclear medicine** radioactive substances known as **radiopharmaceuticals** are administered for either diagnostic or treatment purposes. When used for diagnostic purposes, this is referred to as **nuclear imaging**, and these images document the structure and function of the organ or organs being examined.

- Each radiopharmaceutical contains a *radionuclide tracer*, also known as a *radioactive tracer*, which is specific to the body system being examined.
- Radiopharmaceuticals emit gamma rays that are detected by a gamma-ray camera attached to a computer. These data are used to generate an image showing the pattern of absorption that can be indicative of pathology.

Nuclear Scans

A **nuclear scan**, also known as a *scintigram*, is a diagnostic procedure that uses nuclear medicine technology to gather information about the structure and function of organs or body systems that cannot be seen on conventional x-rays.

Bone Scans

A **bone scan** is a nuclear scanning test that identifies new areas of bone growth or breakdown. The results are obtained after a radionuclide tracer is injected into the bloodstream, and the patient then waits while the material travels through the body tissues. This testing can be done to evaluate damage to the bones, detect cancer that has metastasized (spread) to the bones, and monitor conditions that can affect the bones. A bone scan can often detect a problem days to months earlier than a regular x-ray. Only pathology in the bones absorbs the radionuclide, and these are visible as dark areas on the scan shown in Figure 15.31, which shows bone cancer.

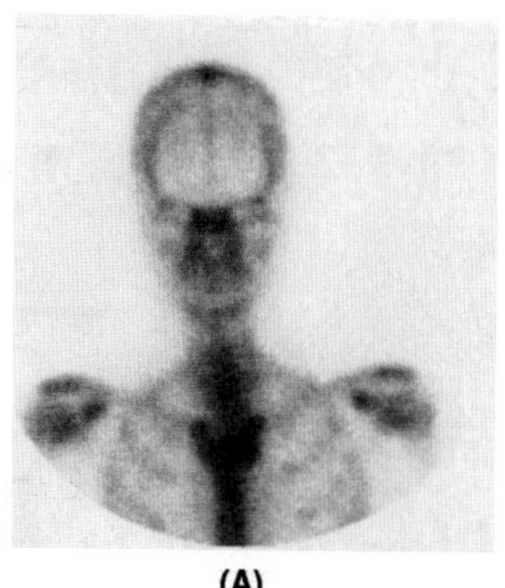

(A)

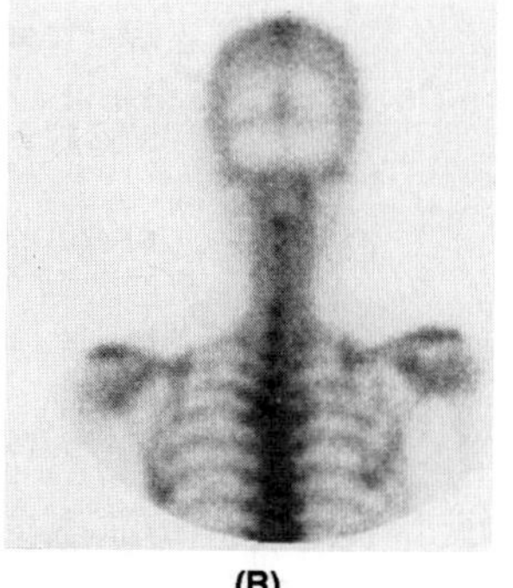

(B)

FIGURE 15.31 A bone scan of the head, shoulders, and upper spine. (A) Anterior view. (B) Posterior view.

Thyroid Scans

For a **thyroid scan**, a radiopharmaceutical containing radioactive iodine is administered. This scan makes use of the thyroid gland's ability to concentrate certain radioactive isotopes to generate images of it. A thyroid scan provides information about the size, shape, location, and relative activity of different parts of the thyroid gland.

Single Photon Emission Computed Tomography

Single photon emission computed tomography, also known as *SPECT*, is a type of nuclear imaging test that produces 3D computer-reconstructed images showing perfusion through tissues and organs. **Perfusion** (per-**FYOU**-zuhn) means the flow of blood through an organ.

- SPECT scanning is used primarily to view the flow of blood through arteries and veins in the brain.
- It is also useful in diagnosing blood-deprived areas of brain following a stroke, and tumors.

Positron Emission Tomography

Positron emission tomography, also known as *PET imaging*, combines tomography with radionuclide tracers to produce enhanced images of selected body organs or areas.

- PET scans of the whole body are often used to detect cancer and to examine the effects of cancer therapy.
- PET scans of the heart are used to determine blood flow to the heart muscle. This procedure helps to evaluate signs of coronary artery disease or to differentiate nonfunctional heart muscle from tissue that would benefit from a procedure such as angioplasty or coronary artery bypass surgery.
- PET scans of the brain are used to evaluate patients who have memory disorders of an undetermined cause, suspected or proven brain tumors, or seizure disorders that are not responsive to medical therapy and are therefore candidates for surgery.

PHARMACOLOGY

Pharmacology is the study of the nature, uses, and effects of drugs for medical purposes (**pharmac** means drug, and **-ology** means study of).

- A **pharmacist** is a licensed specialist who formulates and dispenses prescribed medications.

Prescription and Over-the-Counter Drugs

- A **prescription** drug is a medication that can legally be dispensed only by a pharmacist with an order from a licensed professional such as a physician or dentist. Abbreviations commonly used in prescriptions and drug administration are shown in Table 15.2.
- An **over-the-counter** drug, also known as an *OTC*, is a medication that can be purchased without a prescription.

Generic and Brand-Name Drugs

- A **generic drug** is usually named for its chemical structure and is not protected by a brand name or trademark. For example, *diazepam* is the generic name of a drug frequently used as skeletal muscle relaxant, sedative, and antianxiety agent.
- A **brand-name** drug is sold under the name given the drug by the manufacturer. A brand name is always spelled with a capital letter. For example, *Valium* is a brand name for diazepam.

Terminology Related to Pharmacology

- An **addiction** is compulsive, uncontrollable dependence on a drug, alcohol, or other substance. It can also be a habit, or practice, which cannot be stopped without causing severe emotional, mental, or physiologic reactions.
- An **adverse drug reaction** (ADR), also known as a *side effect*, is an undesirable reaction that accompanies the principal response for which the drug was taken.
- **Compliance** is the patient's consistency and accuracy in following the regimen prescribed by a physician or other health care professional. As used here, *regimen* means directions or rules.
- A **contraindication** is a factor in the patient's condition that makes the use of a medication or specific treatment dangerous or ill advised.
- A **drug interaction** is the result of drugs reacting with each other, often in ways that are unexpected or potentially harmful. Such interactions can also occur when medications are taken along with herbal remedies.
- An **idiosyncratic reaction** (**id**-ee-oh-sin-**KRAT**-ick) is an unexpected reaction to a drug that is peculiar to the individual.

TABLE 15.2

FREQUENTLY USED DRUG ADMINISTRATION ABBREVIATIONS AND SYMBOLS

Abbreviation	Meaning	Abbreviation	Meaning
@	at	q.i.d.	four times a day
ac	before meals	↑	increase
ad lib	as desired	↓	decrease
amt	amount	>	greater than
b.i.d., bid	twice a day	≥	greater than or equal to
$\bar{c}$	with	<	less than
NPO	nothing by mouth	≤	less than or equal to
p.c.	after meals	Rx	prescription
p.o.	by mouth	sig	to be labeled accordingly
p.r.n.	as needed	t.i.d.	three times a day
q.d.	every day	♀	female
q.h.	every hour	♂	male

- A **palliative** (**PAL**-ee-**ay**-tiv) is a substance that eases the pain or severity of the symptoms of a disease, but does not cure it.
- A **paradoxical reaction** is the result of medical treatment that yields the exact opposite of normally expected results. *Paradoxical* means not being normal or the usual kind.
- A **placebo** (plah-**SEE**-boh) is an inactive substance, such as a sugar pill or liquid, that is administered only for its suggestive effects. In medical research, a placebo is administered to one group and the drug being studied is administered to another group.
- In medicine, **potentiation** (poh-**ten**-shee-**AY**-shun) is a drug interaction that occurs when the effect of one drug is increased by another drug, herbal remedy, or other treatment. *Potentiate* means to enhance the effects of a drug.
- An **antipyretic** (**an**-tih-pye-**RET**-ick) is medication administered to prevent or reduce fever (**anti-** means against, **pryet** means fever, and **-ic** means pertaining to). These medications, such as aspirin and acetaminophen, act by lowering a raised body temperature; however, they do not affect a normal body temperature when a fever is not present.
- An **anti-inflammatory** relieves inflammation and pain without affecting consciousness.

Medications for Pain Management

Acute pain generally comes on suddenly as the result of disease, inflammation, or injury to tissues. When the cause of the pain is diagnosed and treated, the pain goes away.

Chronic pain persists over a longer period of time than acute pain and is resistant to most medical treatments. It often causes severe problems for the patient.

Analgesics

The term **analgesic** (**an**-al-**JEE**-zick) refers to the class of drugs that relieves pain without affecting consciousness. These include such drugs as aspirin, acetaminophen, and ibuprofen.

Nonnarcotic analgesics, such as aspirin, are sold over the counter for mild to moderate pain. Prescription pain relievers, sold through a pharmacy under the direction of a physician, are used for more moderate to severe pain.

Narcotic analgesics, such as morphine, Demerol, and codeine are available by prescription only to relieve severe pain. These medications also have a sedative (calming) effect, and can cause physical dependence or addiction.

- **Acetaminophen** (ah-**seet**-ah-**MIN**-oh-fen) is an analgesic that reduces pain and fever, but does not relieve inflammation; however, it does not have the negative side effects of NSAIDS. This substance is basic ingredient found in Tylenol® and its generic equivalents.
- **Nonsteroidal anti-inflammatory drugs**, commonly known as *NSAIDs*, are nonnarcotic analgesics administered to control pain by reducing inflammation and swelling. NSAIDS, such as aspirin and ibuprofen, are available over the counter. Stronger NSAIDs are available by prescription. Medications in this group can cause side effects, including attacking the stomach lining and thinning the blood.
- **Ibuprofen** (eye-byoo-**pro**-fen) is a nonsteroidal anti-inflammatory medicine that is sold over the counter under the brand names of Advil and Motrin. This medication acts an analgesic to relieve the pain of arthritis. It also acts as an antipyretic.
- Although pain management is not their primary roles, **anticonvulsants** and **antidepressants** have been found to be effective as part of some chronic pain management programs. *Anticonvulsants* are traditionally administered to prevent seizures such as those associated with epilepsy. *Antidepressants* are primarily administered to prevent or relieve depression.

Addition Pain Control Methods

- **Pain-relieving creams** are applied topically to relieve pain due to conditions such as osteoarthritis and rheumatoid arthritis. The primary active ingredient in these ointments is *capsaicin*, a chemical found in chili peppers.
- **Transcutaneous electronic nerve stimulation**, also known as *TENS*, is a method of pain control by wearing a device that delivers small electrical impulses, as needed, to the nerve endings through the skin (**trans-** means across, **cutane** means skin, and **-ous** means pertaining to). These electrical impulses cause changes in muscles, such as numbness or contractions, which produce temporary pain relief. The term *transcutaneous* means performed through the unbroken skin.

Methods of Drug Administration

- **Inhalation administration** describes vapors and gases taken in through the nose or mouth and absorbed into the bloodstream through the lungs. One example is the use of a metered-dose inhaler to treat asthma (see Chapter 7) or the gases used for general anesthesia (see Chapter 10).

- **Oral administration** refers to medications taken by mouth to be absorbed through the walls of the stomach or small intestine. These drugs can be in the form of liquids, tablets (pills), or capsules. Medications to be released in the small intestine are covered with an *enteric coating* to prevent them from being absorbed in the stomach.
- **Rectal administration** is the insertion of medication in the rectum either in the form of a suppository or a liquid. A *suppository* is medication in a semisolid form that is introduced into the rectum. The suppository melts at body temperature, and the medication is absorbed through the surrounding tissues.
- **Sublingual administration** is the placement of medication under the tongue where it is allowed to dissolve slowly (**sub-** means under, **lingu** means tongue, and **-al** means pertaining to). Because the sublingual tissues are highly vascular, the medication is quickly absorbed directly into the bloodstream. *Highly vascular* means containing many blood vessels.
- A **topical application** is a liquid or ointment that is rubbed into the skin on the area to be treated. Examples: *cortisone ointment* is applied topically to relieve itching and to speed healing; *antibiotic ointments* are applied over minor wounds to prevent infection.
- A **transdermal** medication is administered from a patch that is applied to unbroken skin (**trans-** means through or across, **derm** means skin, and **-al** means pertaining to). The medication, which is continuously released by the patch, is absorbed through the skin and transmitted to the bloodstream so that it can produce a systemic effect. These multilayered patches are used to convey medications, such as nitroglycerin for angina, hormones for hormone replacement therapy, or nicotine patches for smoking cessation (Figure 15.32).

Parenteral Administration

The term **parenteral** (pah-**REN**-ter-al) means taken into the body, or administered, in a manner other than through the digestive tract. The most common use of parenteral administration is by injection through a *hypodermic syringe* (Figure 15.33).

- A **subcutaneous injection** (SC) is made into the fatty layer just below the skin.
- An **intradermal injection** is made into the middle layers of the skin.
- An **intramuscular injection** (IM) is made directly into muscle tissue.
- An **intravenous injection** (IV) is made directly into a vein. A *peripherally inserted central catheter,*

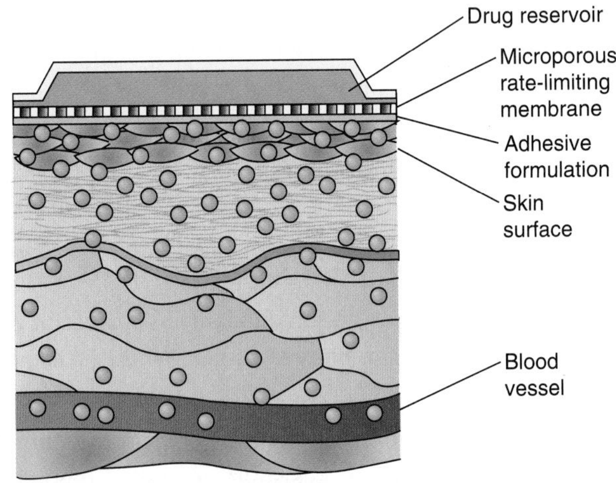

FIGURE 15.32 Transdermal medication administered by a "patch" is released through the intact skin at a controlled rate. This provides timed release into the bloodstream.

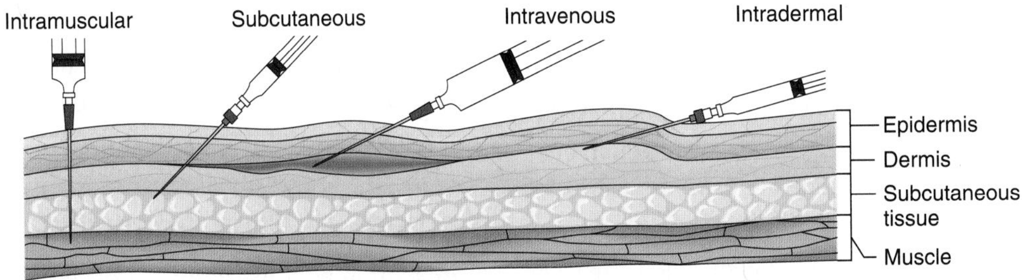

FIGURE 15.33 Types of injections.

commonly known as a *PICC line*, may be used for a patient who will need IV therapy for more than 7 days.

- A **bolus** (**BOH**-lus), also known as a *bolus infusion*, is a single, concentrated dose of drug usually injected into a blood vessel over a short period of time. The term bolus is also used in relation to the digestive system and is discussed in Chapter 8.

ABBREVIATIONS RELATED TO DIAGNOSTIC PROCEDURES AND PHARMACOLOGY

Table 15.3 presents an overview of the abbreviations related to the terms introduced in this chapter. Note: To avoid errors or confusion, always be cautious when using abbreviations.

TABLE 15.3
ABBREVIATIONS RELATED TO THE DIAGNOSTIC PROCEDURES AND PHARMACOLOGY

beats per minute = bpm	**bpm** = beats per minute
blood pressure = BP	**BP** = blood pressure
blood urea nitrogen = BUN	**BUN** = blood urea nitrogen
complete blood count = CBC	**CBC** = complete blood count
endoscopy = endo	**endo** = endoscopy
erythrocyte sedimentation rate = ESR	**ESR** = erythrocyte sedimentation rate
hematocrit = Hct, hct	**Hct, hct** = hematocrit
red blood count = RBC	**RBC** = red blood count
respiratory rate = RR	**RR** = respiratory rate
temperature, pulse, respiration = TPR	**TPR** = temperature, pulse, respiration
white blood count = WBC	**WBC** = white blood count

Career Opportunities

In addition to the medical specialties already discussed, some of the health occupations that involve diagnostic procedures and pharmacology include:

- **Medical laboratory technologist (MT)** or **clinical laboratory technologist:** works under the supervision of a pathologist to study tissues, fluids, and cells of the human body to help determine the presence and/or cause of disease. Specialties include:

  Clinical chemistry

  Blood bank technology and hematology

  Microbiology

  Immunology

- **Medical laboratory technician (MLT):** works under the supervision of an MT or pathologist, performing many of the routine tests that do not require advanced knowledge
- **Histologic technician:** works under the supervision of an MT to cut and stain tissue specimens for microscopic examination
- **Medical laboratory assistant:** prepares specimens for testing, and helps clean and maintain laboratory equipment
- **Pharmacy technician:** works under the supervision of a pharmacist, preparing medications for dispensing to patients, labeling medications, preparing IV solutions, maintaining records, and ordering supplies
- **Radiologic technologist (RT)** or **X-ray technician:** works under the supervision of a radiologist to take x-rays for diagnostic purposes, administer radiation, and use nuclear medicine, ultrasound, and magnetic resonance for the diagnosis and treatment of disease
- **MRI technologist:** an RT with specialized training who works with magnetic resonance imaging
- **Radiation therapy technologist:** prepares cancer patients for treatment and administers prescribed doses of ionizing radiation to specific body parts
- **Sonographer** or **ultrasound technologist:** conducts ultrasound tests. Subspecialties in this field include echocardiography (heart), neurosonography (brain), obstetrics and gynecology, and vascular sonography (blood vessels).

Health Occupation Profile

Medical Technologist

Laurie Howland has been a medical technologist, or clinical laboratory scientist, for over 30 years. *"A love of science and math first led me to the clinical laboratory field. I was fascinated by biology and chemistry labs, wanted an active job where I could do things with my hands, and did not want to be chained to a desk. I can report that my career definitely meets these objectives. I've been pleased with a health care profession that is 'behind the scenes', yet still critical to the care of patients, and always on the leading edge of new treatments and advances in medicine.*

"I've had the opportunity to work in the endocrinology, radioimmunoassay, and chemistry departments. I now focus my efforts on a computer system unique to hospital laboratories. This is a very good profession for full-time or flexible, part-time work. There are also opportunities to stretch beyond the hospital or clinic. I have colleagues who work in the pharmaceutical field and for laboratory instrumentation, computer, and agricultural businesses."

Study Break

Everyone knows that one of the most important *vital signs* is body temperature. One of the most obvious indications of illness is an elevated body temperature, or fever, as the body attempts to kill certain viruses and bacteria that are sensitive to heat.

But is the body always the same temperature?

No. Not every person has 98.6°F as the normal temperature. And most individuals find that their temperature rises during the late afternoon and drops at night. When we go outside, we may lose body temperature when it is cold outside or warm up if it is hot. The body will attempt to equalize this change in temperature through shivering, sweating, and other adjustments to the skin.

Women also have a slight change in body temperature throughout their menstrual cycle. That is why women who are trying to get pregnant will sometimes take a daily temperature reading upon awakening and will try to have intercourse when a dip in body temperature indicates that they may be about to ovulate.

Review Time

Write the answers to the following questions on a separate piece of paper or in your notebook. In addition, be prepared to take part in the classroom discussion.

1. ***Written Assignment:*** Describe the difference between **palpation** and **percussion**.

   Discussion Assignment: What are these techniques used to examine?

2. ***Written Assignment:*** Using terms a physician would understand, identify three conditions a **hematocrit (Hct) test** would be used to diagnose.

   Discussion Assignment: How would you explain to a patient the need for this test?

continues

3. ***Written Assignment:*** Describe the differences between **acetaminophen** and **ibuprofen**.

   Discussion Assignment: Which of these medications would be used to control the pain of conditions such as arthritis?

4. ***Written Assignment:*** Describe the differences between **computed tomography** and **magnetic resonance imaging**.

   Discussion Assignment: Why are some patients uncomfortable about undergoing a closed architecture MRI? What alternative in the design of the equipment might make the patient more comfortable?

5. Dr. Vaughn instructs you to position the patient for a vaginal examination.

   Written Assignment: Name the examination position you would use and describe how the patient would be placed.

   Discussion Assignment: What steps should be taken to maintain the patient's modesty in this examination position?

Optional Internet Activity

The goal of this activity is to help you learn more about medical terminology as it applies to the "real world." Select **one** *of these two options and follow the instructions.*

1. Search for information about a **bone scan**. Write a brief (one- or two-paragraph) report on something new you learned here and include the address of the web site where you found this information.
2. To learn more about **radiology**, go to the web site of the Radiological Society of North America. Write a brief (one- or two-paragraph) report on something new you learned here about careers in this field.

THE HUMAN TOUCH: CRITICAL THINKING ACTIVITY

The following story and questions are designed to stimulate critical thinking through class discussion or as a brief essay response. There are no right or wrong answers to these questions.

The pharmacy was crowded when Jorge Padilla, 21, arrived with his brother, Ramon, 15, to fill Ramon's prescriptions for antibiotics and pain relievers. They didn't like having to wait, but this was their only chance to get these prescriptions filled before Ramon had dental surgery the next day. At least they'd brought books to read, Jorge thought to himself as they took a number. When their number was finally called, a pharmacist hurriedly took the prescription slips and rushed into the back to fill the orders.

Soon the pharmacist returned two bottles of pills in a bag. He gave them to Jorge with brief instructions on how to use them. **"To prevent an infection from the surgery, have your brother start taking the antibiotics today. Be sure to finish all of these pills. Ramon can start taking the pain meds after the surgery. Take one or two every 8 hours as needed, but be careful, because they may make him drowsy or dizzy."**

continues

Jorge paid for the pills and headed home. Jorge gave the bottles to his brother, and Ramon assured him that he had listened carefully to the instructions. Ramon took one of the antibiotics immediately, and about half an hour after taking the pill, he started feeling sleepy and confused. Ramon went to bed early and felt better the next morning. But after he took the second dose of antibiotics, he started feeling dizzy again. But he thought it was just nerves, so they soon left for the surgery.

The procedure went well, and Ramon was home by the end of the day. He was still slightly woozy from the anesthesia, and said he was in a lot of pain despite taking the highest doses of pain relievers that had been prescribed. Jorge didn't know what was wrong. He called the oral surgeon for advice. **"I don't know what to do. The pills aren't helping Ramon's pain, and the antibiotics he took before the surgery made him feel sick. I think something's wrong."** *The dentist asked him to describe the pills, and Jorge called upstairs to find out from Ramon what they look liked.* **"The antibiotics are small, round pills, and the pain relievers are large, oval ones,"** *he replied. The dentist realized that somehow the prescriptions had gotten mixed up, and Ramon had taken the wrong pills.*

Suggested Discussion Topics

1. Discuss what should have been done to prevent the mix-up of the two types of pills.
2. Discuss the responsibility of the pharmacist in verifying that the prescriptions were correctly filled and labeled.
3. Discuss whether the dentist, or a staff member, should have verified before surgery that Ramon was taking the correct pills. Should Ramon's odd behavior made them suspicious about the medication?
4. The dentist prescribed the appropriate medications. Discuss whether the dentist has any responsibility in this mix-up.

STUDENT WORKBOOK AND StudyWARE™ CD-ROM

1. Go to your **Student Workbook** and complete the Learning Exercises for this chapter.

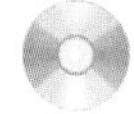

2. Go to the **StudyWARE™ CD-ROM** and have fun with the exercises and games for this chapter.

APPENDIX A

Prefixes, Combining Forms, and Suffixes

Pertaining to

-ac pertaining to
-al pertaining to
-ar pertaining to
-ary pertaining to
-eal pertaining to
-ical pertaining to
-ial pertaining to
-ic pertaining to
-ine pertaining to
-ior pertaining to
-ory pertaining to
-ous pertaining to
-tic pertaining to

Abnormal Conditions

-ago abnormal condition, disease
-esis abnormal condition, disease
-ia abnormal condition, disease
-iasis abnormal condition, disease
-ion condition
-ism condition, state of
-osis abnormal condition, disease

Noun Endings

-a noun ending
-e noun ending
-um singular noun ending
-us singular noun ending
-y noun ending

A

a-	no, not, without, away from, negative
-a	noun ending
ab-	away from, negative, absent
abdomin/o	abdomen
-able	capable of, able to
abort/o	premature expulsion of a nonviable fetus
abrad/o, abras/o	rub or scrape off
abrupt/o	broken away from
abs-	away from
abscess/o	collection of pus, going away
absorpt/o	suck up, suck in
-ac	pertaining to
acanth/o	spiny, thorny
acetabul/o	acetabulum (hip socket)
-acious	characterized by
acne/o	point or peak
acous/o, acoust/o	hearing, sound
acquir/o	get, obtain
acr/o	extremities (hands and feet), top, extreme point
acromi/o	acromion, point of shoulder blade
actin/o	light
acu/o	sharp, severe, sudden
acuit/o, acut/o	sharp, sharpness
acust/o, -acusia, -acusis	hearing, sense of hearing
ad-	toward, to, in the direction of
aden/o	gland
adenoid/o	adenoids
adhes/o	stick to, cling to
adip/o	fat
adnex/o	bound to
adren/o, adrenal/o	adrenal glands
aer/o	air, gas
aesthet/o	sensation, sense of perception
af-	toward, to
affect/o	exert influence on
agglutin/o	clumping, stick together
aggress/o	attack, step forward
-ago	abnormal condition, disease
agor/a	marketplace
-agra	excessive pain, seizure, attack of severe pain
-aise	comfort, ease
-al	pertaining to
alb/i, alb/o, albumin/o	white
albumin/o	albumin, protein
alg/e, algi/o, alg/o, algesi/o	relationship to pain
-algesia, -algesic	painful, pain sense
-algia	pain, painful condition
align/o	bring into line or correct position
aliment/o	to nourish
all/o, all-	other, different from normal, reversal
alopec/o	baldness, mangy
alveol/o	alveolus, air sac, small sac
ambi-	both sides, around or about, double
ambly/o	dull, dim
ambul/o, ambulat/o	walk
ametr/o	out of proportion
-amine	nitrogen compound
amni/o	amnion, fetal membrane
amph-	around, on both sides, doubly
amput/o, amputat/o	cut away, cut off a part of the body
amyl/o	starch
an-	no, not, without
an-, ana-	up, apart, backward, excessive
an/o	anus, ring
-an	characteristic of, pertaining to
-ancy	state of
andr/o	relationship to the male
aneurysm/o	aneurysm
angi/o	blood or lymph vessel
angin/o	angina, choking, strangling
anis/o	unequal
ankyl/o	crooked, bent, stiff
anomal/o	irregularity
ante-	before, in front of
anter/o	before, front
anthrac/o	coal, coal dust
anti-	against
anxi/o, anxiet/o	anxiety, anxious, uneasy
aort/o	aorta
ap-	toward, to
-apheresis	removal
aphth/o	ulcer
apic/o	apex
ap-, apo-	separation, away from, opposed, detached
aplast/o	defective development, lack of development
aponeur/o	aponeurosis (type of tendon)

apoplect/o	a stroke
append/o, appendic/o	appendix
aqu/i, aqu/o, aque/o	water
-ar	pertaining to
arachn/o	spider web, spider
arc/o	bow, arc or arch
-arche	beginning
areat/o	occurring in patches or circumscribed areas
areol/o	little open space
-aria	connected with
arrect/o	upright, lifted up, raised
arter/o, arteri/o	artery
arthr/o	joint
articul/o	joint
-ary	pertaining to
as-	toward, to
asbest/o	asbestos
-ase	enzyme
aspir/o, aspirat/o	to breathe in
asthen-, -asthenia	weakness, lack of strength
asthmat/o	gasping, choking
astr/o	star, star-shaped
at-	toward, to
atel/o	incomplete, imperfect
ather/o	plaque, fatty substance
athet/o	uncontrolled
atop/o	strange, out of place
atres/i	without an opening
atri/o	atrium
attenuat/o	diluted, weakened
aud-, audi/o, audit/o	ear, hearing, the sense of hearing
aur/i, aur/o	ear, hearing
auscult/a, auscult/o	listen
aut/o	self
-ax	noun ending
ax/o	axis, main stem
axill/o	armpit
azot/o	urea, nitrogen

B

bacill/o	rod-shaped bacterium (plural, bacteria)
bacteri/o	bacteria (singular, bacterium)
balan/o	glans penis
bar/o	pressure, weight
bartholin/o	Bartholin's gland
bas/o	base, opposite of acid
bi-	twice, double, two
bi/o	life
bifid/o	split, divided into two parts
bifurcat/o	divide or fork into two branches
bil/i	bile, gall
bilirubin/o	bilirubin
bin-	two by two
-blast	embryonic, immature, formative element
blephar/o	eyelid
borborygm/o	rumbling sound
brachi/o	arm
brachy-	short
brady-	slow
brev/i, brev/o	short
bronch/i, bronchi/o, bronch/o	bronchial tube, bronchus
bronchiol/o	bronchiole, bronchiolus
brux/o	grind
bucc/o	cheek
burs/o	bursa, sac of fluid near joint
byssin/o	cotton dust

C

cadaver/o	dead body, corpse
calcane/o	calcaneus, heel bone
calc/i	calcium, lime, the heel
calci-, calc/o	calcium
calcul/o	stone, little stone
cali/o, calic/o	cup, calyx
call/i, callos/o	hard, hardened and thickened
calor/i	heat
canalicul/o	little canal or duct
canth/o	corner of the eye
capill/o	hair
capit/o	head
capn/o	carbon dioxide, sooty or smoky appearance
capsul/o	little box
carb/o	carbon
carbuncl/o	carbuncle
carcin/o	cancerous
cardi/o, card/o	heart
cari/o	rottenness, decay
carot/o	stupor, sleep
carp/o	wrist bones
cartilag/o	cartilage, gristle

caruncul/o	bit of flesh
cat-, cata-, cath-	down, lower, under, downward
catabol/o	a breaking down
cathart/o	cleansing, purging
cathet/o	insert, send down
caud/o	lower part of body, tail
caus/o, caust/o	burning, burn
cauter/o, caut/o	heat, burn
cav/i, cav/o	hollow, cave
cavern/o	containing hollow spaces
cec/o	cecum
-cele	hernia, tumor, swelling
celi/o, cel/o	abdomen, belly
cement/o	cementum, a rough stone
cent-	hundred
-centesis	surgical puncture to remove fluid
cephal/o, -ceps	head
cera-	wax
cerebell/o	cerebellum
cerebr/o	cerebrum, brain
cerumin/o	cerumen, earwax
cervic/o	neck, cervix (neck of uterus)
cheil/o	lip or lips
cheir/o	hand
chem./i, chem/o, chemic/o	drug, chemical
chir/o	hand
chlor/o	green
chlorhydr/o	hydrochloric acid
chol/e	bile, gall
cholangi/o	bile duct
cholecyst/o	gallbladder
choledoch/o	common bile duct
cholesterol/o	cholesterol
chondr/i, chondr/o	cartilage
chord/o	spinal cord, cord
chore/o	dance
chori/o, chorion/o	chorion, membrane
choroid/o	choroid layer of eye
chrom/o, chromat/o	color
chron/o	time
chym/o	to pour, juice
cib/o	meal
cicatric/o	scar
-cidal	pertaining to killing
-cide	causing death
cili/o	eyelashes, microscopic hair-like projections
cine-	relationship to movement
circ/i	ring or circle
circulat/o	circulate, go around in a circle
circum-	around, about
circumcis/o	cutting around
circumscrib/o	confined, limited in space
cirrh/o	orange-yellow, tawny
cis/o	cut
clasis, -clast	break down
claudicat/o	limping
claustr/o	barrier
clav/i	key
clavicul/o, cleid/o	clavicle, collar bone
climacter/o	crisis, rung of a ladder
clitor/o	clitoris
-clonus	violent action
clus/o	shut or close
-clysis	irrigation, washing
co-	together, with
coagul/o, coagulat/o	clotting, coagulation
coarct/o, coarctat/o	press together, narrow
cocc/i, cocc/o, -coccus	spherical bacteria
coccyg/o	coccyx, tailbone
cochle/o	spiral, snail, snail shell
coher/o, cohes/o	cling, stick together
coit/o	a coming together
col/o	colon, large intestine
coll/a	glue
colon/o	colon, large intestine
colp/o	vagina
column/o	pillar
com-	together, with
comat/o	deep sleep
comminut/o	break into pieces
communic/o	share, to make common
compatibil/o	sympathize with
con-	together, with
concav/o	hollow
concentr/o	condense, intensify, remove excess water
concept/o	become pregnant
conch/o	shell
concuss/o	shaken together, violently agitated
condyl/o	knuckle, knob
confus/o	confusion, disorder

coni/o	dust
conjunctiv/o	conjunctiva, joined together, connected
consci/o	aware, awareness
consolid/o	become firm or solid
constipat/o	pressed together, crowded together
constrict/o	draw tightly together
-constriction	narrowing
contact/o	touched, infected
contagi/o	infection, unclean, touching of something
contaminat/o	render unclean by contact, pollute
contine/o, continent/o	keep in, contain, hold back, restrain
contra-	against, counter, opposite
contracept/o	prevention of conception
contus/o	bruise
convalesc/o	recover, become strong
convex/o	arched, vaulted
convolut/o	coiled, twisted
convuls/o	pull together
copi/o	plentiful
copulat/o	joining together, linking
cor/o	pupil
cord/o	cord, spinal cord
cordi/o	heart
core/o	pupil
cori/o	skin, leather
corne/o	cornea
coron/o	coronary, crown
corp/u, corpor/o	body
corpuscul/o	little body
cort-	covering
cortic/o	cortex, outer region
cost/o	rib
cox/o	hip, hip joint
crani/o	skull
-crasia	a mixture or blending
creatin/o	creatine
crepit/o, crepitat/o	crackling, rattling
crin/o, -crine	secrete
cris/o, critic/o	turning point
-crit	to separate
cry/o	cold
crypt/o	hidden
cubit/o	elbow
cuboid/o	cube-like
culd/o	cul-de-sac, blind pouch
cult/o	cultivate
-cusis	hearing
cusp/i	point, pointed flap
cutane/o	skin
cyan/o	blue
cycl/o	ciliary body of eye, cycle
-cyesis	pregnancy
cyst-, -cyst	bladder, bag
cyst/o	urinary bladder, cyst, sac of fluid
cyt/o, -cyte	cell
-cytic	pertaining to a cell
-cytosis	condition of cells

D

dacry/o	tear, lacrimal duct (tear duct)
dacryocyst/o	lacrimal sac (tear sac)
dactyl/o	fingers, toes
de-	down, lack of, from, not, removal
debrid/e	open a wound
deca-, deci-	ten, tenth
decidu/o	shedding, falling off
decubit/o	lying down
defec/o, defecat/o	free from waste, clear
defer/o	carrying down or out
degenerat/o	gradual impairment, breakdown, diminished function
deglutit/o	swallow
dehisce/o	burst open, split
deliri/o	wandering in the mind
delt/o	Greek letter delta, triangular shape
delus/o	delude, mock, cheat
dem/o	people, population
-dema	swelling (fluid)
demi-	half
dendr/o	branching, resembling a tree
dent/i, dent/o	tooth, teeth
depilate/o	hair removal
depress/o	press down, lower, pressed or sunk down
derma-, dermat/o, derm/o	skin
desic/o	drying
-desis	surgical fixation of bone or joint, to bind, tie together
deteriorat/o	worsening or gradual impairment
dextr/o	right side
di-	twice, twofold, double
dia-	through, between, apart, complete
diaphor/o	sweat
diaphragmat/o	diaphragm, wall across
diastole/o	standing apart, expansion

didym/o	testes, twins, double
diffus/o	pour out, spread apart
digest/o	divide, distribute
digit/o	finger or toe
dilat/o, dilatat/o	spread out, expand
-dilation	widening, stretching, expanding
dilut/o	dissolve, separate
diphther/o	membrane
dipl/o	double
dips/o, -dipsia	thirst
dis-	negative, apart, absence of
dislocat/o	displacement
dissect/o	cutting apart
disseminat/o	widely scattered
dist/o	far
distend/o, distent/o	stretch apart, expand
diur/o, diuret/o	tending to increase urine output
divert/i	turning aside
domin/o	controlling, ruling
don/o	give
dors/i, dors/o	back of body
-dote	what is given
-drome	to run, running
-duct	opening
duct/o	to lead, carry
duoden/i, duoden/o	duodenum, first part of small intestine
-dural	pertaining to dura mater
-dynia	pain
dys-	bad, difficult, or painful

E

e-	out of, from
-e	noun ending
-eal	pertaining to
ec-	out, outside
ecchym/o	pouring out of juice
ech/o	sound
eclamps/o, eclampt/o	flashing or shining forth
ectasia, -ectasis	stretching, dilation, enlargement
ecto-	out, outside
-ectomy	surgical removal, cutting out, excision
-ectopy	displacement
eczemat/o	eruption
-edema	swelling
edem-, edemat/o	swelling, fluid, tumor
edentul/o	without teeth
ef-	out
effect/o	bring about a response, activate
effus/o	pouring out
ejaculat/o	throw or hurl out
electr/o	electricity, electric
eliminat/o	expel from the body
em-	in
emaciat/o	wasted by disease
embol/o	something inserted or thrown in
embry/o	fertilized ovum, embryo
-emesis	vomiting
emet/o	vomit
-emia	blood, blood condition
emmetr/o	in proper measure
emolli/o	make soft, soften
en-	in, within, into
encephal/o	brain
end-, endo-	in, within, inside
endocrin/o	secrete within
enem/o	end in, inject
enter/o	small intestine
ento-	within
eosin/o	red, rosy
epi-	above, upon, on
epidemi/o	among the people, an epidemic
epididym/o	epididymis
epiglott/o	epiglottis
episi/o	vulva
epithel/i, epitheli/o	epithelium
equin/o	pertaining to a horse
-er	one who
erect/o	upright
erg/o, -ergy	work
erot/o	sexual love
eruct/o, eructat/o	belch forth
erupt/o	break out, burst forth
erythem/o, erythemat/o	flushed, redness
erythr/o	red
es-	out of, outside, away from
-esis	abnormal condition, disease
eso-	inward
esophag/o	esophagus
-esthesia, esthesi/o	sensation, feeling
esthet/o	feeling, nervous sensation, sense of perception
estr/o	female
ethm/o	sieve
eti/o	cause
eu-	good, normal, well, or easy

-eurysm	widening
evacu/o, evacuat/o	empty out
ex-	out of, outside, away from
exacerbat/o	aggravate, irritate
exanthemat/o	rash
excis/o	cutting out
excori/o, excoriat/o	abrade or scratch
excret/o	separate, discharge
excruciat/o	intense pain, agony
exhal/o, exhalat/o	breathe out
exo-	out of, outside, away from
exocrin/o	secrete out of
expector/o	cough up
expir/o, expirat/o	breathe out
exstroph/o	turned or twisted out
extern/o	outside, outer
extra-	on the outside, beyond, outside
extreme/o, extremit/o	extremity, outermost
extrins/o	from the outside, contained outside
exud/o, exudat/o	to sweat out

F

faci/o	face, form
-facient	making, producing
fasci/o	fascia, fibrous band
fascicul/o	little bundle
fatal/o	pertaining to fate, death
fauc/i	narrow pass, throat
febr/i	fever
fec/i, fec/o	dregs, sediment, waste
femor/o	femur, thigh bone
fenestr/o	window
fer/o	bear, carry
-ferent	carrying
-ferous	bearing, carrying, producing
fertil/o	fertile, fruitful, productive
fet/i, fet/o	fetus, unborn child
fibr/o	fiber
fibrill/o	muscular twitching
fibrin/o	fibrin, fibers, threads of a clot
fibros/o	fibrous connective tissue
fibul/o	fibula
-fic, fic/o	making, producing, forming
-fication	process of making
-fida	split
filtr/o, filtrat/o	filter, to strain through
fimbri/o	fringe
fiss/o, fissur/o	crack, split, cleft
fistul/o	tube or pipe
flat/o	flatus, breaking wind, rectal gas
flex/o	bend
flu/o	flow
fluor/o	glowing, luminous
foc/o	focus, point
foll/i	bag, sac
follicul/o	follicle, small sac
foramin/o	opening, foramen
fore-	before, in front of
-form, form/o	resembling, in the shape of
fornic/o	arch, vault, brothel
foss/o	ditch, shallow depression
fove/o	pit
fract/o	break, broken
fren/o	device that limits movement
frigid/o	cold
front/o	forehead, brow
-fuge	to drive away
funct/o, function/o	perform, function
fund/o	bottom, base, ground
fung/i	fungus
furc/o	forking, branching
furuncul/o	furunculus, a boil, an infection
-fusion	pour

G

galact/o	milk
gamet/o	wife or husband, egg or sperm
gangli/o, ganglion/o	ganglion
gangren/o	eating sore, gangrene
gastr/o	stomach, belly
gastrocnemi/o	gastrocnemius, calf muscle
gemin/o	twin, double
gen-, gen/o, -gen	producing, forming
-gene	production, origin, formation
-genic, -genesis	creation, reproduction
genit/o	produced by, birth, reproductive organs
-genous	producing
ger/i	old age
germin/o	bud, sprout, germ
geront/o	old age
gest/o, gestat/o	bear, carry young or offspring
gigant/o	giant, very large
gingiv/o	gingival tissue, gums
glauc/o	gray
glen/o	socket or pit
gli/o	neurologic tissue, supportive tissue of nervous system

globin/o, -globulin	protein
globul/o	little ball
glomerul/o	glomerulus
gloss/o	tongue
glott/i, glott/o	back of the tongue
gluc/o	glucose, sugar
glute/o	buttocks
glyc/o, glycos/o	glucose, sugar
glycer/o	sweet
glycogen/o	glycogen, animal starch
gnath/o	jaw
-gnosia	knowledge, to know
-gog, -gogue	make flow
goitr/o	goiter, enlargement of the thyroid gland
gon/e, gon/o	seed
gonad/o	gonad, sex glands
goni/o	angle
gracil/o	slender
grad/i	move, go, step, walk
-grade	go
-gram	a picture or record
granul/o	granule(s)
-graph	a picture or record, machine for recording record
-graphy	the process of producing a picture or record
gravid/o	pregnancy
-gravida	pregnant
gynec/o	woman, female
gyr/o	turning, folding

H

hal/o, halit/o	breath
halluc/o	great or large toe
hallucin/o	hallucination, to wander in the mind
hem/e	deep red iron-containing pigment
hem/o, hemat/o	blood, relating to the blood
hemi-	half
hemoglobin/o	hemoglobin
hepat/o	liver
hered/o, heredit/o	inherited, inheritance
herni/o	hernia
herpet/o	creeping
heter/o	other, different
-hexia	habit
hiat/o	opening
hidr/o	sweat
hil/o	hilum, notch or opening from a body part
hirsut/o	hairy, rough
hist/o, histi/o	tissue
holo-	all
hom/o	same, like, alike
home/o	sameness, unchanging, constant
hormon/o	hormone
humer/o	humerus (upper arm bone)
hydr/o, hydra-	relating to water
hygien/o	healthful
hymen/o	hymen, a membrane
hyper-	excessive, increased
hyp-	deficient, decreased
hypn/o	sleep
hypo-	deficient, decreased
hyster/o	uterus

I

-ia	abnormal condition, disease, plural of -ium
-ial	pertaining to
-ian	specialist
-iasis	abnormal condition, disease
iatr/o	physician, treatment
-iatrics	field of medicine, healing
-iatrist	specialist
-iatry	field of medicine
-ible	capable of, able to
-ic	pertaining to
ichthy/o	dry, scaly
-ician	specialist
icter/o	jaundice
idi/o	peculiar to the individual or organ, one, distinct
-iferous	bearing, carrying, producing
-ific	making, producing
-iform	shaped or formed like, resembling
-igo	attack, diseased condition
-ile	capable of
ile/o	ileum, small intestine
ili/o	ilium, hip bone
illusi/o	deception
im-	not
immune/o	immune, protection, safe
impact/o	pushed against, wedged against, packed
impress/o	pressing into
impuls/o	pressure or pushing force, drive, urging on
in-	in, into, not, without
incis/o	cutting into

incubat/o	incubation, hatching
indurat/o	hardened
-ine	pertaining to
infarct/o	filled in, stuffed
infect/o	infected, tainted
infer/o	below, beneath
infest/o	attack, assail, molest
inflammat/o	flame within, set on fire
infra-	below, beneath, inferior to
infundibul/o	funnel
ingest/o	carry or pour in
inguin/o	groin
inhal/o, inhalat/o	breathe in
inject/o	to force or throw in
innominat/o	unnamed, nameless
inocul/o	implant, introduce
insipid/o	tasteless
inspir/o, inspirat/o	breathe in
insul/o	island
insulin/o	insulin
intact/o	untouched, whole
inter-	between, among
intermitt/o	not continuous
intern/o	within, inner
interstiti/o	the space between things
intestin/o	intestine
intim/o	innermost
intoxic/o	put poison in
intra-	within, inside
intrins/o	contained within
intro-	within, into, inside
introit/o	entrance or passage
intussuscept/o	take up or receive within
involut/o	rolled up, curled inward
iod/o	iodine
-ion	action, process, state or condition
ion/o	ion, to wander
-ior	pertaining to
ipsi-	same
ir-	in
-is	noun ending
ir/i, ir/o, irid/o, irit/o	iris, colored part of eye
is/o	same, equal
isch/o	to hold back
ischi/o	ischium
-ism	condition, state of
iso-	equal
-ist	a person who practices, specialist
-isy	noun ending
-itis	inflammation
-ium	structure, tissue
-ive	performs, tends toward
-ize	to make, to treat

J

jejun/o	jejunum
jugul/o	throat
juxta-	beside, near, nearby

K

kal/i	potassium
kary/o	nucleus, nut
kata-, kath-	down
kel/o	growth, tumor
kera-	horn, hardness
kerat/o	horny, hard, cornea
ket/o, keton/o	ketones, acetones
kines/o, kinesi/o, -kinesia	movement
-kinesis	motion
klept/o	to steal
koil/o	hollow or concave
kraur/o	dry
kyph/o	bent, hump

L

labi/o	lip
labyrinth/o	maze, labyrinth, the inner ear
lacer/o, lacerat/o	torn, mangled
lacrim/o	tear, tear duct, lacrimal duct
lact/i, lact/o	milk
lactat/o	secrete milk
lamin/o	lamina
lapar/o	abdomen, abdominal wall
laps/o	slip, fall, slide
-lapse	to slide, fall, sag
laryng/o	larynx, throat
lat/i, lat/o	broad
later/o	side
lav/o, lavat/o	wash, bathe
lax/o, laxat/o	loosen, relax
leiomy/o	smooth (visceral) muscle
lemm/o	husk, peel, bark
-lemma	sheath, covering
lent/i	the lens of the eye

lenticul/o	shaped like a lens, pertaining to a lens
-lepsy	seizure
lept/o	thin, slender
-leptic	to seize, take hold of
lepto-	small, soft
letharg/o	drowsiness, oblivion
leuk/o	white
lev/o, levat/o	raise, lift up
lex/o, -lexia	word, phrase
libid/o, libidin/o	sexual drive, desire, passion
ligament/o	ligament
ligat/o	binding or tying off
lingu/o	tongue
lipid/o, lip/o	fat, lipid
-listhesis	slipping
lith/o, -lith	stone, calculus
lithiasis	presence of stones
lob/i, lob/o	lobe, well-defined part of an organ
loc/o	place
loch/i	childbirth, confinement
-logy	study of
longev/o	long-lived, long life
lord/o	curve, swayback bent
lumb/o	lower back, loin
lumin/o	light
lun/o, lunat/o	moon
lunul/o	crescent
lup/i, lup/o	wolf
lute/o	yellow
lux/o	to slide
lymph/o	lymph, lymphatic tissue
lymphaden/o	lymph gland
lymphangi/o	lymph vessel
-lysis	breakdown, separation, setting free, destruction, loosening
-lyst	agent that causes lysis or loosening
-lytic	to reduce, destroy

M

macro-	large, abnormal size or length, long
macul/o	spot
magn/o	great, large
major/o	larger
mal-	bad, poor, evil
-malacia	abnormal softening
malign/o	bad, evil
malle/o	malleus, hammer
malleol/o	malleolus, little hammer
mamm/o	breast
man/i	madness, rage
man/i, man/o	hand
mandibul/o	mandible, lower jaw
-mania	obsessive preoccupation
manipul/o	use of hands
manubri/o	handle
masset/o	chew
mast/o	breast
mastic/o, masticat/o	chew
mastoid/o	mastoid process
matern/o	maternal, of a mother
matur/o	ripe
maxill/o	maxilla (upper jaw)
maxim/o	largest, greatest
meat/o	opening or passageway
medi/o	middle
mediastin/o	mediastinum, middle
medic/o	medicine, physician, healing
medicat/o	medication, healing
medull/o	medulla (inner section), middle, soft, marrow
mega-, megal/o	large, great
-megaly	enlargement
mei/o	less, meiosis
melan/o	black, dark
mellit/o	honey, honeyed
membran/o	membrane, thin skin
men/o	menstruation, menses
mening/o, meningi/o	membranes, meninges
menisc/o	meniscus, crescent
mens/o	menstruate, menstruation, menses
menstru/o, menstruat/o	occurring monthly
ment/o	mind, chin
mes-	middle
mesenter/o	mesentery
mesi/o	middle, median plane
meso-	middle
meta-	change, beyond, subsequent to, behind, after or next
metabol/o	change
metacarp/o	metacarpals, bones of the hand
metatars/o	bones of the foot between the tarsus and toes
-meter	measure, instrument used to measure
metr/i, metr/o, metri/o	uterus

-metrist	one who measures
-metry	to measure
micr/o, micro-	small
mictur/o, micturit/o	urinate
mid-	middle
midsagitt/o	from front to back, at the middle
milli-	one-thousandth
-mimetic	mimic, copy
mineral/o	mineral
minim/o	smallest, least
minor/o	smaller
mio-	smaller, less
-mission	to send
mit/o	a thread
mitr/o	a miter, having two points on top
mobil/o	capable of moving
monil/i	string of beads, genus of parasitic mold or fungus
mono-	one, single
morbid/o	disease, sickness
moribund/o	dying
morph/o	shape, form
mort/i, mort/o, mort/u	death, dead
mortal/i	pertaining to death, subject to death
mot/o, motil/o	motion, movement
mu/o	close, shut
muc/o, mucos/o	mucus
multi-	many, much
muscul/o	muscle
mut/a	genetic change
mut/o	unable to speak, inarticulate
mutagen/o	causing genetic change
my/o	muscle
myc/e, myc/o	fungus
mydri/o	wide
mydrias/i	dilation of the pupil
myel/o	spinal cord, bone marrow
myocardi/o	myocardium, heart muscle
myom/o	muscle tumor
myos/o	muscle
myring/o	tympanic membrane, eardrum
myx/o, myxa-	mucus

N

nar/i	nostril
narc/o	numbness, stupor
nas/i, nas/o	nose
nat/i	birth
natr/o	sodium
nause/o	nausea, seasickness
necr/o	death
-necrosis	tissue death
neo-, ne/o	new, strange
nephr/o	kidney
nerv/o, neur/i, neur/o	nerve, nerve tissue
neutr/o	neither, neutral
nev/o	birthmark, mole
nid/o	next
niter-, nitro-	nitrogen
noct/i	night
nod/o	knot, swelling
nodul/o	little knot
nom/o	law, control
non-	no
nor-	chemical compound
norm/o	normal or usual
nuch/o	the nape
nucle/o	nucleus
nucleol/o	little nucleus, nucleolus
nulli-	none
numer/o	number, count
nunci/o	messenger
nutri/o, nutrit/o	nourishment, food, nourish, feed
nyct/o, nyctal/o	night

O

ob-	against
obes/o	obese, extremely fat
obliqu/o	slanted, sideways
oblongat/o	oblong, elongated
obstetr/i, obstetr/o	midwife, one who stands to receive
occipit/o	back of the skull, occiput
occlud/o, occlus/o	shut, close up
occult/o	hidden, concealed
ocul/o	eye
odont/o	tooth
-oid	like, resembling
-ole	little, small
olecran/o	elbow, olecranon
olfact/o	smell, sense of smell
olig/o	scanty, few
-ologist	specialist
-ology	the science or study of
-oma	tumor, neoplasm
om/o	shoulder
oment/o	omentum, fat
omphal/o	umbilical cord, the navel

onc/o	tumor
-one	hormone
onych/o	fingernail or toenail
o/o, oo/o	egg
oophor/o	ovary
opac/o, opacit/o	shaded, dark, impenetrable to light
-opaque	obscure
oper/o, operat/o	perform, operate, work
opercul/o	cover or lid
ophthalm/o	eye, vision
-opia	vision condition
opisth/o	backward
-opsia, -opsis, -opsy	vision, view of
opt/i, opt/o, optic/o	eye, vision
or/o	mouth, oral cavity
orbit/o	orbit, bony cavity or socket
orch/o, orchid/o, orchi/o	testicles, testis, testes
-orexia	appetite
organ/o	organ
orgasm/o	swell, be excited
orth/o	straight, normal, correct
-ory	pertaining to
os-	mouth, bone
-ose	full of, pertaining to, sugar
-osis	abnormal condition, disease
osm/o	pushing, thrusting
-osmia	smell, odor
oss/e, oss/i	bone
ossicul/o	ossicle (small bone)
oste/o, ost/o	bone
-ostomy	surgically creating an opening
-ostosis	condition of bone
ot/o	ear, hearing
-otia	ear condition
-otomy	cutting, surgical incision
ov/i, ov/o	egg, ovum
ovari/o	ovary
ovul/o	egg
ox/i, ox/o, ox/y	oxygen
-oxia	oxygen condition
oxid/o	containing oxygen
oxy/o	the presence of oxygen in a compound

P

pachy-	heavy, thick
palat/o	palate, roof of mouth
pall/o, pallid/o	pale, lacking or drained of color
palliat/o	cloaked, hidden
palm/o	palm of the hand
palpat/o	touch, feel, stroke
palpebr/o	eyelid
palpit/o	throbbing, quivering
pan-	all, entire, every
pancreat/o	pancreas
papill/i, papill/o	nipple-like
papul/o	pimple
par-, para-	beside, near, beyond, abnormal, apart from, opposite, along side of
par/o	to bear, bring forth, labor
-para	to give birth
paralys/o, paralyt/o	disable
parasit/o	parasite
parathyroid/o	parathyroid glands
pares/i	to disable
-paresi	partial or incomplete paralysis
paret/o	to disable
-pareunia	sexual intercourse
pariet/o	wall
parotid/o	parotid gland
-parous	having borne one or more children
paroxysm/o	sudden attack
-partum, parturit/o	childbirth, labor
patell/a, patell/o	patella, kneecap
path/o, -pathy	disease, suffering, feeling, emotion
paus/o	cessation, stopping
-pause	stopping
pector/o	chest
ped/o	child, foot
pedi/a	child
pedicul/o	louse (singular), lice (plural)
pelv/i, pelv/o	pelvic bone, pelvic cavity, hip
pen/i	penis
pend/o	to hang
-penia	deficiency, lack, too few
peps/i, -pepsia, pept/o	digest, digestion
per-	excessive, through
percept/o	become aware, perceive
percuss/o	strike, tap, beat
peri-	surrounding, around
perine/o	perineum
peristals/o, peristalt/o	constrict around
peritone/o	peritoneum
perme/o	to pass or go through

pernici/o	destructive, harmful
perone/o	fibula
perspir/o	perspiration
pertuss/i	intensive cough
petechi/o	skin spot
-pexy	surgical fixation
phac/o	lens of eye
phag/o	eat, swallow
-phage	a cell that destroys, eat, swallow
-phagia	eating, swallowing
phak/o	lens of eye
phalang/o	phalanges, finger and toe
phall/i, phill/o	penis
pharmac/o, pharmaceut/o	drug
pharyng/o	throat, pharynx
phas/o	speech
-phasia	speak or speech
phe/o	dusky
pher/o	to bear or carry
-pheresis	removal
phil/o, -phil, -philia	attraction to, like, love
phleb/o	vein
phlegm/o	thick mucus
phob/o, -phobia	abnormal fear
phon/o, -phonia	sound, voice
phor/o	carry, bear, movement
-phoresis	carrying, transmission
-phoria	to bear, carry, feeling, mental state
phot/o	light
phren/o	diaphragm, mind
-phthisis	wasting away
-phylactic	protective, preventive
-phylaxis	protection
physi/o, physic/o	nature, physical
-physis	to grow
phyt/o, -phyte	plant
pigment/o	pigment, color
pil/i, pil/o	hair
pineal/o	pineal gland
pinn/i	external ear, auricle
pituit/o, pituitar/o	pituitary gland
plac/o	flat plate or patch
placent/o	placenta, round flat cake
plak/o, -plakia	plaque, plate, thin flat layer or scale
plan/o	flat
plant/i, plant/o	sole of foot
plas/i, plas/o, -plasia	development, growth, formation
-plasm	formative material of cells
plasm/o	something molded or formed
-plastic	pertaining to formation
-plasty	surgical repair
ple/o	more, many
-plegia	paralysis, stroke
-plegic	one affected with paralysis
pleur/o	pleura, side of the body
plex/o	plexus, network
plic/o	fold or ridge
pne/o-	breath, breathing
-pnea	breathing
-pneic	pertaining to breathing
pneum/o, pneumon/o	lung, air
pod/o	foot
-poiesis	formation, to make
poikil/o	varied, irregular
pol/o	extreme
poli/o	gray matter of brain and spinal cord
pollic/o	thumb
poly-	many
polyp/o	polyp, small growth
pont/o	pons (a part of the brain), bridge
poplit/o	back of the knee
por/o	pore, small opening
-porosis	lessening in density, porous condition
port/i	gate, door
post-	after, behind
poster/o	behind, toward the back
potent/o	powerful
pract/i, practic/o	practice, pursue an occupation
prandi/o, -prandial	meal
-praxia	action, condition concerning the performance of movements
-praxis	act, activity, practice use
pre-	before, in front of
precoc/i	early, premature
pregn/o	pregnant, full of
prematur/o	too early, untimely
preputi/o	foreskin, prepuce
presby/o	old age
press/o	press, draw
priap/o	penis
primi-	first
pro-	before, in behalf of
process/o	going forth
procident/o	fall down or forward
procreat/o	reproduce

proct/o	anus and rectum
prodrom/o	running ahead, precursor
product/o	lead forward, yield, produce
prolaps/o	fall downward, slide forward
prolifer/o	reproduce, bear offspring
pron/o, pronat/o	bent forward
pros-	before
prostat/o	prostate gland
prosth/o, prosthet/o	addition, appendage
prot/o, prote/o	first
protein/o	protein
proxim/o	near
prurit/o	itching
pseud/o	false
psor/i, psor/o	itch, itching
psych/o	mind
ptomat/o	a fall
-ptosis	droop, sag, prolapse, fall
-ptyal/o	saliva
-ptysis	spitting
pub/o	pubis, part of hip bone
pubert/o	ripe age, adult
pudend/o	pudendum
puerper/i	childbearing, labor
pulm/o, pulmon/o	lung
pulpos/o	fleshy, pulpy
puls/o	beat, beating, striking
punct/o	sting, prick, puncture
pupill/o	pupil
pur/o	pus
purpur/o	purple
purul/o	pus-filled
pustul/o	infected pimple
py/o	pus
pyel/o	renal pelvis, bowl of kidney
pylor/o	pylorus, pyloric sphincter
pyr/o, pyret/o	fever, fire
pyramid/o	pyramid-shaped

Q

quadr/i, quadr/o	four

R

rabi/o	madness, rage
rachi/o	spinal column, vertebrae
radi/o	radiation, x-rays, radius (lateral lower arm bone)
radiat/o	giving off rays or radiant energy
radicul/o	nerve root
raph/o	seam, suture
re-	back, again
recept/o	receive, receiver
recipi/o	receive, take to oneself
rect/o	rectum, straight
recticul/o	network
recuperat/o	recover, regain health
reduct/o	bring back together
refract/o	bend back, turn aside
regurgit/o	flood or gush back
remiss/o	give up, let go, relax
ren/o	kidney
restor/o	rebuild, put back, restore
resuscit/o	revive
retent/o	hold back
reticul/o	network
retin/o	retina, net
retract/o	draw back or in
retro-	behind, backward, back of
rhabd/o	rod, rod-shaped
rhabdomy/o	striated muscle
rheum/o, rheumat/o	watery flow, subject to flow
rhin/o	nose
rhiz/o	root
rhonc/o	snore, snoring
rhythm/o	rhythm
rhytid/o	wrinkle
rigid/o	stiff
ris/o	laugh
roentgen/o	x-ray
rotat/o	rotate, revolve
-rrhage, -rrhagia	bleeding, abnormal excessive fluid discharge
-rrhaphy	surgical suturing
-rrhea	flow or discharge
-rrhexis	rupture
rube-	red
rug/o	wrinkle, fold

S

sacc/i, sacc/o	sac
sacchar/o	sugar
sacr/o	sacrum
saliv/o	saliva
salping/o	uterine (fallopian) tube, auditory (eustachian) tube

-salpinx	uterine (fallopian) tube
san/o	sound, healthy, sane
sangu/i, sanguin/o	blood
sanit/o	soundness, health
saphen/o	clear, apparent, manifest
sapr/o	decaying, rotten
sarc/o	flesh, connective tissue
scalp/o	carve, scrape
scapul/o	scapula, shoulder blade
schiz/o	division, split
scintill/o	spark
scirrh/o	hard
scler/o	sclera, white of eye, hard
-sclerosis	abnormal hardening
scoli/o	curved, bent
-scope	instrument for visual examination
-scopic	pertaining to visual examination
-scopy	visual examination
scot/o	darkness
scrib/o, script/o	write
scrot/o	bag or pouch
seb/o	sebum
secret/o	produce, separate out
sect/o, secti/o	cut, cutting
segment/o	pieces
sell/o	saddle
semi-	half
semin/i	semen, seed, sperm
sen/i	old
senesc/o	grow old
senil/o	old age
sens/i	feeling, sensation
sensitiv/o	sensitive to, affected by
seps/o	infection
sept/o	infection, partition
ser/o	serum
seros/o	serous
sial/o	saliva
sialaden/o	salivary gland
sider/o	iron
sigm/o	Greek letter sigma
sigmoid/o	sigmoid colon
silic/o	glass
sin/o, sin/u	hollow, sinus
sinistr/o	left, left side
sinus/o	sinus
-sis	abnormal condition, disease
sit/u	place
skelet/o	skeleton
soci/o	companion, fellow being
-sol	solution
solut/o, solv/o	loosened, dissolved
soma-, somat/o	body
somn/i, somn/o	sleep
son/o	sound
sopor/o	sleep
spad/o	draw off, draw
-spasm, spasmod/o	sudden involuntary contraction, tightening, or cramping
spec/i	look at, a kind or sort
specul/o	mirror
sperm/o, spermat/o	sperm, spermatozoa, seed
sphen/o	sphenoid bone, wedge
spher/o	round, sphere, ball
sphincter/o	tight band
sphygm/o	pulse
spin/o	spine, backbone
spir/o	to breathe
spirill/o	little coil
spirochet/o	coiled microorganism
splen/o	spleen
spondyl/o	vertebrae, vertebral column, backbone
spontane/o	unexplained, of one's own accord
spor/o	seed, spore
sput/o	sputum, spit
squam/o	scale
-stalsis	contraction, constriction
staped/o, stapedi/o	stapes (middle ear bone)
staphyl/o	clusters, bunch of grapes
-stasis, -static	control, maintenance of a constant level
steat/o	fat, lipid, sebum
sten/o	narrowing, contracted
-stenosis	abnormal narrowing
ster/o	solid structure
stere/o	solid, three-dimensional
steril/i	sterile
stern/o	sternum, the breastbone
stert/o	snore, snoring
steth/o	chest
-sthenia	strength
stigmat/o	point, spot
stimul/o	goad, prick, incite
stol/o	send or place
stom/o, stomat/o	mouth, oral cavity
-stomosis, -stomy	furnish with a mouth or outlet, new opening
strab/i	squint, squint-eyed
strat/i	layer

strept/o	twisted chain
striat/o	stripe, furrow, groove
stric-	narrowing
strict/o	draw tightly together, bind or tie
strid/o	harsh sound
stup/e	benumbed, stunned
styl/o	pen, pointed instrument
sub-	under, less, below
subluxat/o	partial dislocation
sucr/o	sugar
sudor/i	sweat
suffoc/o, suffocat/o	choke, strangle
sulc/o	furrow, groove
super-, super/o	above, excessive, higher than
superflu/o	overflowing, excessive
supin/o	lying on the back
supinat/o	bend backward, place on the back
suppress/o	press down
suppur/o, suppurate/o	to form pus
supra-	above, upper, excessive
supraren/o	above or on the kidney, suprarenal gland
-surgery	operative procedure
sutur/o	stitch, seam
sym-	with, together, joined together
symptomat/o	falling together, symptom
syn-	together, with, union, association
synaps/o, synapt/o	point of contact
syncop/o	to cut short, cut off
-syndesis	surgical fixation of vertebrae
syndesm/o	ligament
syndrom/o	running together
synovi/o, synov/o	synovial membrane, synovial fluid
syphil/i, syphil/o	syphilis
syring/o	tube
system/o, systemat/o	body system
systol/o	contraction

T

tachy-	fast, rapid
tact/i	touch
talip/o	foot and ankle deformity
tars/o	tarsus (ankle bone), instep, edge of the eyelid
tax/o	coordination, order
techn/o, techni/o	skill
tectori/o	covering, roof-like
tele/o	distant, far
tempor/o	temporal bone, temple
ten/o, tend/o	tendon, stretch out, extend, strain
tenac/i	holding fast, sticky
tendin/o	tendon
tens/o	stretch out, extend, strain
terat/o	malformed fetus
termin/o	end, limit
test/i, test/o	testicle, testis
tetan/o	rigid, tense
tetra-	four
thalam/o	thalamus, inner room
thalass/o	sea
thanas/o, thanat/o	death
the/o	put, place
thec/o	sheath
thel/o	nipple
therap/o, therapeut/o	treatment
therm/o	heat
thio-	sulfur
thora/o, thorac/o	chest
-thorax	chest, pleural cavity
thromb/o	clot
thym/o	thymus gland, soul
-thymia	a state of mind
-thymic	pertaining to the mind, relating to the thymus gland
thyr/o, thyroid/o	thyroid gland
tibi/o	tibia (shin bone)
-tic	pertaining to
tine/o	gnawing worm, ringworm
tinnit/o	ringing, buzzing, tinkling
-tion	process, state or quality of
toc/o, -tocia, -tocin	labor, birth
tom/o	cut, section, slice
-tome	instrument to cut
-tomy	process of cutting
ton/o	tension, tone, stretching
tone/o	to stretch
tonsill/o	tonsil, throat
top/o	place, position, location
tors/o	twist, rotate
tort/i	twisted
tox/o, toxic/o	poison, poisonous
trabecul/o	little beam marked with cross bars or beams
trache/i, trache/o	trachea, windpipe
trachel-	neck

tract/o	draw, pull, path, bundle of nerve fibers
tranquil/o	quiet, calm, tranquil
trans-	across, through
transfus/o	pour across, transfer
transit/o	changing
transvers/o	across, crosswise
traumat/o	injury
trem/o	shaking, trembling
tremul/o	fine tremor or shaking
treponem/o	coiled, turning microbe
tri-	three
trich/o	hair
trigon/o	trigone
-tripsy	to crush
-trite	instrument for crushing
trop/o, -tropia	turn, change
troph/o, -trophy	development, nourishment
-tropic	having an affinity for
-tropin	to stimulate, act on
tub/i, tub/o	tube, pipe
tubercul/o	little knot, swelling
tunic/o	covering, cloak, sheath
turbinat/o	coiled, spiral shaped
tuss/i	cough
tympan/o	tympanic membrane, eardrum
-type	classification, picture

U

-ula	small, little
-ule	small one
ulcer/o	sore, ulcer
uln/o	ulna (medial lower arm bone)
ultra-	beyond, excess
-um	singular noun ending
umbilic/o	navel
un-	not
ungu/o	nail
uni-	one
ur/o	urine, urinary tract
-uresis	urination
ureter/o	ureter
urethr/o	urethra
urg/o	press, push
-uria	urination, urine
urin/o	urine or urinary organs
urtic/o	nettle, rash, hives
-us	thing, singular noun ending
uter/i, uter/o	uterus
uve/o	iris, choroid, ciliary body, uveal tract
uvul/o	uvula, little grape

V

vaccin/i, vaccin/o	vaccine
vacu/o	empty
vag/o	vagus nerve, wandering
vagin/o	vagina
valg/o	bent or twisted outward
valv/o, valvul/o	valve
var/o	bent or twisted inward
varic/o	varicose veins, swollen or dilated vein
vas/o	vas deferens, vessel
vascul/o	blood vessel, little vessel
vast/o	vast, great, extensive
vect/o	carry, convey
ven/o	vein
vener/o	sexual intercourse
venter-	abdomen
ventilat/o	expose to air, fan
ventr/o	in front, belly side of body
ventricul/o	ventricle of brain or heart, small chamber
venul/o	venule, small vein
verg/o	twist, incline
verm/i	worm
verruc/o	wart
-verse, -version	to turn
vers/o, vert/o	turn
vertebr/o	vertebra, backbone
vertig/o, vertigin/o	whirling round
vesic/o	urinary bladder
vesicul/o	seminal vesicle, blister, little bladder
vestibul/o	entrance, vestibule
vi/o	force
vill/i	shaggy hair, tuft of hair
vir/o	poison, virus
viril/o	masculine, manly
vis/o	seeing, sight
visc/o	sticky
viscer/o	viscera, internal organ
viscos/o	sticky
vit/a, vit/o	life
viti/o	blemish, defect
vitre/o	glassy, made of glass
voc/i	voice
vol/o	palm or sole

volv/o	roll, turn
vulgar/i	common
vulv/o	vulva, covering

X

xanth/o	yellow
xen/o	strange, foreign
xer/o	dry
xiph/i, xiph/o	sword

Y

-y	noun ending

Z

zo/o	animal life
zygomat/o	cheek bone, yoke
zygot/o	joined together

APPENDIX B

Abbreviations and Their Meanings

Reminders about abbreviations: (1) An abbreviation can have several meanings. (2) A term can have several abbreviations. When in doubt, always verify the meaning of the abbreviation!

A

A2 or A_2	aortic valve closure
A	abnormal; adult; age; allergy; anaphylaxis; anesthesia; anterior; antibody; auscultation
a	accommodation; acid
aa	amino acid
AA, AC	alopecia areata; asthma; asthmatic
AAA	abdominal aortic aneurysm
AAL	anterior axillary line
AAV	adeno-associated virus
A&B	apnea and bradycardia
A/B	acid-base ratio
AB, Ab, ab	abortion
AB, Abnl, abn	abnormal
Ab	antibody
ABC	aspiration, biopsy, cytology
Abd, Abdo	abdomen
ABE	acute bacterial endocarditis
ABG	arterial blood gases
ABP	arterial blood pressure
ABR	auditory brainstem response
abx	antibiotics
ac	acute
AC, ac	anticoagulant; before meals
acc	accident; accommodation
ACD	absolute cardiac dullness; acid-citrate-dextrose; anterior chest diameter; area of cardiac disease
ACE	acute care of the elderly; aerobic chair exercises; angiotensin-converting enzyme
ACG	angiocardiogram; angiocardiography; apex cardiogram
ACH	adrenocortical hormone
ACL	anterior cruciate ligament
ACLS	advanced cardiac life support
ACT	activated coagulation time; anticoagulant therapy
ACTH	adrenocorticotropic hormone
ACU	acute care unit; ambulatory care unit
ACVD	acute cardiovascular disease
AD	admitting diagnosis; advanced directive; after discharge; Alzheimer's disease; right ear
ADC	AIDS dementia complex
ADD	attention deficit disorder
ADE	acute disseminated encephalitis; adverse drug event
ADH	adhesion; antidiuretic hormone
ADHD	attention deficit hyperactivity disorder
ADL	activities of daily life; activities of daily living
ad lib	as desired
adm	admission
ADR	adverse drug reaction
ADS	antibody deficiency syndrome
ADT	admission, discharge, transfer
AE, A/E	above elbow
AED	automated external defibrillation
AF	acid-fast; amniotic fluid; atrial flutter
AF, A fib, AFib	atrial fibrillation
AFB	acid-fast bacilli

AFP alpha-fetoprotein
Ag antigen
AH abdominal hysterectomy
AHD antihypertensive drug; arteriosclerotic heart disease; autoimmune hemolytic disease
AI accidentally incurred; aortic insufficiency; atherogenic index
AID acute infectious disease; artificial insemination donor
AIDS acquired immunodeficiency syndrome
AIH artificial insemination husband
AIHA autoimmune hemolytic anemia
AJ, aj ankle jerk
AK above knee
AKA above-knee amputation
alb albumin
ALD aldosterone
alk alkaline
ALL acute lymphoblastic leukemia; acute lymphocytic leukemia
ALND axillary lymph node dissection
ALP acute lupus pericarditis; alkaline phosphatase
ALS advanced life support; amyotrophic lateral sclerosis; antilymphocytic serum
ALT, alt alternative; altitude
alt dieb alternate days; every other day
alt hor alternate hours
alt noct alternate nights
Am amnion
AMA advanced maternal age; against medical advice; American Medical Association
amb ambulance; ambulatory
AMD age-related macular degeneration
AMI acute myocardial infarction
AML acute myeloblastic leukemia; acute myelocytic leukemia; amyotrophic lateral sclerosis
AMN amniocentesis
amp amplification; ampule; amputate
AMS altered mental status; automated multiphasic screening
amt amount
AN aneurysm; anorexia nervosa
ANA antinuclear antibodies
ANAS anastomosis
anat anatomy
anes, anesth anesthesia; anesthetic
ANLL acute nonlymphocytic leukemia
ANS anterior nasal spine; autonomic nervous system
ant, ANT anterior
ANUG acute necrotizing ulcerative gingivitis
AOD arterial occlusive disease
AODM adult-onset diabetes mellitus
AOM acute otitis media
A & P anatomy and physiology; anterior and posterior; auscultation and percussion
AP abruptio placenta; angina pectoris; anteroposterior; anterior-posterior; appendectomy; appendicitis
APAP acetaminophen
Aph aphasia
APLD aspiration percutaneous lumbar diskectomy
aPTT activated partial thromboplastin time
aq aqueous; water
AR abnormal record; achievement ration; alarm reaction; artificial respiration
ARD acute respiratory disease
ARDS acute respiratory distress syndrome; adult respiratory distress syndrome
ARF acute renal failure; acute respiratory failure
ARI acute respiratory infection
ARM artificial rupture of membranes
ART arthritis; assisted reproductive technology
AS ankylosing spondylitis; aortic stenosis; astigmatism; left ear
ASA acetylsalicylic acid (aspirin)
ASAP as soon as possible
ASCVD arteriosclerotic cardiovascular disease
ASD atrial septal defect
ASH asymmetrical septal hypertrophy
ASHD arteriosclerotic heart disease
ASO administrative services only; arteriosclerosis obliterans
ASS anterior superior spine
AST Aphasia Screening Test; aspartate aminotransferase
As tol as tolerated
AT Achilles tendon
ATP adenosine triphosphate
atr atrophy
AU aures unitas; both ears
AUL acute undifferentiated leukemia
aus, ausc, auscul auscultation
A-V, AV aortic valve; artificial ventilation; arteriovenous; atrioventricular
AVM arteriovenous malfunction

AVN atrioventricular node
AVR aortic valve replacement
A & W alive and well
Ax, ax axilla; axillary
AZT Aschheim-Zondek test

B

B bruit
B/A backache
BA bronchial asthma
Ba barium
BAC blood alcohol concentration
BACT, Bact, bact bacteria; bacterium
BaE barium enema
BAO basal acid output
bas basophils
BBB blood-brain barrier; bundle branch block
BBT basal body temperature
BC bone conduction
BCC basal cell carcinoma
BD bronchodilator
BDT bone density testing
BE barium enema; below elbow
BEAM brain electrical activity map
BED binge eating disorder
BFP biologic false positive
bid, b.i.d. bis in die; twice a day
BID brought in dead
BIL, Bil, Bili bilirubin
bil bilateral
BIN, bin twice a night
BJ Bence Jones
BK below knee
BKA below-knee amputation
Bld blood
BM bone marrow; bowel movement
BMB bone marrow biopsy
BMD Becker's muscular dystrophy; bone mineral density
BMI body mass index
BMR basal metabolic rate
BMT barium meal test; bone marrow transplant
BNO bladder neck obstruction
BNR bladder neck resection
BOM bilateral otitis media
BP Bell's palsy; bedpan; bathroom privileges; blood pressure
BPD borderline personality disorder
BPH benign prostatic hyperplasia; benign prostatic hypertrophy
BPM beats per minute
bpm breaths per minute
BP&P blood pressure and pulse
BPPV benign paroxysmal positional vertigo
BR, Br bed rest; bronchitis
BRBPR bright red blood per rectum
BRO, Bronch bronchoscope; bronchoscopy
BRP bathroom privileges
BS blood sugar; bowel sounds; breath sounds
BSE breast self-examination
BSO bilateral salpingo-oophorectomy
BT bleeding time
BUN blood urea nitrogen
BV bacterial vaginosis; blood volume
Bx, bx biopsy

C

C1 through C7 cervical vertebrae
C centigrade; Celsius; cholesterol; convergence; cyanosis
C. chlamydia
c centimeter
$\bar{c}$ with
$\underline{c}$ without
Ca calcium
CA, Ca cancer; cardiac arrest; carcinoma; chronological age
CAB coronary artery bypass
CABG coronary artery bypass grafting
CAD computer-assisted diagnosis; coronary artery disease
CAL calcitonin
cal calorie
cap, caps capsule
CAPD continuous ambulatory peritoneal dialysis
card cath cardiac catheterization
CAT cataract
cath catheter; catheterization; catheterize
caut cauterization
CAVH continuous arteriovenous hemofiltration
CBC, cbc complete blood count
CBF capillary blood flow; coronary blood flow
CBI continuous bladder irrigation
CBR complete bedrest

CBS chronic brain syndrome
CC chief complaint; colony count; cardiac cycle; cardiac cauterization; creatinine clearance
cc cubic centimeter (1/1,000 liter)
CCA circumflex coronary artery
CCCR closed chest cardiopulmonary resuscitation
CCE cholecystectomy
CCPD continuous cycle peritoneal dialysis
CCr creatinine clearance
CCU coronary care unit
CD communicable disease; contact dermatitis; Crohn's disease
CDC calculated date (day) of confinement; Centers for Disease Control and Prevention
CDE common duct exploration
CDH congenital dislocation of the hip
CEA carotid endarterectomy
CEPH cephalic
CF complete fixation; counting fingers; cystic fibrosis
CFS chronic fatigue syndrome
CGL chronic granulomatous leukemia
C gl with correction; with glasses
CH chromosome
CHB complete heart block
CHD congenital heart defects; coronary heart disease
CHF congestive heart failure
CHO carbohydrate
chol cholesterol
chole cholecystectomy
CI conjunctivitis; coronary insufficiency
cib food
CID cytomegalic inclusion disease
CIR, CIRR cirrhosis
CIRC, circum circumcision
CIS carcinoma in situ
CIT conventional insulin treatment
CK creatine kinase
ck check
Cl, cl clinic; chloride
CL cholelithiasis; chronic leukemia; cirrhosis of the liver; cleft lip; corpus luteum
CLD chronic liver disease
CLL chronic lymphocytic leukemia
cl liq clear liquid
cm centimeter (1/100 meter)
cm^3 cubic centimeter
CME cystoid macular edema
CMG cystometrogram
CML chronic myelocytic leukemia
CMM cutaneous malignant melanoma
CMV controlled mechanical ventilation; cytomegalovirus
CNS central nervous system; cutaneous nerve stimulation
C/O, c/o complains of
CO carbon monoxide; coronary occlusion; coronary output
CO_2 carbon dioxide
COD cause of death
COH carbohydrate
COL colonoscopy
COLD chronic obstructive lung disease
comp compound
cond condition
contra against
COPD chronic obstructive pulmonary disease
CP cardiopulmonary; cerebral palsy
CPA carotid phonoangiograph
CPAP continuous positive airway pressure
CPC clinicopathologic conference
CPD cephalopelvic disproportion
CPE cardiopulmonary edema
CPK creatine phosphokinase
CPN chronic pyelonephritis
CPPB continuous positive-pressure breathing
CPR cardiopulmonary resuscitation
CPS cycles per second
CR closed reduction; complete response; conditioned reflex
CRC colorectal carcinoma
CRD chronic respiratory disease
creat creatinine
CRF chronic renal failure
CRP C-reactive protein
CRPS complex regional pain syndrome
CRYO cryosurgery
C & S culture and sensitivity
CS central supply; complete stroke; conditioned stimulus; Cushing's syndrome
CSAP cryosurgical ablation of the prostate
C-section cesarian section
CSF cerebrospinal fluid
CSO craniostenosis
CSR central supply room; Cheyne-Stokes respiration
CT computed tomography
CTCL cutaneous T cell lymphoma

CTD cumulative trauma disorders
CTR carpal tunnel release
CTS carpal tunnel syndrome
cu cubic
CUC chronic ulcerative colitis
CUG cystourethrogram
CV cardiovascular
CVA cardiovascular accident; cerebrovascular accident
CVD cardiovascular disease
CVL central venous line
CVP central venous pressure; Cytoxan, vincristine, prednisone
CVS chorionic villus sampling
CWP childbirth without pain
Cx cervix
CX, CXR chest x-ray film
cysto cystoscopic examination; cystoscopy
cyt cytology; cytoplasm

D

D diopter; dorsal
d day
DAT diet as tolerated
db, dB decibel
D & C dilation and curettage
D/C, d/c diarrhea/constipation
DCC direct-current cardioversion
DCIS ductal carcinoma in situ
DCR direct cortical response
D/D, DD, DDx, Ddx differential diagnosis
D & E dilation and evacuation
debr debridement
Dg, dg diagnosis
del delivery
DES diethylstilbestrol
DEXA dual energy x-ray absorptiometry
DF dorsiflexion
DG, dg diagnosis
DGE delayed gastric emptying
DHFS dengue hemorrhagic fever shock syndrome
DI diabetes insipidus
Diag, diag diagnosis
DIC diffuse intravascular coagulation
diff differential diagnosis
diopt, Dptr diopter
DIP distal interphalangeal
diph diphtheria
disch discharge
DJD degenerative joint disease
DKA diabetic ketoacidosis
DL danger list
DLE discoid lupus erythematosus
DM dermatomyositis; diabetes mellitus; diastolic murmur
DMD Duchenne's muscular dystrophy
DNA deoxyribonucleic acid
DNR do not resuscitate
DNS deviated nasal septum
DOA dead on arrival
DOB date of birth
DOC date of conception
DOE dyspnea on exertion
DOMS delayed-onset muscle soreness
DOT directly observed therapy
DPT diphtheria-pertussis-tetanus
DQ developmental quotient
DR diabetic retinopathy; digital radiography; doctor
dr dram; dressing
DRD developmental reading disorder
DRE digital rectal exam
DRG diagnosis-related group
DRP diabetic retinopathy
D/S dextrose in saline
DS Down syndrome
DSA digital subtraction angiography
DSD dry sterile dressing
dsg dressing
DT diphtheria and tetanus toxoids
DT, DT's, DTs delirium tremens
DTP diphtheria, tetanus toxoids, and pertussis vaccine
DTR deep tendon reflex
du decubitus ulcer
DUB dysfunctional uterine bleeding
DVA distance visual acuity
DVI digital vascular imaging
DVT deep vein thrombosis
D/W dextrose in water
DX, Dx diagnosis
DXA dual x-ray absorptiometry

E

E encephalitis; enema; etiology
e epinephrine; estrogen

EBL estimated blood loss
EBP epidural blood patch
EBV Epstein-Barr virus
ECC endocervical curettage; extracorporeal circulation
ECCE extracapsular cataract extraction
ECG electrocardiogram; electrocardiography
ECHO echocardiogram; echocardiography
E coli *Escherichia coli*
ECT electroconvulsive therapy
ED effective dose; emergency department; epidural; erythema dose; erectile dysfunction
EDA epidural anesthesia
EDC estimated date (day) of confinement
EDD end-diastolic dimension
EDS Ehlers-Danlos syndrome
EDV end-diastolic volume
EECG electroencephalography
EEE eastern equine encephalomyelitis
EEG electroencephalogram; electroencephalo graphy
EENT eye, ear, nose, and throat
EFM electronic fetal monitor
EGD esophagogastroduodenoscopy
EIA enzyme immunoassay
EIB exercise-induced bronchospasm
Ej elbow jerk
EKG electrocardiogram; electrocardiography
ELISA enzyme-linked immunosorbent assay
elix elixir
EM electron microscope; emmetropia; erythema multiforme
emb embolism
EMG electromyogram; electromyography
EMP emphysema
EMR educable mentally retarded; electronic medical record; eye movement record
EMS early morning specimen; electromagnetic spectrum
EN, endo endoscopy
Endo endometriosis
ENG electronystagmography
ENT ear, nose, and throat
EOG electro-oculogram
EOM extraocular muscles; extraocular movement
Eos, eosins eosinophils
EP ectopic pregnancy; evoked potential
EPF early pregnancy factor; exophthalmos-producing factor
Epi, EPI epinephrine
epi, epil epilepsy
epid epidemic
epis episiotomy
EPO erythropoietin
EPR electron paramagnetic resonance; emergency physical restraint
EPS extrapyramidal symptoms; exophthalmos-producing substance
ER emergency room; epigastric region
ERCP endoscopic retrograde cholangiopancreatography
ERPF effective renal plasma flow
ERT estrogen replacement therapy; external radiation therapy
ERV expiratory reserve volume
ESD end-systolic dimension
ESPF end-stage pulmonary fibrosis
ESR erythrocyte sedimentation rate
EST electric shock therapy
ESRD end-stage renal disease
ESWL extracorporeal shock-wave lithotripsy
ESV end-systolic volume
ET embryo transfer; enterically transmitted; esotropia; eustachian tube
et and
ETF eustachian tube function
ETI endotracheal intubation
etiol etiology
ETT endotracheal tube; exercise tolerance test
EU Ehrlich units; emergency unit; etiology unknown
EV esophageal varices
EWB estrogen withdrawal bleeding
ex excision; exercise
exam examination
exp expiration
ext extraction; external
Ez eczema

F

F Fahrenheit
FA fluorescein angiography; fluorescent antibody; fructosamine test
FAS fetal alcohol syndrome
FB foreign body
FBS fasting blood sugar
FCD fibrocystic disease
FDP fibrin-fibrinogen degradation products
FECG fetal electrocardiogram

FEF	forced expiratory flow
FESS	functional endoscopic sinus surgery
fet	fetus
FEV	forced expiratory volume
FFA	free fatty acids
FH	family history
FHR	fetal heart rate
FHS	fetal heart sounds
FHT	fetal heart tones
FIA	fluorescent immunoassay; fluoroimmuno assay
Fluor	fluoroscopy
fMRI	functional magnetic resonance imaging
FMS	fibromyalgia syndrome
FNA	fine-needle aspiration
FOBT	fecal occult blood test
FPG	fasting plasma glucose
fr	French (catheter size)
FRC	functional residual capacity
FROM	full range of motion
FS	frozen section
FSH	follicle-stimulating hormone
FSP	fibrin-fibrinogen split products
FSS	functional endoscopic sinus surgery
FT	family therapy
FTND	full-term normal delivery
FTT	failure to thrive
FU, F/U	follow-up; follow up
FUO	fever of unknown origin
FX, Fx	fracture

G

G	gingiva; glaucoma; glycogen
g	gram; gravida (pregnancy)
GA	gastric analysis; general anesthesia
ga	gallium
GAD	generalized anxiety disorder
GB	gallbladder
GBM	glomerular basement membrane
GBS	gallbladder series; Guillain-Barré syndrome
G-Cs	glucocorticoids
GC	gonorrhea
GCG	glucagon
G&D	growth and development
GD	Graves' disease
GDM	gestational diabetes mellitus
GE	gastroenteritis
GER	gastroesophageal reflux
GERD	gastroesophageal reflux disease
GFR	glomerular filtration rate
GG	gamma globulin
GGT	gamma-glutamyl transferase
GH	growth hormone
GHb	glycohemoglobin
GI	gastrointestinal
GIFT	gamete intrafallopian transfer
GIT	gastrointestinal tract
glau, glc	glaucoma
GLTT	glucose tolerance test
gm	gram
GN	glomerulonephritis
GP	general practice
gr	grain
grav I	pregnancy one; primigravida
GS	general surgery
GSW	gunshot wound
GT	glucose tolerance
GTT	glucose tolerance test
gtt	drops
GU	genitourinary
GVHD	graft-versus-host disease
GxT	graded exercise test
GYN, Gyn	gynecology

H

H	hydrogen; hypodermic; hyperopia
h	hour
H & H	hemoglobin and hematocrit
HA	hemolytic anemia; histamine
HAA	hepatitis associated antigen; hepatitis Australia antigen
halluc	hallucination
HASHD	hypertensive arteriosclerotic heart disease
HAV	hepatitis A virus
HB	heart block; hemoglobin; hepatitis B; His bundle
Hb	hemoglobin
HBE	His bundle electrocardiogram
HbF	fetal hemoglobin
HBGM	home blood glucose monitoring
HBP	high blood pressure
HbS	sickle cell hemoglobin
HBV	hepatitis B virus
HC	Huntington's cholera
HCD	heavy-chain disease
HCG	human chorionic gonadotropin
HCl	hydrochloric acid
HCL	hairy cell leukemia

HCT, Hct, hct hematocrit
HCV hepatitis C virus
HCVD hypertensive cardiovascular disease
HD hearing distance; heart disease; hemodialysis; hip disarticulation; Hodgkin's disease; Huntington's disease
HDL high-density lipoproteins
HDN hemolytic disease of the newborn
HDS herniated disk syndrome
HE hereditary elliptocytosis; hyperextension
He helium; hemorrhage
HEENT head, eyes, ears, nose, throat
HEM hematuria
HEM, hemo hemophilia; hemodialysis
hemat hematocrit
hemi hemiplegia
HF heart failure
HG hypoglycemia
Hg mercury
HgA1c glycohemoglobin test
Hgb hemoglobin
HGE human granulocytic ehrlichiosis
HH hiatal hernia
HIE hypoxic ischemic encephalopathy
Hi, his histamine
HIS, Histo, histol histology
HIV human immunodeficiency virus
H & L heart and lungs
HL Hodgkin's lymphoma
HLA human leukocyte antigen
HLR heart-lung resuscitation
HM hand motion; Holter monitor
HMD hyaline membrane disease
HMO health maintenance organization
hmt hematocrit
HNP herniated nucleus pulposus
HO hyperbaric oxygen
HOB head of bed
H & P history and physical
HP hemipelvectomy; hyperparathyroidism
HPN hypertension
HPO hypothalamic-pituitary-ovarian
HPS hantavirus pulmonary syndrome
HPV human papilloma virus
HR heart rate
hr hour
HRT hormone replacement therapy
HS hamstring; heavy smoker; herpes simplex; hospital stay
hs, h.s. at bedtime; hour of sleep
HSG hysterosalpingogram
HSV herpes simplex virus
HSV-1 oral herpes simplex virus type 1
HSV-2 herpes simplex virus type 2
HT Hashimoto's thyroiditis; hormone therapy
ht height; hematocrit
HTO high tibial osteotomy
HV hallux valgus; hospital visit
HVD hypertensive vascular disease
HVT hyperventilation
Hx history
hypo hypodermic
HYS hysteroscopy
HZ herpes zoster
Hz hertz

I

I intensity of magnetism; iodine
IABP intra-aortic balloon pump
IACP intra-aortic counterpulsation
IADH inappropriate antidiuretic hormone
IASD interatrial septal defect
IBC iron-binding capacity
IBD inflammatory bowel disease
IBS irritable bowel syndrome
IC inspiratory capacity; intermittent claudication; interstitial cystitis
ICCE intracapsular lens extraction
ICCU intensive coronary care unit
ICD implantable cardioverter defibrillator
ICF intracellular fluid
ICP intracranial pressure
ICS ileocecal sphincter; intercostal space
ICSI intracytoplasmic sperm injection
ICT indirect Coombs' test; insulin coma therapy
ICU intensive care unit
I & D incision and drainage
ID infectious disease; intradermal
IDC infiltrating ductal carcinoma; invasive ductal carcinoma
IDD insulin-dependent diabetes
IDDM insulin-dependent diabetes mellitus
IDK internal derangement of the knee
IDS immunity deficiency state
IEMG integrated electromyogram
IF interferon; interstitial fluid

IFG	impaired fasting glucose
Ig	immunoglobulin
IgA	immunoglobulin A
IgD	immunoglobulin D
IgE	immunoglobulin E
IgG	immunoglobulin G
IgM	immunoglobulin M
IGT	impaired glucose tolerance
IH	infectious hepatitis; inguinal hernia
IHD	ischemic heart disease
IL	interleukin
ILC	infiltrating lobar carcinoma; invasive lobular carcinoma
ILD	interstitial lung diseases
IM	infectious mononucleosis; intramuscular
IMAG	internal mammary artery graft
IMF	idiopathic myelofibrosis
IMI	immunofluorescence
IMV	intermittent mandatory ventilation
inf	inferior; infusion
Inflam, Inflamm	inflammation
I & O	intake and output
IO	intestinal obstruction; intraocular
IOD	iron-overload disease (hemochromatosis)
IOL	intraocular lens
IOP	intraocular pressure
IPF	idiopathic pulmonary fibrosis
IPG	impedance plethysmography
IPPB	intermittent positive-pressure breathing
IQ	intelligence quotient
irrig	irrigation
IS	impingement syndrome; intercostal space
ISG	immune serum globulin
isol	isolation
IT	immunotherapy
ITP	idiopathic thrombocytopenic purpura
IU	international unit
IUD	intrauterine device
IUP	intrauterine pressure
IV	intravenous; intravenously
IVC	inferior vena cava
IVCP	inferior vena cava pressure
IVD	intervertebral disk
IVDA	intravenous drug abuse
IVF	in vitro fertilization
IVFA	intravenous fluorescein angiography
IVP	intravenous pyelogram
IVSD	interventricular septal defect
IVU	intravenous urogram

J

j, jaund	jaundice
jct	junctions
JOD	juvenile-onset diabetes
JRA	juvenile rheumatoid arthritis
Jt	joint
JVP	jugular venous pressure; jugular venous pulse

K

K	potassium
KB	ketone bodies
KCF	key clinical findings
KCl	potassium chloride
KD	knee disarticulation
KE	kinetic energy
kg	kilogram
kj	knee jerk
KO	keep open
KOH	potassium hydrochloride
KS	Kaposi's sarcoma
KUB	kidneys, ureters, bladder
KVO	keep vein open

L

l	liter
L1 through L5	lumbar vertebrae
L & A	light and accommodation
LA	left atrium
lab	laboratory
lac	laceration
LAD	left anterior descending
LAP	laparoscopy; leucine aminopeptidase
lap	laparotomy
lar, lx	larynx
laryn	laryngitis; laryngoscopy
laser	light amplification by stimulated emission of radiation
LASIK	laser in situ keratomileusis
lat	lateral
LAVH	laparoscopically assisted vaginal hysterectomy
LB	large bowel; low back
lb	pound
LBBB	left bundle branch block
LBP	low back pain

LBW low birth weight
LBBX left breast biopsy and examination
LCIS lobular carcinoma in situ
L & D labor and delivery
LDD light-dark discrimination
LDL low-density lipoproteins
LE left eye; life expectancy; lower extremity; lupus erythematosus; lymphedema
LES lower esophageal sphincter
lg large
LH luteinizing hormone
LHBD left heart bypass device
LHF left-sided heart failure
lig ligament
liq liquid
litho lithotripsy
LLE lower left extremity
LLL left lower lobe
LLQ left lower quadrant
LLSB left lower sternal border
L/min liters per minute
LMP last menstrual period
LNMP last normal menstrual period
LOC level of consciousness; loss of consciousness
LOM limitation of motion; loss of motion
LOS length of stay
LP light perception; lumbar puncture; lumbo-peritoneal
LPF low-power field
LPS lipase
LR light reaction
LRDKT living related donor kidney transplant
LRT lower respiratory tract
LSB left sternal border
lt left
LTB laryngotracheobronchitis
LTC long-term care
LTH lactogenic hormone; luteotropic hormone
LUE left upper extremity
LUL left upper lobe
LUQ left upper quadrant
LV left ventricle
LVH left ventricle hypertrophy
lymphs lymphocytes

M

M meter; murmur; myopia
MABS monoclonal antibodies
MAO maximal acid output; monoamine oxidase
MAR multiple antibiotic resistant
MBC maximal breathing capacity
MBD minimal brain damage
mc millicurie
mcg microgram
MCH mean corpuscular hemoglobin
MCHC mean corpuscular hemoglobin concentration
MCT mean circulation time
MCV mean corpuscular volume
MD macular degeneration; medical doctor; muscular dystrophy
MDS myelodysplastic syndrome
MDR-TB multidrug-resistant tuberculosis
ME middle ear
MED minimal effective dose; minimal erythema dose
men meningitis; menstruation
men, mgtis meningitis
mEq milliequivalent
MET metastasis
met metastasize
M & F mother and father
MFT muscle function test
mg milligram
MG myasthenia gravis
mgm milligram
MH malignant hyperpyrexia; malignant hyperthermia; marital history
MHC mental health care
MI mitral insufficiency; myocardial infarction
MICU medical intensive care unit; mobile intensive care unit
MID multi-infarct dementia
MIDCAB minimally invasive direct coronary artery bypass
MIP maximal inspiratory pressure
ml, mL milliliter
MLD manual lymph drainage; minimum lethal dose
MM multiple myeloma; malignant melanoma
mm millimeter
mm Hg millimeters of mercury
MND motor neuron disease
MNT medical nutrition therapy
MO morbid obesity
MODY maturity-onset diabetes of the young
MOM milk of magnesia
mono monocytes

MP	metacarpal-phalangeal
MPD	myofascial pain dysfunction
MR	mental retardation; metabolic rate; mitral regurgitation
MRA	magnetic resonance angiography
MRD	medical record department
MRI	magnetic resonance imaging
MS	mitral stenosis; multiple sclerosis; musculoskeletal
MSH	melanocyte-simulating hormone
MTD	right eardrum
MTS	left eardrum
MTX	methotrexate
MV	mitral valve
MVP	mitral valve prolapse
MY, Myop	myopia
myel	myelogram
myop	myopia

N

N & T	nose and throat
NA	not applicable; numerical aperture
Na	sodium
NaCl	sodium chloride
NAD	no acute disease; no apparent distress
NB	newborn
N/C	no complaints
NCV	nerve conduction velocity
NED	no evidence of disease
NEG, neg	negative
Neph	nephron
neuro	neurology
NF	National Formulary; necrotizing fasciitis; neurofibromatosis
N/G	nasogastric (tube)
ng	*Neisseria gonorrhoeae*
NGF	nerve growth factor
NGU	nongonococcal urethritis
NHL	non-Hodgkin's lymphoma
NI	nuclear imaging
NICU	neurologic intensive care unit
NIDDM	non-insulin-dependent diabetes mellitus
NK cell	natural killer cell
NKA	no known allergies
NLP	neurolinguistic programming
N & M	nerves and muscles; night and morning
NM	nuclear medicine
nm	neuromuscular
NMR	nuclear magnetic resonance
No	number
noc, noct	night
NOFTT	nonorganic failure to thrive
NP	nasopharynx
NPC	no point of convergence
NPO	nothing by mouth
NR	no response
NREM	no rapid eye movements
NS	nephrotic syndrome; normal saline; not stated; not significant; not sufficient
NSAID	nonsteroidal anti-inflammatory drug
NSR	normal sinus rhythm
nst	nystagmus
NSU	nonspecific urethritis
Nt	neutralization
NTD	neural tube defect
NTG	nitroglycerin
N & V	nausea and vomiting
NVA	near visual acuity
NVD	nausea, vomiting, and diarrhea; neck vein distention
NVS	neural vital signs
NYD	not yet diagnosed
ny	nystagmus

O

OA	osteoarthritis
OAB	overactive bladder
OB	obstetrics
OB-GYN	obstetrics and gynecology
obl	oblique
OBS	organic brain syndrome
Obs	obstetrics
OC	office call; oral contraceptive
OCC	occasional
OCD	obsessive compulsive disorder
OCT	oral contraceptive therapy
OD	overdose; right eye (oculus dexter)
od	once a day
OGN	obstetric-gynecologic-neonatal
OGTT	oral glucose tolerance test
oint	ointment
OJD	osteoarthritic joint disease
OM	otitis media
OME	otitis media with effusion
OMR	optic mark recognition
OOB	out of bed
O & P	ova and parasites
OP	oropharynx; osteoporosis; outpatient

OPA	oropharyngeal airway
OPD	outpatient department
Ophth	ophthalmic
OPT	outpatient
OPV	oral poliovirus vaccine
OR	operating room
ORIF	open reduction internal fixation
ORT	oral rehydration therapy
Orth	orthopedics
OS	left eye (oculus sinister)
os	mouth
OSA	obstructive sleep apnea
OT	occupational therapy; old tuberculin
OTC	over-the-counter
Oto	otology
OU	each eye (oculus unitas)
oz	ounce
OXT	oxytocin

P

P	percussion; phosphorus; physiology; posterior; presbyopia; progesterone; prolactin; pulse
P & A	percussion and auscultation
PA	pernicious anemia; physician's assistant; polyarteritis; posteroanterior; pulmonary artery
PA, pa	pathology
PAC	premature atrial contraction
PACAB	port-access coronary artery bypass
PADP	pulmonary artery diastolic pressure
PAMP	pulmonary arterial mean pressure
Pap	Papanicolaou smear
PAR	perennial allergic rhinitis; postanesthetic recovery
PARA (P_1)	full-term infants delivered
paren	parenterally
PASP	pulmonary artery systolic pressure
PAT	paroxysmal atrial tachycardia
Path	pathology
Pb	presbyopia
PBC	primary biliary cirrhosis
PBI	protein-bound iodine
PBP	progressive bulbar palsy
PBT_4	protein-bound thyroxine
PC	pheochromocytoma; prostate cancer
p.c.	after meals
PCA	prostate cancer
PCKD, PKD	polycystic kidney disease
PCNL	percutaneous nephrolithotomy
PCO, PCOS	polycystic ovary syndrome
PCP	*Pneumocystis carinii* pneumonia
PCT	plasmacrit time
PCU	progressive care unit
PCV	packed cell volume
PD	interpupillary distance; Parkinson's disease; peritoneal dialysis; postural drainage
PDA	patent ductus arteriosus
PDD	pervasive developmental disorder
PDL	periodontal ligament
PE	physical examination; preeclampsia
PEA	pulseless electrical activity
Peds	pediatrics
PEEP	positive end-expiratory pressure
PEF	peak expiratory flow rate
PEG	pneumoencephalogram; pneumoencephalography
PEL	permissible exposure limit
per	by; through
PERLA	pupils equally reactive (responsive) to light and accommodation
PERRLA	pupils equal, round, reactive to light and accommodation
PET	positron emission tomography; preeclamptic toxemia
PFT	pulmonary function test
PG	pregnant; prostaglandin
PGH	pituitary growth hormone
PGL	persistent generalized lymphadenopathy
PH	past history; personal history; public health
pH	acidity; hydrogen ion concentration
PHN	postherpetic neuralgia
PI	present illness
PICU	pulmonary intensive care unit
PID	pelvic inflammatory disease
PIF	peak inspiratory flow
PIH	pregnancy-induced hypertension
PK	pyruvate kinase; pyruvate kinase deficiency
PKD	polycystic kidney disease
PKR	partial knee replacement
PKU	phenylketonuria
PL	light perception
pl	placenta
PLC	platelet count
PLMS	periodic limb movements in sleep

PLS primary lateral sclerosis
PLTS platelets
PM evening or afternoon; physical medicine; polymyositis; postmortem
PMA progressive muscular atrophy
PMDD premenstrual dysphoric disorder
PMH past medical history
PMI point of maximal impulse
PMN polymorphonuclear neutrophils
PMP past menstrual period; previous menstrual period
PMR physical medicine and rehabilitation; polymyalgia rheumatica
PMS premenstrual syndrome
PMT premenstrual tension
PMVS prolapsed mitral valve syndrome
PN peripheral neuropathy; postnatal
PN, Pn, PNA, pneu, pneum pneumonia
PND paroxysmal nocturnal dyspnea; postnasal drip
PNH postnatal headache
Pno pneumothorax
PNP peripheral neuropathy
PNS parasympathetic nervous system; peripheral nervous system
PO, p.o. by mouth; orally; phone order; postoperative
POC products of conception
polys polymorphonuclear leukocytes
POMR problem-oriented medical record
POS polycystic ovary syndrome
pos positive
post-op postoperatively
PP placenta previa; postpartum; postprandial (after meals); pulse pressure
ppb parts per billion
PPBS postprandial blood sugar
PPD purified protein derivative
ppm parts per million
PPS postperfusion syndrome; postpolio syndrome; progressive systemic sclerosis
PPT partial prothrombin time
PPV positive-pressure ventilation
PR peripheral resistance; pulse rate
Pr presbyopia; prism
pr by rectum
PRA plasma renin activity
PRC packed red cells
PRE progressive restrictive exercise
preg pregnant
preop preoperative
prep prepare
PRK photorefractive keratectomy
p.r.n. as needed
proct proctology
prog, progn prognosis
PROM passive range of motion; premature rupture of membranes
pro time prothrombin time
PRRE pupils round, regular, and equal
Prx prognosis
PS, Ps psoriasis
PSA prostate-specific antigen
PSS progressive systemic sclerosis; physiologic saline solution
psych psychiatry
PT paroxysmal tachycardia; physical therapy; prothrombin time
pt patient; pint
PTA percutaneous transluminal angioplasty
PTE pulmonary thromboembolism
PTC percutaneous transhepatic cholangiography
PTCA percutaneous transluminal coronary angioplasty
PTD permanent and total disability
PTE parathyroid extract; pulmonary thromboembolism
PTH parathyroid hormone; parathormone
PTSD posttraumatic stress disorder
PTT partial thromboplastin time; prothrombin time
PU peptic ulcer; pregnancy urine; prostatic urethra
PUD peptic ulcer disease; pulmonary disease
pul pulmonary
P & V pyloroplasty and vagotomy
PV peripheral vascular; plasma volume; polycythemia vera
PVC premature ventricular contraction
PVD peripheral vascular disease
PVE prosthetic valve endocarditis
PVOD peripheral vascular occlusive disease
PVS persistent vegetative state
PVT paroxysmal ventricular tachycardia
pvt private
PWB partial weight-bearing
PWP pulmonary wedge pressure
Px prognosis

Q

q every
qd, q.d. every day
qh, q.h every hour
q 2 h every 2 hours
QID, qid, q.i.d. four times a day
qm every morning
qn every night
qns quantity not sufficient
qod every other day
qoh every other hour
QOL quality of life
qs quantity sufficient
qt quart; quiet
q.q. each
quad quadrant; quadriplegia; quadriplegic

R

R rectal; respiration; right
RA refractory anemia; rheumatoid arthritis; right arm; right atrium
rad radiation absorbed dose
RAF rheumatoid arthritis factor
RAI radioactive iodine
RAIU radioactive iodine uptake determination
RAS reticular activating system
RAST radioallergosorbent
RAT radiation therapy
RBBB right bundle branch block
RBC red blood cell; red blood count
RBCV red blood cell volume
RBE relative biologic effects
RCA right coronary artery
RD respiratory distress; retinal detachment
RDA recommended daily allowance
RDS respiratory distress syndrome
RE right eye
reg regular
rehab rehabilitation
rem roentgen-equivalent-man
REM sleep rapid eye movement sleep
RER renal excretion rate
resp respiration
RF renal failure; respiratory failure; rheumatoid factor; rheumatic fever
RFS renal function study
RH right hand
RHD rheumatic heart disease
Rh neg Rhesus factor negative
Rh pos Rhesus factor positive
RIA radioimmunoassay
RICE rest, ice, compression, elevate
Rick rickettsia
RIST radioimmunosorbent
RK radial keratotomy
RL right leg
RLC residual lung capacity
RLD related living donor
RLE right lower extremity
RLL right lower lobe
RLQ right lower quadrant
RLS restless legs syndrome
RM respiratory movement
RMD repetitive motion disorder
RML right mediolateral
RMSF Rocky Mountain spotted fever
RNA ribonucleic acid
RND radical neck dissection
R/O rule out
ROA radiopaque agents
ROM range of motion; rupture of membranes
ROP retinopathy of prematurity
ROPS rollover protection structures
ROS review of systems
ROT right occipitis transverse
RP radiopharmaceuticals; Raynaud's phenomenon; relapsing polychondritis; retrograde pyelogram
RPF renal plasma flow
RPG retrograde pyelogram
rpm revolutions per minute
RPO right posterior oblique
RPR rapid plasma reagin
RQ respiratory quotient
R & R rate and rhythm
RR recovery room; respiratory rate
RSD repetitive stress disorder
RSDS reflex sympathetic dystrophy syndrome
RSHF right-sided heart failure
RSI repetitive stress injuries
RSR regular sinus rhythm
RSV right subclavian vein
RT radiation therapy; renal transplantation; respiratory therapy
rt right; routine
RTA renal tubular acidosis
rt lat right lateral

rtd retarded
RU roentgen unit; routine urinalysis
RUE right upper extremity
RUL right upper lobe
RUQ right upper quadrant
RV residual volume; right ventricle
RVG radionuclide ventriculogram
RVH right ventricular hypertrophy
RVS relative value schedule
RW ragweed
Rx prescription; take; therapy; treatment

S

s̄ without
S-A sinoatrial node
S & A sugar and acetone
SA salicylic acid; sinoatrial; sperm analysis; surgeon's assistant
SAAT serum aspartate aminotransferase
SAB spontaneous abortion
SACH self-assessed change in health
SAD seasonal affective disorder
SAH subarachnoid hemorrhage
SAL sensorineural activity level; sterility assurance level; suction-assisted lipectomy
Sal, Salm salmonella
SALP salpingectomy; salpingography; serum alkaline phosphatase
Salpx salpingectomy
SAM self-administered medication program
SARS severe acute respiratory syndrome
SAS short arm splint; sleep apnea syndrome; social adjustment scale; subarachnoid space
SB small bowel; spina bifida; stillbirth; suction biopsy
SBE subacute bacterial endocarditis
SBO small bowel obstruction
SC, sc subcutaneous
SC Snellen chart; spinal cord
SCA sickle cell anemia
SCC squamous cell carcinoma
SCD sudden cardiac death
schiz schizophrenia
SCI spinal cord injury
SCID severe combined immune deficiency
SCT sickle cell trait
SD septal defect; shoulder disarticulation; spontaneous delivery; standard deviation; sudden death
SDAT senile dementia of Alzheimer's type
SDM standard deviation of the mean
SDS sudden death syndrome
sec second
sed rate sedimentation rate
seg segmented neutrophils
SEM scanning electron microscopy
semi half
SES subcutaneous electric stimulation
sev sever; severed
SF scarlet fever; spinal fluid
SG serum globulin; skin graft
SGA small for gestational age
SH serum hepatitis; sex hormone; social history
sh shoulder
SI saturation index
SICU surgical intensive care unit
SIDS sudden infant death syndrome
sig let it be labeled
SIRS systemic inflammatory response syndrome
SIS saline infusion sonohysterography
SISI short increment sensitivity index
SLE St. Louis encephalitis; systemic lupus erythematosus
SLND sentinel lymph node dissection
SLPS serum lipase
SM simple mastectomy
sm small
SMA sequential multiple analysis
SMAC sequential multiple analysis computer
SMG senile macular degeneration
SMR submucous resection
SMRR submucous resection and rhinoplasty
SNR signal-to-noise ratio
SNRI serotonin and norepinephrine reuptake inhibitor
SNS sensory nervous system; sympathetic nervous system
SO salpingo-oophorectomy
SOAP symptoms, observations, assessments, plan; subjective, objective, assessment, plan
SOB shortness of breath
SOM serous otitis media
SONO sonography
SOP standard operating procedure
sos if necessary
spec specimen
SPECT single photon emission computerized tomography
SPF skin protective factor; sun protective factor

sp gr specific gravity
SPP suprapubic prostatectomy
SPR scanned projection radiography
SQ subcutaneous
SR sedimentation rate; stimulus response; system review
SRS smoker's respiratory syndrome
ss half
SS signs and symptoms; Sjögren's syndrome; soap solution
SSE soap suds enema
SSRI selective serotonin reuptake inhibitor
SSU sterile supply unit
ST esotropia; sclerotherapy
staph staphylococcus
stat immediately
STD sexually transmitted disease; skin test dose
STH somatotropic hormone
STK streptokinase
strab strabismus
strep streptococcus
STS serologic test for syphilis
STSG split thickness skin graft
subcu, sub-Q subcutaneous
SUI stress urinary incontinence
supp suppository
surg surgical; surgery
SVC superior vena cava
SVD spontaneous vaginal delivery
SVG saphenous vein graft
SVN small volume nebulizer
SX symptom reduction
Sx symptoms
Sz seizure

T

T temperature; thrombosis
T1 through T12 thoracic vertebrae
T3 triiodothyronine
T4 thyroxine
T & A tonsillectomy and adenoidectomy
TA, TAB therapeutic abortion
tab tablet
TACT target air-enema computed tomography
TAF tumor angiogenesis factor
TAH total abdominal hysterectomy
TAH-BSO total abdominal hysterectomy with bilateral salpingo-oophorectomy
TAO thromboangiitis obliterans
TB tuberculosis
TBD total body density
TBF total body fat
TBG thyroxine-binding globulin
TBI thyroxine-binding index
TBW total body weight
TCD transcranial doppler
TCDB turn, cough, deep breathe
TCP time care profile
TD total disability; transdermal
TDM therapeutic drug monitoring
TDT tone decay test
TE tetanus; tonsillectomy
TEE transesophageal echocardiography
temp temperature
TEN toxic epidermal necrolysis
TENS transcutaneous electrical nerve stimulation
TES treadmill exercise score
TFS thyroid function studies
TGA transposition of great arteries
THA total hip arthroplasty
THR total hip replacement
TIA transient ischemic attack
TIA-IR transient ischemic attack incomplete recovery
TIBC total iron-binding capacity
TID, tid, t.i.d. times interval difference; three times a day
tinct tincture
TJA total joint arthroplasty
TKA total knee arthroplasty
TKO to keep open
TKR total knee replacement
TLC tender loving care; total lung capacity
TLE temporal lobe epilepsy
TM temporomandibular; tympanic membrane
TMD temporomandibular disease; temporomandibular disorder
TMJ temporomandibular joint
TMs tympanic membranes
Tn normal intraocular tension
TND term normal delivery
TNF tumor necrosis factor
TNI total nodal irradiation
TNM tumor, nodes, metastases
TO telephone order
top topically

TP testosterone propionate; total protein
TPA, tPA tissue plasminogen activator; *Treponema pallidum* agglutination
TPBF total pulmonary blood flow
TPI *Treponema pallidum* immobilization
TPN total parenteral nutrition
TPR temperature, pulse, respiration
TPUR transperineal urethral resection
TR tuberculin residue
tr tincture
trach trachea; tracheostomy
TRBF total renal blood flow
TRH thyrotropin-releasing hormone
Trich trichomonas
TS Tourette syndrome
TSD Tay-Sachs disease
TSE testicular self-examination
TSH thyroid-stimulating hormone
TSP total serum protein
TSS toxic shock syndrome
TST thallium stress test; tuberculin skin test
TT thrombin time
TTH thyrotropic hormone
TULIP transurethral ultrasound-guided laser-induced proctectomy
TUMT transurethral microwave therapy
TUR transurethral resection
TURP transurethral resection of prostate; prostatectomy
TV tidal volume; tricuspid valve
TVH total vaginal hysterectomy
TW tap water
TWE tap water enema
Tx traction; treatment

U

U units
U/A, UA urinalysis
UB urinary bladder
UC ulcerative colitis; urine culture; uterine contractions
UCD usual childhood diseases
UCG urinary chorionic gonadotropin; uterine chorionic gonadotropin
UCR unconditioned reflex
UE upper extremity
UFR uroflowmeter; uroflowmetry
UG upper gastrointestinal; urogenital
UGI upper gastrointestinal
UK unknown
UL upper lobe
ULQ upper left quadrant
umb umbilical; umbilicus
UN urea nitrogen
ung ointment
UOQ upper outer quadrant
UPP urethral pressure profile
UR upper respiratory
ur urine
URD upper respiratory disease
URI upper respiratory infection
urol urology
URQ upper right quadrant
URT upper respiratory tract
US ultrasonic; ultrasonography
USP United States Pharmacopeia
UTI urinary tract infection
UV ultraviolet
UVJ ureterovesical junction

V

V ventral; visual acuity
VA vacuum aspiration; visual acuity
vag vaginal
VAS vasectomy
VB viable birth
VBAC vaginal birth after cesarean
VBP ventricular premature beat
VC acuity of color vision; vena cava; vital capacity
VCUG voiding cystourethrogram
VD venereal disease
VDG venereal disease, gonorrhea
VDH valvular disease of heart
VDRL Venereal Disease Research Laboratory
VDS venereal disease, syphilis
VE visual efficiency
Vent, ventr ventral
VEP visual evoked potential
VER visual evoked response
VF ventricular fibrillation; visual field; vocal fremitus
V fib ventricular fibrillation
VG ventricular gallop
VH vaginal hysterectomy
VHD valvular heart disease; ventricular heart disease
VI volume index

vit cap	vital capacity
VLDL	very-low-density lipoprotein
VP	venipuncture; venous pressure
V & P	vagotomy and pyloroplasty
VPC	ventricular premature contraction
VPRC	volume of packed red cells
VS, vs	vital signs
VSD	ventricular septal defect
VTAs	vascular targeting agents
VV	varicose veins
VVF	vesicovaginal fistula
VZV	varicella-zoster virus (chickenpox)

W

W	water
WA	while awake
WB	weight-bearing; whole blood
WBC	white blood cell; white blood count
W/C, w/c	wheelchair
wd	wound
WD, w/d	well-developed
WDWN	well-developed, well-nourished
wf	white female
w/n	well-nourished
WNL	within normal limits
w/o	without
WR, W.r.	Wassermann reaction
wt	weight
w/v	weight by volume

X

X	xerophthalmia
x	multiplied by; times
XDP	xeroderma pigmentosum
XM	cross-match
XR	x-ray
XT	exotropia
XU	excretory urogram

Y

y/o	year(s) old
YOB	year of birth
yr	year

Z

Z	atomic number; no effect; zero
zyg	zygote

INDEX

Note: Page numbers in **boldface** indicate tables/figures.

A

B

C

D

E

F

G

H

J

K

L

M

N

O

P

Q

R

S

T

U

V

W

X

Y

Z

License Agreement for Delmar Cengage Learning

IMPORTANT! READ CAREFULLY: This End User License Agreement ("Agreement") sets forth the conditions by which Delmar Learning will make electronic access to the Delmar Learning-owned licensed content and associated media, software, documentation, printed materials, and electronic documentation contained in this package and/or made available to you via this product (the "Licensed Content"), available to you (the "End User"). BY CLICKING THE "I ACCEPT" BUTTON AND/OR OPENING THIS PACKAGE, YOU ACKNOWLEDGE THAT YOU HAVE READ ALL OF THE TERMS AND CONDITIONS, AND THAT YOU AGREE TO BE BOUND BY ITS TERMS, CONDITIONS, AND ALL APPLICABLE LAWS AND REGULATIONS GOVERNING THE USE OF THE LICENSED CONTENT.

1.0 SCOPE OF LICENSE

1.1 Licensed Content. The Licensed Content may contain portions of modifiable content ("Modifiable Content") and content which may not be modified or otherwise altered by the End User ("Non-Modifiable Content"). For purposes of this Agreement, Modifiable Content and Non-Modifiable Content may be collectively referred to herein as the "Licensed Content." All Licensed Content shall be considered Non-Modifiable Content, unless such Licensed Content is presented to the End User in a modifiable format and it is clearly indicated that modification of the Licensed Content is permitted.

1.2 Subject to the End User's compliance with the terms and conditions of this Agreement, Delmar Learning hereby grants the End User, a nontransferable, nonexclusive, limited right to access and view a single copy of the Licensed Content on a single personal computer system for noncommercial, internal, personal use only. The End User shall not (i) reproduce, copy, modify (except in the case of Modifiable Content), distribute, display, transfer, sublicense, prepare derivative work(s) based on, sell, exchange, barter or transfer, rent, lease, loan, resell, or in any other manner exploit the Licensed Content; (ii) remove, obscure, or alter any notice of Delmar Learning's intellectual property rights present on or in the Licensed Content, including, but not limited to, copyright, trademark, and/or patent notices; or (iii) disassemble, decompile, translate, reverse engineer, or otherwise reduce the Licensed Content.

2.0 TERMINATION

2.1 Delmar Learning may at any time (without prejudice to its other rights or remedies) immediately terminate this Agreement and/or suspend access to some or all of the Licensed Content, in the event that the End User does not comply with any of the terms and conditions of this Agreement. In the event of such termination by Delmar Learning, the End User shall immediately return any and all copies of the Licensed Content to Delmar Learning.

3.0 PROPRIETARY RIGHTS

3.1 The End User acknowledges that Delmar Learning owns all rights, title and interest, including, but not limited to all copyright rights therein, in and to the Licensed Content, and that the End User shall not take any action inconsistent with such ownership. The Licensed Content is protected by U.S., Canadian and other applicable copyright laws and by international treaties, including the Berne Convention and the Universal Copyright Convention. Nothing contained in this Agreement shall be construed as granting the End User any ownership rights in or to the Licensed Content.

3.2 Delmar Learning reserves the right at any time to withdraw from the Licensed Content any item or part of an item for which it no longer retains the right to publish, or which it has reasonable grounds to believe infringes copyright or is defamatory, unlawful, or otherwise objectionable.

4.0 PROTECTION AND SECURITY

4.1 The End User shall use its best efforts and take all reasonable steps to safeguard its copy of the Licensed Content to ensure that no unauthorized reproduction, publication, disclosure, modification, or distribution of the Licensed Content, in whole or in part, is made. To the extent that the End User becomes aware of any such unauthorized use of the Licensed Content, the End User shall immediately notify Delmar Learning. Notification of such violations may be made by sending an e-mail to delmar.help@cengage.com.

5.0 MISUSE OF THE LICENSED PRODUCT

5.1 In the event that the End User uses the Licensed Content in violation of this Agreement, Delmar Learning shall have the option of electing liquidated damages, which shall include all profits generated by the

End User's use of the Licensed Content plus interest computed at the maximum rate permitted by law and all legal fees and other expenses incurred by Delmar Learning in enforcing its rights, plus penalties.

6.0 FEDERAL GOVERNMENT CLIENTS

6.1 Except as expressly authorized by Delmar Learning, Federal Government clients obtain only the rights specified in this Agreement and no other rights. The Government acknowledges that (i) all software and related documentation incorporated in the Licensed Content is existing commercial computer software within the meaning of FAR 27.405(b)(2); and (ii) all other data delivered in whatever form, is limited rights data within the meaning of FAR 27.401. The restrictions in this section are acceptable as consistent with the Government's need for software and other data under this Agreement.

7.0 DISCLAIMER OF WARRANTIES AND LIABILITIES

7.1 Although Delmar Learning believes the Licensed Content to be reliable, Delmar Learning does not guarantee or warrant (i) any information or materials contained in or produced by the Licensed Content, (ii) the accuracy, completeness or reliability of the Licensed Content, or (iii) that the Licensed Content is free from errors or other material defects. THE LICENSED PRODUCT IS PROVIDED "AS IS," WITHOUT ANY WARRANTY OF ANY KIND AND DELMAR LEARNING DISCLAIMS ANY AND ALL WARRANTIES, EXPRESSED OR IMPLIED, INCLUDING, WITHOUT LIMITATION, WARRANTIES OF MERCHANTABILITY OR FITNESS FOR A PARTICULAR PURPOSE. IN NO EVENT SHALL DELMAR LEARNING BE LIABLE FOR: INDIRECT, SPECIAL, PUNITIVE OR CONSEQUENTIAL DAMAGES INCLUDING FOR LOST PROFITS, LOST DATA, OR OTHERWISE. IN NO EVENT SHALL DELMAR LEARNING'S AGGREGATE LIABILITY HEREUNDER, WHETHER ARISING IN CONTRACT, TORT, STRICT LIABILITY OR OTHERWISE, EXCEED THE AMOUNT OF FEES PAID BY THE END USER HEREUNDER FOR THE LICENSE OF THE LICENSED CONTENT.

8.0 GENERAL

8.1 Entire Agreement. This Agreement shall constitute the entire Agreement between the Parties and supercedes all prior Agreements and understandings oral or written relating to the subject matter hereof.

8.2 Enhancements/Modifications of Licensed Content. From time to time, and in Delmar Learning's sole discretion, Delmar Learning may advise the End User of updates, upgrades, enhancements and/or improvements to the Licensed Content, and may permit the End User to access and use, subject to the terms and conditions of this Agreement, such modifications, upon payment of prices as may be established by Delmar Learning.

8.3 No Export. The End User shall use the Licensed Content solely in the United States and shall not transfer or export, directly or indirectly, the Licensed Content outside the United States.

8.4 Severability. If any provision of this Agreement is invalid, illegal, or unenforceable under any applicable statute or rule of law, the provision shall be deemed omitted to the extent that it is invalid, illegal, or unenforceable. In such a case, the remainder of the Agreement shall be construed in a manner as to give greatest effect to the original intention of the parties hereto.

8.5 Waiver. The waiver of any right or failure of either party to exercise in any respect any right provided in this Agreement in any instance shall not be deemed to be a waiver of such right in the future or a waiver of any other right under this Agreement.

8.6 Choice of Law/Venue. This Agreement shall be interpreted, construed, and governed by and in accordance with the laws of the State of New York, applicable to contracts executed and to be wholly preformed therein, without regard to its principles governing conflicts of law. Each party agrees that any proceeding arising out of or relating to this Agreement or the breach or threatened breach of this Agreement may be commenced and prosecuted in a court in the State and County of New York. Each party consents and submits to the nonexclusive personal jurisdiction of any court in the State and County of New York in respect of any such proceeding.

8.7 Acknowledgment. By opening this package and/or by accessing the Licensed Content on this Web site, THE END USER ACKNOWLEDGES THAT IT HAS READ THIS AGREEMENT, UNDERSTANDS IT, AND AGREES TO BE BOUND BY ITS TERMS AND CONDITIONS. IF YOU DO NOT ACCEPT THESE TERMS AND CONDITIONS, YOU MUST NOT ACCESS THE LICENSED CONTENT AND RETURN THE LICENSED PRODUCT TO DELMAR LEARNING (WITHIN 30 CALENDAR DAYS OF THE END USER'S PURCHASE) WITH PROOF OF PAYMENT ACCEPTABLE TO DELMAR LEARNING, FOR A CREDIT OR A REFUND. Should the End User have any questions/comments regarding this Agreement, please contact Delmar Learning at delmar.help@cengage.com.